Urethral Reconstructive Surgery

CURRENT CLINICAL UROLOGY

ERIC A. KLEIN, MD, SERIES EDITOR

For other titles published in the series, go to
www.springer.com/humana
select the subdiscipline
search for your title

Urethral Reconstructive Surgery

Edited by
Steven B. Brandes, M.D., FACS

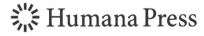 Humana Press

Editor
Steven B. Brandes MD, FACS
Washington University School of Medicine
Saint Louis, MO
USA
brandess@wustl.edu

Series Editor
Eric A. Klein, MD
Professor of Surgery
Cleveland Clinic Lerner College of Medicine
Head, Section of Urologic Oncology
Glickman Urological and Kidney Institute
Cleveland, OH

ISBN: 978-1-58829-826-3   e-ISBN: 978-1-59745-103-1
DOI: 10.1007/978-1-59745-103-1

Library of Congress Control Number: 2008929547

Cover illustrations: (*Clockwise from top*) Postoperative urethrogram with widely patent bulbar urethra and characteristic shelf-like
appearance, after a dorsal, augmented anastomotic urethroplasty (Fig. 13.14; *see* discussion on p. 149); long bulbar urethral stricture
with tight proximal segment and an adjacent, distal portion of affected urethra (Fig. 13.5; *see* complete caption on p. 145); buccal
mucosal graft augmented by a gracilis muscle flap, in the repair of a prostato-rectal fistula (Fig. 22.11; *see* complete caption on
p. 260); retrograde urethrogram showing restenosis by hypertrophic tissue within tandem placed Urolume stents in the bulbar urethra
(Fig. 8.3; *see* discussion on p. 88); and bulbar urethral mobilization for dorsal placement of a buccal mucosal graft urethroplasty (Fig.
11.21; *see* complete caption on p. 128).

Printed on acid-free paper

9 8 7 6 5 4 3 2 1

springer.com

Preface

Urethral reconstructive surgery can often be complex, time consuming, and demanding. Most urologists today have had little exposure or experience with urethral surgery during their training or in practice. This general lack of exposure, and thus lack of knowledge, has led to the popularity of temporizing procedures such as urethrotomy and dilation. Most urologists treat strictures by a "reconstructive ladder" approach, where definitive urethroplasty is only considered after successive failed dilations or urethrotomies. Furthermore, major textbooks in urology only devote a cursory view of urethral reconstructive surgery. Clearly, the gap in contemporary urology training and textbooks needs to be bridged.

The following volume aims to enlighten urologists in a practical manner on how to evaluate and manage complex urethral problems and how to end the cycle of just performing short-lived, temporizing procedures. The chapters initially lay a groundwork on the anatomy and blood supply of the urethra and genital skin, as well as the practical aspects of wound healing and applicable plastic surgical techniques. The chapters then focus on the etiologies for urethral strictures and the methods for evaluating their extent and degree. The remaining chapters are a practical and comprehensive review, with concentrations in each of the typical surgical techniques that are currently employed in the reconstructive armamentarium. In addition, chapters focus on managing surgical complications and particularly difficult and unusual problems, such as Lichen Sclerosus, the irradiated urethra, hypospadias "cripple," panurethral strictures, failed urethroplasty, urethral stent extraction, postprostatectomy strictures, and follow-up strategies. The promise of tissue engineering trends and "off the shelf" graft repair are also detailed. We have been diligent to make our text broad, as well as specific, so that the reader will have a comprehensive review of adult urethral reconstructive surgery. We also have condensed into a chapter, pre and intraoperative decision making - imparting skills and experience that often takes years of practice to develop. We also hope that we have made a text that is visually appealing, so that it can function as a sort of surgical atlas. Overall, we have striven to make our text evidence based, as well as a distillation of the knowledge, clinical experience, and surgical acumen of current leading world experts and their historical predecessors. Enjoy.

Steven B. Brandes, MD, FACS

Introduction

"Cure occasionally, relieve often, console always."
Ambroise Pare (1510–1590)

Over the years, I have often been asked by Urology Residents in training and by my patients for words of wisdom about surgery. Their most frequent question being, "what are the best aphorisms about surgery you have heard over the years?" When it comes to education and learning, the following comes to mind.

"Hear and you forget
See and you remember
Do and you understand"

I hope this text will give you the principles and basic fund of knowledge to at least remember what to do when it comes to urethral reconstructive surgery. I leave it in the good reader's hands to put into practice what we have written. Only by your own experience will you eventually understand.

The next aphorism that comes to mind is one not just for the operating room, but a general rule for life.

"Think fast and move slow."

The best and quickest surgeons I have known over the years all seemed not to be moving quickly at all. They never rushed or seemed anxious. They seemed very even keeled in motion and in temperament. They utilized paucity of motion, and when they did move or cut something, it was with great deliberation and accuracy. No motion was ever wasted. Moreover, while they seemed not to be doing much or moving much, before you realized, the surgery was completed or the organ was removed. As to their thought process, they were always thinking quickly and numerous steps ahead;

always moving forward and not deterred by unanticipated events during the surgery.

Aside from thinking quickly and moving slowly, what makes a good and quick surgeon is having a sound surgical plan, knowing how to properly expose the surgical field ("for a monkey could do the surgery as long as you set it up for him and made the intra-operative decision making"), and thinking about the next and multiple steps ahead. It is said that what makes a chess player a grand champion is his ability to think multiple steps into the future and his ability for anticipation and contingency plans for those future moves. The same holds for surgery – good hands make a good surgeon, but what makes a great surgeon is a beautiful mind, a quick wit and great decision making skills.

So, dear reader I will leave you with another parting word of wisdom about good surgical principles:

"Selection is the silent partner of the surgeon."

In other words, often times, it is more important to know when not to operate and who not to operate on, than being able to do the surgery. Timing of surgery, the quality of the tissues, and the protoplasm of the patient will often determine the surgical outcomes more then the so-called "quality" of the surgery. In other words, no matter how good the reconstruction looks at the end of the surgery, if it all falls apart or fails postoperatively, it typically has more to do with selection and timing then any perceived lack of technical skill. In other words, as my mentor would often say, in his Texan drawl, "well, you can't make a silk purse out of a sow's ear".

Steven B. Brandes, MD, FACS

Contents

Preface.. v

Introduction... vii

Contributors xiii

1   **Genital Skin and Urethral Anatomy** 1
    Peter A. Humphrey

2   **Vascular Anatomy of Genital Skin and the Urethra:**
    Implications for Urethral Reconstruction... 9
    Steven B. Brandes

3   **Lichen Sclerosus**.. 19
    Ramón Virasoro and Gerald H. Jordan

4   **Imaging of the Male Urethra**... 29
    Christine M. Peterson, Christine O. Menias, and Cary L. Siegel

5   **Techniques in Tissue Transfer: Plastic Surgery for the Urologist**................... 43
    Thomas A. Tung and Christopher M. Nichols

6   **Epidemiology, Etiology, Histology, Classification, and Economic Impact**
    of Urethral Stricture Disease.. 53
    Steven B. Brandes

7   **Urethrotomy and Other Minimally Invasive Interventions**
    for Urethral Stricture.. 63
    Chris F. Heyns

8   **Endourethral Prostheses for Urethral Stricture**.. 85
    Daniel Yachia and Zeljko Markovic

9   **Fossa Navicularis and Meatal Reconstruction**... 97
    Noel A. Armenakas

10   **Stricture Excision and Primary Anastomosis for Anterior Urethral Strictures**................ 107
    Reynaldo G. Gomez

11   **Buccal Mucosal Graft Urethroplasty**.. 119
    Guido Barbagli

12 **Lingual Mucosa and Posterior Auricular Skin Grafts** 137
Steven B. Brandes

13 **Augmented Anastomotic Urethroplasty** 141
Neil D. Sherman and George D. Webster

14 **Penile Skin Flaps for Urethral Reconstruction** 153
Sean P. Elliott and Jack W. McAninch

15 **Panurethral Strictures** 165
Steven B. Brandes

16 **The Combined Use of Fasciocutaneous, Muscular and Myocutaneous Flaps
    and Graft Onlays in Urethral Reconstruction** 171
Leonard N. Zinman

17 **Posterior Urethral Strictures** 189
Daniela E. Andrich and Anthony R. Mundy

18 **Staged Urethroplasty** 201
Michael Coburn

19 **Complications of Urethroplasty** 213
Hosam S. Al-Qudah, Osama Al-Omar, and Richard A. Santucci

20 **Postprostatectomy Strictures** 229
James K. Kuan and Hunter Wessells

21 **Urethral Stricture and Urethroplasty in the Pelvic Irradiated Patient** 241
Kennon Miller, Michael Poch, and Steven B. Brandes

22 **Complex Rectourinary and Vesicoperineal Fistulas** 251
Steven B. Brandes

23 **Reconstruction of Failed Urethroplasty** 269
Steve W. Waxman and Allen F. Morey

24 **Urethral Stent Complications and Methods for Explantation** 277
Steven B. Brandes

25 **Reoperative Hypospadias Surgery and Management of Complications** 285
Douglas E. Coplen

26 **Use of Omentum in Urethral Reconstruction** 297
Steven B. Brandes

27 **Female Urethral Reconstruction** 303
Jason Anast, Steven B. Brandes, and Carl Klutke

28 **Follow-up Strategies After Urethral Stricture Treatment** 315
Chris F. Heyns

29 **General Technical Considerations and Decision Making
    in Urethroplasty Surgery** 323
Steven B. Brandes

30 **Tissue Engineering of the Urethra** 337
Anthony Atala

**31 History of Urethral Stricture and Its Management
    From the 18th to 20th Century** 347
    Steven B. Brandes and Chris F. Heyns

Index 355

Contributors

Hosam S. Al-Qudah, MD
Division of Urology, Department of General
Surgery, Jordan University of Science and
Technology, School of Medicine, Irbid, Jordan

Osama Al-Omar, MD
Department of Urology, Wayne State University
School of Medicine and Detroit Receiving
Hospital, Detroit, MI, USA

Jason Anast, MD
Division of Urologic Surgery, Department of Surgery,
Washington University School of Medicine,
Saint Louis, MO, USA

Daniela E. Andrich, MD
Institute of Urologic Surgery at the Middlesex
Hospital, University of London, London, UK

Noel A. Armenakas, MD
Department of Urology, Cornell Weill Medical
School, New York, NY, USA

Anthony Atala, MD
Department of Urology, Wake Forest University,
Institute for Regenerative Medicine, Winston-
Salem, NC, USA

Guido Barbagli, MD
Department of Medicine and Surgery,
University of Vita Salute-San Raffaele and
Center for Reconstructive Urethral Surgery,
Arezzo, Italy

Steven B. Brandes, MD, FACS
Division of Urologic Surgery, Department of
Surgery, Washington University School of
Medicine, Saint Louis, MO, USA

Michael Coburn, MD
Scott Department of Urology, Baylor College
of Medicine and Ben Taub General Hospital,
Houston, TX, USA

Douglas E. Coplen, MD
Division of Urology, Department of Surgery,
Washington University School of Medicine and
St. Louis Children's Hospital,
Saint Louis, MO, USA

Sean P. Elliott, MD
Department of Urologic Surgery, University of
Minnesota, Minneapolis, MN, USA

Reynaldo G. Gomez, MD
Urology Service, Hospital del Trabajador,
Santiago, Chile

Chris F Heyns, MB, ChB, PhD
Department of Urology, University of Stellenbosch
and Tygerberg Hospital, Cape Town,
South Africa

Peter A. Humphrey, MD, PhD
Anatomic and Molecular Pathology, Department
of Pathology, Washington University School of
Medicine, Saint Louis, MO, USA

Gerald H. Jordan, MD, FACS, FAAP · Adult and
Pediatric Genitourinary Reconstructive Surgery
Program, Eastern Virginia Medical School,
Norfolk, VA, USA

Carl Klutke, MD
Division of Urologic Surgery, Department of
Surgery, Washington University School of
Medicine, Saint Louis, MO, USA

James K. Kuan, MD
Department of Urology, University of Washington,
and Harborview Medical Center, Seattle, WA, USA

Zeljko Markovic, MD
Institute of Radiology, Central Clinic of Serbia,
University of Belgrade, Belgrade, Serbia

Jack W. McAninch, MD
Department of Urology, University of California
San Francisco, San Francisco, CA, USA

Christine O. Menias, MD
Mallinckrodt Institute of Radiology, Washington
University School of Medicine, Saint Louis, MO,
USA

Kennon Miller, MD
University Urological, Brown Medical School,
Rhode Island Hospital, Providence, RI, USA

Allen F. Morey, MD, FACS
Department of Urology, University of Texas,
Southwestern Medical School and Parkland
Memorial Hospital, Dallas, TX, USA

Anthony R. Mundy, MS, FRCP, FRCS
Institute of Urology at the Middlesex Hospital,
University of London, London, UK

Christopher M. Nichols, MD
Division of Plastic and Reconstructive Surgery,
Department of Surgery, Washington University
School of Medicine, Saint Louis, MO, USA

Christine M. Peterson, MD
Mallinckrodt Institute of Radiology, Washington
University School of Medicine, Saint Louis, MO,
USA

Michael Poch, MD
Department of Urology, Brown Medical School,
Rhode Island Hospital, Providence, RI, USA

Richard A. Santucci, MD
Department of Urology, Wayne State University
School of Medicine and Detroit Receiving
Hospital, Detroit, MI, USA

Neil D. Sherman, MD
Division of Urology, University of Medicine and
Dentistry of New Jersey – New Jersey Medical
School, Newark, NJ, USA

Cary L. Siegel, MD
Mallinckrodt Institute of Radiology,
Washington University School of Medicine,
Saint Louis, MO, USA

Thomas A. Tung, MD
Division of Plastic and Reconstructive Surgery,
Department of Surgery, Washington University
School of Medicine, Saint Louis, MO, USA

Ramon Virasoro, MD
Division of Urology, Center for Medical
Education and Clinical Research (CEMIC),
Buenos Aires, Argentina

Steve W. Waxman, MD
Department of Urology, Brooke Army Medical
Center, Fort Sam Houston, TX, USA

George D. Webster, MB, FRCS
Division of Urology, Duke University School of
Medicine, Durham, NC, USA

Hunter Wessells, MD, FACS
Department of Urology, University of Washington
School of Medicine and Harborview Medical
Center, Seattle, WA, USA

Daniel Yachia, MD
Department of Urology, Hillel Yaffe Medical
Center, Hadera, Israel

Leonard N. Zinman, MD
Institute of Urology, Tufts University School of
Medicine, Lahey Clinic Medical Center, Boston,
MA, USA

1
Genital Skin and Urethral Anatomy

Peter A. Humphrey

Contents

1. Female Genital Skin.. 1
2. Female Urethra.. 3
3. Male Genital Skin 3
4. Male Urethra 5
References.. 7

Summary   An intimate knowledge of genital skin and urethral anatomy is essential for successful surgical management of male and female urethral strictures, fistulas and other anomalies. Of particular importance for urethral reconstruction is the prepuce, a mixture of skin and mucosa and anatomically divided into five layers – epidermis, dermis, Dartos, lamina propria, and epithelium. The urethra is divided into the anterior (bulbar, pendulous and fossa navicularis) and the posterior (membranous and prostatic). Urethral epithelium transitions from urothelial (transitional cell) (proximal), to pseudo-stratified or stratified columnar (distal), and then onto squamous (meatus). Location of the urethra within the spongiosum is also clinically important, where the more proximal (bulbar) the more eccentric and ventral.

Keywords   Genital skin, prepuce, male urethra, anatomy, histology, female urethra, urothelial

1. Female Genital Skin

The female external genitalia may be defined as including the mons pubis, clitoris, labia majora, labia minora, vulvar vestibule and vestibulovaginal bulbs, urethral meatus, hymen, Bartholin's and Skene's glands and ducts, and vaginal introitus (**Fig. 1.1** [1]). The appearance of the female skin varies with age (2). Age-related changes occurring with puberty include hair growth on the mons pubis and lateral labia majora during puberty, increase in size (as the result of increased adipose tissue) and pigmentation of the labia and clitoral enlargement. After menopause, there is a degree of hair loss, and thinning (atrophy) of the epithelial lining of the vulvar skin. Histologically, the entire vulva, with the exception of the vulvar vestibule, is covered by a keratinized, stratified squamous epithelium (**Fig. 1.2**).

The clitoris consists of two crura and a glans. The crura comprise erectile tissue, which is characterized by cavernous veins and small muscular arteries. The glans is composed of squamous mucosa with a dense vascular dermis and a large number of sensory receptors, including numerous Pacinian corpuscles (1,3). Of relevance to this textbook on the urethra, the clitoris has been described as being intimately related to the perineal urethra (4), with the urethra surrounded by the erectile tissue complex (clitoris), with the clitoral body directly anterior to the urethra, which is flanked by clitoral bulb and crura (4).

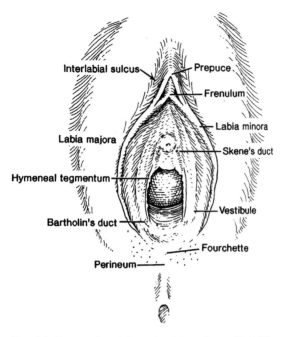

FIG. 1.1. Topography of the vulva (From Stacey E. Mills (ed) (2007) Histology for Pathologists, 3rd, Lippincott, Williams and Williams, Philadelphia, chapter 39)

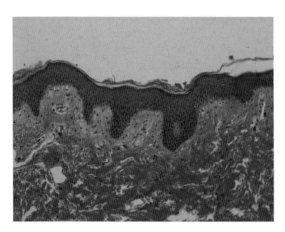

FIG. 1.2. Normal keratinized squamous epithelium of the vulva

The skin of the labia majora, in addition to lateral hair follicles, harbors sebaceous glands, which can be found with or without associated hair follicles (1). Sweat glands of apocrine and merocrine (eccrine) types also are present. The sulcus between the labia majora and minora has mammary-like glands. Deep in the dermis is a thin smooth muscle layer, beneath which is adipose tissue. There are abundant nerve endings and touch receptors, such as Meissner's corpuscles. The labia minora, unlike the labia majora, does not typically have skin appendages, although in the lateral aspects sweat and the sebaceous glands may be found (1). The subepithelial tissue is a vascular connective tissue, without fat.

The skin of the vulvar vestibule, which is bounded medially by external portion of the hymeal ring, posteriorly and laterally by the line of Hart, and anteriorly by the clitoral frenulum, has a nonkeratinizing squamous epithelium. Within the vestibule are the vaginal opening, openings of the major vestibular glands (Bartholin's glands) and minor vestibular glands, openings of the paired Skene's glands, and opening of the urethral orifice (1). Bartholin glands are tubuloalveolar glands with acini having simple, columnar mucous-secreting epithelium. Bartholin gland ducts open on the posterolateral aspect of the vestibule and distally have a transitional epithelium that merges with the surface squamous epithelium of the vestibule. The minor vestibular glands, which are also mucus-producing, ring the vestibule. Skene's glands are paraurethral, being located immediately adjacent to and posterolateral to the urethra. Skene's glands are no greater than 1.5 cm in length and are lined by a pseudostratified mucus-secreting columnar epithelium. Skene's glands are thought to be a prostate gland homologue, and often express prostate-specific antigen and prostatic acid phosphatase. The transitional cell (urothelial) lining of the urethral orifice (meatus urinarius) urethra is in continuity with squamous epithelium of the vestibule. The vulvar aspect of the hymen is lined by a glycogen-rich nonkeratinizing stratified squamous epithelium, underneath which lies a fibrovascular stroma with some touch and pain receptors (1).

Lymphatic drainage from the vulva is to femoral and inguinal lymph nodes, with a notable exception being the existence of a second lymphatic pathway from the glans clitoris (1,5,6). In this latter route, the lymphatic channels join the lymphatics of the urethra, traverse the urogenital diagram, and merge with the lymphatic plexus on the anterior surface of the urinary bladder, with subsequent drainage to interiliac, obturator, and external iliac nodes.

Arterial blood supply to the vulva is from the femoral artery to superficial and deep external pudendal arteries and internal iliac arteries to internal pudendal arteries. There are separate blood supplies to the clitoris, from the deep arteries of the

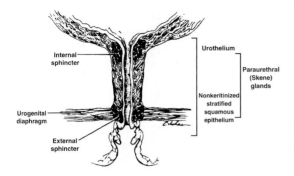

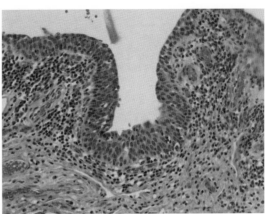

Fig. 1.3. Anatomy of the female urethra (From: Carroll PR, Dixon CN (1997) Surgical management of urethral carcinomas. In Current Genitourinary Cancer Surgery. Crawford D and Das S (eds.), Williams & Wilkins, Baltimore)

Fig. 1.4. Lining of the proximal female urethra: urotherlium, shown with chronic inflammation

clitoris, and vestibule and Bartholin's gland areas via the anterior vaginal artery. Venous blood drainage is mainly via the bilateral internal iliac veins, which drains into the external iliac venous system (1).

Innervation of the vulva is mostly via the anterior and posterior labial nerves, which are branches of the ilioinguinal nerve and pudendal nerve, respectively (1,7). The clitoris and vestibule receive nerve supply from the dorsal nerve of the clitoris and the cavernous nerves of the clitoris (1,7).

2. Female Urethra

The female urethra is about 4 cm in length (**Fig. 1.3**) in its course from the urinary bladder neck to the vaginal vestibule (8–10). Paraurethral glands are found along the periphery. Distally, the ducts from the glands (Skene's glands) empty near the external urethral meatus (**Fig. 1.4**). The proximal one-third of the female urethra is lined by urothelium and the distal two-thirds by nonkeratinized stratified squamous epithelium. There is a richly vascular underlying submucosa. The mucosa and submucosa are surrounded by a thick layer of inner longitudinal smooth muscle that runs from the urinary bladder to the external meatus. A thin layer of circular smooth muscle is outside the longitudinal layer. The striated urethral sphincter is found along the distal two-thirds of the female urethra (9–11). The skeletal muscle fibers are embedded in connective tissue and admixed with smooth muscle. The urethra is suspended beneath the pubis by a pubourethral ligament composed of an anterior suspensory ligament of the clitoris, a posterior pubourethral ligament of endopelvic fascia

and an intermediate ligament representing a fusion of those two (12). Somatic innervation to the urethral sphincter muscle is from pudendal and pelvic somatic nerves. Branches of the pudendal artery supply the urethra (and perineum). Lymphatic drainage of the anterior (distal third) of the female urethra drains preferentially into the superficial inguinal lymph nodes, while drainage from the posterior urethra (the proximal two-thirds) is into a combination of three pelvic lymphatic channels (10). These flow underneath the clitoris to the external iliac nodes, along the internal pudendal artery to the obturator lymph nodes, and to the presacral lymph nodes (10).

3. Male Genital Skin

Male genital skin includes the cutaneous lining of the penis and scrotum. The skin of the penis includes epithelium and lamina propria, which overlay the corpora cavernosa, corpus spongiosum, and pendulous urethra (**Fig. 1.5**). The microanatomy of the penile skin can be discussed based upon consideration of distal anatomy, including glans, coronal sulcus and foreskin and of a proximal portion, the corpus or shaft (**Figs. 1.6, 1.7**) (13,14). The glans and coronal sulcus are covered by a thin, partially keratinized squamous epithelium. The glans and coronal sulcus surface is actually a mucosa, rather than skin, since no adnexal or glandular structures are present. The glans lamina propria separates the corpus spongiosum from the epithelium. Its thickness varies from 1 mm (at the corona) to 2.5 mm (near the meatus). Histologically, the lamina propria is comprised of fibrous and

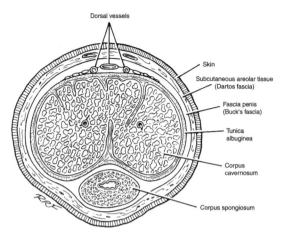

FIG. 1.5. Cross section of the penis (From Quartey JFM (1997) Microcirculation of Penile Scrotal Skin. Atlas of Urologic Clinics of NA 5(1), pg 2.)

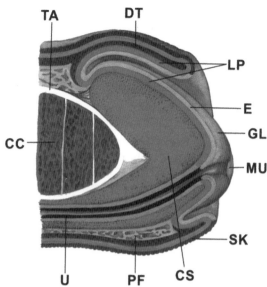

FIG. 1.7. Distal portion of penis including glans (GL), coronal sulcus, and foreskin. (E, epithelium; LP, lamina propria; CS, corpus spongiosum; TA, tunica albuginea; CC, corpus cavernosum; DT, dartos; SK, skin; U, urethra; MU, meatus urethralis; PF, penile or Buck's fascia) (From Stacey E. Mills (ed) (2007) Histology for Pathologists, 3rd, Lippincott, Williams and Williams, Philadelphia, chapter 38)

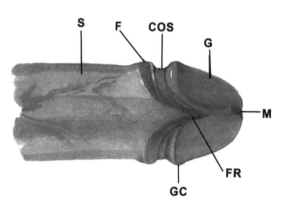

FIG. 1.6. Penile anatomy: Distal portion includes glans (G), coronal sulcus (COS), and foreskin, whereas proximal portion includes corpus or shaft (S), (M) urethral meatus, (GC) glans corona, and (FR) frenulum). (From Stacey E. Mills (ed) (2007) Histology for Pathologists, 3rd, Lippincott, Williams and Williams, Philadelphia, chapter 38)

vascular tissue, with the vascularity being less prominent compared to the underlying corpus spongiosum. The coronal sulcus lamina propria is essentially a prolongation of the foreskin and glans lamina propria.

The foreskin, or prepuce, is a mixture of skin and mucosa that is basically an extension of the skin of the shaft and normally covers most of the glans, with an inner mucosal surface of the foreskin covering the coronal sulcus and glans surface *(13,14)*. Grossly, the skin surface is dark and wrinkled while the opposite mucosal lining exhibits a pink to tan coloration.

Histologically, there are five layers to the foreskin: the epidermis, dermis, Dartos, lamina propria, and epithelium. The skin is made up of epidermis with keratinized stratified squamous epithelium and dermis with connective tissue containing blood vessels, nerve endings, Meissner (touch), and Vater-Panini (deep pressure and vibration) corpuscles, with a few hair structures and sebaceous and sweat glands. The Dartos is the middle component of the foreskin and has smooth muscle fibers surrounded by elastic fibers, with numerous nerve endings. The lamina propria is a loose fibrovascular and connective tissue with free nerve endings and genital corpuscles. The squamous epithelium of the mucosa surface of the foreskin is in continuity with the glands and coronal sulcus mucosal epithelium and is the same structurally. The skin of the penile shaft overlies the Dartos, Buck's fascia, tunica albuginea, corpora cavernosa, and corpus spongiosum (**Fig. 1.5**). It is rugged and elastic and comprises an epidermis and dermis. The epidermis is thin, with slight keratinization and basal layer pigmentation. Hair follicles are present and are more frequent in the proximal shaft. Only a few sebaceous and sweat glands can be found.

Lymphatics of the glans drain into superficial and deep inguinal lymph nodes, whereas lymphatics of the foreskin and skin of the shaft drain into superficial inguinal nodes *(14)*. The blood supply of the skin is supplied by external pudendal blood vessels *(15)*. Venous blood of penile skin flows into a subdermal venous plexus, which drains into several veins at the base of the penis *(15)*. Innervations of the glans and foreskin are by terminal branches of the dorsal nerve of the penis *(13)*.

Skin of the scrotum is pigmented, hair-bearing, and loose with numerous sebaceous and sweat glands. Depending on patient age and tone of the underlying smooth muscle, the surface is smooth to highly folded and wrinkled, with transverse rugae. The epidermis is thin, and along with the dermis, overlies the Dartos layer of smooth muscle. A subcutaneous fat (adipose) layer is lacking. The anterior scrotum is supplied by the external pudendal blood vessels and the posterior scrotum is supplied by the internal pudendal blood vessels *(15)*. Venous drainage for anterior scrotum is via the anterior scrotal subdermal venous plexus that converges at the neck of the scrotum to join the external pudendal vein. The subdermal venous plexus of the posterior scrotal wall drains into the perineal vein to join the internal pudendal vein *(15)*. Lymphatic drainage is to the superficial inguinal lymph nodes. The scrotum has a complex pattern of innervation *(16)*. The main supply is via scrotal branches of the perineal nerve, a branch of the pudendal nerve. Other contributions come from the inferior pudendal branch of the femoral cutaneous nerve and the genital branch of genitofemoral nerve and anterior cutaneous branches of the iliohypogastric and ilioinguinal nerves *(16)*.

4. Male Urethra

The male urethra may be divided into proximal (posterior) and distal (anterior) segments. The proximal segment comprises prostatic and membranous portions, whereas the distal segment is made up of bulbous and penile (pendulous) segments (**Fig. 1.8**). The prostatic urethra is 3–4 cm in length, is formed at the bladder neck, turns anteriorly 35 degrees at its midpoint (the urethral angle), and exits the prostate at the apex, where it is continuous with the membranous urethra. The urethral angle divides the prostatic

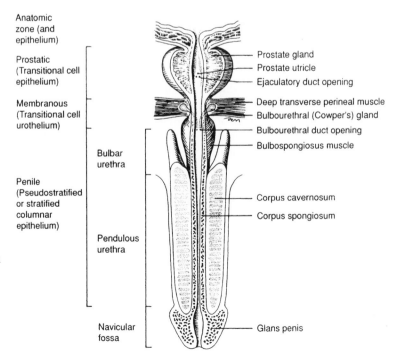

FIG. 1.8. Anatomy of male urethra (From Carroll PR, Dixon CN (1997) Surgical management of urethral carcinomas in Current Genitourinary Cancer Surgery. Crawford and Das S (ed); Williams & Wilkins, Baltimore)

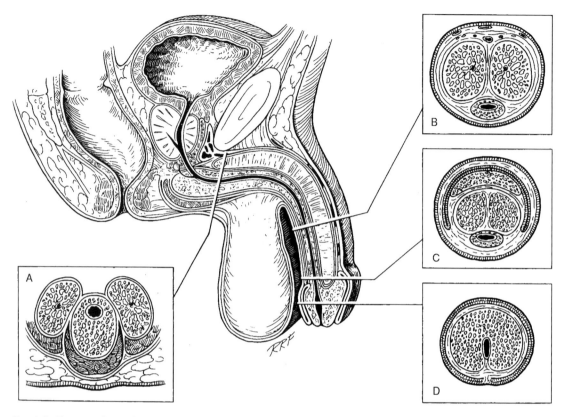

FIG. 1.9. Cross sections of the anterior urethra. (A) The bulbous urethra. (B) Penile shaft. (C) Coronal margin. (D) Glans (From Complications of interventional techniques for urethral stricture. In Complications of Interventional Techniques. (1996) Carson CC (ed), Igaku-Shoim, New York, pg 89)

urethra into proximal (so-called preprostatic) and distal (so-called prostatic) segments. The transition zone of the prostate wraps around the proximal urethra. The main prostatic ducts from this zone drain into posterolateral recesses of the urethra at a point just proximal to the urethral angle. Beyond the angle, ejaculatory ducts and ducts from the central prostatic zone empty at the posterior urethral protuberance known as the verumontanum. At the apex of the verumontanum, the slit-like orifice of the prostatic utricle, a 6-mm mullerian remnant, which is a sac-like structure, may be found. Ducts from the peripheral zone of the prostate empty into posterior urethral recesses in grooves in a double row from the verumontanum to the prostatic apex. Histologically, the surface epithelial lining of the prostatic urethra is predominately urothelial (transitional cell), although prostatic epithelium also may be found.

The membranous urethra, at 2 to 2.5 cm in length, is the shortest segment of the male urethra. It is lined by stratified/pseudostratified columnar epithelium and surrounded by skeletal muscle fibers of the urogenital diaphragm (external urethral sphincter).

The bulbous urethra is 3 to 4 cm in length, has a larger luminal caliber than the prostatic or membranous urethra, and extends in the root of the penis within the bulb of the corpus spongiosum from the distal margin of urogenital diagram to the penile urethra (**Fig. 1.9**). The lining epithelium is identical to that of the membranous urethra, being of a stratified/pseudostratified type. The ducts of Cowper's (bulbourethral) glands, which are embedded in the urogenital diagram, open into the posterior aspect of the bulbous urethra. Mucin-secreting Littre's glands can also be found in the walls of the bulbous urethra (**Fig. 1.10**).

The penile urethra is of about 15 cm in length and extends to the tip of the glans penis at the urethral meatus. It is surrounded in its entire length by the corpus spongiosum (**Fig. 1.2**). The distal 4

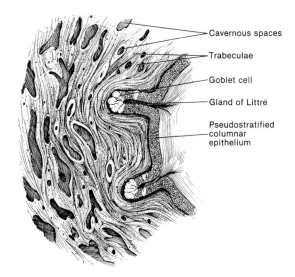

FIG. 1.10. Anatomy of the epithelium and glands of the penile urethra (From: Hinman F, Jr. (1993) Atlas of Urosurgical Anatomy, Philadelphia. WB Saunders, pg 447)

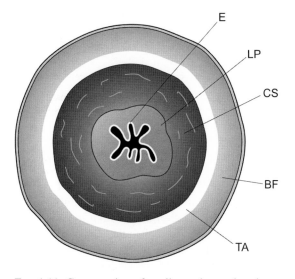

FIG. 1.11. Cross section of penile urethra and periurethral tissues. Diagrammatic cross section. E, epithelium; LP, lamina propria; CS, corpus spongiosum; TA, tunica albuginea; BF, Buck's fascia

to 6 cm of the prostatic urethra is a saccular dilation, termed the fossa navicularis, that terminates at the urethral meatus. Recesses called lacunae of Morgagni, which extend into Littre's glands, are found in the lateral walls of the penile urethra.

There are five anatomical levels of the distal (anterior) urethra (**Fig. 1.11**): urethral epithelium, lamina

propria, corpus spongiosum, tunica albuginea, and Buck's fascia *(13,17)*. Most of the penile urethral lining is a stratified/pseudostratified columnar epithelium, whereas the distal penile urethra, including the fossa navicularis, is lined by ciliated stratified columnar epithelium or stratified nonkeratinizing squamous epithelium. The lamina propria of the penile urethra is fibroconnective tissue with elastic fibers and scattered, longitudinally oriented smooth muscle.

Lymphatic drainage of the prostate and bulbomembranous urethra is into obturator and external iliac nodes, whereas the drainage from the penile urethra is into the superficial inguinal nodes. Urethral innervation is mainly by the dorsal nerve of the penis. Branches of the perineal nerve can supply the periurethral area in some men *(13)*.

References

1. Wilkinson EJ, Hardt NS (2007) Vulva. In: Mills SE (ed) Histology for pathologists, vol 3. Lippincott Williams and Wilkins, Philadelphia, pp 983–997
2. Farage M, Maibach K (2000) Lifetime changes in the vulva and vagina Arch Gynecol Obstet 273:195–202
3. O'Connel HE, Sanjeevan KV, Hutson JM (2005) Anatomy of the clitoris. J Urol 176:1109–1195
4. O'Connell HE, Hutson JM, Anderson CR, Plenter RJ (1998) Anatomical relationship between urethra and clitoris J Urol 159:1892–1987
5. Wilkinson EJ (1994) Benign diseases of the vulva. In: Kurman RJ (ed) Blaustein's pathology of the female genital tract. Springer-Verlag, New York, 4, pp 31–86
6. Parry-Jones E (1963) Lymphatics of the vulva J Obstet Gynecol Br Commun 70:756–765
7. Yucel S, DeSouza A Jr, Baskin LS (2004) Neuroanatomy of the human female lower urogenital tract J Urol 172:191–195
8. Reuter VE (1997) Urethra. In: Bostwick DG, Eble JN (eds) Urologic surgical pathology. Mosby, St. Louis, pp 435–454
9. Brooks JD (2002) Anatomy of the lower urinary tract and male genitalia In: Walsh PC (ed) Campbell's urology. Saunders, Philadelphia, 8, pp 41–80
10. Carroll PR, Dixon CM (1992) Surgical anatomy of the male and female urethra Urol Clin N Am 19:339–346
11. Oelrich TM (1983) The striated urogenital sphincter muscle in the female Anat Rec 205:223–232
12. Milley PS, Nichols DH (1971) The relationship between the pubo-urethral ligaments and the urogenital diaphragm in the human female Anat Rec 170:281–284
13. Velazquez EF, Barreto JE, Cold CJ, Cubilla AL (2007) Penis and distal urethra. In: Mills SE (ed)

Histology for pathologists. Lippincott Williams and Wilkins, Philadelphia, 3, pp 983–997

14. Young RH, Srigley JR, Amin MB, Ulbright TM, Cubilla AL (2000) The penis. In: Tumors of the prostate gland, seminal vesicles, male urethra, and penis. Armed Forces Institute of Pathology, Washington, DC, pp 403–488

15. Quartey JKM (1997) Microcirculation of penile and scrotal skin. Atlas of Urol Clin N Am 5:1–9

16. Yucel S, Baskin LS (2003) The neuroanatomy of the human scrotum: surgical ramifications BJU Int 91:393–397

17. Young RH, Srigley JR, Amin MB, Ulbright TM, Cubilla AL (2000) The male urethra. In: Tumors of the prostate gland. Seminal vesicles, male urethra and penis. Armed Forces Institute of Pathology, Washington, DC, pp 367–402.

2
Vascular Anatomy of Genital Skin and the Urethra: Implications for Urethral Reconstruction

Steven B. Brandes

Contents

1. Penile Anatomy: Gross 9
2. Penile Skin Arterial Blood Supply.. 10
3. Scrotal Skin Blood Supply.. 12
4. Venous Drainage of the Penile Skin.. 13
5. Venous Drainage of the Scrotum 13
6. Genital Flap Selection... 14
7. Blood Supply of the Urethra (Corpus Spongiosum).. 14
    7.1. Arterial Blood Supply 14
    7.2. Venous Drainage 17
References... 18

Summary An intimate knowledge of the penile skin blood supply is essential to successfully mobilize and construct a fasciocutaneous onlay flap for "substitution" urethral reconstruction. For successful anastomotic urethroplasty, an intact and adequate dual urethral arterial blood supply is essential. The key vascular feature of the urethra and the reason that it can be mobilized extensively and divided is its unique bipedal blood supply. The proximal and distal ends of the urethra are supplied by two arterial blood supplies, the proximal urethra in an antegrade fashion, and the distal, retrograde. The common penile artery, a branch of the internal pudendal, first branches into the bulbar and circumflex cavernosal arteries (supplying the proximal corpus spongiosum), and then bifurcates into the central cavernosal arteries and into the dorsal artery of the penis. The dorsal artery arborizes and penetrates into the glans penis, and then flows retrograde into the spongiosum. Thus, the corpus spongiosum has two blood supplies, proximally the bulbar and circumflex arteries, and distally, arborizations of the dorsal penile artery.

Keywords External pudendal artery, internal pudendal artery, bipedal blood supply, circumflex vessels, arterial plexus.

1. Penile Anatomy: Gross

The penis is covered with an elastic layer of skin that has no subcuticular adipose layer. Beneath the penile skin is the Dartos fascia, a layer of loose areolar subcutaneous tissue. The Dartos is devoid of fat and slides freely over the underlying Buck's fascia. The Dartos of the penis is contiguous with Scarpa's fascia of the abdominal wall, in which run the superficial nerves, lymphatics, and blood vessels. Beneath the Dartos fascia lies the superficial lamina (or lamella) of Buck's fascia. Buck's fascia covers in one envelope the tunica albuginea (outer longitudinal fibers) of the two corpora cavernosa, and the tunica of the corpus spongiosum. In the scrotum, the embryologic equivalent of Buck's fascia is the external spermatic fascia.

When one develops a fasciocutaneous penile skin island flap of genital skin, as one does with an Orandi (vertical flap) or a McAninch/Quartey (circular transverse) flap, we take advantage of the natural anatomical cleavage planes of the superficial layers of the penis. The main two distinct cleavage (relatively avascular) planes are between the skin and the Dartos fascia, whereas the other is between the Dartos fascia and Buck's fascia. Buck's fascia is fairly adherent to the underlying longitudinal fibers of the tunica albuginea and much more difficult to separate. In Peyronie's disease surgery, tunica plaque incision and grafting demands developing that difficult plane between the outer longitudinal layer of tunica albuginea and the overlying Buck's fascia.

2. Penile Skin Arterial Blood Supply

The blood supply to the skin of the penis and the anterior scrotal wall are from the external pudendal arteries. The blood supply to the posterior aspects of the scrotum is from posterior scrotal arteries, which is a branch of the perineal artery, which is a further branch of the internal pudendal arteries *(5)* (**Fig. 2.1**).

Branching off the medial aspect of the femoral artery are the superficial/ superior branches and the deep/inferior branches of the external pudendal artery. These superficial external pudendal branches pass from lateral to medial, in a variable pattern, across the femoral triangle, and within Scarpa's fascia (a loose membrane of superficial fascia; **Fig. 2.2**).

After giving off scrotal branches to the anterior scrotum, the superficial external pudendal artery cross the spermatic cord and enter the base of the penis as posterolateral and anterolateral axial branches. Together with interconnecting, perforating branches, they form an arterial network within the Dartos fascia. The Dartos fascia is not really the blood supply; it is more accurate to visualize the fascia as a trellis and the blood supply as

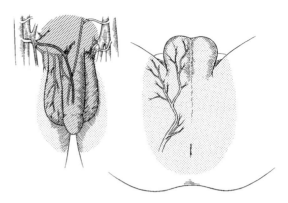

FIG. 2.1. The relative areas of arborization of the superficial external pudendal artery and the perineal/labial scrotal arborization. Cross-hatched area is based predominantly on the superficial external pudendal artery. The dotted area is based primarily on the perineal/labial scrotal arterial blood supply. There are areas of overlap on the scrotum. (From Jordan GH (ed) (1997) Reconstruction for urethral stricture, Atlas of Urol Clin NA 5(1))

the vine entwined on the trellis. At the base of the penis, branches from the axial penile arteries form a subdermal plexus which supplies the distal penile skin and prepuce (**Fig. 2.3**). There are perforating connections between the subcutaneous and subdermal arterial plexuses. These connections typically are minimal and very fine and, thus, a relatively avascular plane can be developed between the Dartos and Buck's fascia. Because the fascial plexus is the true blood supply to the penile skin flaps that we use in urethral reconstruction, the flaps are considered axial, penile skin island flaps that therefore can be mobilized widely and transposed aggressively. When developing a penile skin island flaps, it is often important to preserve the lateral and base aspects of the flap pedicle, because the arborizations of the superficial external pudendal arteries pass onto the penile shaft from lateral to medial. The pedicles can be kept large and mobilized extensively and reliably, enough so to even reach the perineum and proximal urethra. Occasionally, between the two layers, there is a large communication or perforating branch that needs to be ligated and divided. At the subcorona, the axial penile arteries continue onto the foreskin as preputial arteries, as well as send perforating arterial branches which pierce Buck's fascia to anastomose with the dorsal arteries *(5)* (**Fig. 2.4**).

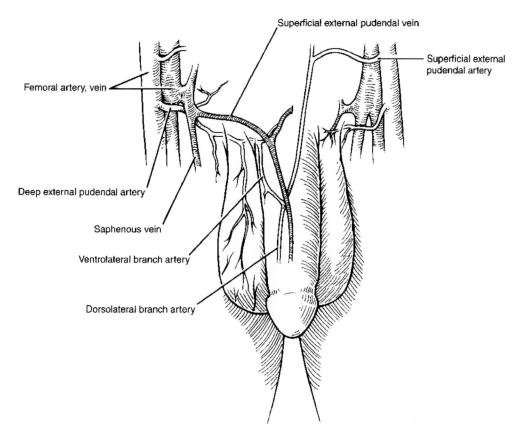

FIG. 2.2. The superficial external pudendal blood supply (to penile and anterior scrotal skin). (From Jordan GH (ed) (1997) Reconstruction for urethral stricture, Atlas of Urol Clin NA 5(1))

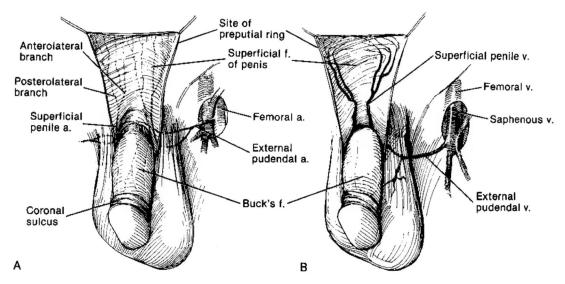

FIG. 2.3. Preputial blood supply. (A), Arterial supply. (B), Venous drainage (From Hinman F, Jr (1993) Atlas of Urosurgical Anatomy, Philadelphia, WB Saunders)

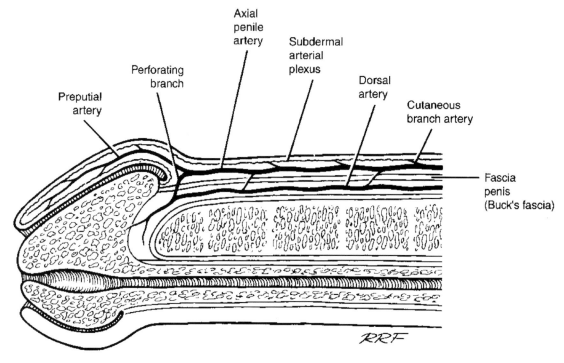

FIG. 2.4. Cross-sectional view of penile skin arterial plexuses; subdermal, subcutaneous, dorsal arterial. (From Jordan GH (ed) (1997) Reconstruction for urethral stricture, Atlas of Urol Clin of NA 5(1))

3. Scrotal Skin Blood Supply

The anterior aspect of the scrotum is supplied by anterior scrotal arteries, which are branches of the external pudendal artery. At the cephalad end (top) of the scrotum, they give off branches superficially to form a subdermal plexus that continue along the caudal aspect of the anterior scrotum to anastomose with the posterior scrotal arteries.

The blood supply to the posterior aspect of the scrotum is from several scrotal arteries, which are branches of the perineal artery, which is a superficial terminal branch of the internal pudendal artery (**Fig. 2.5**). The perineal artery emanates from Alcock's canal to pierce the posterolateral corner of the perineal membrane and then runs anteriorly, along the superficial fascia, in a groove between the bulbospongiosus and ischiocavernosus muscles. The scrotal arteries also give off branches to form a subdermal arterial plexus that anastomose at the apex of the scrotum with anterior scrotal arteries from the other side (**Fig. 2.1**). Furthermore, along the central scrotal septum, there are additional

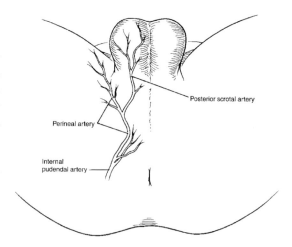

FIG. 2.5. The perineal artery/labial-scrotal blood supply. (From Jordan GH (ed) (1997) Reconstruction for urethral stricture, Atlas of Urol Clin of NA 5(1))

intercommunications between the anterior and posterior scrotal arteries.

Scrotal skin island flaps, based on a fascial flap of tunica Dartos can be efficient for mobilizing skin island to the bulbar urethra, the pedicle is

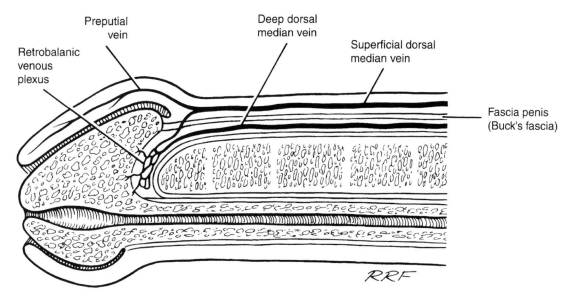

FIG. 2.6. Deep and superficial dorsal median veins arising from the retrobalanic venous plexus. (From Jordan GH (ed) (1997) Reconstruction for urethral stricture, Atlas of Urol Clin of NA 5(1))

often too short to reach anterior urethra. The facial pedicle can also be oriented posteriorly, by extending a "∩"-shaped incision onto the perineum (as in the Blandy flap for perineal urethrostomy).

4. Venous Drainage of the Penile Skin

Between the proximal–posterior aspects of the glans penis and the distal ends of the corpora cavernosal bodies is the retrobalanic venous plexus. From this venous plexus arise two branches of veins, the deep dorsal median and the superficial dorsal median (**Fig. 2.6**). The deep dorsal median vein runs posterior to Buck's fascia, while the superficial dorsal median vein pierces Buck's fascia subcoronally to run in the superficial layer of the Dartos fascia. Typically, there are no large connections between the deep (subdermal) venous plexus and the superficial (subcutaneous) veins (**Fig. 2.6**). However, occasionally the circumflex or deep dorsal median veins connect to the superficial veins in the subcutaneous tissue, or the superficial dorsal median vein branch off directly from the deep dorsal median vein, instead of the more typical origin in the retrobalanic venous plexus.

The superficial veins can also run dorsolateral, lateral, and/or ventrolateral. Running with the axial dorsal penile arteries are venae comitantes. The veins in the prepuce, however, are small and multiple and are distributed without particular orientation. These veins then join together to drain into one or two of the large superficial veins or continue independently, to the base of the penis, that drain through the inferior external pudendal vein into the saphenous vein (**Fig. 2.3B**). At the base of the penis, the large communicating veins, the venae comitantes, and the subdermal venous plexuses all combine in variable patterns to form the external pudendal veins, which further empty into the long saphenous veins or directly into the femoral vein.

5. Venous Drainage of the Scrotum

The anterior scrotal veins and the veins that drain the anterior scrotal subdermal venous plexus coalesce at the base of the scrotum to drain into the external pudendal vein. The posterior scrotal veins combine with the veins of the subdermal venous plexus of the posterior scrotal wall and drain into the perineal vein. The perineal vein then pierces the posterolateral corners of the perineal membrane to join the internal pudendal vein within Alcock's canal.

6. Genital Flap Selection

Genital skin island flaps are versatile for anterior urethral reconstruction. A thorough knowledge of the anatomy and specific tissue characteristics and adhering to the surgical principles of tissue transfer can result in long term success. The specific skin island flap that is selected should be based on specific physical characteristics. Sought after characteristics for such island flaps are: 1) skin for harvest is from an area of natural skin redundancy, 2) the skin at the donor site is elastic or redundant enough to be closed, 3) the skin island is thin and hairless, 4) the island of skin is long and wide enough to bridge the entire stricture, 5) the vascular pedicle to the skin island is reliable, long, and robust.

7. Blood Supply of the Urethra (Corpus Spongiosum)

A detailed knowledge of the arterial blood supply of the corpus spongiosum is essential to perform stricture excision and primary anastomosis urethral surgery.

7.1. Arterial Blood Supply

The key feature and the reason that the urethra can be mobilized extensively, divided, and then sewn back together is that it has a unique dual blood supply. The distal and proximal ends of the urethra are supplied by two arterial blood supplies, the proximal urethra in an antegrade fashion, and the distal urethra in a retrograde fashion. The internal pudendal artery branches into the perineal artery and posterior scrotal artery and then continues distally as the common penile artery (**Fig. 2.7**). The common penile artery branches into the bulbar arteries and circumflex cavernosal arteries (which both supply the proximal corpus spongiosum). The common penile artery then bifurcates into the central cavernosal arteries (also known as the deep artery of the corpus cavernosum) and into the dorsal artery of the penis (**Fig. 2.8**). The dorsal artery of the penis arborizes and penetrates into the spongy tissue of the glans penis. From the glans penis, the blood flows retrograde into the corpus spongiosum. The corpus spongiosum thus has two blood supplies, proximally by the bulbar and circumflex cavernosal arteries, and distally by arborizations of the dorsal penile artery. There are also perforators between the ventral corpora cavernosa and the corpus spongiosum. These perforators, however, are neither constant nor reliable in their distribution. When the urethra is mobilized and transected for anastomotic urethroplasty, adequate distal blood supply and retrograde flow is essential. Within the corpus spongiosum there are typically two or three urethral arteries. Based on recent ultrasonography studies, contrary to common belief, the urethral

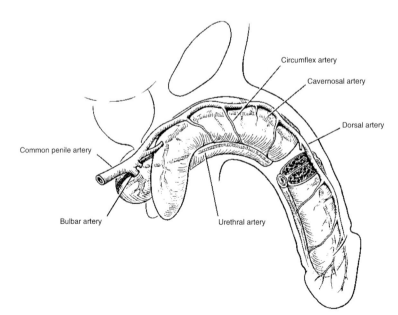

Circumflex artery

Cavernosal artery

Dorsal artery

Common penile artery

Bulbar artery   Urethral artery

FIG. 2.7. Urethral and penile arterial blood supply. (From Jordan GH (ed) (1997) Reconstruction for urethral stricture, Atlas of Urol Clin of NA 5(1))

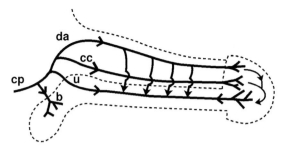

FIG. 2.8. Bipedal arterial blood supply of the urethra (cp, common penile; da, dorsal artery of the penis; cc, central cavernosal; u, urethral; b, bulbar artery)

arteries are not typically located at the 3- or 9-o'clock positions (1). Urethral arteries, in contrast, have a variable position, and the location varies with near equal distribution around the clock, among patients (**Fig. 2.9**). The arteries can be close to the urethral lumen epithelium, especially in patients who have undergone prior urethral procedures. Although researchers suggest that urethral stricture patients who undergo urethrotomy, the direction for the incision can be determined by the preoperative ultrasound artery location, we have not found this to be particularly helpful. Rather, urethrotomy location probably does not matter so much as it is not too deep into the spongiosum, yet deep enough to allow the epithelium open up and re-scar in an open position.

If the urethra is overly mobilized distally or the patient has a known severe hypospadias, retrograde distal blood flow can be severely compromised.

Here, anastomotic urethroplasty can result is proximal urethral ischemia and re-stricture. Such patients with compromised dual blood supply are thus often better served with substitution urethroplasty (**Fig. 2.10**). The other situation where the proximal urethra is at risk for ischemic necrosis with excision and primary anastomosis (EPA) surgery is the unusual situation where the bulbar arteries, as well as the common penile circulation have been disrupted and, thus, bipedal blood flow is inadequate (**Fig. 2.11**).

Urethral ischemic necrosis or ischemia refers to recurrence of stricture of the anterior and proximal urethra after Excision and primary anastomosis (EPA) urethral surgery. Such ischemic strictures are particularly difficult to manage because often they are very long and either have a very narrow caliber or completely obliterate the proximal anterior urethra. In contrast, technical error strictures are typically short, annular and easily amenable to internal urethrotomy. Jordan et al. (2), upon reviewing all their failed posterior urethroplasties after pelvic fracture, observed that patients who developed the severe complication of proximal urethral necrosis all seemed to have one or more of the same characteristics; namely, previous histories of pelvic fracture associated with vascular injuries, were children, were elderly, had a cold or decreased sensate glans penis, decreased erections, or failed prior posterior urethroplasty. They further studied these patients with nocturnal penile tumescence studies and, if abnormal, with penile ultrasound and Doppler and of those, if abnormal, with pudendal angiography. They concluded

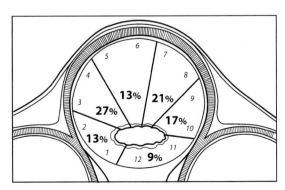

Bulbar Urethra

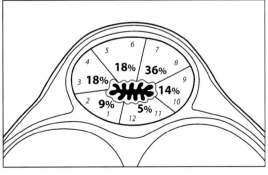

Pendulous Urethra

FIG. 2.9. Distribution of the location of the urethral arteries in the bulbar and pendulous urethra. (Redrawn after Ref. *[1]*)

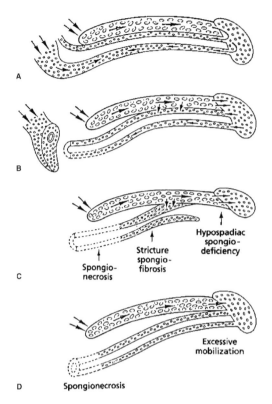

FIG. 2.10. Vascular principles of anastomotic urethroplasty. After division of the bulbar arteries, blood supply of the proximal bulbar urethra relies on the retrograde blood supply along its spongy tissue (A) and (B). Ischemic necrosis of the proximal mobilized urethra can result when the retrograde blood supply is compromised, such as occurs with hypospadias (C), incidental spongiofibrosis, or division of distal collateral vessels by excessive mobilization of the penile urethra (D). (From Yu G, Miller HC (2996) Critical operative maneuvers in urologic surgery. Mosby, St. Louis)

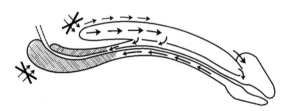

FIG. 2.11. The illustration shows that, in bilateral internal pudendal complex obliteration ("X" marks), there can be insufficient blood supply to the proximal urethra with an anastomotic urethroplasty. Hatched marks demonstrate "ischemic necrosis" of the proximal urethra after EPA surgery

that ischemic urethral necrosis was most likely, when on angiography, there was bilateral injury to the deep internal pudendal artery-common penile arterial system, without distal reconstitution. In other words, because the bulbar arteries and the common penile circulation are disrupted in this situation, there is inadequate retrograde and antegrade urethral blood flow for anastomotic urethroplasty. Such extreme vascular injuries after pelvic fracture are exceedingly rare (4).

Jordan et al. (2) suggest that patients who lack adequate bipedal blood supply of the urethra should be considered for penile revascularization before posterior urethroplasty. An algorithm for evaluating and managing patients at risk for ischemic necrosis is detailed in Fig. 2.12. When possible, a bilateral end to side anastomosis of inferior epigastric artery to dorsal penile artery should be performed (Fig. 2.13). Impotent patients with bilateral pudendal complex injury with distal reconstruction also may have insufficient blood flow not allowing for normal erections (4). In our experience with penile revascularization and refractory impotence after pelvic fracture, in young patients with few comorbidities, revascularization helps to resolve penile numbness and "coldness" and enables erection with intracavernosal injections or intraurethral alprostadil. In general, after pelvic fracture, aside from neurologic or venous problems, for normal erectile function or a normal response to pharmacotherapy, patients need at least one intact internal pudendal complex. According to Jordan et al. (2), all patients with risk factors for urethral ischemic necrosis who undergo successful penile revascularization before anastomotic urethroplasty have successful urethral reconstructions. Successful penile revascularization means here that at 3 to 6 months after revascularization, peak systolic arterial blood flows are in the normal range. In summary, all patients with ischemic urethral necrosis, when studied, have bilateral injuries to the pudendals without reconstitution. Lack of reconstitution, however, only predisposes, not guarantees, that the urethra will experience necrosis after EPA.

The other place where antegrade and retrograde blood flow preservation with EPA urethroplasty is important is the postprostatectomy incontinent patient who also has a urethral stricture. When stress incontinence is severe, it often is treated with an artificial urinary sphincter, where a cuff is placed

FIG. 2.12. Algorithm for identifying patients for potential
urethral ischemic stenosis after
posterior urethroplasty, and
after urethral disruption injury.
(From Jordan GH (ed) (1997)
Reconstruction for urethral
stricture, Atlas of Urol Clin of
NA 5(1))

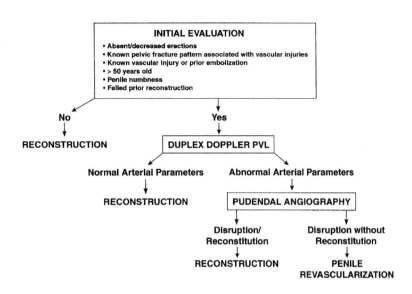

FIG. 2.12. Algorithm for identifying patients for potential urethral ischemic stenosis after posterior urethroplasty, and after urethral disruption injury. (From Jordan GH (ed) (1997) Reconstruction for urethral stricture, Atlas of Urol Clin of NA 5(1))

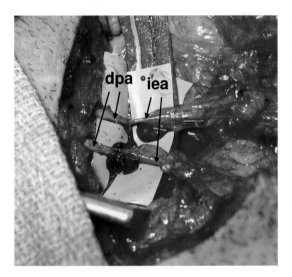

FIG. 2.13. Revascularization of the penis with bilateral end to side inferior epigastric artery (iea) to the dorsal penile artery (dpa)

blood flow. In maintaining the bulbar arteries, there should be adequate antegrade blood flow to the urethra proximal to the cuff. It seems logical that a vessel sparing technique could improve spongiosal vascularity and bulk underneath the cuff, and thus possibly decrease the risk of cuff erosion. Jordan et al. *(3)* have described an elaborate technique for sparing these vessels.

The other place where maximizing the bipedal blood supply of the urethra is important is when a bulbar or membranous urethral stricture is associated with a distal urethra with compromised blood supply (such is the case with patients with hypospadias, distal urethral spongiofibrosis). Because the retrograde blood flow is compromised with such distal urethral conditions, it is important to try to isolate and preserve the antegrade blood flow of the bulbar arteries, and consider either a pedicle skin island flap for the distal urethral stricture or a staged approach.

around the urethra and compresses it circumferentially. In our experience, the cuff erosion rate is high after anastomotic urethroplasty. Perseveration of the bulbar arteries, however, can help maintain the blood supply of the urethra proximal to the cuff, which might otherwise be compromised by cuff compression and occlusion of retrograde urethral

7.2. Venous Drainage

The venous drainage of the corpus spongiosum is predominantly the venous drainage of the glans panis and the other deep structures, namely via the periurethral veins, circumflex veins and the deep and superficial dorsal veins (**Fig. 2.14**).

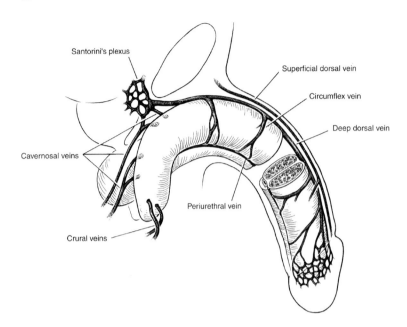

Santorini's plexus

Superficial dorsal vein

Circumflex vein

Deep dorsal vein

Cavernosal veins

Periurethral vein

Crural veins

FIG. 2.14. The venous drainage of the urethra and penis. (From Jordan GH (ed) (1997) Reconstruction for urethral stricture, Atlas of Urol Clin of NA 5(1))

References

1. Chiou RK, Donovan IM, Anderson JC, Matamoros A Jr, Wobig RK, Taylor RJ (1998) Color Doppler ultrasound assessment of urethral anatomy artery location: Potential implications for technique of visual internal urethrotomy (OIU). J Urol 159: 796–799
2. Jordan GH, Colen LB (2007) Penile revascularization after pelvic trauma: current rationale and results. Cont Urol 19:24–33
3. Jordan GH, Eltahawy EA, Virasoro R (2007) The technique of vessel sparing excision and primary anastomosis for proximal bulbous urethral reconstruction. J Urol 177:1799–1802
4. Levine FJ, Greenfield AJ, Goldstein I (1990) Arteriographically determined occlusive disease within the hypograstric cavernous bed in impotent patients following blunt perineal and pelvic trauma J Urol 144:1147–1153
5. Quartey JKM (1997) Microcirculation of penile and scrotal skin, In: Jordan GH (ed) Reconstruction for urethral stricture, Atlas of Urol Clin of NA 5(1).

3
Lichen Sclerosus

Ramón Virasoro and Gerald H. Jordan

Contents

1. Introduction... 19
2. Historical Aspects 20
3. Etiology.. 20
    3.1. Koebner Phenomenon 20
    3.2. Genetic Susceptibility and Autoimmunity... 21
    3.3. Oxidative Stress 21
    3.4. Infectious... 22
4. LS and Squamous Cell Carcinoma (SCC).. 22
5. Histology.. 22
6. Clinical Presentation 23
7. Management.. 24
    7.1. Medical Treatment 25
    7.2. Surgical Management... 25
Editorial Comment.. 26
References.. 26

Summary Lichen Sclerosus is a chronic inflammatory disorder of the skin. Incidence in the western world is 1:300. In men, LS peaks between the 30 to 50 years. Both genders can be affected, although genital involvement is much more common in women. Possible etiologies for LS are the Koebner phenomenon, genetic susceptibility and autoimmunity, oxidative stress, and infection. Clinical presentation is usually white patches that seem to coalesce into "plaques" that can affect the prepuce and glans. It is not clear whether LS spreads by direct extension into the fossa navicularis and a portion of the anterior urethra, or if urethral involvement is secondary to LS induced meatal stenosis and subsequent "Littritis". The classic radiographic appearance of LS anterior urethral stricture is a saw-toothed pattern. Surgical management of LS is primarily by staged urethroplasty.

Keywords Skin disorder, Koebner phenomenon, urethral stricture, staged urethroplasty.

1. Introduction

Lichen sclerosus (LS) is a chronic inflammatory disorder of the skin of unknown origin. No specific mechanism of disease has been elucidated, although substantial advances in characterizing the immunological basis of other disease processes may eventually characterize the pathogenesis of LS. There are several acquired scarring disorders of the skin associated with pathology of the basement-membrane, such as mucous membrane pemphigoid, that may be shown to be related *(1)*.

The reported incidence of LS in the western population is 1 in 300 *(2)*; however, the worldwide prevalence

From: *Current Clinical Urology: Urethral Reconstructive Surgery*
Edited by: S.B. Brandes © Humana Press, Totowa, NJ

may be substantially different. LS has been described in Africans *(3,4)*, Asians *(5)*, and other dark-skinned races, which may bias the prevalence because of the analyzed population. Most current publications come from Europe and the United States.

The peak ages of recognition in women are bimodal, with many cases noted before puberty, but another peak presenting in postmenopausal women *(6)*. In men, LS seems to peak between the ages of 30 to 50 years; however, incidences of LS has been described in people of all ages, from infants to the elderly *(6)*.

Both genders have been affected, although genital involvement is far more frequent in women, with a female to male ratio with genital involvement of 10:1 *(7)*.

In the past, the genital involvement with lichen sclerosus was called balanitis xerotica obliterans (BXO), and much of the older literature reflects that previous designation. Any area of the skin may be involved; however, the prevalence of involvement of the genitalia in the male and female is estimated to be 85% to 98 % of total cases *(8)*.

LS is believed to possibly be premalignant. The incidence of squamous cell carcinoma associated with vulvar lichen sclerosus averages between 4% and 6% *(9)*. In men, the association between LS and penile cancer ranges from 2.3% to 9.3% *(10–13)*. The true risk of malignancy remains to be determined. The problem is that few studies analyze the complete population followed with lichen sclerosus versus those that develop squamous cell carcinoma in previously determined lesions.

2. Historical Aspects

The term BXO was first applied by Stühmer in 1928 *(14)* and, as mentioned, is now considered to be just the genital manifestation of LS. Freeman and Laymon showed that BXO and LS were probably the same process *(15,16)*. The first report of what was probably LS was published by Weir in 1875, where he described a case of vulvar and oral "ichthyosis" *(17)*. Hallopeau reported in 1887 a case of trunk, forearm, and vulvar lichenification consistent with LS, and suggested the name of "lichen plans atrophique" *(18)*. Darier in 1892 described the typical histological characteristics of

what he called lichen planus scleréux, which later was renamed lichen sclerosus et atrophicus *(19)*. Since those initial reports, a number of names were then proposed to the entity we recognize as LS as follows: Kartenblattförmige sklerodermie ("playing card" or "cardboard-like" scleroderma *[20]*); Weissflecken Dermatose ("white spot disease" *[21]*); lichen albus *(22)*, lichen planus sclerosus et atrophicus *(23)*, dermatitis lichenoides chronica atrophicans *(24)*, and kraurosis vulvae *(25)*. Histologically, not all cases of LS are atrophic and, thus, Friedrich suggested that the term atrophicus was not accurate *(26)*. In 1976, the International Society for the Study of Vulvar Disease unified the nomenclature devising a new classification system and proposed the term lichen sclerosus *(27)*.

3. Etiology

As mentioned previously, the cause of LS is not known. A number of various mechanisms have been proposed. The Koebner phenomenon relates the development of LS to trauma to the affected area. It has been proposed that the etiology may be that of an autoimmune disease. Sanders hypothesized that reactive oxidative stress contributes to the sclerotic, immunologic, and carcinogenic processes in LS *(28)*. An infectious cause with the organism Borrellia burgdorferi implicated has been proposed. That has been called into question as the organism has not been able to be uniformly demonstrated in the lesions.

3.1. Koebner Phenomenon

Stühmer originally described LS as a postcircumcision phenomenon *(14)* and, clearly, LS has appeared in scars, both in the genitalia and other sites *(29)*. Patients have been described to develop lesions in areas exposed to radiotherapy *(30)*, ultraviolet (sunburn *[31]*), or thermal injury. These associations have led to the proposal that LS is a manifestation of the isomorphic or Koebner phenomenon, in which a patient with latent dermatoses, because of histological and immunologic alterations, may then develop the disease as the result of a stimulus. In this case, trauma would cause a lesion to develop in what would appear to be a clinically unaffected area.

3.2. Genetic Susceptibility and Autoimmunity

The theory that LS has a genetic origin is based on the observation of a familial distribution of cases, being reported in identical twins *(32,33)* and nonidentical twins *(34)* with coexistence of dermatosis. Concomitant appearance of the disease in mothers and daughters has also been published *(35)*.

Studies on the human leukocyte antigen (HLA) have suggested a genetic component in patients afflicted with LS. The major histocompatibility complex (MHC), a group of genes located in the short arm of chromosome 6, codes for the HLA antigens that influence cellular and humoral responses, determining an individual's susceptibility to inflammatory diseases. There are two isotypes of HLA molecules: HLA class I (A, B, C) and HLA class II (DR, DQ, DP). Class I and class II HLA gene clusters are located in different loci of the MHC, and between them are found several other genes with relevance to immune functions, such as tumor necrosis factors α and β (TNF-α, TNF-β). The major histocompatibility antigen complex determines an individual's susceptibility to inflammatory diseases by influencing cellular and humoral responses. Reports have described a disease association of LS with HLA class II antigens, specifically DQ7–DQ9. Several studies have shown what appears to be correlation with the DQ7 and DQ1R.

Men with LS have been found to have significantly greater incidences of autoimmune-related disorders and autoantibodies than control populations *(36,37)*. Azurdia et al. *(38)* found two cases (3%) with another autoimmune disease (alopecia areata and vitiligo) in more than 58 men with clinically (33%) or histologically proven (67%) lichen sclerosus *(38)*. Ten percent of the same population had a first-degree relative with an autoimmune disease. A not statistically significant increased frequency of DR11, DR12, and DR7 was also found in the same cohort *(38)*.

The association with various autoimmune disorders, which would include diabetes mellitus, alopecia areata, vitiligo, thyroid disease, and pernicious anemia, might suggest an immunologic component to the development of LS *(39–41)*.

Other entities presumed to be of autoimmune origin, such as psoriasis, eczema, primary billiary cirrhosis, mystic, lupus erythematous, and rheumatic polymyalgia, have all been described in association with LS *(40–45)*. The finding of thyroid antimicrosomal antibodies and gastric parietal cell antibodies has also been shown to be more frequent in patients with LS *(46,47)*.

Sanders speculates that a specific humoral immune response of circulating autoantibodies in LS could be the result of DNA damage by reactive oxygen species (ROS), causing changes at a macromolecular level *(28)*. Thus, defective apoptosis and delayed apoptotic cell clearance would lead to interaction of apoptotic cells and ROS resulting in neoepitope formation and subsequent autoimmunity *(28)*.

Oyama et al. *(48)* have recently described a specific autoantibody response to extracellular matrix protein 1 (ECM-1), an 85-kDa glycoprotein with important functions in skin physiology and homeostasis, which is located between the dermis and the epidermis. The mechanism of synthesis of these autoantibodies is not understood. It has been proposed that there is defective apoptosis with a delay in apoptotic cell clearance *(28)*. ECM1 has a role in epidermal differentiation and, at the dermis level, it binds to perlecan, the major heparan sulphate proteoglycan, acting as "biological glue" *(49)*. Mutation of the ECM1 gene results in lipoid proteinosis (Urbach-Wiethe disease); a rare autosomal-recessive genodermatosis that shares both clinical and histologic features with lichen sclerosus *(50)*. It is characterized by papules/nodules, indurated plaques, and sometimes ulcerated lesions involving primarily the skin and mucous membranes. Extracellular matrix protein 1 may also have a role in other acquired skin disorders and physiological skin changes including aging, wound healing, and scarring, although this remains to be determined *(49)*.

3.3. Oxidative Stress

Sanders et al. *(28)* hypothesize that oxidative stress contributes to the sclerotic, immunological, and carcinogenic processes in LS. A physiological balance between free radicals and antioxidant substances is maintained by cell antioxidant enzyme systems: copper-zinc superoxide dismutase (CuZnSOD); manganese superoxide dismutase (MnSOD); and catalase. Both CuZnSOD and MnSOD convert superoxide anions (O_2^-) into peroxide (H_2O_2), using O_2 and hydrogen as substrate. H_2O_2 is then divided into water and O_2 by catalase. ROS occurs when this equilibrium is altered; thus, there is augmentation of free radical formation, or antioxidant deficiency, or both. The resultant production of ROS causes oxidative injury of structural lipids and proteins at the cell membrane level, as well as at the DNA and sulfur-containing enzyme level. There are very sensitive markers of DNA damage, and Sanders demonstrated an increase in these markers and epidermal keratinocytes and dermal fibroblasts in the LS patient group when compared with controls (28).

3.4. Infectious

Acrodermatitis chronica atrophicans (ACA) is a dermatosis associated with *Borrellia burgdorferi*. Coexistence of ACA and morphea (localized scleroderma) has been published in 10% of cases (51). Associations of morphea with LS, as well as transition between the two entities, have been described (51,52). Aberer et al. (53) were the first to propose *B. burgdorferi* as the cause of morphea. Several articles followed their work with controversial results about the possible association of *B. burgdorferi* and morphea and LS.

In a review of the English, French and German literature from 1983 to 2000, Weide et al. (54) investigated the role of *B. burgdorferi* in the pathogenesis of morphea and LS by serology, immunohystology, culture, lymphocyte stimulation and DNA detection with polymerase chain reaction. They concluded that *B. burgdorferi* does not play a part in the pathogenesis of morphea or LS.

4. LS and Squamous Cell Carcinoma (SCC)

Although extragenital LS does not carry a risk for malignant transformation, the relationship of anogenital LS and SCC is more controversial. The association between LS and malignant lesions on the genitoanal skin has been well established in women and has been reported in 3% to 6% of patients with vulvar involvement (9). In men this association is more controversial. Nasca et al. (11) presented

5 (5.8%) cases of penile malignant lesions in 86 uncircumcised white patients with a long-standing diagnosis of lichen sclerosus. Three patients had SCC, 1 patient developed erythroplasia of Queyrat (CIS), and the other verrucous carcinoma (VC). Interestingly, four of the five patients tested positive for HPV 16 with protein chain reaction, which is contrary to reports from other authors, who report a lack of association with HPV induced-SCC and lichen sclerosus (13). In a subsequent report, Nasca et al. (12) presented three additional cases that developed squamous cell carcinoma in the same series, making a total of 8 penile malignancies in 86 patients with LS (9.3%); which suggests a considerable risk to develop epithelial malignancy in patients with long-standing LS (12).

Depasquale et al. (10) reported an incidence of 2.3% of SCC in a series with long-term follow up of men with genital lichen sclerosus. Twelve patients, of 522 with genital LS, developed squamous cell carcinoma; five were uncircumcised and the other seven had undergone circumcision (10). Recently, Barbagli and associates (13) presented their experience with 130 patients with long-standing LS diagnosis. They reported 11 cases (8.4%) of penile carcinoma arising from previous lichen sclerosus lesions.

Although malignant changes are an accepted complication of other dermatoses, there is not consensus whether LS represents a premalignant condition or just appears concomitantly with squamous cell carcinoma. There is, on the other hand, general agreement that close surveillance should be done in patients with long-standing LS, advising prompt biopsies of any suspicious lesions, since early treatment of penile carcinoma carries a high success rate.

5. Histology

The histology of LS is not one of pathognomonic features, but rather one of global histologic appearance (**Fig. 3.1A and B**). There are clearly other entities, with potential malignant significance, which share many of these features. The histologic features can vary within the stages of the LS process, the severity of lesions, and after effective treatment (55,56).

At the epithelial level, there is an effacement of the crests with epidermal thinning. Hydropic degeneration (vacuolization) of the basal keratinocytes and

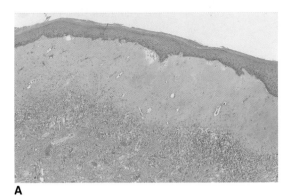 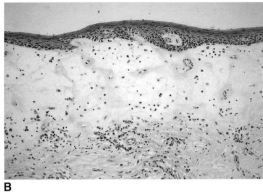

A   **B**

FIG. 3.1. (A) LS with hyperkeratosis, atrophic epidermis, edema, and homogenization of the papillary dermis with band-like mononuclear inflammatory infiltrate immediately beneath (hematoxylin and eosin, magnification 100x). (B) High-power view with thick hyperkeratotic layer, focal interface changes and pigment incontinence (hematoxylin and eosin, magnification 40x)

inflammation and disruption of the basal membrane are common findings. When vacuolization is intense, there is disruption at the level of the dermis or the epidermis with consequent bulla formation, usually associated with mechanical trauma (e.g., scratching). There is also edema and homogenization of the collagen of the superficial dermis, with reduction of the elastic fibers, vascular stasis, and the deposition of glicosaminglycans. Additionally, perivascular mononuclear infiltrates are noted and the absence of melanocytes is noteworthy. These histologic findings along with edema produce the typical "white-patch appearance" of the lesions which are recognized as lichen sclerosus. In quiescent cases, it is common to observe an alternation of atrophic areas with epidermal hyperplasia; and the edema of the acute phase is replaced by collagen sclerosus *(56)*.

6. Clinical Presentation

As mentioned previously, the most commonly affected areas, in both males and females are the genitalia and perineum *(2)*. The lesions start as white patches that seem to coalesce into "plaques" **(Fig. 3.2)**. In men, this often affects the prepuce, forming a sclerotic white ring creating a phimosis *(57)*. When the glans is involved, it may have a mottled appearance. It is, in the author's experience, not unusual for patients to sometimes present just with perimeatal involvement, and the perimeatal area will appear white and scarred.

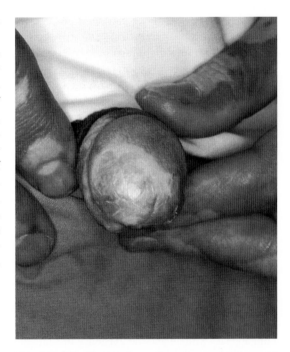

FIG. 3.2. LS affecting the entire glans and subcoronal skin in a 30-yr-old man with resultant meatal stenosis and difficulty voiding. Note a well-defined line between healthy penile skin and atrophic/discolored tissue. (From Lynch PJ, Edwards L (1994) Genital dermatology. Churchill Livingstone, New York, p. 153)

With progression, the lesions tend to obliterate the coronal sulcus. The frenulum becomes retracted in the scarring process and eventually the meatus can be almost obliterated by the scar *(55)*. It is not agreed

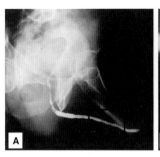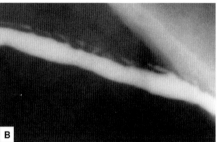

Fig. 3.3. (A) and (B), Urethrogram demonstrating the typical long and "saw-toothed" urethral stricture pattern of LSA, along with dilation of the glands of Littre

upon as to whether LS progresses into the fossa navicularis and a portion of the anterior urethra, or whether the involvement of the urethra may all be secondary to the initial involvement at the level of the meatus with the development of meatal stenosis and high pressure voiding. It is not at all unusual for the process to involve only a portion of the anterior urethra, and possibly may reflect the distribution of the glands of Littre in a given patient.

The classic appearance of male anterior urethral stricture associated with LS is that of a saw-toothed appearance throughout the involved area, with an area of perfectly normal anterior urethra proximally (**Fig. 3.3**). Patients present with both local as well as voiding symptoms. Itching is frequently reported, loss of glans sensation is likewise reported, and erections are often painful because of the scar limitation and limitation of the expansion of the penile skin due to scarring, particularly the area of the frenulum. Voiding complaints such as dysuria, urethral discharge, and obstructive lower urinary tract symptoms are frequent.

At cystoscopy, the meatus is narrow, often times displaced ventrally, even in patients who have not had meatotomy previously. The urethral epithelium appears whitish and the existence of filamentous white tissue which can be easily passed with the cystoscope is usual *(55)*. If one uses a pediatric cystoscope, usually the area of involvement can be traversed, with the sudden appearance of absolutely normal urethral epithelium, and on contrast studies what appears to be normally compliant tissues. However, in the multiply instrumented patient, and the patient with urethral stricture secondary to LS, is usually a multiply instrumented patient, the preservation of a normal proximal urethra is not a given.

7. Management

There is no best practice guideline for the management of the patient with genital LS and, in particular, anterior urethral stricture disease secondary to genital involvement with LS. All management is based on nonrandomized series, and local expert opinion.

The association with malignancy of the glans has been discussed previously. It is not the author's feelings that all patients need a biopsy. It is of paramount importance to rule out premalignant and malignant lesions that can be confused with lichen sclerosus, such as erythroplasia of Queyrat, Lichen Planus, and leukoplakia, all of them with distinctive histologic features *(55)*. What seems to be hallmark with the suspicion of malignancy, is the patient with "genital lichen sclerosus" that "behaves abnormally." In our experience, the vast majority of patients, even with significantly inflamed lichen sclerosus, can have their disease process quieted with the use of local application of super potent steroids (0.05% clobetasol propionate cream) and antibiotics. The use of antibiotics initially was done because of the proposed infectious etiology. Both doxycycline and the fluoroquinolones share the property of having excellent tissue accumulation of the antibiotic. Whether it is the antibiotic effect or an effect of the antibiotic being present in the skin is not clear. However, the experience of many who deal with LS would suggest that most cases can be treated with this combination. Thus, if the patient's inflamed status does not settle down with such a regimen, this raises a red flag that these patients should be biopsied. The problem with biopsy is that the findings of squamous cell carcinoma of the glans can be very elusive. We have had a number of patients who have been biopsied, with a biopsy read as benign, who continue to have problems, were rebiopsied, and eventually read as consistent with squamous cell carcinoma of the penis. We have also had other patients, where the biopsy has been consistently read as benign and, later shifted to a therapy more compatible with the treatment of superficial squamous cell carcinoma of the glans (i.e., topical 5FU cream), where the process has responded. Again, concern should be about the patient who "doesn't act right." The opinions regarding urethral reconstruction are discussed below under section 7.2 and in chapter 18, Stage Urethroplasty, in this text.

7.1. Medical Treatment

Nonsurgical management of these patients can certainly be undertaken. As mentioned, these patients are treated with a superpotent steroid and antibiotic. Our regimen consists of super steroids two to three times a day for 6–8 wk with patients who present acutely and an initiation of antibiotic therapy at suppressive levels. The patient is reassessed at 6 wk to 3 mo. If the process has settled, the patient is voiding adequately and, his urinalysis reflects sufficient voiding, then the patient is followed.

Recently, the use of topical tacrolimus has been proposed in an effort to avoid late atrophy and further damage to an already thinned and fragile skin as a result of the inflammatory process of lichen sclerosus *(58)*. Luesley and Downey present the first series of histologically confirmed LS treated with macrolactams. Sixteen women were enrolled and 60% responded to treatment, and two patients had complete remission. They state that this observational study would justify a larger phase II study to accurately quantify the response to this topical alternative *(58)*.

7.2. Surgical Management

Surgical managements that are proposed are circumcision, repeated meatal dilation, meatotomy, and obviously urethral reconstruction. Circumcision is no guarantee that the LS process will settle and not progress. Depasquale and Bracka *(10)* presented a high success rate with circumcision. Of 522 patients with LS diagnosis, they treated 287 with circumcision alone. Of the 287 patients who had been circumcised, 276 (92%) needed no further treatment and were considered "cured."

Other surgeons have also reported good long-term results with circumcision in lichen sclerosus patients.

Meatal dilation can certainly buy time; meatotomy is seldom a long-term fix. Whether it is the Koebner phenomenon that dooms meatotomy to failure or just the fact that LS is a "skin disease" is not clear. When there is meatal or perimeatal compromise, more aggressive therapy is required. Patients with meatal and perimeatal involvement frequently have developed panurethral stricture disease, probably the result of a combination of disease progression and high pressure voiding against meatal stenosis. The trauma of repeated dilations cannot be underestimated.

Conservative methods to manage urethral strictures, such as internal urethrotomy and frequent dilations, have proven to achieve poor results in urethral strictures associated with lichen sclerosus. Several meatoplasty techniques have been proposed in the past, with variable functional and cosmetic results *(56–64)*. In a recent review of our series of strictures of the meatus and fossa navicularis, corrected with the ventral transverse skin island elevated on a dartos fascial flap, 12 patients (34 %) had LS. LS recurred at the fossa or meatus in 6 patients (50 %), with a mean follow-up of 8.9 years, and a median of 8.3 years (in press).

Early on, we applied this technique to every patient with a fossa stricture; in fact we believed it was the solution for those patients with a meatal stricture secondary to LS *(65)*. With better understanding of the physiopathology of LS, we know that the process can recur in the flap. Venn and Mundy *(66)* published a 100% recurrence of the inflammatory process when using genital skin for the repair of fossa navicularis stricture with LS/BXO. We had a 50% flap recurrence in our series (in press), and an explanation of this lower number could be that not all of them had true LS/BXO, because we did not biopsy all of the patients. After 2001 we stopped using this technique for LS/BXO, and since then, we have been treating LS fossa navicularis strictures with primary or staged buccal mucosa graft onlay; preliminary results are encouraging (data not published). Recent debate around the proper tissue for reconstruction of the meatus and fossa navicularis in patients with LS involvement needs to be clarified with long term results of buccal mucosa procedures *(67–69)*. For further details on urethroplasty surgical technique for LS, see chapters 11 and 18 in this volume.

Editorial Comment

On the bassis of our clinical experience and on reports by Mundy, Braka, and others, our standard surgical practice for LSA strictures is to avoid local genital skin, because in the long term, such surgeries progressively fail. We feel that foreskin or genital skin used for a flap, may be infected by nonvisible LSA and eventually lead to disease recurrence in the urethra. Although some authors do report good success with local genital skin flaps for LSA, we feel this is more the exception then the rule. Surgical therapy must be tailored to the site affected, the extent that the tissue is involved, and patient preference. For strictures that involve the urethral meatus, we usually perform a wide meatotomy, followed by long-term topical high-potency steroid or tacrolimus therapy. Strictures that involve the fossa navicularis or the penile urethra we manage either by a two-stage urethroplasty (with either a buccal graft or split thickness skin graft) or a one-stage urethroplasty with a dorsal buccal or posterior auricular skin graft. At the time of surgery, wide surgical margins are demanded in order to ensure that all infected LSA tissue is removed. Furthermore, all LSA patients require long-term follow-up because the disease can progressively relapse and because of some rare, yet controversial concerns for potential malignant transformation.—S.B. Brandes.

References

1. Bernard P, Prost T, Durepaire N, et al. (1992) The major cicatricial pemphigoid antigen is a 180-KD protein that shows immunologic cross-reactivity with the bullous pemphigoid antigen J Invest Dermatol 99:174–179
2. Wallace HJ (1971) Lichen sclerosus et atrophicus. Trans St John's Dermatol Soc 57:9–30
3. Dogliotti M, Bentley-Phillips CB, Schmaman A (1974) Lichen sclerosus et atrophicus in the Bantu Br J Dermatol 91:81–85
4. Jacyk WK, Isaac F (1979) Lichen sclerosus et atrophicus in Nigerians J Natl Med Assoc 71:387–388
5. Datta C, Dutta SK, Chaudauri A (1993) Histopathological and immunological studies in a cohort of balanitis xerotica obliterans J Indian Medical Assoc 91:146–148
6. Tasker GL, Wojnarowska F (2003) Lichen sclerosus. Clin Exp Dermatol 28:128–33
7. Meffert JJ, Davis BM, Grimwood RE (1995) Lichen Sclerosus J Am Acad Dermatol 32:393–416
8. Powell J and Wojnarowska F (1999) Lichen sclerosus. Lancet 353:177–183
9. Walkden V, Chia Y, Wojnarowska F (1997) The association of squamous cell carcinoma of the vulva and lichen sclerosus: implications for management and follow up J Obstet Gynecol 17:551–553
10. Depasquale I, Park AJ, Bracka A (2000) The treatment of balanitis xerotica obliterans BJU Int 86:459–465
11. Nasca MR, Innocenzi D, Micali G. (1999) Penile cancer among patients with genital lichen sclerosus J Am Acad Dermatol 41:911–914
12. Micali G, Nasca MR, Innocenzi D (2001) Lichen sclerosus of the glans is significantly associated with penile carcinoma. Sex Transm Infect 77:226
13. Barbagli G, Palminteri E, Mirri F, et al. (2006) Penile carcinoma in patients with genital lichen sclerosus: a multicenter survey J Urol 175:1359–1363
14. Stühmer A. Balanitis xerotica obliterans (post operationem) und ihre beziehungem zur Kraurosis glandis et preaeputii. Penis Arch Derm Syph (Berlin) 156:613–623
15. Freeman C, Laymon CW (1941) Balanitis xerotica obliterans. Arch Dermatol Syphilol 44:547–561
16. Laymon CW, Freeman C. (1944) Relationship of balanitis xerotica obliterans to lichen sclerosus et atrophicus. Arch Dermatol Syphilol 49:57–59
17. Weir RF (1875) Icthyosis of the tongue and vulva. NY State J Med 246.
18. Hallopeau H (1889) Lichen plan scléreux. Ann Derm Syph (2nd series) 20:447–449
19. Darier J. (1892) Lichen plan scléreux. Ann Derm Syph 23:833–837
20. Unna PG (1894) Kartenblattförmige sklerodermie. Lehrbuch der speziell path. Anatomie (8 lief) Berlin: A Hirschwald, 112
21. Westberg F (1901) Ein Fall von mit weissen flecken Einherhehender, bisher nicht bekannten. Dermatose Monatschr Prakt Dermatol 33:355–361
22. Von Zombusch LR (1906) Über Lichen albus, eine bisher unbeschrieben Erkrankung. Arch Dermatol Syph (Berlin) 82:339
23. Montgomery FH, Ormsby OS (1907) "White spot disease" (morphea guttata) and lichen planus sclerosus et atrophicus. J Cutan Dis 25:1–16
24. Csillag J (1909) Dermatitis lichenoides chronica atrophicans. Ikonographia Dermatol 4:147
25. Breisky A (1885) Über Kraurosis vulvae. Z Heilkr 6:69

26. Friedrich EG (1976) Lichen sclerosus. J Reprod Med 17:147–154
27. Friedrich EG (1976) New nomenclature for vulvar disease Obstet Gynecol 47:122–124
28. Sander CS, Ali I, Dean D, et al. (2004) Oxidative stress is implicated in the pathogenesis of lichen sclerosus. Br J Dermatol 151:627–635
29. Pass CJ (1984) An unusual variant of lichen sclerosus et atrophicus: delayed appearance in a surgical scar. Cutis 33:405–406
30. Cockerell EG, Knox JM, Rogers SF (1960) Lichen sclerosus et atrophicus. Obstet Gynecol 15:554–559
31. Milligan A, Graham-Brown RA, Burns DA (1988) Lichen sclerosus et atrophicus following sunburn. Clin Exp Dermatol 13:36–37
32. Fallic ML, Faller G, Klauber GT (1997) Balanitis xerotica obliterans in monozygotic twins. Br J Urol 79:810
33. Thomas RHM, Kennedy CT (1986) The development of lichen sclerosus et atrophicus in monozygotic twin girls. Br J Dermatol 114:277–279
34. Cox NH, Mitchell JNS, Morley Wn (1986) Lichen sclerosus et atrophicus in non-identical female twins. Br J Dermatol 115:743–746
35. Shirer JA, Ray MC (1987) Familial occurrence of lichen sclerosus et atrophicus. Arch Dermatol 123:485–488
36. Meyrick Thomas RH, Ridley CM, Black MM, et al. (1983) The association between lichen sclerosus et atrophicus and autoimmune related diseases in males. Br J Dermatol 109:661–664
37. Meyrick Thomas RH, Ridley CM, Black MM, et al. (1984) The association between lichen sclerosus et atrophicus and autoimmune related disease in males: an addendum (letter). Br J Dermatol 111:371–372
38. Azurdia MR, Luzi G, Byren I, et al. (1999) Lichen sclerosus in adult men: a study to HLA association and susceptibility to autoimmune disease. Br J Dermatol 140:79–83
39. Garcia-Bravo B, Sánchez-Pedrero P, Rodríguez-Pichardo A, et al. (1988) Lichen sclerosus et atrophicus. A study of 76 cases and their relation to diabetes. J Am Acad Dermatol 19:482–485
40. Faergemann J (1979) Lichen sclerosus et atrophicus generalisata, alopecia areata, and polymyalgia rheumatica found in the same patient. Cutis 23:757–758
41. Cunliffe WJ, Newell DJ, Hall R, et al. (1968) Vitiligo, thyroid disease, and autoimmunity. Br J Dermatol 80:135–139
42. Ditkowsky SP, Falk AB, Baker N, et al. (1956) Lichen sclerosus et atrophicus in childhood. Am J Dis Child 91:52–54
43. Panet-Raymond G, Dirard C. (1972) Lichen sclerosus et atrophicus. Can Med J 106:1332–1334
44. Lewis GM. (1961) Scleroderma: Lichen sclerosus et atrophicus? Arch Dermatol 84:146–148
45. Kahana M, Levy A, Schewach-Millet M, et al. (1985) Appearance of lupus erythematous in a patient with lichen sclerosus et atrophicus of the elbows (Letter). J Am Acad Dermatol 12:127–129
46. Goolamali SK, Barnes EW, Irvine WJ, et al. (1974) Organ-specific antibodies in patients with lichen sclerosus. Br Med J 4:78–79
47. Poskitt L, Wojnarowska F (1993) Lichen sclerosus as a cutaneous manifestation of thyroid disease (letter). J Am Acad Dermatol 28:665
48. Oyama N, Chan I, Neill SM, et al. (2003) Autoantibodies to extracellular matrix protein 1 in lichen sclerosus Lancet 362:118–123
49. Chan I. (2004) The role of extracellular matrix protein 1 in human skin. Clin Exp Dermatol 29:52–56
50. Hamada T. (2002) Lipoid proteinosis Clin Exp Dermatol 27:624–629
51. Buechner SA, Winkelmann RK, Lautenschlager S, et al. (1993) Localized scleroderma associated with Borrelia burgdorferi infection. Clinical, histologic, and immunohistochemical observations. J Am Acad Dermatol 29:190–196
52. Shono S, Imura M, Ota M, et al. (1991) Lichen sclerosus et atrophicus, morphea and coexistence of both diseases. Histological studies using lectins. Arch Dermatol 127:1352–1356
53. Aberer E, Neumann R, Stanek G (1995) Is localized scleroderma a Borrelia infection (letter)? Lancet ii:278
54. Weide B, Waltz T, Garbe C (2000) Is morphea caused by Borrelia burgdorferi? A review. Br J Dermatol 142:636–644
55. Akporiaye LE, Jordan GH, Devine CJ Jr. (1997) Balanitis xerotica obliterans (BXO). AUA Updates Series 16:162
56. Virasoro R, Kahn AG, Secin FP (2003) Balanitis xerotica obliterante. Rev Arg de Urol 68:125–130
57. Chalmers RJG, Burton PA, Bennet RF (1984) Lichen sclerosus et atrophicus. Arch Dermatol 120:1025–1027
58. Luesley D, Downey G (2006) Topical tacrolimus in the management of lichen sclerosus BJOG 113:832–834
59. Cohney BC (1963) A penile flap procedure for the relief of meatal stricture Br J Urol 35:182
60. Blandy JP, Tresidder GC (1967) Meatoplasty Br J Urol 39:633
61. Brannen GE (1976) Meatal reconstruction. J Urol 116:319
62. Devine CJ Jr (1986) Surgery of the urethra. In: Walsh PC, Gittes RF, Perlmutter AD, et al. (eds) Campbell's urology, ed 5. WB Saunders, Philadelphia, p 2853

63. De Sy WA (1984) Aesthetic repair of meatal stric-
    ture. J Urol 132:678
64. Duckett, J. W. (1980) Transverse preputial island flap
    technique for repair of severe hypospadias. Urol Clin
    North Am 7:423
65. Jordan GH (1987) Reconstruction of the fossa navic-
    ularis. J Urol 138:102
66. Venn SN, Mundy AR (1998) Urethroplasty for
    balanitis xerotica obliterans. Br J Urol 81:735
67. Armenakas NA, Morey AF, McAninch JW (1998)
    Reconstruction of resistant strictures of the fossa
    navicularis and meatus. J Urol 160:359
68. Nahas BW, Hart AJ (1999) Letter to the editor. Re:
    Reconstruction of resistant strictures of the fossa
    navicularis and meatus. J Urol 161:924
69. Bracka A (1999) Letter to the editor. Re: Reconstruction
    of resistant strictures of the fossa navicularis and
    meatus. J Urol 162:1389

4
Imaging of the Male Urethra

Christine M. Peterson, Christine O. Menias, and Cary L. Siegel

Contents

1. Introduction.. 29
2. Conventional Urethrography.. 30
   2.1. Normal Anatomy 30
3. Retrograde Urethrography 31
4. Voiding Cystourethrography... 31
5. Stricture Characteristics and Extent.. 33
6. Sonourethrography.. 34
7. Magnetic Resonance Imaging... 37
8. Voiding CT Urethrography 39
Editorial Comment.. 39
References.. 42

Summary The most common methods for imaging the male urethra are retrograde urethrography (RUG) and voiding cystourethrography (VCUG). In order to formulate a proper management plan, an accurate and well executed study is essential to determine stricture presence, number, location, degree and length. Conventional urethrography is performed under fluoroscopy with the hip tilted and the penis placed on slight stretch. Inadequate oblique images will underestimate "true" stricture length. VCUG is most valuable for assessing the posterior urethra, the proximal extent of stenoses, and their functional significance. Other modalities, such as MRI, CT and sonourethrography have an important, yet limited role in urethral evaluation. MRI has particular value in evaluating the pelvic fracture patient with associated urethral disruption injury. Sonourethrography is particularly accurate at determining true bulbar urethral stricture length. Detailed here-in are such imaging techniques and the imaging characteristics of both the normal and abnormal male urethra.

Keywords retrograde urethrography, voiding cystourethrography, sonourethrography, magnetic resonance imaging.

1. Introduction

There are a number of different imaging techniques that may be used in imaging the male urethra. The most widespread methods include retrograde urethrography (RUG) and voiding cystourethrography (VCUG). However, other modalities, such as ultrasound, magnetic resonance imaging (MRI), and computed tomography, have been used as adjuncts.

Accurate diagnosis of stricture presence, number, location, and length is of paramount importance in planning appropriate treatment. Although RUG and VCUG are often sufficient for this purpose, ultrasound and MRI can be useful in certain situations, such as the evaluation of spongiofibrosis and the periurethral tissues. The purpose of this chapter is to review the different imaging modalities used

From: *Current Clinical Urology: Urethral Reconstructive Surgery*
Edited by: S.B. Brandes © Humana Press, Totowa, NJ

in studying the male urethra, including their techniques and indications. Normal and abnormal anatomy will be illustrated, with special attention to pre- and post-operative imaging of urethral stricture disease.

2. Conventional Urethrography

RUG and VCUG are the most commonly used techniques for male urethral imaging. They are readily available and can be safely and relatively quickly performed. The information they provide is usually sufficient to direct patient care. Serious complications are rare, and the procedure is usually well tolerated by patients.

2.1. Normal Anatomy

The anterior urethra consists of a distal pendulous or penile segment and a proximal bulbar segment. The pendulous urethra is a smooth and featureless structure that widens focally near the meatus at the fossa navicularis. It is separated from the bulbar urethra at the penoscrotal junction, a natural bend that occurs in the urethra where it is bound superiorly by the suspensory ligament of the penis. The bulbar urethra is also smooth in contour and assumes a cone or funnel shape proximally at the bulbomembranous junction. Visualization of the bulbar cone is very important in the evaluation of a bulbomembranous junction abnormality, as an abnormal appearance of the cone is highly associated with membranous urethral involvement in disease (**Fig. 4.1 [1]**).

The posterior urethra consists of a distal membranous segment which, as it traverses the muscular urogenital diaphragm, becomes the narrowest portion of the normal urethra. More proximally, the prostatic urethra can be seen extending from the bladder neck to the membranous segment. A small longitudinally oriented mound of smooth muscle, the verumontanum, is present along the dorsal aspect of the prostatic urethra and can be seen as a filling defect during fluoroscopic studies. Its distal end marks the proximal aspect of the membranous urethra (2). Useful anatomic landmarks to identify the membranous urethra are the inferior margins of the obturator foramina (**Fig. 4.2 [3]**). It is particularly important to identify the exact location of the

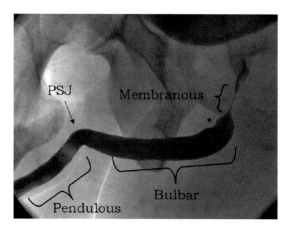

FIG. 4.1. Normal RUG. The tip of the Foley catheter can be seen in the fossa navicularis, as well as an air bubble which was introduced during the exam. The segments of the urethra are labeled. Note the natural bend in the urethra at the penoscrotal junction (PSJ), separating the pendulous and bulbar segments. Note the indentation in the anterior surface of the proximal bulbar urethra caused by the musculus compressor nuda (asterisk), composed of fibers of the bulbocavernous muscle which wrap anterior to the urethra.(*1*)

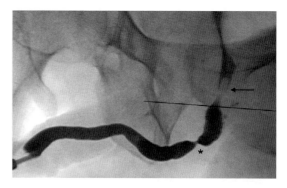

FIG. 4.2. Bony landmark for the membranous urethra. An imaginary line drawn near the inferior margin of the obturator foramina intersects the bulbomembranous junction of the urethra. This is most useful when urethral anatomy is distorted by trauma or stricture, precluding identification of the different portions of the urethra by morphology alone. Note the verumontanum (arrow), a filling defect in the posterior urethra whose distal end marks the proximal extent of the membranous urethra. There is a severe stricture of the bulbar urethra in this patient (asterisk).

membranous urethra, as this is where the urogenital diaphragm and external sphincter are located. In the trauma setting, injury to the external sphincter may affect urinary continence.

3. Retrograde Urethrography

The RUG is most useful for evaluation of the anterior urethra from the external meatus to the proximal bulbar portion. To perform the procedure, the patient is placed supine on the fluoroscopy table and then rolled up slightly onto one hip (approximately to a 45-degree angle), with the dependent thigh flexed so that an oblique view of the lengthened urethra can be obtained (**Fig. 4.3**). Attention to proper patient positioning is extremely important to lengthen the urethra and avoid overlap of the urethra and foreshortening of any strictures that may be present (**Fig. 4.4**).

The glans penis is cleansed with the use of a sterile technique, and a contrast administration device is inserted into the meatus. A small Foley catheter with the balloon gently inflated with 1–1.5 mL of air in the fossa navicularis until the catheter is secure generally serves this purpose well. Other devices include a suction catheter. Sterile iodinated contrast is then injected into the urethra with the use of gentle pressure to avoid extravasation. In men with a patulous external meatus, a soft clamp or gauze tied around the external meatus may be used to stabilize the catheter in the fossa navicularis.

Because the anterior urethra is distended during the RUG, this examination is most useful for interrogation of the anterior segment. The number, location, and severity of strictures can be well delineated. Although the posterior urethra is opacified during most examinations, its distention is usually poor after contrast passes through the relatively narrow membranous urethra. To improve visualization of the posterior urethra, the patient can be instructed to void during the examination, distending the posterior segment. Alternatively, autourethrography, where the patient injects the contrast himself after a catheter has been placed, has been shown to increase distention of the posterior urethra. It also may result in a less uncomfortable exam, with less risk of contrast intravasation *(4)*.

4. Voiding Cystourethrography

The VCUG often is performed in conjunction with retrograde urethrography and is especially useful in assessing the posterior urethra. In contrast to the RUG, opening of the bladder neck and distention of the posterior urethra are achieved during VCUG *(5)*. During normal voiding, the membranous urethra distends slightly, while remaining the narrowest part of the urethra. As the membranous urethra

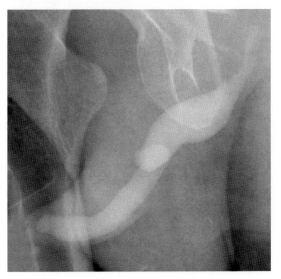

FIG. 4.3. Importance of proper patient positioning during RUG. In this patient who has not been placed in an oblique enough position, the distal bulbar and proximal pendulous urethra overlap, thereby foreshortening and obscuring any strictures that may be present.

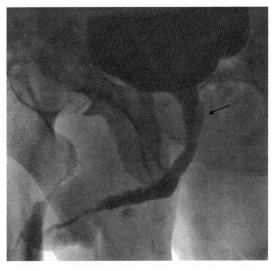

FIG. 4.4. VCUG. With voiding the bladder neck opens and the prostatic urethra is distended. Note the faint filling defect posteriorly in the prostatic urethra due to the verumontanum (arrow).

widens, the cone of the bulbar urethra becomes less apparent and is infrequently seen *(1)*.

To perform a VCUG, the bladder is filled with contrast either through the urethra in a retrograde fashion, an indwelling Foley catheter, or a suprapubic catheter. Rarely, a VCUG may be performed when contrast has been injected intravenously and the bladder has been allowed time to fill. The patient is positioned in much the same way as during a RUG, and instructed to void into a canister. This is more easily accomplished if the fluoroscopy table is tilted upwards so that the patient is in a standing position. Images of the urethra are then obtained during voiding (**Fig. 4.5**).

Occasionally, normal anatomic structures are opacified during RUG or VCUG and should not be confused with areas of extravasation. Examples of such structures include the glands of Littre, the prostate gland, and Cowper's glands and ducts. Opacification of the glands of Littre is often associated with urethral inflammation and stricture disease *(3)*. The musculus compressor nuda muscle may also be apparent, and should not be confused with a stricture (**Figs. 4.6** to **4.8**).

RUG and VCUG usually are safely and quickly performed, with little risk to the patient. Complications are extremely rare but may occur if there is venous intravasation of contrast in either a

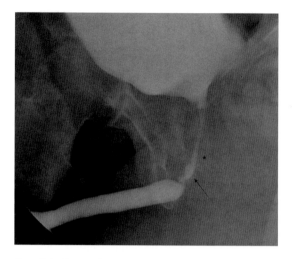

FIG. 4.6. Cowper's glands and ducts. Opacification of these structures is often, but not always, associated with urethral strictures or inflammation. In this case, a stricture of the bulbomembranous junction is present. Remembering that Cowper's glands (asterisk) are located in the urogenital diaphragm, at the same level as the membranous urethra, and that the ducts (arrow) empty into the proximal bulbar urethra can be useful anatomic landmarks, as in this case.

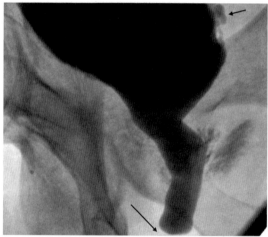

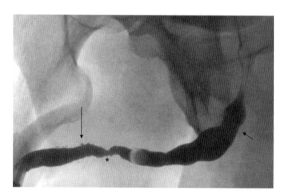

FIG. 4.5. Musculus compressor nuda and glands of Littre. The musculus compressor nuda creates a normal muscular indentation along the anterior aspect of the proximal bulbar urethra is frequently seen during retrograde urethrography and should not be mistaken for a stricture (arrow). Note the true strictures in the pendulous urethra, immediately distal to an air bubble in the urethral lumen (asterisk). There is also filling of the glands of Littre (long arrow) in the pendulous urethra, commonly associated with prior episodes of urethral infection or inflammation.

FIG. 4.7. Prostate gland. There are multiple tiny openings in the prostatic urethra from the prostatic ducts. These may become opacified during RUG, leading to visualization of the prostate gland itself. When this occurs, the pattern of glandular enhancement assumes a feathery appearance as illustrated above. There is a severe stricture of the membranous urethra (long arrow) causing dilatation of the prostatic urethra. Also note the bladder diverticula (short arrow), suggestive of longstanding bladder obstruction.

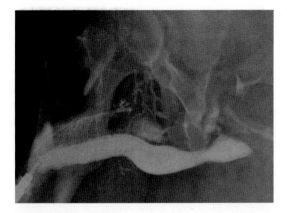

FIG. 4.8. Venous intravasation. If contrast is injected during RUG with excessive force or against a stricture that creates a pressure head, the urethral mucosa may be violated, leading to passage of contrast into the corpora spongiosum and the highly vascular corpora cavernosum.[1,13] The contrast is then taken up by the penile venous system. This may predispose the patient to bacteremia or a contrast reaction, if the patient is allergic to iodinated contrast.

patient with a contrast allergy or in a patient with active infection, as a contrast reaction or bacteremia may result (**Fig. 4.9**).

5. Stricture Characteristics and Extent

Urethral strictures are most commonly the result of trauma, including iatrogenic injury. In the past, urethral strictures were most commonly caused by infection. However, as AIDS awareness has increased since the early 1980s, infectious strictures have become less frequent (3). In nonindustrialized countries, chlamydia, gonorrhea, and tuberculosis are the most common agents to result in urethral stricture, whereas in the industrialized world, it is more commonly lichen sclerosus.

Strictures caused by instrumentation tend to occur at the membranous segment, because of its relatively narrow diameter, and the peno-scrotal junction, where the urethra is fixed by the suspensory ligament of the penis. They are usually short in length and smooth in contour. Traumatic

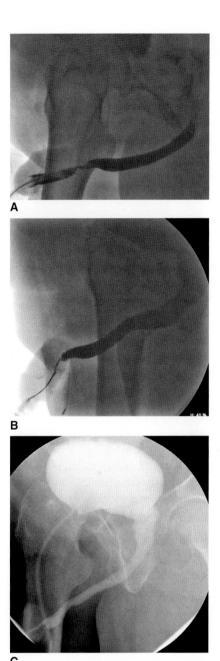

FIG. 4.9. Pendulous stricture. Preoperative RUG (A) and VCUG (B) demonstrate a proximal pendulous and distal bulbar urethral stricture with associated subtle filling of the glands of Littre. Note that the distal margin of the stricture is not defined during VCUG due to poor distention of the urethra distal to the stricture. A post urethroplasty VCUG (C) shows only mild residual narrowing of the distal pendulous urethra with no leakage of contrast.

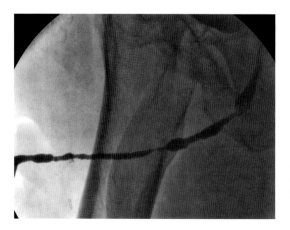

FIG. 4.10. Anterior urethral stricture. A long segment stricture involves the entire course of the anterior urethra, which is diffusely irregularly narrowed.

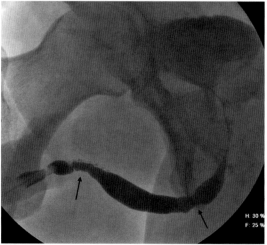

A

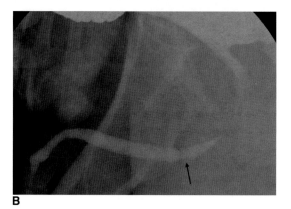

B

FIG. 4.11. Anterior urethral strictures. RUG (A) and VCUG (B) show strictures of both the pendulous and distal bulbar urethra (arrows) with associated filling of Cowper's glands and the glands of Littre. Note that the strictures are more apparent on the retrograde examination due to the superior distention of the anterior urethra that is attained during RUG.

stricture are also typically short, focal, and smooth contoured but involve the bulbar urethra. In contrast, infectious strictures are irregular in contour, several centimeters in length, and often multifocal and involve the anterior urethra.

Not only is urethral imaging crucial in detailing the characteristics and extent of stricture disease before therapy, but it is also extremely useful in the evaluation of the post-operative patient to assess response to therapy as well as possible complications. (**Figs. 4.10** to **4.17**).

6. Sonourethrography

A less frequently used method of imaging the urethra is sonourethrography. Introduced in the mid 1980s, it is an accurate tool for the diagnosis and characterization of strictures, particularly of the bulbar urethra. The examination is usually performed during the installation of sterile saline into the urethra in a retrograde fashion with the use of a small Foley catheter with its balloon inflated in the fossa navicularis or using a tipped syringe, much in the same way as a RUG. A high-frequency (7.5 MHz) linear transducer is then placed on the ventral surface of the penis and oriented along the course of the pendulous and bulbar urethra. The probe may have to be repositioned more posteriorly onto the perineum to visualize the bul-

bar urethra. Although less frequently performed, transperineal scans may be obtained to image the posterior urethra. Some authors have advocated the use of an endorectal probe for imaging the posterior urethra, but this is seldom necessary (**Figs. 4.18** and **4.19** *[6]*).

The advantage of sonourethrography lies in its ability to determine stricture length, especially in the bulbar urethra, with a high degree of accuracy. Because the probe can be oriented along the course

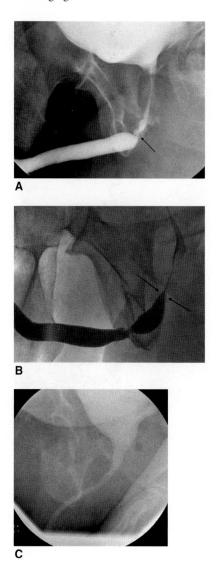

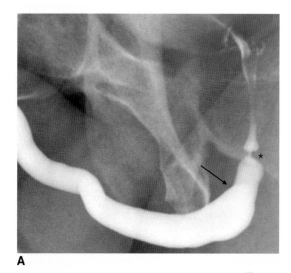

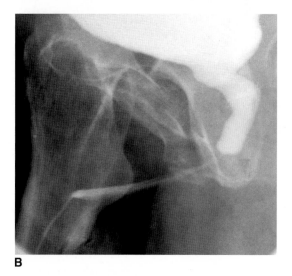

FIG. 4.12. Anterior urethral stricture. (A) RUG showing a severe stricture of the proximal bulbar urethra (arrow) with filling of Cowper's glands. Note the loss of the normal bulbar cone, shown in a different patient in (B) (arrow), indicating involvement of the bulbomembranous junction. Post urethroplasty image (C) showing the normal post-operative appearance of the urethra.

FIG. 4.13. Posterior urethral stricture. A focal stenosis of the membranous urethra is seen with both RUG (A) and VCUG (B) (asterisk). The cone of the bulbar urethra is preserved during the RUG (arrow), indicating that the proximal bulbar urethra is not involved in the stricture. There is distention of the prostatic urethra during voiding (B), due to the severe membranous urethral stricture.

of the urethra, there is less tendency to foreshorten the length of a stricture than with RUG. Several authors have demonstrated the superiority of ultrasound in determining bulbar urethral stricture length, which is an important factor in treatment planning (7–10). Short strictures may be amenable to excision and primary anastomosis, whereas longer strictures may necessitate urethroplasty. In addition, sonourethrography may provide information about the soft tissues surrounding the urethra including the degree of spongiofibrosis surrounding the stenotic portions of the lumen (8,9,11). As fibrosis develops, the urethra becomes less distensible compared with the surrounding normal

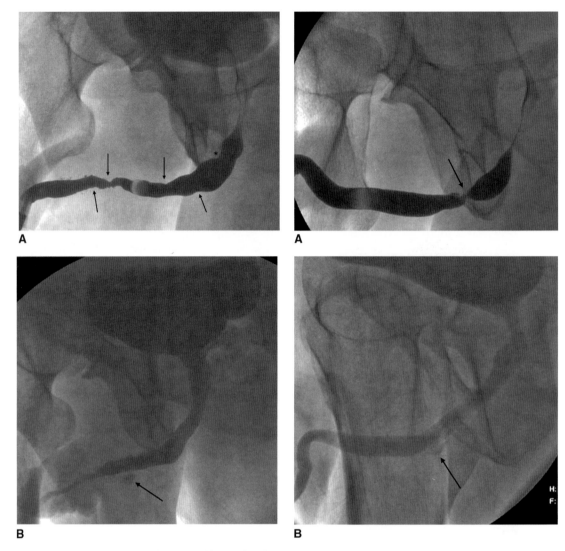

FIG. 4.14. Anterior urethral strictures. RUG (A) showing multiple strictures involving the pendulous and distal bulbar urethra (arrows). Note the normal appearance of the musculus compressor nuda (asterisk) and filling of the glands of Littre. A post-urethroplasty VCUG (B) demonstrates a small contrast leak at the operative site (arrow).

FIG. 4.15. Anterior urethral stricture. There is a focal stricture of the distal bulbar urethra seen on this retrograde exam (A) (arrow). A small contrast leak is seen arising from the operative site of this post-urethroplasty VCUG (B).

tissues, which is illustrated during the sonourethrogram *(5,10)*. This information cannot be provided by conventional RUG/VCUG and is relevant as the severity of periurethral fibrosis is proportional to the frequency of stricture recurrence and may dictate treatment. Areas of periurethral fibrosis appear as hyperechogenicity of the tissues of the spongiosa surrounding the urethra *(12)*. The length and depth of fibrosis may also be measured with ultrasound. The disadvantages of sonourethrography include its limited availability, cost, limited evaluation of the posterior urethra, and the high level of technical expertise necessary to be able to perform and interpret the exam.

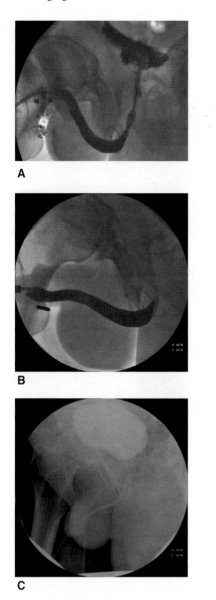

A

B

C

FIG. 4.16. Bulbomembranous disruption. Pericatheter RUG (A) in a patient with pelvic trauma reveals no gross abnormality. A standard retrograde exam performed two months later shows normal opacification of the anterior urethra, but no filling of the posterior urethra (B). A voiding exam performed after urethroplasty shows resolution of the stricture and no leakage of contrast (C).

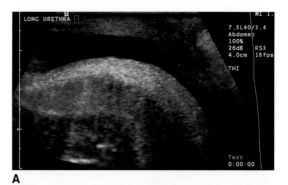

A

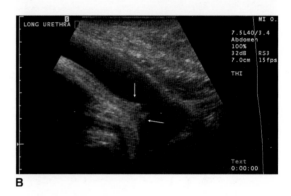

B

FIG. 4.17. Sonourethrogram. The pendulous urethra (A) is normal in caliber and distends uniformly after saline administration. However, there is a mound of tissue along the dorsal aspect of the bulbar urethra (arrows in B) causing a mild stricture. Note that the most superficial surface of the urethra closest to the transducer corresponds to the ventral surface.

7. Magnetic Resonance Imaging

MRI is infrequently used in the evaluation of the male urethra. It is not widely available and is an expensive and technically difficult examination to perform. In most cases, little information is gained beyond that provided by more conventional imaging methods. However, MRI may provide useful information in certain clinical situations, particularly posterior urethral trauma and in the evaluation of the periurethral soft tissues.

Techniques used vary from institution to institution, and often depend on the preferences of the performing radiologist. Both T1- and T2-weighted sequences are necessary for full evaluation of the urethra. Intravenous contrast may be used and is useful in determining the amount of active periurethral inflammation which may be observed in patients with spongiofibrosis, because inflamed tissue tends to take up contrast material. Injection of sterile saline into the urethra is variably performed *(13,14)*.

In general, axial and coronal images are most useful for evaluation of the posterior urethra,

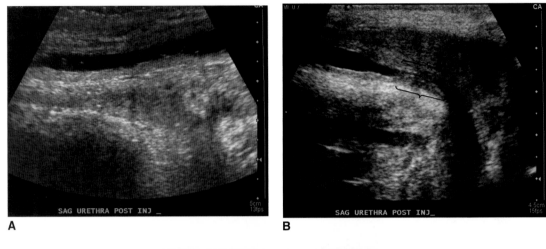

A   B

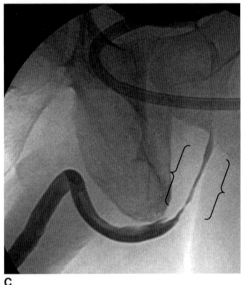

C

FIG. 4.18. Sonourethrogram. Normal distention of the pendulous urethra (A). Long segment of the bulbar urethra which fails to distend (B), corresponding to the stricture seen during pericatheter retrograde urethrography (C).

whereas sagittally oriented images are most useful for the anterior urethra *(15)*. A phased array coil is placed over the perineum, and a small field of view is used.

If detailed urethral anatomic information is desired, contrast may be injected into the urethra prior to imaging. This may be performed using a dilute gadolinium mixture (1:200 dilution yields good urethral opacification) which is injected into the urethra using a Foley catheter in the same manner as with a RUG or sonourethrogram. An MRI-compatible clamp is then placed on the distal end of the penis and fat-saturated T1-weighted images are then acquired. This protocol has several advantages over simply injecting saline and obtaining T2-weighted images. First, fat-saturated T1-weighted sequences are usually faster to obtain than most high-resolution T2 sequences, thus minimizing scanning time and leakage of contrast from the urethra around the catheter. Also, any fluid containing structure will appear hyperintense on T2-weighted images, which may be confound evaluation of periurethral fluid collections and make it impossible to differentiate collections which communicate with the urethra from those that do not. In contrast, only the urethra and collections or structures which communicate with the urethra will be hyperintense on fat-saturated T1 sequences (**Figs. 4.20** to **4.22**).

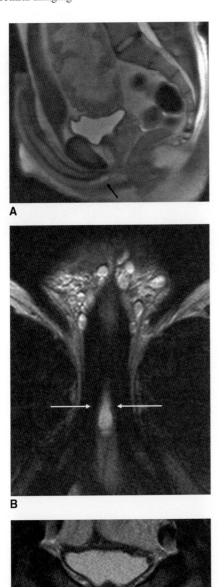

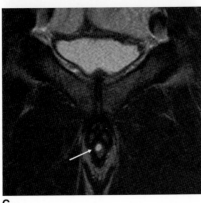

FIG. 4.19. Penile MRI. Sagittal (A), axial (B), and coronal (C) T2 weighted images of the penis in a patient with hematuria following penile trauma. There is a small T2 hyperintense fluid collection along the proximal corpora spongiosum (arrows). In this case, intraurethral contrast was not administered, making the distinction between contusion and a fluid-filled cavity communicating with the urethra difficult.

In addition to cases of possible active periurethral inflammation, MRI may also be useful in studying patients with traumatic posterior urethral injury *(5)*. The periurethral soft tissues are included in the imaging field, and information about the location of the prostate gland and pelvic hematoma may be obtained *(1,15)*.

8. Voiding CT Urethrography

Few centers have used multidetector CT for evaluation of the urethra. Benefits of CT include a very rapid scanning time and the ability to perform multiplanar reformatting to lengthen the urethra and determine stricture length and location accurately. For this examination to be performed, the bladder may be filled in an antegrade fashion by administering intravenous (IV) contrast in conjunction with oral or IV hydration and using an appropriately long scan delay time to allow distention of the bladder with contrast and urine. Alternatively, the bladder may be filled through a Foley catheter, which is then removed before scanning. The patient is then placed on the scanner table and instructed to signal when he is beginning to void. This then triggers the initiation of the scan *(16)*.

There are several drawbacks to this seldom used technique. First, it is unlikely to provide information about the urethra that cannot be obtained using a less expensive and more conventional technique. Second, the anterior urethra may not be fully distended during voiding, which may limit evaluation of anterior urethral disease. There are also the standard risks when IV contrast is administered: nephrotoxicity and contrast allergy. If the patient triggers the scan but does not actually initiate a full voiding stream, then adequate opacification of the urethra will not be achieved, and the scan may have to be repeated, thus greatly increasing the gonadal radiation dose. Finally, the wait time for initiation of voiding while the patient is occupying the scanner may be impractical in centers with limited CT resources.

Editorial Comment

In the treatment of urethral stricture disease, overall stricture length and location, as well as etiology, dictates the surgical technique to be used. Thus, a

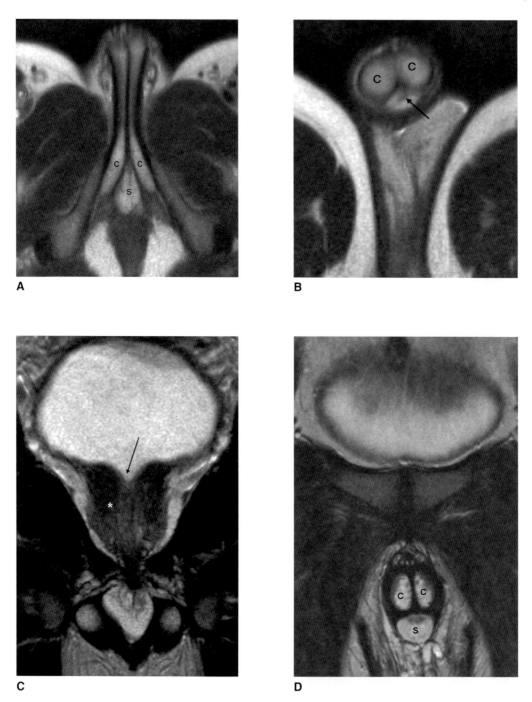

Fig. 4.20. Normal penile MRI. A. Axial T1 weighted image through the base of the penis shows the proximal corpora spongiosum (S) flanked by the corpora cavernosa (C). B. Slightly more caudally, the paired cavernosa and the
spongiosa are seen in the penile shaft. A faintly hypointense structure, the urethra, is present within the spongiosum
(arrow). C and D. Coronal images demonstrate the bladder neck and prostate gland (arrow and asterisk in C), and the
penile base with the central spongiosum (S) and paired cavernosa (C).

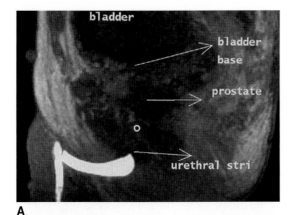

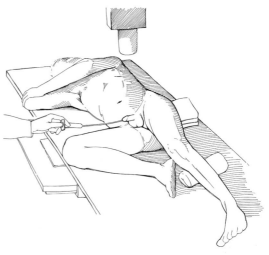

FIG. 4.22. Proper oblique positioning for retrograde ure-thrography. (From Armenakas NA, McAninch JW (1996) Acute anterior urethral injuries: Diagnosis and initial man-agement, in McAninch (ed) Traumatic and Reconstructive Urology. Philadelphia, Saunders, pg. 547).

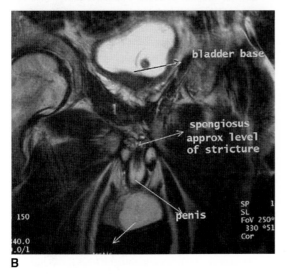

FIG. 4.21. MR urethrogram. Sagittal (A) and coronal (B) images obtained after intraurethral administration of gadolinium demonstrate an abrupt termination of the contrast column in the proximal bulbar urethra with widening of the space between the bulbar urethra and the bladder base in this patient with a post-traumatic urethral disruption.

well-performed retrograde urethrogram to demon-strate the distal aspect and a voiding cystourethrogram to demonstrate the proximal part of the stricture are essential in order to formulate a surgical plan (**Fig. 4.22**). The typical intraoperative method for retro-grade urethrography we employ is illustrated in **Fig. 4.23**. Dynamic contrast imaging is the best evalua-tion approach despite the advent of newer imaging modalities. Both studies are commonly needed to fully assess stricture length, location, caliber, and

the functional significance of the stricture. Although accurate for determining pendulous urethral stricture length, they can at times underestimate the true bul-bar urethral length.

Cystoscopy and transperineal urethral ultra-sound can further complement the investigations. Admittedly, previously we often performed ure-thral ultrasounds to help determine the true stricture length of bulbar urethral strictures. However, over the years, as our surgical experience has grown, we have found the ultrasound was often not neces-sary, and we were easily able to make the manage-ment decision preoperatively or intraoperatively. Sonography of bulbar strictures accurately corre-sponds to the true intra-operative length. When the bulbar stricture length as noted on urethrography is 11–25 mm, sonography can help with treatment decision making. Strictures on sonography shorter then 25 mm can be treated by an anastomotic ure-throplasty whereas those longer then 25 mm typi-cally require a graft or flap for reconstruction. The advantage of using sonography then is, by deter-mining true stricture length preoperatively, then graft or flap mobilization can be performed first in the supine position. In so doing, time in lithotomy and subsequent positioning complications can be limited.

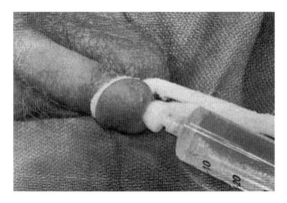

FIG. 4.23. RUG technique with cone tipped catheter and penis on stretch (Courtesy J Gelman).

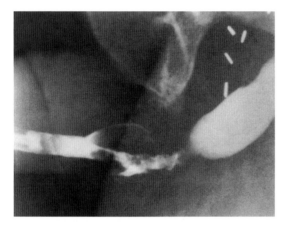

FIG. 4.24. Voiding urethrogram of bulbar urethral stricture due to primary squamous cell carcinoma.

The other evaluation method that we have used more frequently over the years is evaluation under anesthesia, where the radiographic images and cystoscopy from above and below can be performed in a controlled setting, and further enable an accurate evaluation of both stricture length and degree of stenosis. Although not addressed in this chapter, strictures in the bulbar urethra that recur quickly after urethrotomy in the middle aged or elderly patient, or have a very ratty or moth-eaten appearance on urethrography should be considered for urethral biopsy to rule out primary malignancy (**Fig. 4.24**). Where urethral ultrasound still has a particular role is for the more inexperienced urethral surgeon, for whom ultrasound can at times help determine if adjunctive procedures are needed. When dealing with reconstructive urethral surgery, it is always better to make the surgical plan and a contingency plan prior to the operation, then to try to

make the decision making intra-operatively, and on the cuff. Well-performed radiographic and endoscopic imaging are essential to formulate of a sound surgical plan. If you do not have a dedicated GU radiologist in your institution who can insure good quality control, we recommend that the urologist perform all the retrograde urethrograms and voiding cystourethrograms him- or herself.—S.B. Brandes

References

1. Rosen, McAninch (1996) Preoperative staging of the anterior urethral stricture: traumatic and reconstructive urology. Philadelphia, Saunders, pp 551–564
2. Pavlica, Menchi, Barozzi (2003) New imaging of the anterior male urethra. Abdom Imaging 28:180–186
3. Kawashima et al (2004) Imaging of urethral disease: a pictorial review. Radiographics 24:195–216
4. Kirshy et al (1991) Autourethrography. Radiology 180:443–445
5. Gallentine, Morey (2002) Imaging of the male urethra for stricture disease. Urol Clin N Am 29:361–372
6. Shabsigh, Fishman, Krebs (1987) The use of transrectal longitudinal real-time ultrasonography in urodynamics. J Urol 138:1416–1419
7. Gluck et al (188) Sonographic urethrogram. Comparison to roentgenographic techniques. J Urol 140:1404–1408
8. McAninch, Laing, Jeffery (1988) Sonourethrography in the evaluation of urethral strictures: a preliminary report. J Urol 139:294–297
9. Gupta et al (1993) Sonourethrography in the evaluation of anterior urethral strictures: correlation with radiographic urethrography. J Clin Ultrasound 21:231–239
10. Pushkarna, Bhargava, Jain (2000) Ultrasonographic evaluation of abnormalities of the male anterior urethra. Ind J Radiol Imag 10:2:89–91
11. Eaton, Richenberg (2005) Imaging of the urethra. Curr Status Imaging 17:139–149
12. Choudhary, et al (2004) A comparison of sonourethrography and retrograde urethrography in evaluation of anterior urethral strictures. Clin Radiol 59:736–742
13. Pavlica, Barozzi, Menchi (2003) Imaging of male urethra. Eur Radiol 13:1583–1596
14. Dixon, McAninch (1996) Preoperative Staging of Posterior Urethral Disruptions, in McAninch (ed) Traumatic and reconstructive urology. Philadelphia, Saunders, pp 377–384
15. Ryu, Kim (2001) MR imaging of the male and female urethra. Radiographics 21:1169–1185
16. Chou et al (2005) CT voiding urethrography and virtual urethroscopy preliminary study with 16-MDCT. AJR Am J Roentgenol 184:1882–1888

5
Techniques in Tissue Transfer: Plastic Surgery for the Urologist

Thomas A. Tung and Christopher M. Nichols

Contents

1. Introduction 44
2. Assessment 44
3. Management Options 44
   3.1. Secondary Intention 44
   3.2. Primary Repair 45
   3.3. Graft Reconstruction 45
   3.4. Flap Reconstruction 47
4. Flap Techniques 48
   4.1. Sliding Advancement Flap 48
   4.2. Rotation/Transposition Flaps 49
   4.3. Tubed Flaps 50
   4.4. Pedicled Muscle Flaps 50
   4.5. Free Flaps 51
   4.6. Adjunctive Techniques 51
References 52

Summary The art and science of tissue transfer has evolved over centuries. Management options for reconstructing tissue defects, in degree of complexity, range from secondary intention to primary repair, to graft reconstruction, to flap reconstruction. Graft success id dependent on a well-vascularized host bed, rapid onset of imbibition, good apposition and immobilization, and rapid onset of inosculation. Flaps are primarily categorized by both their blood supply and their method of transfer. Random flaps do not have a defined or named blood supply. Axial flaps rely on a specific and defined vessel. Axial flaps are further divided by the course of the vascular pedicle that supplies the overlying tissue – namely musculocutaneous, fascio-cutaneous or neurocutaneous. Penile skin island flaps are fascio-cutaneous flaps, based on a pedicle of Dartos and anterior lamina of Buck's fascia. Flaps are also defined by the method of transfer – advancement, rotation, interpolation. Penile skin flaps are island and axial flap type. Flaps can be further categorized as local or distant flaps based on their proximity to the recipient site. Other flap techniques utilized for urologic reconstruction include: sliding advancement flap, rotation/transposition flap, tubed flap, pedicled muscle flap, and free flaps.

Keywords graft, imbibition, inosculation, flaps, primary repair, secondary intention

From: *Current Clinical Urology: Urethral Reconstructive Surgery*
Edited by: S.B. Brandes © Humana Press, Totowa, NJ

1. Introduction

The art and science of tissue transfer has evolved over centuries, with origins dating back three millennia to the Indian tile maker caste, who introduced skin grafts for nasal reconstruction *(1)*. Early physicians subsequently built upon this knowledge with the development of rotational forehead flaps. The European Renaissance brought forth further innovation with the addition of sliding and pedicle flaps to the French and Italian literature *(2)*. Subsequent refinements and advances were forged in the chaos and trauma of the World Wars with the development of split-thickness grafts, the concept of composite flaps, and extensive application of pedicled flaps and an understanding of the concept of vascular territories or angiosomes *(3)*. The 1970s marked the inception of the free tissue transfer. This novel technique vastly expanded the horizon of the reconstructive surgeon with myriad novel reconstructive options. The 1980s heralded the development of fasciocutaneous flaps and further broadened the reconstructive armamentarium *(4)*. At the same time, tissue culture and bioengineering techniques were creating a new array of allogenic, xenogenic, and synthetic reconstructive alternatives. Current innovations in reconstructive surgery will likely add even more rungs to the reconstructive ladder as surgeons and scientists refine techniques of tissue engineering, immune modulation, and transplantation *(5)*. As we enter this new millennium, all of the strides of the past combine with the promise of the future to provide the reconstructive surgeon with a vast array of options to offer patients with complex tissue defects. This is especially relevant for the reconstructive urologic surgeon who is often faced with complex defects of delicate and specialized tissues.

2. Assessment

Every patient and every wound has different requirements for healing. When considering a defect, the reconstructive surgeon must take all of these factors into consideration to balance the maximum likelihood of successful reconstruction with the least morbid intervention. Urethral

defects warrant special consideration due to the specialized nature of these tissues (see Chapter 1 by P. Humphrey in this volume) and the need to preserve a watertight, mucosalized conduit for the elimination of urine as well as a layer of coverage to repair any exterior skin defect.

As in any surgical undertaking, the first step in the reconstruction of any defect is a careful and detailed assessment of the patient through history and physical examination. This information can then be used in conjunction with a meticulous evaluation of the wound to choose the most appropriate reconstructive option. Critical points to elucidate are any underlying factors that may pose a threat to the patient or the success of the reconstruction and that may preclude the selection of a particular reconstructive technique. For example, patients with severe cardiopulmonary embarrassment should not be considered for a lengthy operation such as a free tissue transfer just as patients who are keloid formers should not have a skin graft harvested from an aesthetically sensitive area. The patient's historical information should also be reviewed for factors that can be optimized before intervention to increase success, such as nutritional deficiency and anemia.

Once the relevant historical data have been accrued and the defect carefully evaluated, the reconstructive plan can then be designed. When choosing a reconstructive option, it is useful to use the "reconstructive ladder" to select the intervention that has the best qualities to repair the defect coupled with the minimum amount of donor morbidity to the patient.

3. Management Options

3.1. Secondary Intention

The first and least invasive rung of the reconstructive ladder is healing by secondary intention. In accordance with the Hippocratic Oath, the reconstructive surgeon is compelled to consider the option of watchful waiting and local wound care, although the applicability of this technique is clearly less relevant in urethral defects, which lead to the extravasation of urine and impaired wound healing, fistula formation, strictures. Also healing by secondary intention will lead to significant wound contraction, which is likely to be detrimental to urethral function. Nonetheless, secondary intention remains an important option in the reconstructive gamut and is especially applicable when used in conjunction with other reconstructive interventions. Because of the great capacity of mucosal surfaces to remucosalize after injury and to epithelialize raw surfaces that are transposed into a mucosal area, nonepithelial tissue transfer, in conjunction with urinary diversion, may be sufficient to reconstruct a urethral defect. Thus a component of a complex reconstruction may rely on healing by secondary intention.

3.2. Primary Repair

The next rung on the reconstructive ladder is primary repair. If sufficient local tissue exists, devitalized tissues can be débrided and wound edges may be mobilized and directly coapted to repair the defect. It is crucial to stay within the limitations of the tissue available when attempting primary closure. Attempts to force tissues beyond their limits of tension or blood supply to avoid a more complex reconstruction will inevitably result in reconstructive failure and cause further iatrogenic damage to the wounded tissues. This is especially relevant to urethral reconstruction where attempts to "short change" the urethra may cause more significant morbidity in the form of urethral strictures or fistulas (6,7), which are discussed in more detail in other sections of this text.

3.3. Graft Reconstruction

Ascending the reconstructive ladder further constitutes the use of grafts. Grafts involve the transfer of nonvascularized tissue from a donor area into a recipient bed, where they undergo a well-described series of events that lead to revascularization and engraftment (**Table 5.1**). Disruption of these processes will lead to graft failure. The first phase of engraftment is known as plasmatic imbibition. During this time, the

TABLE 5.1. Conditions for Graft Success.

1. Well-vascularized host bed
2. Rapid onset of plasmatic imbibition
3. Good apposition and immobilization of graft
4. Rapid onset of inosculation

transferred tissue derives nutrition and eliminates metabolic wastes by "drinking" from the exudate in the host wound bed. Diffusion of nutrients, oxygen, and metabolic wastes occurs passively back and forth across the concentration gradient from the graft to the wound bed (8). This process sustains the graft for approximately the first 48 h after grafting. Subsequent to this period, inosculation, the second phase of engraftment begins. The inosculatory process involves the formation of anastomotic connections between host and graft vasculature, leading to direct vascular continuity between the host bed and the graft. In conjunction with this process, capillary ingrowth is also occurring from the host bed into the graft (9). New vessels invade the graft and establish the definitive vasculature that will ensure the long term survival of the graft. Whether the pre-existing vessels in the graft act as conduits for ingrowth and become re-endothelialized, or entirely new vessels form, or both, remains an area of ongoing research and debate.

Graft survival can be adversely affected by several local factors. The primary cause of graft failure is fluid accumulation under the graft. Hematoma or seroma formation between the graft and recipient bed disrupts the delicate interface required for plasma imbibition. This can be prevented by creating perforations in the graft (pie crusting) to allow for egress of any fluid that may accumulate. Meshing a graft similarly allows any fluid under the graft to escape, and has the added benefit of allowing the graft to be expanded to cover more surface area. Expanded meshed grafts however, yield a net like scar pattern upon healing. A bolster dressing or vacuum assisted closure device may also help the graft to conform closely to the underlying tissue, thus precluding the accumulation of fluid (10). A bolster dressing serves a dual purpose; it also holds the graft securely in place to prevent any shearing from occurring. Shearing of graft from the recipient bed disrupts the neovascularization from the host bed to the graft and impedes graft take. Infection may also lead to graft loss and can be prevented by meticulous debridement and preparation of the wound bed to ensure that it is clean and able to support the graft.

There are several types of grafts available that can be categorized by the type of tissue transferred. Skin grafts are by far the most common type of grafts. They may be harvested from a variety of locations and tend to retain the properties of their donor area. In urethral reconstruction, the thin hairless genital skin (penile or preputial skin) is very well suited for reconstruction *(6)*. The palpebral donor area can also provide an excellent source of thin skin.

Skin grafts may be further subdivided into split-thickness (STSG) and full-thickness (FTSG) skin grafts. STSGconsist of the epidermis and a small portion of the dermis. FTSG contain the entire dermis and epidermis. Because of the differences in graft composition, FTSG and STSG have several important differences. FTSG display significantly more primary contraction, whereas STSG tend to contract more secondarily. Primary contraction is the contraction that occurs immediately after the graft is separated from the surrounding tissue. Because of the significant proportion of elastic dermal tissue in a FSTG, this contraction is approximately 40% of the original volume, whereas a STSG which has minimal dermal components will only undergo primary contraction of approximately 10% *(11,12)*. Secondary contraction occurs after the graft has been transferred to the recipient site as the wound heals. FTSG demonstrate minimal secondary contraction, whereas STSG contract significantly in direct proportion to the amount of dermis they contain. Secondary contraction is caused primarily by the action of myofibroblasts, which is diminished by the presence of a dermal layer *(13,14)*. A second important distinction between FTSG and STSG is the durability of the graft and, once again, this distinction is attributable to the incorporation of the dermal layer.

A STSG is harvested at a depth of 0.005–0.022 inches at the level of the subepidermal or intradermal vascular plexus. In contrast, a FTSG is harvested with the entire dermis at the level of the subdermal vascular plexus (**Fig. 5.1**). A STSG will survive more readily on a less vascular recipient bed for two reasons: The more superficial vascular plexuses have smaller and more numerous vascular channels available for anastomosis and also the STSG contains less bulk and thus requires less influx of nutrition and egress of waste. These properties combine to make STSGs more resistant to hypoxia and congestion upon transfer. The converse is true in terms of mechanical durability; the dermal layer of a FTSG allows it to be much stronger and more resistant to tearing than a thin STSG in the long term once it has healed.

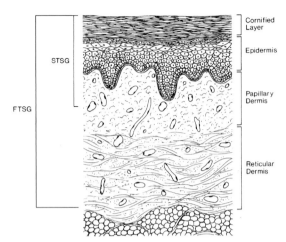

FIG. 5.1. Layers of the skin. Split-thickness skin grafts include a variable amount of dermis. Full-thickness grafts are taken with all the dermis (From Yu GW and Miller HC (1996) Critical maneuvers in urologic surgery, Mosby, St. Louis, p. 255)

Mucosal grafts deserve special mention in the context of urethral reconstruction. These grafts can provide an excellent source of specialized epithelial tissue for urethral lining *(15)*. Mucosal grafts are analogous to skin grafts but supply a secretory epithelium rather than a cornified squamous epithelium. Mucosal grafts are available from several donor areas including bladder epithelium, buccal or palatal mucosa, and nasal septal mucosa. These grafts are essentially harvested as FTSG and exhibit similar contractile properties. However, they tend to come from areas with numerous microvascular channels and thus have more robust circulation then true FTSGs. An important consideration in mucosal graft transfer is desiccation. These grafts, especially bladder mucosa, need to be kept well moistened during the transfer process to prevent damage to the epithelial surface, and should not be transferred to external areas.

Dermal grafts are created from FTSG that are subsequently denuded of their epithelium, which yields a graft with vascular channels available for inosculation and vascular ingrowth on both sides, thus making them ideal as a buried graft (**Fig. 5.2**) *(16)*. Dermal grafts will not epithelialize, however, and will require STSG coverage once vascularized if placed in an external location. Dermal allografts also are commercially available in the form of processed cadaveric dermis and synthetic dermal substitutes and offer the advantage of sparing the patient any donor site morbidity.

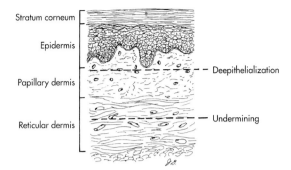

Stratum corneum

Epidermis

Papillary dermis — Deepithelialization

Reticular dermis — Undermining

FIG. 5.2. Deepitheliazation and undermining technique. Dermal grafts consist of dermis denuded of epithelium. (From YU GW and Miller HC (1996) Critical maneuvers in urologic surgery, Mosby, St. Louis, p. 227)

Graft reconstruction of a tubular structure such as the urethra requires special preparation of the graft. Reconstruction of partial defects may be accomplished by patching with a flat piece of graft. However, bolstering of the graft is challenging as it must be accomplished from inside the tube and may be placed over a catheter. It is also crucial that it is anchored outward to the surrounding tissues so that it can make firm contact with the recipient tissues that will provide its vasculature. Through and through quilting sutures may be required to accomplish this. For circumferential urethral defects, a tubular graft will be required for reconstruction. This can be achieved by fashioning a flat graft into a tube or by using a tubular donor structure. Urethral gaps may require the use of specialized grafts to restore length and continuity to the urethra (7). Multiple autologous materials have been investigated for this application, including tunica vaginalis, small intestinal submucosa, colonic mucosa, and peritoneum. Vein (17) or appendix (18) grafts may also provide a potential source of tubular conduit material to span urethral defects.

3.4. Flap Reconstruction

Flaps represent the next level of the reconstructive ladder. They consist of tissue that is transferred to a new location but maintains its own blood supply and does not rely on the recipient site for survival. Flaps are incredibly versatile and may be used to transfer healthy vascularized tissue into a wound defect that cannot support a graft.

In contrast to grafts in which sensibility relies on neural ingrowth from the recipient site and is typically quite poor, sensation as well as vascularity may be transposed using a flap if the neural elements are included (19,20). However, in the case of distant flaps, the original cortical connections remain and reeducation may be required to interpret the stimuli. Also, erogenous sensation may only be achieved through direct nerve anastomosis to the pudendal nerve branches (21).

Flaps may be composed of skin, fat, fascia, muscle, bone, or specialized tissues and may contain one component or be designed as a composite of multiple tissue types. Muscle or fascial flaps may also be useful in conjunction with grafts because they provide a healthy, vascular recipient bed for engraftment. Flaps are primarily categorized based on both their blood supply and method of transfer. Many other subcategories of flaps also exist.

By blood supply, flaps may be either random or axial (**Fig. 5.3**). Random flaps do not have a defined or named blood supply and rely on the random inclusion of many small arteries and veins in their base, or pedicle. In contrast, axial flaps are designed on a specific vessel that is known to vascularize the flap territory (angiosome [3,20]). Axial flaps may transfer an entire angiosome and, thus, are limited only by the extent of the feeding vessel. Random flaps are constrained by the arbitrary vascular plexus contained in the pedicle and have limited length to width ratios (traditionally 3:1). Axial flaps may be further subdivided based on the nature and course of the vascular pedicle that supplies the overlying tissue. The flap may be classified as a musculocutaneous (the pedicle is contained within a muscle), fasciocutaneous (the pedicle is contained within a fascial septum), or even neurocutaneous (the pedicle is based on the vasa nervorum that travel with a cutaneous nerve [5]). The penile skin island flaps that are used for urethral reconstruction are fasciocutaneous flaps, where the vascular pedicle is contained within a trellis of Dartos fascia and the anterior lamina of Buck's fascia of the penis.

Flaps are also defined by their method of transfer. Advancement flaps are moved parallel to the long axis of their pedicle. Rotation flaps, in contrast, are transposed perpendicular to the long axis of their pedicle. Interpolation flaps are transposed from an area that is not directly adjacent to the defect, such that the pedicle must be tunneled under the intervening tissues. Island flaps

RANDOM/RANDOM CUTANEOUS PATTERN SKIN FLAPS

AXIAL/ARTERIAL PATTERN SKIN FLAPS

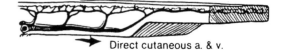

Direct cutaneous a. & v.

1. Peninsular Axial Pattern Flap

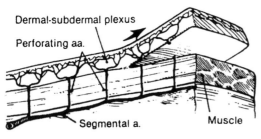

Dermal-subdermal plexus

Perforating aa.

Segmental a.   Muscle

1. Random Cutaneous Flap

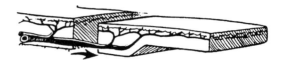

2. Island Axial Pattern Flap

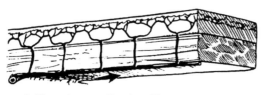

2. Myocutaneous Random Flap

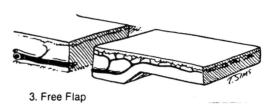

3. Free Flap

Fig. 5.3. Classification of skin flaps according to their blood supply

are flaps that are transferred based only on their vascular pedicle without a cuff of surrounding tissue and are by definition axial flaps. Penile skin flaps used for urethral reconstruction are thus both the island and axial flap type. Although this technique dramatically improves the mobility of the flap, great care must be taken to protect the vascular pedicle which will be more prone to kinking and twisting. Additionally, flaps may be further categorized as local or distant flaps based on their proximity to the recipient site. Distant flaps may be direct, by means of positioning. For example, a random thigh skin flap raised to cover a distal penile defect. They may be tubed, such that the pedicle of the flap is fashioned into a tube to form a bridge of tissue that allows transfer of the distal portion of the flap over an intervening segment of tissue, such as a tubed superficial inferior epigastric artery flap to carry abdominal tissue into a penile wound. These types of flaps will require secondary procedures approximately 3 weeks after inset to divide their attachments to the donor site. Microvascular free flaps are also defined as distant flaps which are completely harvested from

their donor site based on their axial vessels. These vessels are then reattached to suitable vessels in the region of the recipient defect to reestablish perfusion of the flap tissues, such as a free radial forearm flap transferred to the femoral vessels to recreate a urethra in a penile reconstruction. Microvascular free tissue transfer constitutes the topmost rung in the reconstructive ladder.

4. Flap Techniques

There are a myriad of ingenious flap designs, some examples of specific reconstructive flaps have been chosen to illustrate the principles of flap transfer. This is by no means an exhaustive list as the design of a flap is truly only limited by the tissue available, and the skill and ingenuity of the reconstructive surgeon.

4.1. Sliding Advancement Flap

Advancement flaps usually are designed as random flaps that are advanced directly into an adjacent defect. Sufficient skin laxity in the donor area is required for advancement into the defect. Several adjunctive techniques can be used to improve the mobility and reach of an advancement flap.

Mobility can be improved by judiciously undermining the tissues of the donor area. Small triangles of redundant tissue at the base of the flap (Burrow's triangles) tend to bunch as the flap is advanced, these can be excised to improve flap reach and prevent dog ears from forming (**Fig. 5.4**). A specific type of advancement flap which is commonly employed in reconstruction is the V to Y advancement flap (**Fig. 5.5**) in which a 'V'-shaped area of tissue is advanced as required into a defect and closed as a "Y." The converse of this technique is also possible in a Y to V advancement. These techniques eliminate the formation of dog ears and allow direct linear closure. Another example of an advancement technique is a bipedicle advancement flap. In this case the flap is based at the superior and inferior pole and advanced laterally, like a bucket handle. This allows a double blood supply to the flap but it will require the donor area to be skin grafted for closure.

4.2. Rotation/Transposition Flaps

Rotation flaps are designed to move in an arc to cover an adjacent defect (**Fig. 5.6**). Rotation flaps typically are circular or semicircular in nature. Once

again, skin laxity is required in the donor area to allow the flap to reach its destination, reach can be improved by local undermining) and a cautious back cut at the tightest point of the base of the flap. The base of a rotation flap will tend to bunch as it rotates through its arc and as a consequence the flap will shorten; thus, the flap should be designed larger then the defect to be covered in order to compensate for this tendency. A clever variant of a rotation flap is a bilobed flap. This rotation flap is designed with two progressively smaller lobes, which allows the large lobe to fill the defect, the smaller lobe to fill the harvest site of the larger lobe, and the harvest site of the smaller lobe to be closed primarily (**Fig. 5.7**).

A transposition flap is similar to a rotation flap in principle, but it is designed geometrically as a quadrilateral which pivots directly into an adjacent defect. The resultant linear defect can then be closed directly as a straight line. An excellent

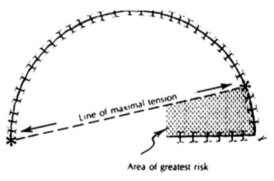

Fig. 5.6. Rotation flaps are typically circular or semicircular in nature

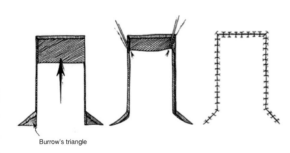

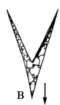

Burrow's triangle

Fig. 5.4. Burrow's triangles and island advancement skin flap

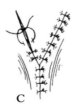

A	B	C

Fig. 5.5. V–Y, advancement flap

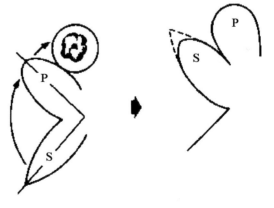

Fig. 5.7. Rotation flaps are designed with two progressively smaller lobes

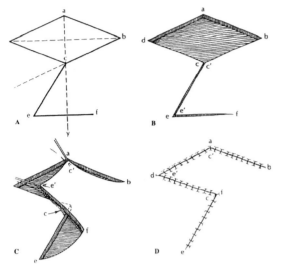

FIG. 5.8. Rhomboid flap

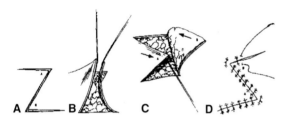

FIG. 5.9. Z-plasty

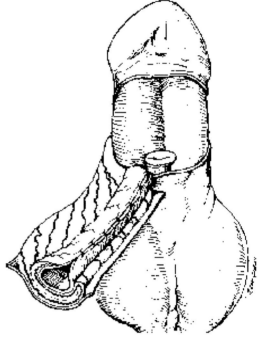

FIG. 5.10. Tubed flap

example of a transposition flap is a rhomboid flap (**Fig. 5.8**). The use of multiple transposition flaps in concert can also be a useful reconstructive technique. The quintessential example of this is the Z-plasty (**Fig. 5.9**). A Z-plasty is essentially a double triangular transposition flap. The flaps are oriented along the line of greatest tension in the shape of a "Z" and transposed with each other to yield an "S." This serves to relax the tension, which was along the long axis of the "Z" and distribute it into the more lax transverse axis.

4.3. Tubed Flaps

Tubed flaps are interpolation flaps that are designed to span intact tissue to transpose non adjacent tissue into a defect (**Fig. 5.10**). These flaps are created by rolling a transposition flap into a tube, which allows it to temporarily span intervening tissue until it engrafts in the recipient area, at which point the tubed pedicle may

be divided. Historically, "walking" tubed flaps were used to sequentially march tissue from a distant location into a defect. This practice has been abandoned since the advent of microvascular free tissue transfer. However, tubed flaps remain useful when ready sources of nearby donor tissue are available through positioning, as in genital reconstruction. Thigh and lower abdominal skin may easily be tubed and carried into a penile or urethral defect. However, historically, onlay flaps tend to have a higher success rate o and more durable results then tube grafts when it comes to urethral reconstruction.

4.4. Pedicled Muscle Flaps

The vascular supply of a muscle allows it to be transferred and in some cases, to carry overlying skin to a defect. Muscle flaps that are useful and typically employed in genital reconstruction include the gracilis and rectus abdominus flaps. The gracilis flap is fed by a proximal pedicle from the medial circumflex femoral artery and is readily transferred to the genitalia for reconstruction (22). It may carry muscle bulk and skin, and it can remain sensate through branches of the obturator nerve. (See the Chapter 22 by Brandes, for a more detailed description of the gracilis anatomy and harvest method.) The rectus abdominus muscle is also strategically located for genital reconstruction; it may be based on its inferior pedicle from the inferior epigastric vessels to carry muscle and skin to the genitals.

4.5. Free Flaps

Free tissue transfer is the most complex and most versatile operation in reconstruction. Many donor sources are available based on the desired tissue characteristics. Muscle flaps can provide bulk, while fascial or fasciocutaneous can provide a thinner more pliable construct. The anterolateral thigh flap is an example of a versatile fasciocutaneous flap (**Fig. 5.11**) *(23)*. It is based on a septocutaneous branch from the descending branch of the lateral circumflex femoral artery, and can provide a significant amount (8 × 25 cm) of thin pliable skin. It may also be neurotized via the lateral femoral cutaneous nerve. An important caveat in the use of the anterolateral thigh flap is that it is not ideal in obese patients. They have large subcutaneous fat deposits which make the flap too thick and very difficult to harvest.

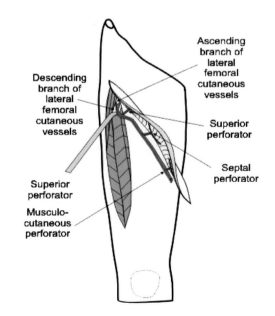

Descending branch of lateral femoral cutaneous vessels

Superior perforator

Musculo-cutaneous perforator

Ascending branch of lateral femoral cutaneous vessels

Superior perforator

Septal perforator

FIG. 5.11. Free Flap

4.6. Adjunctive Techniques

There are some adjunctive therapies to the traditional reconstructive ladder that deserve mention as well. These techniques are very useful in increasing the utility, reach, and success of conventional tissue transfer methods. Negative pressure dressings are very helpful devices to help improve the local wound characteristics before definitive closure. A negative pressure dressing can be used to temporarily cover a wound in patients who are not yet medically stable enough to undergo reconstruction. These dressings are also beneficial in cleaning an infected wound bed after debridement but before reconstruction to ensure that no infection remains. Additionally, the negative pressure milieu created by the dressing combats retraction of the wound edges and contributes to the formation of vascular granulation tissue. In some cases, this process can convert a wound that originally would have required flap reconstruction into one that can be closed with a simpler graft. Negative pressure dressings are also excellent skin graft bolsters; they conform well to irregular surfaces and prevent shearing and fluid accumulation *(24)*.

Delay of flaps is another helpful adjunct to tissue transfer. A delay procedure may improve the blood flow and potentially expand the vascular territory of a flap. Delaying a flap is the practice of dividing a portion of the vascular supply to the flap at a primary procedure before actual flap transfer and while the flap remains in situ. This stimulates increased blood flow to be diverted to the flap through the planned pedicle and improves the vascularity of the flap. It is also thought that delay can lead to the recruitment of additional flap territory beyond the original angiosome by the dilation of vascular channels (choke vessels) between the territories in response to the delay *(25)*. The exact mechanism of action of delay remains controversial but may include partial sympathectomy leading to vascular dilation, vascular reorientation, and improved flap tolerance to hypoxia. Delay procedures are typically performed 1–2 wk before definitive flap transfer.

Tissue expansion is also very helpful in increasing the utility and range of a flap. To achieve expansion, an expandable implant with an access port is placed beneath the area of the proposed flap. The implant is then periodically inflated with saline to stretch the overlying tissues. Once the desired dimensions have been achieved the expander is removed and the expanded flap is transferred in to the defect. Tissue expansion also has the added benefit of producing a delay type effect in the expanded tissues, with improved vascularity. The body also forms a capsule in response to the expander, which has its own vascular network. The drawbacks of tissue expansion include the risk of implant exposure or infection, which will then require removal of the expander and setback reconstruction. In addition, some patients are embarrassed by the contour changes produced by the expander during the expansion process [26]).

References

1. Ratner D (1998) Skin grafting. From here to there (review). Dermatol Clin 16:75–90
2. Hauben DJ, Baruchin A, Mahler A (1982) On the History of the free skin graft Ann Plastic Surg 9:242–245
3. Taylor GI, Palmer JH (1987) The vascular territories (angiosomes) of the body: experimental study and clinical applications Br J Plast Surg 40:113–141
4. Lamberty BG, Cormack GC (1990) Progress in flap surgery: greater anatomical understanding and increased sophistication in application World J Surg 14:776–785
5. Mathes SJ (2006) Plastic Surgery. 2 ed. Saunders Elsevier, Philadelphia.
6. Wessells H, McAninch JW (1998) Current controversies in anterior urethral stricture repair: free-graft versus pedicled skin-flap reconstruction World J Urol 16:175–180
7. Zinman L (2000) Optimal management of the 3- to 6-centimeter anterior urethral stricture Curr Urol Reports 1:180–189
8. Converse JM, Uhlschmid GK, Ballantyne Jr DL. (1969) Plasmatic circulation" in skin grafts. The phase of serum imbibition Plastic Reconstr Surg 43:495–499
9. Converse JM, et al. (1975) Inosculation of vessels of skin graft and host bed: a fortuitous encounter Br J Plastic Surg 28:274–282
10. Blackburn JH, 2nd, et al. (1998) Negative-pressure dressings as a bolster for skin grafts Ann Plastic Surg 40:453–457
11. Brown D, Garner W, Young VL(1990) Skin grafting: dermal components in inhibition of wound contraction Southern Med J 83:789–795
12. Corps BV (1969) The effect of graft thickness, donor site and graft bed on graft shrinkage in the hooded rat. Br J Plastic Surg 22:125–133
13. Rudolph R (1979) Inhibition of myofibroblasts by skin grafts. Plastic Reconstr Surg 63:473–480
14. Rudolph R, et al. (1977) Control of contractile fibroblasts by skin grafts. Surg Forum 28:524–525
15. Gupta NP, et al. (2004) Dorsal buccal mucosal graft urethroplasty by a ventral sagittal urethrotomy and minimal-access perineal approach for anterior urethral stricture. BJU Int 93:1287–1290
16. Hendren WH, Keating MA (1988) Use of dermal graft and free urethral graft in penile reconstruction. J Urol 140:1265–1269
17. Zhang F, et al. (2001) Reconstruction of ureteral defects with microvascular vein grafts in a rat model. J Reconstr Microsurg 17:179–183
18. Koshima I, et al. (1999) Free vascularized appendix transfer for reconstruction of penile urethras with severe fibrosis. Plastic Reconstr Surg 103:964–969
19. Yap LH, et al. (2005) Sensory recovery in the sensate free transverse rectus abdominis myocutaneous flap. Plastic Reconstr Surg 115:1280–1288
20. Taylor GI, M.P. Gianoutsos, and S.F. Morris (1994) The neurovascular territories of the skin and muscles: anatomic study and clinical implications (see comment). Plastic Reconstr Surg 94:1–36
21. Levine LA, L.S. Zachary, and L.J. Gottlieb (1993) Prosthesis placement after total phallic reconstruction. J Urology 149:93–98
22. Kayikcioglu A (2003) A new technique in scrotal reconstruction: short gracilis flap Urology 61:1254–1256
23. Kuo YR, et al. (2001) Free anterolateral thigh flap for extremity reconstruction: clinical experience and functional assessment of donor site. Plastic Reconstr Surg 107:1766–1771
24. Venturi ML, et al. (2005) Mechanisms and clinical applications of the vacuum-assisted closure (VAC) Device: a review. Am J Clin Dermatol 6:185–194
25. Dhar SC, Taylor GI (1999) The delay phenomenon: the story unfolds. Plastic Reconstr Surg 104:2079–2091
26. Manders EK, et al. (1984) Soft-tissue expansion: concepts and complications. Plastic Reconstr Surg 74:493–507

6
Epidemiology, Etiology, Histology, Classification, and Economic Impact of Urethral Stricture Disease

Steven B. Brandes

Contents

1. Epidemiology 53
    1.1. Demographics 53
    1.2. Incidence 54
    1.3. Signs and Symptoms of Urethral Stricture 54
2. Histology/Pathology 54
3. Stricture Classification 55
4. Stricture Characteristics and Etiology 56
    4.1. Etiology 56
    4.2. Stricture Etiology by Location of the Stricture 58
5. Consequences of Untreated Strictures 59
6. Economic Impact 60
References 61

Summary Urethral stricture is a common urologic problem, with the highest prevalence in underdeveloped countries. Urethral strictures have a significant economic impact and burden. Economics and resource availability can influence stricture treatment. Detailed here-in is the epidemiology of anterior urethral strictures as to demographics, incidence, and signs and symptoms. Histology and pathology are addressed; in particular, the fibrotic process of spongiofibrosis and the changes in collagen, smooth muscle and extracellular matrix. Various classification schema for staging anterior and posterior urethral strictures are detailed. Etiology of infectious/ inflammatory (attention to the paraurethral glands) and traumatic/ischemic strictures are also elaborated.

Keywords histology, epidemiology, classification, etiology, economic burden

1. Epidemiology

1.1. Demographics

In the United States, urethral stricture disease appears to be more common in the elderly and in African Americans. Stricture incidence increases gradually with increasing age, particularly for those older than 55. Furthermore, at urban/inner city hospitals, strictures are 2.6 times as common as in the community hospital population. Potential explanations are that patients with urethral stricture commonly are referred to university centers for definitive care, or that the indigent population is more disposed to stricture from either infection or trauma. In non-industrialized countries, urethral stricture is more commonly infectious or inflammatory in origin and, thus, typically affects a much-younger populace and with more frequency then in the West (1).

From: *Current Clinical Urology: Urethral Reconstructive Surgery*
Edited by: S.B. Brandes © Humana Press, Totowa, NJ

1.2. Incidence

The true incidence of urethral stricture disease can only be estimated. However, in the United States, male urethral strictures occur at rates as high as 0.6% in susceptible populations and results in more than 5000 inpatient visits across the United States per year. Between 1992 and 2000, more than 1.5 million office visits were made for male urethral strictures *(1)*. However, by most measures, stricture prevalence appears to have decreased over time. Potential explanations for such decreases in numbers are the overall decrease of stricture incidence and the increasingly successful use of anastomotic and substitution urethroplasty. Emergency room visits by male Medicare patients with urethral strictures accounted for 6.9 per 1000,000 visits in 2001. For ambulatory surgery center visits for stricture, there appears to be a bimodal distribution in peak incidence: patients <10 years and >35 years. Among current practicing U.S. urologists, only 6–20 (median, 11) cases of urethral stricture are treated per year (**Table 6.1**). In many nonindustrialized counties with limited medical resources, male urethral stricture disease remains highly prevalent. Definitive therapy often is not feasible for most because of the lack of adequate hospital facilities or adequate operating rooms.

1.3. Signs and Symptoms of Urethral Stricture

As the urethral lumen gradually strictures down, obstructive voiding symptoms worsen and in an insidious pattern. Typical symptoms include weak

TABLE 6.1. Number of patients with urethral strictures treated in 2004 by surveyed U.S. Urologists.

Number	Frequency	Percentage
None	3	0.7
1–5	54	12.5
6–10	140	32.5
11–20	132	30.6
>20	59	13.7
No response	43	10
Total	431	100

Reprinted from Bullock TL, Brandes SB (2007) Adult anterior urethral strictures: a national practice patterns survey of board certified urologists in the United States. J Urol 177:685–690.

urinary stream, straining to void, hesitancy, incomplete emptying, urinary retention, post-void dribbling, and urinary tract infections. Other fairly common symptoms can include urinary frequency, nocturia, dysuria, or occasionally suprapubic pain. These symptoms can also suggest bladder outlet obstruction from an enlarged prostate or prostate inflammation. Recurrent epididymitis in a young person or the signs or symptoms of recurrent prostatitis should trigger an evaluation for an undiagnosed urethral stricture. Moreover, patients who present with Fournier's gangrene must undergo and evaluation for the presence of a urethral stricture, especially when associated with urinary extravasation or perineal abscess. Obstructed ejaculation suggests stricture and is an important cause of infertility. Meatal strictures have a deviated or splayed urinary stream. Palpation of the urethra often can reveal firm areas consistent with spongiofibrosis/periurethral scarring. (See the chapter 28 on urethral stricture follow-up for detailed methods for investigating the degree and extent of urethral strictures by such noninvasive methods as flow rate, ultrasound, or AUS symptom score.)

2. Histology/Pathology

In general, a urethral stricture is a fibrotic process with varying degrees of spongiofibrosis that results in poorly compliant tissue and decreased urethral lumen caliber. The normal urethra is a lined mostly by pseudostratified columnar epithelium. Beneath the basement membrane there is a connective tissue layer of the spongiosum rich in vascular sinusoids and smooth muscle. The connective tissue is composed of mainly fibroblast and an extracellular matrix that contains collagen, proteoglycans, elastic fibers and glycoproteins. The most dramatic histologic changes of urethral strictures occur in the connective tissue. Strictures are the consequence of epithelial damage and spongiofibrosis.

Scott and Foote *(2)* showed that, after trauma, the epithelium became ulcerated and covered with stratified columnar cells. The stricture itself was noted to be rich in myofibroblasts and giant multinucleated giant cells. Both were felt to be related to stricture formation and collagen production. An increase in collagen results in fibrosis. Singh and Blandy *(3)* showed in rat urethral stricture experiments that the total amount of collagen increases in urethral stricture, resulting in dense fibrotic tissue with decreased smooth muscle and thus elasticity. In contrast, Baskin *(4)* did not demonstrate an increase in collagen but rather a change in subtype distribution, in favor of type III collagen. The change in the ratio of type I to III collagen was associated with a decrease in urethral elasticity and compliance.

Calvacanti et al. *(5)* analyzed 15 urethral strictures managed by anastomotic urethroplasty. They noted that, with collagen replacement, there was a complete loss of the relationship between smooth muscle, extracellular matrix, and sinusoids in the peri lumen. Fibrosis of the tissue and reduction in vascular density was greatest when the etiology was trauma. Etiology of stricture did not play a role in the content of smooth muscle or collagen in the peripheral corpus spongiosum. Increase in collagen subtype was noted in the perilumen with type II and in the spongiosum with type I. Stricture also had fewer elastic fibers. Overall, urethral strictures are characterized by marked changes in the extracellular matrix. Bastos et al. *(6)* noted that concentration of elastic fibers are high in the spongiosum and explains in part its high degree of extensibility. In urethral stricture, particularly of traumatic etiology, the scar is dense, hypovascular, and reduced in elastic fibers.

3. Stricture Classification

An anterior urethral stricture is a scar of the urethral epithelium and commonly extends into the underlying corpus spongiosum. The scar (stricture) is composed of dense collagen and fibroblasts and, thus, contracts in all directions, shortening urethral length an narrowing luminal size. Strictures are usually asymptomatic until a lumen size below 16F. (See chapter 28 in this volume for more details.)

In 1983, Devine et al. *(7)* proposed a classification of urethral strictures based on the extent of spongiosal fibrosis (**Fig. 6.1**). Jordan and Devine *(8)* subsequently outlined a treatment algorithm with types of surgery or urethrotomy based on the classification stage. For class D or greater, where spongiosal fibrosis was full thickness, they recommended open urethroplasty. The concept of selecting treatment based on the extent of spongiosal fibrosis is sound; however, it

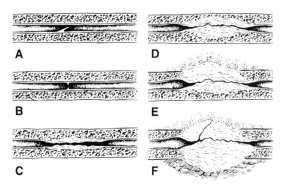

Fig. 6.1. Devine classification of urethral stricture disease according to the anatomy of the stricture. (A) Stricture with no spongio-fibrosis and an epithelial flap. (B) Epithelial scar with minimal spongio-fibrosis. (C–E) Progressive spongiofibrosis. (F) Spongio-fibrosis occupies the entire corpus spongiosum and potential fistula formation. (From Schlossberg SM, Jordan GH (2005) Urethral stricture. In: Rakel RE and Bope ET (eds) Conn's current therapy. Elsevier, Amsterdam)

is not clinically practical unless one has an accurate and reliable noninvasive means to evaluate the degree of fibrosis. Conventional urethrography can only detail luminal narrowing and not the character of the underlying tissue. Physical examination (palpation of urethral induration) and urethroscopy (elasticity of the tissue and the color of the epithelium) can be helpful surrogates for underlying fibrosis, but the extent of reliably predicting such is limited. Ultrasonography has promise as a modality for assessing fibrosis. However, by its very nature, sonography is operator dependent and clinical stratification of strictures then by this means is very subjective, which can often time not be reproducible. Excessive probe external compression can result in a false urethral lumen narrowing. The spongiosum in generally hypoechoic and with increasing fibrosis it has been suggested by Chiou et al. *(9)* that increased echogenicity, at times calcifications, and lack of blood flow on color Doppler suggests fibrosis. McAninch *(10)* first proposed in 1988 a sonographic appearance of the urethral stricture staging system, which ranged from normal to severe, based on the degree of lumen occlusion (**Fig. 6.2**).

Later, combining the sonographic findings of spongiosal involvement with the length of the urethral

Normal

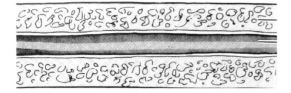

Mild < 1/3 Lumen occluded

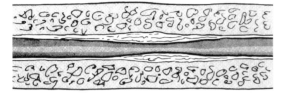

Moderate 1/3-1/2 Lumen occluded

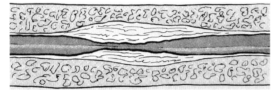

Severe > ½ Lumen occluded

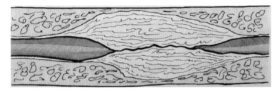

Fig. 6.2. Ultrasound classification of the degree of urethral occlusion, after McAninch and later modified by Chiou (From Ref. *[10]*).

stricture, Chiou et al. *(9)* categorized urethral strictures into five categories:

   I: Short stricture (<2.5 cm) with minimal spongiosal tissue involvement
  II: Short stricture with moderate (some normal spongiosal tissue in the periphery) spongiosal tissue involvement
 III: Short stricture with extensive (full thickness) spongiosal tissue involvement.
  IV: Long (>2.5 cm) or multiple strictures with moderate spongiosal tissue involvement
   V: Long (>2.5 cm) or multiple with extensive spongiosal tissue involvement.

Unfortunately, we have not have the same success with assessing fibrosis sonographically as Chiou

et al. and thus we do not feel that ultrasound is the modality of choice to assess spongiofibrosis. We have found that the best correlation with fibrosis to be the extent of lumen narrowing and the length of stricture. Longer and narrower strictures tend to have more spongiofibrosis. The recent advent of extended field-of-view ultrasound technology produces good images that can help to better assess stricture length and location because the images look like a urethrogram. The lack of blood flow on color Doppler, however, may have more value as a predictor of spongiofibrosis. The less blood flow noted, the more spongiofibrosis suggested.

Barbagli *(11)* has proposed a classification schema for LSA inflammatory strictures and of the disease process when it involves the penis and urethra. His proposal is as follows:

Stage 1: LSA only involves the foreskin
Stage 2: LSA involves the foreskin, the coronal sulcus and meatus
Stage 3: The foreskin, glans, and external meatus are effected, as well as an associated stricture of the fossa navicularis and anterior urethra. At times, the infectious process spreads to the glands of Littre and the patient develops a pan urethral stricture.
Stage 4: An associated premalignant or cancerous lesion is also present.

Pansadoro et al. *(12)* have proposed a classification of prostatic urethral strictures. However, classification is clinically not significant because they suggested that all injuries are best managed in the same fashion, by bladder neck incision. The grading system is as follows: Type I: Fibrous tissue involves the bladder neck only, termed "bladder neck contracture." Type II: Stricture is localized to the median part of the prostatic fossa, with open bladder neck and spared verumontanum. Type III: Complete prostatic urethral obliteration.

4. Stricture Characteristics and Etiology

4.1. Etiology

Most present-day anterior urethral strictures in industrialized countries are the result of occult or recognized blunt external perineal trauma (e.g., straddle

TABLE 6.2. Meta-analysis of anterior urethral stricture etiology *(12)*.

Investigator	Stricture (n)	Cause (n)			
		Idiopathic	Iatrogenic	Inflammatory	Traumatic
Wessells and McAninch	40	5	12	13	10
Wessells et al.	25	0	11	9	5
Andrich and Mundy	83	35	38	7	1
Santucci et al.	168	64	24	12	68
Elliot et al.	60	37	9	7	7
Andrich et al.	162	38	84	23	17
Fenton et al.	194	65	63	38	28
Total (%); included only bulbar strictures	732	244 (33)	241 (33)	109 (15)	136 (19)

injury) or instrumentation (e.g., traumatic catheter placement/removal, chronic indwelling Foley catheter, or transurethral surgery). A recent meta-analysis of the literature shows that most anterior stricture are iatrogenic (33%), idiopathic (33%) and, to a lesser extent, trauma (19%) and inflammation (15%; see **Table 6.2** for details). The site of the stricture also varies considerably in different reports, which may further account for some of the differences in treatment outcome. Bulbar (posterior) strictures are the most common (44% to 67% of patients), followed by penile (anterior) strictures in 12% to 39%, mixed (posterior plus anterior) in 6% to 28%, external meatal or submeatal (0% to 23%), membranous (0% to 20%), and prostatic (0% to 4%).

Inflammatory strictures, such as secondary to gonococcal urethritis, are relatively very uncommon today. However, there is no apparent relationship between nonspecific urethritis (chlamydia and ureaplasma urealyticum) and subsequent stricture development. At the turn of the century or in contemporary undeveloped countries, more than 90% of strictures are inflammatory, and commonly involve the bulbar and pendulous urethra. Gonococcal urethral strictures occur because of abscesses that form in the paraurethral glands of Littre (**Fig. 6.3**). The abscess then affects the surrounding corpus spongiosum and heals by fibrosis and scarring. The paraurethral glands are in greatest concentration in the bulbar urethra and it is the bulb then where most inflammatory stricture occurs (**Fig. 6.4**), In the bulb, the glands extend deeply into the corpus spongiosum and are distributed circumferentially around the urethra. The membranous and the penile urethra (except for a short segment proximal to the meatus) lack glands, whereas the penoscrotal junction has a few sparse and small glands. It is inter-

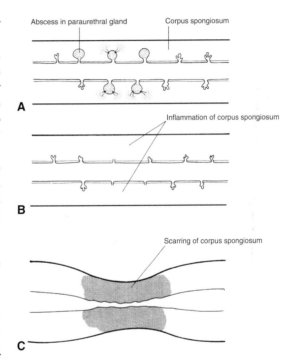

FIG. 6.3. (A) Acute gonococcal inflammation of the paraurethral glands bursts out into the corpus spongiosum to produce inflammation (B), which heals by scarring and, thus, (C) lumen stenosis and spongiofibrosis. (From Blandy JP, Fowler C (1996) Urethra and penis inflammation. In: Urology. Blackwell Science, Oxford, p. 476)

esting to note that most mammals except humans and guinea pigs lack paraurethral mucous glands. With downstream urethral stenosis, infected urine can accumulate under pressure and extravasate into the corpus spongiosum and result in spongiofibrosis. As a result, a relatively short stricture can slowly progress or "creep" proximally (upstream) (**Fig. 6.5**). Long tortuous strictures, in particular those

SITES OF INFLAMMATORY
STRICTURES

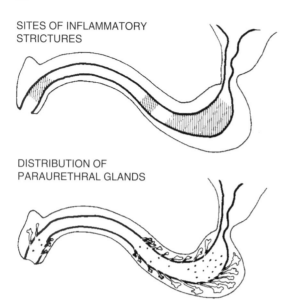

DISTRIBUTION OF
PARAURETHRAL GLANDS

FIG. 6.4. Paraurethral glands are most numerous in the distal pendulous and in the mid/proximal bulb. Inflammatory strictures commonly occur in the same location as the higher concentration of paraurethral glands. (From Singh M, Blandy JP (1976) The pathology of urethral stricture. J Urol 115:673–676)

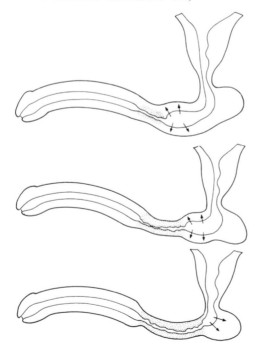

FIG. 6.5. Inflammatory stricture tends to "creep up" the urethra as infected urine is forced into the corpus spongiosum upstream of a stricture. (From Blandy JP, Fowler C (1996) Urethra and penis inflammation. In: Urology. Blackwell Science, Oxford, p. 477)

associated with fistulas or periurethral abscesses or tuberculous prostatitis, are associated in the developing world with tuberculosis of the urethra. In the classic animal experiments of the 1970s by John Blandy, urine extravasation exacerbates the post-traumatic inflammatory process that in some cases leads to complete stenosis of the urethra. Urinary diversion is thus essential to help prevent the severe periurethral fibrocytic reaction that can be seen.

In Western countries today, the most common cause for inflammatory strictures is lichen sclerosus et atrophicus (LSA), which starts out as affecting only the glans, meatus, and preputial skin. Metal stenosis can also lead to high pressure voiding as with GC, and eventually inflammation or infection of the periurethral glands ('Littritis'). Potentially, pan-urethral stricture disease can occur in this manner. LSA is a common cause of phimosis and thus is often temporally apparent after circumcision. (See Chapter 3 by Virasoro and Jordan in this volume detailing the etiology and histology of LSA.)

4.2. Stricture Etiology by Location of the Stricture

Strictures that involve the fossa navicularis are typically the result of inflammatory (33–47%) and iatrogenic (33–37%) causes. In Fenton et al. *(13)*, mean stricture lengths in the anterior urethra were longest in the pendulous urethra at 6.1 cm, shortest in the bulbar urethra at 3.1 cm, and in the fossa navicularis at 2.6 cm. That pendulous strictures were long underscores the customary need for substitution urethroplasty for pendulous strictures, whereas for bulbar strictures, which are typically much shorter, are often amenable to an anastomotic urethroplasty or an augmented anastomosis. For their series, most urethral strictures were idiopathic (34%), iatrogenic (32%), inflammatory (20%) or traumatic (14%).

Etiology of iatrogenic stricture is typically caused by instrumentation. Such strictures are mostly to the result of transurethral resection (41%), prolonged catheterization (36.5%) and, to a lesser degree, cystoscopy (12.7%), prior hypospadias (6.3%), and radical prostatectomy surgery (3.2%). Such strictures are the result of an ischemic insult from the traumatic passage of large instruments into the urethra during transurethral surgery or by prolonged catheterization (particularly when a larger bore catheter is used). Such iatrogenic urethral strictures typically occur at sites of greatest compression and ischemia, namely points of urethral fixation or lumen narrowness (the membranous-proximal bulb, penoscrotal junction and the fossa-meatus; **Fig. 6.6**). Thus, when prolonged catheterization is needed, for short durations, a 16-Fr catheter is advocated, whereas for extended time periods, an SP tube is often placed.

Iatrogenic strictures appear to occur after trauma from faulty catheterization, the inflammatory response provoked by the catheter material, or avascular necrosis (compressive ischemia), such as from a large catheter. From animal experiments, it is clear that different catheter materials result in differing local tissue reactions and destruction (from best to worst: silicone, plastic, latex, and rubber). Furthermore, instrumentation strictures occur in predictable locations of urethral fixation and narrowing. Traumatic urethral strictures tend to be short and in the bulbar urethra. Most are due to a straddle injury. Idiopathic strictures also can be short and common (up to 38%). So called idiopathic stricture are probably the cause of unrecognized childhood perineal trauma. Baskin and McAninch *(14)* noted that it can take years from the time of the perineal trauma to the advent of significant stricture.

5. Consequences of Untreated Strictures

A review of U.S. 2001 Medicare data notes that urethral stricture patients annually have high rates of UTI (42%) and urinary incontinence (11%). Common complications from untreated urethral stricture disease can result in minor-to-severe complications, among them urethral discharge, urinary tract infection, stones, chronic prostatitis or epididymitis, periurethral abscess (a rupture of an infected glands of Littre outside the spongiosum), urethral diverticulum (an abscess that forms but does not communicate with the overlying skin and often results in a outpouching, where a urethral stone may often form), and urethral cancer (historically, one-third to one-half of men with urethral cancer have a history of stricture disease. Other complications can include urethro-cutaneous fistula, where as long as there is a distal stricture, the urinary fistula will persist. When a maze of fistula channels link, it is often referred to as a "watering pot perineum." Urine extravasation of urine into the perineum or scrotum typically is confined by Colle's fascia (**Fig. 6.7**) and can result in devastating sequela. Infected hypertonic urine is particularly virulent and can cause fat and fascia necrosis of the scrotum, penis, and perineum, or even abdominal wall, as in Fournier's gangrene.

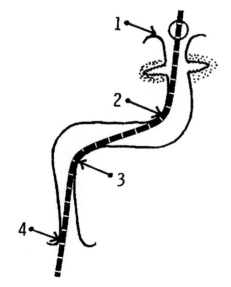

FIG. 6.6. Locations of ischemic urethral strictures from instrumentation. Note strictures occur at the sites of bowstring compression-like effects by a rigid instrument placed per urethra. (From Edwards LE, Lock R, Jones P (1983) Post catheterization urethral strictures. A clinical and experimental study. Br J Urol 55:53–56)

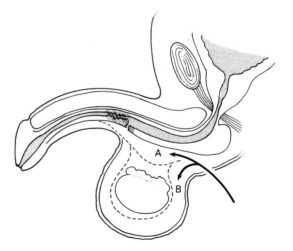

FIG. 6.7. (A, B) Neglected stricture and subsequent extravasation of urine into both compartments of Colles' fascia. (From Blandy JP, Fowler C (1996) Urethra and penis inflammation. In: Urology. Blackwell Science, Oxford, p 477)

Because infections travel along predictable fascial planes, the testes, deep to the tunica vaginalis are never involved. Chronic infection is associated with squamous cell carcinoma in the body. Long-standing recurrent strictures in the elderly and in the bulb should be suspected of having cancer.

6. Economic Impact

Urethral stricture remains a common urological problem, with the highest prevalence in some third-world countries, which have limited resources and can least afford the costs of treatment and follow-up of patients with recurrent strictures. Although urethroplasty is the "gold standard," urethral dilation and urethrotomy remain attractive treatment options, particularly in the nonindustrialized word. In such less-developed settings of the world, there is often a lack of surgical facilities and adequately trained staff relative to the large case load.

As an example of the economics of stricture care in underdeveloped counties, Ogbonna (15) reported on 134 patients treated during a 3-year period in Nigeria, where the incidence of urethral stricture disease is high and where the short-term goal of providing some treatment to most may override the sometimes conflicting long-term aim of minimizing recurrence rates. The overall recurrence rate was 22%. A combination of direct vision internal urethrotomy (DVIU) plus intermittent self catheterization had a recurrence rate of 17% and a recurrence free period similar to that after urethroplasty. They concluded that DVIU was 10 times cheaper, 10 times faster to perform, and offered the surgeon better protection from human immunodeficiency virus bodily fluid exposure than did urethroplasty. Self-catheterization significantly increased the recurrence-free period after DVIU. The author emphasized the importance of preoperative recognition of strictures with a high risk of recurrence after DVIU, so that they can be selected for primary urethroplasty.

In these times of health care fiscal restraint and managed care, the emphasis is to determine cost savings methods without compromising care. In industrialized countries, the costs of medical care are mostly in equipment, operating theater time, and hospitalization. Thus, from a cost to the overall medical system model, for industrial-ized countries, urethrotomy is more expensive than urethroplasty, due to its high failure rate and need for repeat treatment. Greenwell et al. (16) reviewed 126 patients in the United Kingdom who were followed for a mean of 25 months after DVIU and found that 48% required more than one endoscopic retreatment (mean, 3.13 each), 40% performed biweekly intermittent self catheterization, and 6% required urethroplasty. They calculated that the most cost-effective strategy was initial urethrotomy or urethral dilation followed by urethroplasty in patients with recurrent stricture, which yielded a total cost per patient of UK 5866 pounds sterling ($8799 dollars per patient). The costs for urethrotomy were $3375 compared with $7522 for one-stage urethroplasty and $15,555 for two-stage urethroplasty. They concluded that this financially based strategy concurs with evidence based best practice for urethral stricture management.

Rourke and Jordan (17) compared the costs of DVIU and anastomotic urethroplasty for a 2-cm bulbous urethral stricture. The cost minimization decision analysis model that they used predicted that treatment with DVIU was more costly ($17,747 per patient) than immediate urethroplasty ($16,444 per patient). Treatment with DVIU became more favorable when the long-term risk of stricture recurrence after DVIU was less than 60%. The authors concluded that, from a fiscal standpoint, open urethroplasty should be considered over urethrotomy in the majority of clinical circumstances. Wright et al. (18) used decision analysis to determine the cost-effectiveness of different management strategies for short, bulbar urethral strictures 1 to 2 cm in length. Urethroplasty as the primary therapy was cost-effective only when the expected success rate of the first DVIU was less than 35%. The most cost-effective approach was one DVIU before urethroplasty. The authors recommended urethroplasty for strictures recurring after a single urethrotomy, and for longer strictures when the success rate of urethrotomy is expected to be less than 35%.

In the United States, for the fiscal year of 2000, the estimated annual expenditures for male urethral stricture disease was $191 million, or a yearly individual average cost of disease at $6000 (1). These costs are substantially less then more common urologic conditions, such as nephrolithiasis, which had a economic burden of $2.1 billion in 2000. During the last two decades, total costs for managing urethral strictures appear to have peaked in 1998 at 207 million. Ambulatory surgeries comprise the majority (70%) of urethral stricture treatment costs. Economics may also be influencing the way that urethral strictures are managed. Bullock and Brandes *(19)*, in a U.S. nationwide survey of U.S. urologists, noted that 33% would perform successive urethrotomies on a resistant stricture, while only 29% would refer to a specialist. 2006 Medicare physician reimbursement payments for anterior urethroplasty is a paltry $735.62, for urethrotomy with steroid injection $377.56, and office cystoscopy and dilation $296.46. There is an obvious financial disincentive to performing urethroplasty in the United States. Clearly, the stricture patient who is managed by only dilation or urethrotomy is a life-long repeat customer. Urethroplasty, on the other hand, is often a time-consuming, complex surgery that can achieve cure and thus be lost source of repeat revenue.

References

1. Santucci RA, Joyce GF, Wise M (2007) Male urethral stricture disease. J Urol 177:1667–1674
2. Scott TM and Foote J (1980) Early events in stricture formation in the guinea pig urethra. Urol Int 35:334–339
3. Singh M, Blandy JP (1976) The pathology of urethral stricture. J Urol 115:673–676
4. Baskin LS, Constantinescu SC, Howard PS, Mcaninch JW, Ewalt DE, Duckett JW, Snyder HM, Macarak EJ (1993) Biochemical characterization and quantitation of the collagenous components of urethral stricture tissue. J Urol 150:642–647
5. Calvacanti AG, Costa WS, Baskin LS, McAninch JA, Sampaio FJ (2007) A morphometric analysis of bulbar urethral strictures BJU Int 100(2):397–402
6. Bastos AL, Silva EA, Silva Costa W, Sampaio FJ (2004) The concentration of elastic fibers in the male urethra during human fetal development. BJU Int 94(4):620–623
7. Devine CJ, Devine PD, Felderman TP, Burns CN (1983) Classification and standardization of urethral strictures. J Urol A 325
8. Jordan GH, Devine PC (1988) Management of urethral stricture disease. Clin Plast Surg 15:493–505
9. Choiu RK, Anderson JC, Tran T, Patterson RH, Wobig R, Taylor RJ (1996) Evaluation of urethral strictures and associated abnormalities using high resolution and color Doppler ultrasound. Urology 47:102–107
10. McAninch JW, Laing FC, Jeffrey RJ (1988) Sonourethrography in the evaluation of urethral stricture: A preliminary report. J Urol 139:294–297
11. Barbagli et al (2004) Lichen sclerosus of the male genitalia and urethral stricture diseases. Urol Int 73(1):1–5
12. Pansadoro V, Emiliozzi P (1999) Iatrogenic prostatic urethral strictures: classification and endoscopic treatment Urology 53:784–789
13. Fenton AS, Morey AF, Aviles R, Garcia CR (2005) Anterior urethral strictures: etiology and characteristics.Urology 65(6):1055–8
14. Baskin LS and McAninch JW (1993) Childhood urethral injuries: perspectives on outcome and treatment. Br J Urol. 72(2):241–6.
15. Ogbonna BC (1998) Managing many patients with a urethral stricture: a cost-benefit analysis of treatment options. Br J Urol. 81(5):741–4
16. Greenwell TJ et al (2004) Repeat urethrotomy and dilation for the treatment of urethral stricture are neither clinically effective nor cost-effective. J Urol. 172(1):275–7
17. Rourke KF, Jordan GH (2005) Primary urethral reconstruction: the cost minimized approach to the bulbous urethral stricture. J Urol 173(4):1206–10
18. Wright JL et al (2006) What is the most cost-effective treatment for 1 to 2-cm bulbar urethral strictures: societal approach using decision analysis. Urology 67(5):889–93
19. Bullock TL, Brandes SB (2007) Adult anterior urethral strictures: a national practice patterns survey of board certified urologists in the United States. J Urol 177:685–690

7

Urethrotomy and Other Minimally Invasive Interventions for Urethral Stricture

Chris F. Heyns

Contents

1. Dilation 64
2. Urethrotomy 66
3. Direct Vision Internal Urethrotomy 66
4. Laser Urethrotomy 68
5. Core-Through Urethrotomy 69
6. Endoscopic Urethroplasty 70
7. Anesthesia 70
8. Antibiotics... 70
9. Catheterization 70
    10.1. Dilation 71
    10.2. DVIU 71
    10.3. TUR of Scar Tissue After DVIU 72
    10.4. CTU 72
11. Results.. 72
12. Risk Factors for Recurrence... 73
    12.1. Age of the Patient 73
    12.2. Symptoms at Presentation... 73
    12.3. Etiology... 73
    12.4. Previous Stricture Treatment 74
    12.5. Periurethral Scarring 74
    12.6. Length of the Stricture 74
    12.7. Caliber or Diameter of the Stricture 74
    12.8. Site of the Stricture 74
    12.9. Number of Strictures... 75
    12.10. Instrument Used, Number, and Location of Incisions 75
    12.11. Complications During the Procedure.. 75
    12.12. Perioperative Infection... 75
    12.13. Type of Catheter Used 75
    12.14. Duration of Catheterization 75
    12.15. Length of Follow-Up 75
    12.16. Repeated Treatment 75
13. Prevention of Recurrence.. 75
    13.1. TUR of Fibrous Callus.. 75
    13.2. Hydraulic Self-Dilation.. 76
    13.3. Clean Intermittent Self-Catheterization 76
    13.4. Clinic Dilation.. 76

From: *Current Clinical Urology: Urethral Reconstructive Surgery*
Edited by: S.B. Brandes © Humana Press, Totowa, NJ

    13.5. Steroids 77
    13.6. Halofuginone 77
    13.7. Botulinum Toxin 77
    13.8. Mitomycin-C 77
    13.9. Brachytherapy 77
14. Indications for Dilation or DVIU 77
Editorial Comment 78
References 80

Summary The minimally invasive interventions most often used for treating urethral strictures are dilation and direct vision internal urethrotomy (DVIU), which are equally effective for the initial treatment of strictures. The reported success rate with DVIU varies from 66% to 90%, and declines progressively with longer follow-up. The recurrence rate is higher with previously treated, long (>2 cm), multiple strictures, penile compared with bulbar strictures, and those with perioperative infection. Specific contraindications to DVIU include suspicion of urethral carcinoma, bleeding diathesis, and active infection. The rate of stricture recurrence may be decreased by teaching the patient to do hydraulic self-dilation or clean intermittent self-catheterization, or by performing regular follow-up dilation in a clinic setting.

The advantages of dilation and DVIU are that they can be performed under local anesthesia in an outpatient setting, with a low complication rate (<10%) and virtually no risk of mortality. Because dilation does not require special endoscopic equipment or operating room facilities, it is the procedure of choice where facilities for DVIU are not available.

The optimal indications for dilation or DVIU are single, bulbar strictures shorter than 2 cm, with no inflammatory changes and no previous treatment. A second DVIU for early stricture recurrence (at 3 months) is of limited value in the short term (24 months) but of no value in the long term (48 months), whereas a third repeated dilation or DVIU is of no value. There is some evidence that DVIU is being used excessively and inappropriately because of its simplicity and ease of repetition, and because there is a lack of familiarity with urethroplasty.

Keywords Urethra, Stricture, Dilation, Urethrotomy, Minimally Invasive, Urethroplasty

1. Dilation

The urethra can be dilated with metal sounds or bougies (e.g., Lister's or Béniqué's), urethral catheters of increasing size, filiforms and followers, Amplatz dilators, or an inflatable balloon. The goal of dilation is to stretch the scar tissue without producing more scarring. Forceful dilation until bleeding occurs implies that the stricture has been torn rather than stretched, and healing is likely to occur with even more fibrosis (1–6). The need for nontraumatic dilation gave rise to the statement: "The skill of the urologist is measured by his gentleness" (7).

The least-traumatic way of dilating the urethra is to use multiple treatment sessions. In former years, some hospitals treating large numbers of men with urethral strictures had "dilation clinics," where these men came for weekly and later monthly serial dilations. Although this is a relatively safe and easy form of management, the logistics and cost implications were considerable, leading to the abandonment of this treatment option.

Metal dilators with curved tips are very effective, but they must be used with extreme caution, because it is very easy to make a false passage (**Fig. 7.1**). The operator has to learn by experience the skill of passing the tip of the dilator up to the stricture and then swiveling it around so that the curve of the tip conforms to the curve of the bulbar urethra. If resistance is met, the exertion of force easily results in urethral trauma and a false passage. The thinner the dilator, the easier it is for the tip to make a false passage. Therefore, it is best to start with a large- or medium-sized dilator, gently sounding the urethra up to the stricture, and then trying serially smaller dilators until one of them is passed through the stricture. Thereafter, serially larger dilators are passed through the stricture, keeping in mind that the objective is to stretch the fibrosis, not to tear open the whole urethra and cause torrential bleeding. It is usually adequate to dilate the urethra to 20F or 24F.

Filiform dilators are safer because they do not easily make a false passage, but it is difficult to pass the filiform leader if the stricture is narrow or its opening is not in the center of the lumen. The easiest technique is to pass the filiform leader under direct vision with a rigid urethroscope or flexible cystoscope. Alternatively, if the straight tip leader cannot be passed, one can try one of the variety of spiral tips, twirling it in the hope of finding the stricture opening, or one can continue gently passing multiple straight filiforms to fill up the urethra, eventually allowing one of them to pass through the stricture (**Fig. 7.2A,B**).

Balloon dilation may be the least traumatic form of dilation, but it requires fluoroscopy for proper placement of the balloon and may require flexible cystoscopy to pass a guide wire through the stricture so that the balloon can be advanced into the stricture area *(8,9)*.

Stormont and associates *(10)* reported a retrospective review of 199 nonrandomized patients with newly diagnosed, short, single bulbar strictures treated with dilation or **direct** vision internal urethrotomy (DVIU). The success rate at 3 yr was 65% for dilation and 68% for DVIU, indicating that they were equally effective as initial treatment of bulbar urethral stricture *(10)*. However, there were some differences in etiology and presentation between these two groups; therefore, treatment selection bias cannot be excluded.

Steenkamp and associates *(1)* performed a prospective, randomized comparison of filiform dilation and DVIU in 210 men with urethral strictures. At 36 months' follow-up, the recurrence rate was 16% greater in the dilation than in the DVIU group and, at 48 months, it was 10% greater in the dilation group, but these differences were not statistically significant *(1)*. These studies indicate that dilation and DVIU are equally

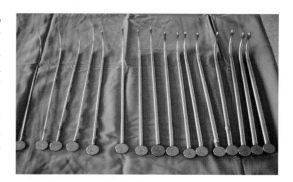

FIG. 7.1. Metal (Lister's) dilators

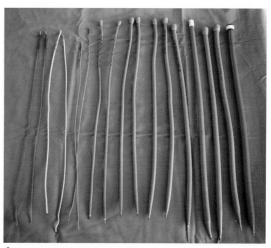

A

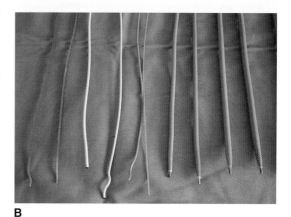

B

FIG. 7.2. Filiform dilators – leaders and followers

FIG. 7.3. Stricture recurrence after internal urethrotomy (A) or dilation (B). Note no statistically significant difference at 48 months follow-up *(1)*

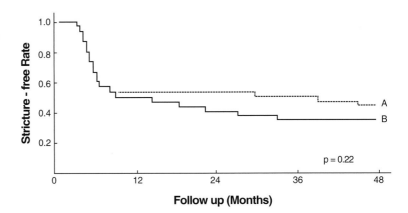

p = 0.22

Follow up (Months)

efficacious as initial treatment of male urethral strictures (**Fig. 7.3**) *(11)*.

2. Urethrotomy

The Otis urethrotome can not be passed if the stricture is <16 F (**Fig. 7.4**). In these cases, a small ureteral catheter may be passed and left in place for 3 to 4 d to dilate the stricture. It has been suggested that Otis internal urethrotomy (IU) should be performed in the 12-o'clock position, with the urethrotome opened to a maximum size of 45 F *(2)*. However, there is some concern that opening the Otis device to its full extent of 45 F may cause tearing rather than cutting of the stricture, with a less favourable outcome *(2)*. Some authors advocate performing Otis IU up to 35F in the 12-o'clock position *(12)*.

The success rate of Otis IU has been reported as 82% at a follow-up of 29 months *(2)*. However, these patients probably did not have very severe strictures, because the Otis urethrotome can not be passed through strictures less than about 16 F in diameter. The results reported after Otis IU followed by 3–6 wk of silicone urethral catheter drainage are similar to those after DVIU *(13)*.

Otis IU has been advocated for the prevention of urethral stricture after transurethral resection of the prostate (TURP) *(14)*. The reported incidence of stricture formation following TURP preceded by Otis urethrotomy (varying from less than 1% to 14%) appears to be substantially less than the 10% to 21% reported to occur after TURP without pretreatment *(15)*. In a prospective trial of Otis

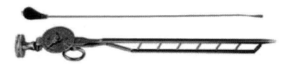

Otis Urethrotome

FIG. 7.4. Otis urethrotome

urethrotomy to 30F with a 2-mm deep incision at the 12-o'clock position, versus urethral dilation to 26/30F prior to (TURP), the incidence of stricture was 0 in the Otis urethrotomy and 10% in the dilation group *(16)*. Schultz and associates *(15)* reported a randomized clinical trial to study the prevention of strictures after TURP. Urethral catheter dilation was performed by insertion of a 22F latex Foley catheter for 24 h, and then substituting it for a 24F catheter for 24 h, with final dilation to 25.5F with metal dilators before TURP. IU to 33F was performed with a Mauermayer urethrotome. Strictures developed in 16% of patients treated by catheter dilation and 4% who had undergone IU. However, it may be that inserting a catheter 2 d before TURP caused urinary tract infection or injured the urethra, causing the higher stricture rate in the catheter dilation group.

3. Direct Vision Internal Urethrotomy

The technique of cold-knife DVIU is relatively simple (**Fig. 7.5**). The urethrotome with a 0- or 12-degree telescope and a 19F or 21F sheath is

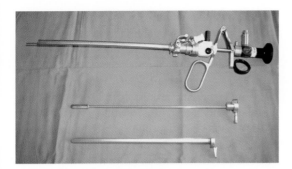

FIG. 7.5. Sachse urethrotome

inserted through the external meatus and advanced under vision up to the stricture. It is, of course, important to keep the blade withdrawn. The irrigation fluid should be isotonic (normal saline is ideal, unless electrodiathermy is to be used) because if there is extravasation it minimizes tissue damage and avoids the risk of hyponatremia.

Through the side-channel of the urethrotome, a 5F ureteric catheter or guide wire is inserted through the stricture, preferably all the way into the bladder. The stilet of the ureteric catheter should be removed because if it is too rigid, it may become stuck against the verumontanum, prostate, or bladder neck. If the stricture is very short, and if the operator is experienced, the stricture may be incised without a guide wire, but there is a real risk of cutting a false passage and even ending up in the rectum. The knife blade (which may be straight, semi-circular of curved) is extended along the upper surface of the guide wire and incisions are made by tilting and slightly withdrawing the urethrotome. Care should be taken not to cut through the ureteric catheter used as guide wire.

As the stricture is opened up, the urethrotome is advanced and further incisions are made until the full thickness of the stricture has been divided up to the normal proximal urethra. It is important to enter the bladder and perform a quick but thorough cystoscopy, because on occasion stones or even a bladder tumor may be discovered (1,17). If there is severe bleeding from the incised urethra, hemostasis may be obtained with a Bugbee or ball electrode, but this is rarely necessary (13,18).

A transurethral catheter is usually inserted after DVIU. It is advisable to fill the bladder before removing the urethrotome, so that when the catheter is inserted, the efflux of irrigation fluid shows that the catheter tip is inside the bladder before the balloon is inflated. When there is difficulty in negotiating the catheter, the urethrotome is passed under vision, the telescope is removed, and a ureteral catheter or firm guide wire is introduced through the urethrotome sheath, which is then withdrawn. The catheter tip is cut off and it is threaded over the ureteral catheter or guide wire.

Alternatively, a urethrotome with a half-round sheath can be introduced into the bladder. The telescope is removed and the catheter is guided through the urethrotome sheath, which is withdrawn, leaving the catheter indwelling. The only drawback is that the urethrotome sheath usually does not take a catheter larger than 16F (19). A curved metal catheter introducer may be used to insert the transurethral catheter, provided the operator is sufficiently experienced, because there is a real risk of making a false passage with the rigid introducer (20).

If no guide wire can be passed, but the patient has a suprapubic cystostomy, the bladder can be filled with methylene blue and by forcefully pressing on the full bladder, while the irrigation inflow through the urethroscope is turned off, it is often possible to see where the methylene blue squirts or billows through the track and then to incise the stricture, following the "blue route."

A pediatric cystoscope or a ureteroscope is useful if the stricture is difficult to negotiate, especially when there is gross displacement after severe pelvic fracture or if the stricture is complicated by a false passage, fistula or calculi. An 8F or 10F pediatric cystoscope is used to traverse the urethral stricture under direct vision, the optical system is then removed and a 5F or 3F ureteral catheter is passed via the sheath into the bladder and used as a guide to perform the DVIU (6).

To deal with long strictures without using a guidewire, Matsuoka et al. (21) passed a semirigid ureteroscope with an outer diameter of 6F at the tip through the stricture under direct vision. The ureteroscope was then pulled back while an incision was made using a holmium:YAG laser at the 10-o'clock and 2-o'clock positions to a diameter of 17F. The ureteroscope was then replaced by a 17F urethrotome and an antegrade incision was similarly made up to 21F to 22F.

Most reports describe doing a simple incision at the 12-o'clock position, because it minimizes the risk of severe hemorrhage due to incising the corpus cavernosum *(1,4,13,22–26)*. Some authors feel that the 12-o'clock incision is not ideal because the dorsal aspect of the corpus spongiosum is usually thinner than the ventral aspect and there is less room for spongiosal tissue supported healing after urethrotomy. Repeated incision at the 12-o'clock position may lead to the formation of dense fibrotic tissue with no supportive healthy spongiosal tissue beneath it, which increases the risk of stricture recurrence. Repeat deep incisions at the same area of the urethra may also increase the risk of injury to the periurethral structures *(27)*.

Some authors maintain that urethrotomy at only the 12-o'clock position is not adequate, because almost all strictures are circular. For this reason, they advocate the use of multiple incisions made close together through the entire thickness of the stricture wall. The first incision is performed at the most favorable site, whether it be at the 6-, 9-, or 12-o'clock position. Multiple incisions are made close together radially, and the stricture is incised over its entire circumference. If hemorrhage occurs the operation is interrupted, and as a precaution the urethra is compressed from the outside for at least 3 minutes after every operation. Control urethroscopy is performed after 2–3 wk, and stricture remnants are removed in this second session. However, it appears that the recurrence rate after multiple incisions does not differ markedly from series in which a single incision was used *(19,28)*.

Some authors advocate using cuts at the 4- and 8-o'clock positions because the spongiosum is thicker; therefore, incisions are more likely to reach healthy spongiosum *(29,30)*. Others use incisions at the 6- and 12-o'clock, or laterally at the 5- and 7-o'clock positions *(31)*.

It has been suggested that DVIU for anastomotic stricture after radical prostatectomy should be performed at the 4- and 8-o'clock positions to avoid injury to the rectum. The scar tissue is incised down to bleeding vessels and hemostasis is obtained with a 5F Bugbee electrode only when there is major arterial bleeding. Urinary continence can be preserved by not extending the urethrotomy distal to the area of scarification into the functioning sphincteric mechanism *(18,32)*. Alternatively, incisions can be made at the 3- and 9-o'clock positions *(33)*.

Color Doppler ultrasound may be useful to evaluate the length and diameter of the stricture and the extent of spongiofibrosis, and also to locate the urethral arteries. This enables the selection of areas free of arteries and allows incision through fibrotic layers without cutting through the full thickness of the corpus spongiosum *(27,34)*. Ultrasound of the distal male urethra is performed by disinfecting the glans and the meatus, instilling 10 to 12 mL of 0.9% saline solution into the urethra, placing a penile clamp on the patient, and asking him to contract the pelvic muscles to prevent the saline solution from escaping into the bladder. The penis is placed with its dorsal side on the lower abdominal wall, making the urethra and corpus spongiosum accessible to the 7-MHz ultrasound scanner, with gelatin applied as contact medium *(35,36)*.

Contrary to the belief that the urethral arteries are located at the 3- and 9-o'clock position, color Doppler ultrasonography has shown that there is no predictable pattern for their anatomy. In normal men, the site of the urethral arteries varies among individuals, but the symmetry of arteries is maintained. In men with urethral stricture, there is a loss of symmetry in all cases, and in some men with a dense stricture the urethral arteries can not be detected on ultrasound *(37)*.

The value of ultrasound was assessed in a prospective randomized trial where 562 men with inflammatory urethral stricture (<1.5 cm) were divided in two groups: 319 cases where the DVIU technique was adapted to the ultrasound features of the stricture zone, and 243 cases who underwent DVIU with a "classical" 12-o'clock incision. At a mean follow-up of about 39 months, the recurrence rate was 45% in the first and 52% in the second group. The authors suggested that the high recurrence rate after DVIU is caused by inadequate incision, and that urethral ultrasound could improve the DVIU technique by better location of the fibrosis area *(38)*. However, it remains unproven whether using ultrasound to adapt the DVIU technique will result in a clinically significant improvement of treatment outcomes *(27)*.

4. Laser Urethrotomy

Several different types of laser have been used for DVIU, including potassium-titanyl-phosphate (KTP-532), argon, diode, neodymium:yttrium-aluminum-garnet (Nd:YAG), and holmium:YAG (Ho:

YAG) laser *(39–45)*. Initially, it was thought that circumferential laser ablation of stricture fibrosis would lead to a lower recurrence rate *(39)*. However, the reported success rates with laser are comparable with those of conventional cold-knife DVIU and also decline with follow-up over longer periods *(39,46,47)*. Examples of reported success rates are 90% after 6–12 mo and 75% after 27 mo, or 76%, 67%, and 52% after 6, 12, and 24 mo, respectively *(42)*. There are no prospective, randomized comparisons of laser and cold-knife DVIU. The success rate with laser IU was greaer in patients with previously untreated strictures than after previous cold-knife DVIU (e.g., 79% vs 13%) *(41)*. In pediatric patients a high success rate of 89% has been reported, but the follow-up was relatively short *(43)*.

5. Core-Through Urethrotomy

In 1978, Sachse first attempted DVIU in patients with impassable strictures and, in 1983, Gonzalez and associates described optical urethrotomy and transvesical endoscopy of the proximal urethra for the treatment of complete occlusion of the membranous urethra *(48)*. This procedure has become known as core-through urethrotomy (CTU) or "cut to the light," because it involves coring a channel through the blocked site toward the light of an endoscope introduced via a suprapubic tract and through the bladder neck to the proximal end of the occluded urethra *(19,20,49)*. Some authors perform urethroscopy 3 wk after CTU and then resect residual fibrotic tissue with a standard 24F adult resectoscope *(50)*.

The "cut for the light" approach is possible only if there is a short area of occlusion with a thin membrane separating the ends of the urethra *(50)*. When there is a long obliterated segment, various techniques can be used to guide the urethrotome while cutting from the distal to the proximal urethra. These techniques include transrectal digital guidance with a Béniqué bougie in the proximal urethra *(19,50)*, C-arm fluoroscopy on an X-ray screening table *(50,51)*, and transrectal ultrasonography combined with a suprapubic cystoscope or nephroscope placed via the bladder neck *(50,52)*.

Perforation of the occluded urethra can be performed with a thin trocar introduced through the ure-throtome from below the stricture *(19,49)*, a 19-gauge sternal guide wire passed through the working channel of a 19F cystoscope with the curved tip angled upward *(33)* or an Evrim bougie, which is passed through the cystostomy tract—it has a curved end and a built-in channel of 1.5 mm in diameter for a sliding needle exiting at its tip *(51)*. All types of laser (KTP-532, Nd: YAG and Ho:YAG) have been used to vaporize the obliterating tissue *(53)*.

The reported success rates of CTU have varied considerably, from 0% to 100% *(53,54)*. Examples of the reported success rates are 35% cured after one procedure, 65% required 1 to 9 (mean, 3) additional urethrotomies *(19)*; favorable results in 40% after the first, and in 54% after a second procedure *(33,55)*; 58% were voiding satisfactorily after a mean follow-up of 2 yr *(56)*; in 70% voiding stabilized 1 year after the initial procedure *(50)*; success was obtained in 80% *(20)*.

Some authors have reported excellent results with laser CTU for obliterative posttraumatic urethral strictures *(53,57)*. After laser CTU, the requirement for subsequent DVIU (40% to 67%) and failure rate (3% to 42%) appear to be fairly comparable with the rates (57% to 66% and 10% to 30%, respectively) after open surgical repair *(53)*.

CTU is more likely to be successful if the stricture length is 2 cm or less, the proximal urethra is not displaced or kinked, there is no active infection at the site, and if there has been no previous urethral manipulation (e.g., "railroading"), severe distraction injuries, or associated false passage *(20,53)*. Koraitim *(54)* found successful results after DVIU for posterior urethral strictures complicating pelvic fracture only when there was a genuine stricture with no loss of urethral continuity.

A comparison of CTU with perineal anastomotic urethroplasty for strictures of the posterior urethra after pelvic fracture showed that operating time and blood loss were lower in the endoscopic group, but there were no other significant differences in morbidity or invasiveness. After DVIU, all patients required multiple secondary procedures, whereas normal voiding was achieved in all patients after perineal urethroplasty, although 22% required a single DVIU within 3 mos after surgery. The authors concluded that DVIU offers no compelling advantage over open urethroplasty for the delayed treatment of posttraumatic posterior urethral strictures *(58)*.

6. Endoscopic Urethroplasty

Petterson and associates *(59)* described tying a skin graft to a Foley catheter positioned with the graft over the raw area where DVIU had just been performed. However, with this technique movement between the graft and its bed could not be eliminated, potentially compromising graft take *(60)*.

Chiou *(61)* reported good results with endo-urethroplasty after CTU in patients with strictures following pelvic fracture distraction injuries of the urethra. After CTU and resection of the scarred urethral segment endo-urethroplasty was performed by grafting the raw area with a free patch of full thickness foreskin fixed to a catheter *(56,61)*.

In an attempt to eliminate movement between the graft and its bed, Naudé *(60)* designed purpose specific instruments for the carrying of a full-thickness penile skin graft at the site of the stricture after DVIU. An ultrathin full-thickness penile skin graft or buccal mucosa is tubularized over a balloon device with the epithelial surface facing inward, and endoscopically placed needles are used to fix the graft in position. Naudé reported an overall graft take of 95% and urethral patency in 100% of inflammatory and iatrogenic strictures, in 50% of established strictures after pelvic fracture, and in 75% of patients with urethral rupture treated 2–3 wk after the injury. Endoscopic skin-graft urethroplasty is not recommended in patients with established strictures after pelvic fracture distraction injuries of the urethra, or in anterior urethral strictures, because penile elongation during erection would compromise the graft take *(60)*. The need for procedure-specific instruments and the intricacy of the operation may be factors responsible for the lack of its widespread application *(44)*. Endoscopic urethroplasty using small intestinal submucosa (SIS) as a substitute for skin in patients with bulbar strictures proved unsuccessful, because the SIS grafts were resorbed without stimulating the necessary tissue regeneration *(62)*.

7. Anesthesia

DVIU was originally performed under general or spinal anesthesia *(13,39)*. However, just as with dilation, DVIU can be performed under local anesthesia, using 10 mL of 2% lidocaine (lignocaine) or mepivacaine instilled into the urethra *(1,11,28,29)*. After urethroscopy, a second dose of 10 mL of 2% lidocaine can be administered and 10 min allowed to elapse before performing DVIU. Intracorpus spongiosum anesthesia can be performed by injecting 3 mL of 1% lidocaine into the glans penis. This produces anesthesia lasting for about 1.5 h, allowing DVIU in an outpatient setting *(30)*.

8. Antibiotics

Pain and Collier *(17)* found that stricture recurrence after DVIU was increased when there was postoperative infection that was not treated with antibiotics, while the recurrence rate in patients with infection receiving antibiotics perioperatively was not significantly different from that in patients without infection. They recommended that prophylactic antibiotics should be given with the premedication and continued until the catheter is removed.

Most authors report using antibiotics with DVIU *(18,63)*. The type of antibiotic prophylaxis has varied from sulfonamides *(13)* to first-generation cephalosporins *(6)*, co-trimoxazole *(29)*, gentamycin *(1,11)*, and nitrofurantoin *(12)* or oral quinolones *(64)*. On the other hand, some authors reported using no prophylactic antibiotics when performing CTU for complete urethral occlusion *(19)*. The recommended duration of antibiotic treatment varies from a single preoperative dose *(1,11)* to continuous treatment until 24 h after catheter removal, which could be from 5 to 7 d *(2,6,32,64)*.

9. Catheterization

The size of the transurethral catheter inserted after DVIU has varied from 14F to 24F, but there is no real evidence that the catheter size has a significant effect on stricture recurrence rates *(1,2,4,12,13, 17–19,24,26,30,32,33,47,52,56,65)*. Use of a 24F catheter has been recommended after CTU for urethral obliteration *(49,50,53,56)*.

Silicone catheters were shown to be superior to conventional catheters when used after DVIU *(12)*. Although some authors have used PVC *(17)* or latex catheters *(26)*, most have reported using silicone or silicone-coated catheters. Some authors believe that the silicone stenting catheter should have multiple sideholes to drain blood and secretions (63).

Sachse suggested that a urethral catheter should be left postoperatively for 10 to 14 d. (66). Some authors recommend that the duration of catheterization should be adapted to the characteristics of the stricture, with no catheter drainage for short (less than 1 cm) strictures, and 5–7 d for long, fibrotic, or multiple strictures and when a false passage has been made (6). Inserting a catheter may have the disadvantages of preventing the drainage of blood and secretions and promoting infection, which may result in delayed healing and stricture recurrence (2,28). It has been suggested that transurethral catheterization for less than 3 d, or using a suprapubic catheter, may lead to lower recurrence rates (13,25,67). However, it seems unlikely that prolonged catheter drainage improves the outcome (22). The duration of catheterization may simply reflect case selection, with short catheterization used for simple strictures which have lower recurrence rate, and longer catheterization used for complicated strictures, which have a greater recurrence rate.

The reported duration of catheterization has varied from 1 d to 3 mo. Earlier studies reported catheterization for as long as 6 wk (12,68). However, most studies have reported catheterization for 1 to 4 d (1,2,13,17,18,24,30,32,46,47,64,65,69).

Longer periods have been used for more complicated procedures: 5 d after DVIU for failed previous urethroplasty (23), 8 d after DVIU and TUR of fibrous callus (63), and 2 wk to 3 mo after CTU for an obliterated urethra—this long period is thought to permit urethral mucosal regeneration (19,20,31,33,49,50,52,53,56).

10. Complications

10.1. Dilation

Stormont and associates (10) reported in a retrospective, nonrandomized study that DVIU compared to urethral dilation resulted in a greater incidence of post-procedure cystitis (5% versus 3%), epididymitis (5% vs 3%) and penile hemorrhage (8% vs 2%), with total complications 18% for DVIU and 8% for dilation. Steenkamp and associates (1) performed a prospective, randomized study of dilation and DVIU

and reported complications in 14% of the dilation and 11% of DVIU group. Failure to perform the procedure occurred in 13% of DVIU and 18% of dilation patients. The causes of failure were difficult or tight stricture, hemorrhage, false passage, extravasation, pain, breakage of the blade and, in the dilation group, knotting or breaking of the filiform leader or bending of the filiform follower (1). It should be noted that these procedures were performed under local anesthesia (intra-urethral instillation of lignocaine gel); therefore, the procedure failure rates of 13% to 18% would probably have been lower under general or spinal anesthesia.

10.2. DVIU

The relative safety of DVIU has been documented, with morbidity rates as low as 8% to 9% (10). Minor complications usually occur in less than 10% of cases (25), although a complication rate as high as 27% has been reported (31). In an early study by Pain and Collier peri-operative infection occurred in 38% of cases (17).

Examples of complication rates after DVIU in various studies are the following: pyrexia 5%, septicemia 2%, extravasation 3%, bleeding 3%, retention 2%, blocked catheter 2%, DVT 1% (17); hemorrhage 3%, urinary sepsis 2%, septicemia 1%, scrotal abscess 0.7%, extravasation 0.7%, epididymo-orchitis 0.7% (6); urethral bleeding 11%, extravasation 3% and chordee 1% (26); hemorrhage 3.4% to 4%, fever 2.2% to 1%, epididymitis 1%, incontinence 0.5% (25). In the pediatric population, urethralgia and urethral diverticulum occurred in 2% of children after laser DVIU (31).

Erectile dysfunction (ED) is reported by some authors to be a complication of DVIU in 2–11% of cases (70,71). It is presumably caused by direct severance of the cavernous nerve with the cutting blade by incising at the 3- and 9-o'clock positions, late fibrosis after extravasation and infection, or by DVIU of long and dense strictures causing a shunt between the corpora cavernosa and corpus spongiosum. In a study of 68 patients without erectile problems, only one (1.5%) complained about ED after DVIU (71).

Rare complications include high flow priapism, or a urethral-internal pudendal artery fistula, which can be treated with embolization (72–74). Rarely, severe bleeding and life-threatening septicaemia may occur, requiring active fluid resuscitation and ventilation *(34)*. After Otis urethrotomy to 45F, complications occurred in 8% of patients, hemorrhage requiring blood transfusion in 4%, bacteremia in 3%, and incontinence in 1% *(2)*.

10.3. TUR of Scar Tissue After DVIU

Transurethral resection (TUR) of scar tissue after DVIU (Guillemin's technique) leads to a greater complication rate. After IU alone, epididymitis occurred in 7.5%, scrotal edema in 15% and stenosis of the urethral meatus in 5%. After DVIU plus TUR of fibrous tissue the complications consisted of epididymitis in 10%, scrotal edema in 12.5%, perineal hematoma in 20%, and extravasation of the irrigating fluid in 40%. All complications were successfully managed with oral antibiotics and anti-inflammatories. The scrotal edema, perineal hematoma and extravasation of the irrigating fluid were totally absorbed within 8 d *(63)*.

10.4. CTU

Complication rates of CTU for urethral obliteration include: hematuria 9%, symptomatic urinary tract infection 7%, extravasation of blood or irrigation fluid into the perineum 3%, which resolved spontaneously, stress incontinence 0.6%; knife breakage 6.5% (the blade was easily retrieved with bladder biopsy forceps through the urethrocystoscope), and urethrotome handle breakage in one case with a long occlusion and extensive fibrosis *(19)*. CTU for obliterated urethra may also lead to formation of a false passage and damage to the rectum. In one study, CTU for complete posterior urethral obliteration with TUR of fibrotic tissue led to severe hemorrhage requiring transfusion as well as hyponatremia from irrigant absorption in 2 of 10 patients *(50)*.

11. Results

In the early 1980s, the reported "immense success" of the Sachse urethrotomy was reflected in a dramatic decrease in the number of urethroplasties being performed worldwide *(6,78)*. It was stated that, in cases of short and/or proximal strictures, the 2-yr cure rate was well above 80%, which was identical to what the best open urethroplasty could offer *(13)*. DVIU became the initial treatment of choice for most strictures of the male urethra *(6)*.

The reported success rate with DVIU varies from 66% to 90%, depending on the series *(10,11,22,25,28)*. In some literature reviews the success rates vary from 56% to 95% *(26)*; 35% to 60% *(63)*; 70–80% or 40–50% *(13,79)*. In the pediatric population similar success rates have been reported *(31,80)*; DVIU for strictures after hypospadias repair has a success rate of 21–40% *(81)*.

It soon became clear that the length of follow-up was the most important parameter for recurrence. Boccon-Gibod and Le Portz considered 56% of their patients cured at 6 mo, 43% at 1 yr, and only 25% at 2 yr. *(13)*. Albers and associates found a 95% success rate at 6 mo and only 55% at 38 mo *(25)*. Giannakopoulos and associates reported success rates of 55% at 6 mo and 35% at 2 yr *(63)*. Studies have confirmed the possibility of recurrence long after DVIU and showed that after 5 yr the success rate was only 25% to 36% *(26,82)*.

Some authors believe that with each repeated urethrotomy the fibrotic process becomes less virulent and the stricture is more readily overcome *(6)*. They believe that with repeated DVIU or dilatation most strictures (up to 85%) eventually "stabilize" within 1 yr and require no further treatment *(6,50)*. Holm-Nielsen and associates reported an overall "cure rate" of 77% at 2 yr of followup, but the cure rate after each individual operation was less than 50% *(22)*. Albers and associates reported that approximately 90% of patients were cured with up to two urethrotomies at a follow-up of longer than 3 yr *(25)*. In the pediatric population the success rate after initial DVIU was 36%, a second DVIU improved the success rate to 58% and the overall success rate after more than two urethrotomies was 71% *(80)*.

Most studies have reported that, if stricture recurrence occurs after DVIU, it occurs very soon after the procedure, within 3 to 9 mo *(4,17,24,64)*. In one study the mean time to recurrence was somewhat longer (16 mo; range, 0.5 to 132) *(79)*. In pediatric patients the time to recurrence varied from a median of 8 to a mean of 26 mo *(31,80)*.

Pansadoro and Emiliozzi *(26)* noted stricture recurrence within 12 mo after DVIU in 56% of their patients, at 12–24 mo in a further 26%, at 24–36 months in 8%, at 36–60 months in 7%, and after 60 months in 6%. Steenkamp and associates *(1)* found that after dilatation or DVIU the risk of stricture recurrence was greatest at 6 mo, and very small after 12 mo (**Fig. 7.6**). The median time to recurrence was 12 mos after DVIU and 6 mo after dilation. However, strictures can recur up to 8 yr after DVIU, therefore follow-up to 10 yr is recommended *(11)*.

Albers and associates *(25)* reported that a high recurrence rate correlated with a short time to recurrence (average 18 mo), whereas a low recurrence rate correlated with a long time to recurrence (average 35 mo). Heyns and associates *(11)* reported a similar finding, with a median time to recurrence of 21 mo after two treatments and 4.5 mo after three treatments, where the risk of recurrence was greater after three compared with two treatments (**Fig. 7.7**). Albers and associates *(25)* found that the time to stricture recurrence was shorter

with post-TUR strictures (mean, 18 mo) than with idiopathic strictures (mean, 35 months). Mandhani and associates *(77)* reported a mean recurrence-free duration of 13 mos vs 45 mo in cases of treatment failure and success, respectively. After CTU for complete obliteration of the posterior urethra, stricture recurrence occurred at 1 wk to 3 mo *(52)*. After Otis IU failures were usually apparent by 2 to 3 mo after the catheter was removed (the catheter was kept in for 6 weeks after IU *(12)*.

12. Risk Factors for Recurrence

The following factors have been investigated with regard to their effect on the risk of stricture recurrence after DVIU:

12.1. Age of the Patient

One study reported a "cure rate" of 85% in men younger than 60, and 71% in men older than 60 yr of age *(22)*. However, most studies found no correlation between the recurrence rate and the age of the patient *(13,25,31,80)*.

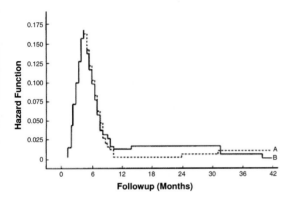

FIG. 7.6. Risk of first stricture recurrence after urethrotomy (A) or dilation (B). Stricture recurrences are greatest at 6 months, and slight after 12 months *(1)*

12.2. Symptoms at Presentation

One study reported a greater recurrence rate in men who had had symptoms for several years *(2)*. Another study found a marginal statistical significance for a greater risk of recurrence in men presenting with complications such as retention or infection *(1)*. However, most studies did not comment on this or found no significant correlation *(80)*.

12.3. Etiology

One study reported that traumatic strictures had a greater rate of recurrence *(4)*. Two studies found that post-TUR or inflammatory strictures occurring after long-term catheterization or genital infection had a higher risk of recurrence than traumatic and iatrogenic strictures *(13,25)*. One study found a greater recurrence rate in iatrogenic compared with infective or traumatic strictures *(22)*, but another study reported the opposite, with the best results obtained in iatrogenic strictures *(63)*. Several studies found no relationship between the stricture etiology and the risk of recurrence *(1,2,26,80)*.

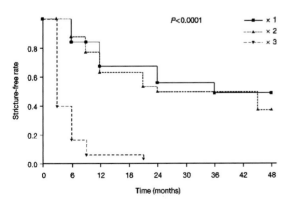

FIG. 7.7. Stricture free rate after dilation or internal urethrotomy in patients never treated before randomization. Time to stricture recurrence is shorter after successive urethrotomies *(1)*

12.4. Previous Stricture Treatment

Most authors reported that the recurrence rate was greater with previously treated strictures *(22,26,64)*. The success rate for previously untreated strictures was 47% vs 0% in those with a recurrent bulbar stricture *(26)*. The success rate was 75% for primary and 45% for secondary treatment *(63)*. However, several studies found that previous stricture treatment had no effect on the risk of recurrence *(1,2,13,17,86,87)*.

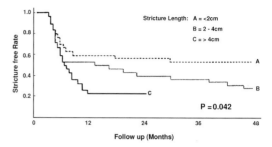

FIG. 7.8. Association between stricture length and stricture recurrence after dilation or urethrotomy *(1)*

12.5. Periurethral Scarring

Several studies have shown that the risk of recurrence was greater for strictures with significant periurethral scarring *(1,4,11,17,36,83,86,87)*.

12.6. Length of the Stricture

Many studies did not report the stricture length, possibly because it is difficult to measure accurately and reliably. The reported stricture length has varied considerably, for example a median length of 1.6 cm (range, 1 to 6.5 cm) in one study *(26)* and a mean length of 2.4 cm (range, 0.5 to 10 cm) in another *(1)*. Many studies have found that the recurrence rate is lower with short strictures and higher with long strictures *(4,6,11,13,25,26,64,83)*. A few studies reported no correlation between the stricture length and the risk of recurrence *(2,82)*.

Examples of the reported differences are: short strictures (<5 mm) had an 85% success rate at 2 yr *(13)*; the cure rate was 55% in short strictures <5 mm and 39% in those >10 mm in length *(22)*; the recurrence rate was 28% for strictures less than 1 cm compared with 51% for longer strictures *(25)*; the success rate was 71% for strictures shorter than 10 mm and 18% for longer strictures *(26)*; the success rate was 80% at 12 months for strictures shorter than 1 cm *(63)*. In pediatric cases the recurrence rate for strictures less than 1 cm was 7% and for long strictures it was 50% *(80)*.

Steenkamp and associates *(1)* reported that the recurrence rate at 12 mo was approximately 40% for strictures shorter than 2 cm and 80% for those longer than 4 cm. For strictures 2–4 cm in length, the recurrence rate increased from

approximately 50% at 12 months to 75% at 48 mo. For each 1 cm increase in the length of the stricture the risk of recurrence was increased by 1.22 (95% confidence interval 1.05 to 1.43) **(Fig. 7.8)** *(1)*.

12.7. Caliber or Diameter of the Stricture

Very few studies have reported on the stricture diameter, which may be due to the inherent difficulties of estimating the caliber *(10)*. One study found that the success rate was 69% for strictures more than 15F in caliber and 34% for those less than 15F *(26)*. Mandhani and associates *(77)* found that the percentage narrowing of the bulbar urethral lumen at the stricture site (as measured by retrograde urethrography) was a useful predictor of DVIU outcome. Mean percentage narrowing was significantly greater with treatment failure (70% versus 49%). A cutoff of 74% for urethral narrowing predicted the outcome with 78% probability.

12.8. Site of the Stricture

Several studies reported a lower recurrence rate in bulbar compared with penile strictures, which may be explained by better vascularization of the proximal urethra *(11,13,25,26,63,64)*. One study found a marginal statistical significance with a higher recurrence rate of penile strictures *(1)*. Another study reported that penile strictures recurring after DVIU were significantly longer than those not recurring: 3.9 vs 1.5 cm *(79)*. In contrast, one study found that strictures in the bulbar region recurred more commonly *(17)*. A few studies found no relationship between stricture location and the risk of recurrence *(2,80)*.

12.9. Number of Strictures

Several studies found that the recurrence rate is lower with single compared with multiple strictures *(6,11,25,26,64)*. Examples of the difference are: the recurrence rate was 28% for single strictures compared with 51% for multiple strictures *(25)*; the success rate was 50% in single versus 16% in multiple strictures *(26)*; the success rate was 60% to 70% with a single stricture versus 35% to 50% for cases with multiple strictures *(63)*. However, a few studies found no correlation between the number of strictures and the risk of recurrence *(1,17,80)*.

12.10. Instrument Used, Number, and Location of Incisions

Two studies in children found no relationship between these factors and the risk of recurrence *(31,80)*.

12.11. Complications During the Procedure

One study found a marginal statistical significance for the higher recurrence rate in patients where complications occurred during the procedure *(1)*.

12.12. Perioperative Infection

Several studies have reported a higher recurrence rate with perioperative infection, especially if it was untreated *(1,13,17,86,87)*. However, a few studies found no relationship between infection and the risk of recurrence *(22,26)*.

12.13. Type of Catheter Used

There appears to be no relationship between the type of catheter used and the risk of recurrence, possibly because most recent studies have used silicone catheters *(13)*.

12.14. Duration of Catheterization

Some studies showed that the risk of recurrence was increased if postoperative catheter drainage was longer than 3 d *(13,25)*. However, other studies showed no relationship *(22,31,80)*.

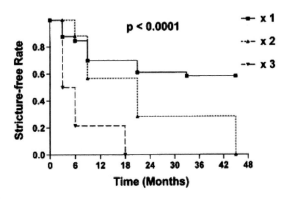

FIG. 7.9. Kaplan-Meier estimate of stricture-free rate after 1, 2 or 3 times repeated dilation or internal urethrotomy (regardless of stricture treatment before randomization) *(1)*

12.15. Length of Follow-Up

There is a clear correlation between the duration of follow-up and the risk of recurrence, with most recurrences occurring within 6 to 12 mo after DVIU *(13,63)*. In pediatric patients the length of follow-up was the most important risk factor for recurrence: 19% at 6 mo and 65% after 4 yr *(80)*.

12.16. Repeated Treatment

Pansadoro and Emiliozzi *(26)* commented that repeated DVIU did not improve the success rate, and that a third urethrotomy failed in all patients. In a prospective, randomized study, Heyns and associates *(11)* found that after a single dilation or DVIU not followed by re-stricturing at 3 mo, the Kaplan-Meier estimated stricture-free rate was 55% to 60% at 24 mo, and 50% to 60% at 48 mo (**Fig. 7.9**). After a second dilation or DVIU for stricture recurrence at 3 mo, the stricture-free rate was 30% to 50% at 24 mo and 0 to 40% at 48 mo. After a third dilation or DVIU for stricture recurrence, at 3 and 6 mo, the stricture-free rate at 24 mo was 0.

13. Prevention of Recurrence

13.1. TUR of Fibrous Callus

Giannakopoulos and associates *(63)* randomized 80 patients with single, short, iatrogenic, bulbar strictures to group A, 40 patients who underwent

DVIU with a cold-knife incision at the 12-o'clock position and group B, 40 patients who underwent cold-knife incisions at the 11- and 1-o'clock positions, followed by TUR of all scar tissues (Guillemin's technique). Group A obtained good results in 95%, 85%, 55%, 45% and 25% at 6, 12, 24, 36, and 60 mo, respectively; group B obtained good results in 98%, 95%, 90%, 80%, and 70% at 6, 12, 24, 36, and 60 mo, respectively. The differences between the two groups were statistically significant after 24 mo. In the literature Guillemin's technique has been reported with good 5-yr results of between 75% and 80% (63). TUR of the fibrous callus reduced recurrence from 75% to 30% after 5 years of follow-up (64).

13.2. Hydraulic Self-Dilation

Hydraulic self-dilation is performed by the patient, who compresses the urethra intermittently during micturition so that dilation of the whole urethra occurs. Some authors have advocated using this for 3 to 6 mo, beginning 15 d after DVIU (4,13,17,26). Hjortrup and associates (2) did not recommend hydraulic self-dilation after Otis IU, because they believe that extravasation of infected urine could lead to recurrent stricture.

13.3. Clean Intermittent Self-Catheterization

Several open, uncontrolled studies using clean intermittent self-catheterization (CISC) after DVIU (twice weekly for 1 mo, then once weekly, or once daily for 1 wk, then once weekly or once monthly) reported no stricture recurrence in patients who continued performing CISC for 6 to 8.5 months (24,88–90). Bødker and associates randomized 28 men to DVIU and CISC for 3 mo (treatment group) and 33 to DVIU only (observation group). CISC was performed by the patient twice weekly for 1 mo and then once weekly for the next 2 mo after the DVIU using a 16F or 18F catheter with Nélaton point, which was left in for 5 min. Treatment results were not significantly different, with new stricture occurring in 78% and 82%, respectively, at 4 mo. The authors concluded that CISC after DVIU should

be continued for a long duration, possibly permanently (24).

In a controlled study CISC was superior to no adjuvant treatment (91). Harriss et al. (92) reported an approximately 14% recurrence rate in patients who performed CISC for longer than 12 mo compared with 40% in those with only 6 months of catheterization. In a nonrandomized study CISC twice a month for a mean of 17 months gave a 12% recurrence rate, compared with 27% for the entire study group, but the minor complication rate (mainly bleeding) was 50% (25). In one study, 9% of patients discontinued CISC after DVIU because of urethral hemorrhage (24).

After CTU and resection of scar tissue, the patient can be taught self-dilation using a balloon dilator with gradually decreasing frequency for the next few months (50). CISC has not been reported to be significantly beneficial in long, follow-up randomized studies because the recurrence rate approximates that of the control group after termination of catheterization (64). The long-term result of CISC was not significantly different from that of DVIU alone, with a 78% and 82% recurrence rate following the two methods (24,56).

13.4. Clinic Dilation

Tunc and associates randomized men with bulbomembranous urethral strictures shorter than 2 cm recurring after DVIU to observation alone, or urethral dilation with Béniqué dilators (maximal 21F) beginning 10 d after DVIU, weekly for 1 mo, once after 3 and 6 mo, then once a year. Stricture recurred within 12 mo in 56% in the observation group and in 11% in the dilation group (64). This confirms the efficacy of the "dilation clinics" which were quite common in former years, but adopting this form of management has significant logistical and cost implications. It is basically the same as CISC, except that the patients themselves do not manage the dilation (24).

Gnanaraj and associates (93) reported a nonrandomized study of 78 patients who performed regular intermittent self-catheterization and 49 who underwent regular outpatient dilation after DVIU. Patients on self-calibration had slightly narrower strictures (4.8 vs 5.7F) but there was no significant difference in stricture length (1.5 vs 1.7 cm) and duration of follow-up (22 vs 24 months). Self calibration resulted in a lower restricture rate (5%) compared with regular urethral dilation (16%). Self-dilation with a stainless steel chopstick has been described *(94)*.

13.5. Steroids

Sachse claimed good results with longer strictures by using weekly intrauretrhal installations of steroid jelly, kept in place by a specially designed ribbon, which is wrapped around the glans penis *(4)*. In a recent study, triamcinolone was instilled intraurethrally after removal of the catheter in all patients after YAG laser DVIU *(47)*.

13.6. Halofuginone

Halofuginone, an oral inhibitor of type I collagen synthesis, has been investigated in animals and has shown promising results for decreasing scar formation after urethrotomy. In an experimental study with rabbits, a diet containing oral halofuginone (which has antifibrotic effects) was effective in limiting the occurrence of de novo and recurrent urethral stricture after DVIU. The authors suggested that the effect of halofuginone to prevent stricture recurrence should be tested in humans *(101)*.

13.7. Botulinum Toxin

Khera et al. *(92)* recently did a small pilot study of three patients that underwent urethrotomy and scar injection by botulinum toxin type A (Botox) and found that two of the three had substantially decreased scar reformation. Botox has been used in cosmetic surgery to decrease scar appearance for facial wounds effectively, by blocking vesicle transport of acetylcholine, reducing underlying muscle tension, and thus decreasing scar formation.

13.8. Mitomycin-C

MMC inhibits fibroblast proliferation and is effective in preventing scar formation. In an experimental rat model intra-urethral irrigation with low

dose MMC appeared to be effective in preventing fibrosis after DVIU *(102)*.

13.9. Brachytherapy

Endourethral brachytherapy has been reported as a safe method that can reduce urethral restricture *(103)*. Intraurethral brachytherapy with 192-iridium in 17 patients with recurrent urethral stricture after DVIU or TUR of scar showed a restricture rate of 7% at a mean follow-up of 20 mo *(104)*. Endourethral brachytherapy in patients with recurrent bulbar strictures (n = 9), bladder neck stenosis after TURP (n = 3), anastomotic stricture after radical prostatectomy (n = 2), or penile urethral stricture (n = 1) showed a recurrence free rate of 46% at a median follow-up 22 mo, whereas in 40%, the treatment was considered to be unsuccessful. Prospective randomized studies are required to assess the efficacy of this technique *(105)*.

14. Indications for Dilation or DVIU

Successful treatment depends more on appropriate case selection than on the technicalities of any particular procedure. Koraitim has pointed out that DVIU and the various types of urethroplasty should be regarded not as competing modalities, but as different complementary techniques available for the cure of different types of strictures, each with its own indications and limitations *(54,83)*.

It has been suggested that DVIU is being used excessively and inappropriately because of its simplicity and ease of repetition, and because there is a lack of familiarity with major urethral reconstruction techniques *(79,109)*. It is important to emphasize that optimal treatment requires appropriate case selection. Although urethroplasty for a urethral stricture is technically much more difficult than an endoscopic procedure, this should not be an excuse for performing an unsuitable procedure rather than referring the patient to someone who is proficient in urethroplasty *(98–104)*.

The advantages of dilation and DVIU are that they can be performed under local anesthesia in an outpatient setting (with obvious cost reduction compared to urethroplasty), they have a low complication rate and virtually no risk of mortality, so they are attractive options in elderly patients who are unfit for anesthesia and open urethroplasty *(13,22,29,30)*.

Because dilation does not require special endoscopic equipment or operating room facilities, and the results are equivalent to those of DVIU, dilation is the procedure of choice where the instrumentation, theatre facilities and technical skills required for DVIU are not available. The optimal indications for dilation should be the same as those for DVIU *(1)*.

The ideal indications for DVIU are strictures shorter than 2 cm, with no inflammatory changes, and no previous dilation or DVIU *(1,4)*. DVIU is an alternative to urethroplasty in patients with high comorbidity who are not suitable for open reconstruction *(47)*. In patients with stricture recurrence after previous perineal or transpubic urethroplasty for posterior strictures, DVIU as a complementary treatment may achieve good results in 60% to 80% of cases *(23)*.

DVIU for posterior urethral strictures after pelvic fracture injury is indicated only if the stricture is limited in length, circumference and depth, but not if there is a dense stricture extending into the periurethral tissues or involving the entire circumference *(2,110)*.

If an anastomotic stricture after radical prostatectomy is immature (presenting within 8 weeks) the procedure of choice may be to perform filiform and follower dilation with placement of an indwelling urethral catheter for 48 to 72 h, and subsequent optical DVIU 2 to 6 wk later. In patients who present with mature anastomotic strictures, most can be treated successfully with 1 endoscopic incision *(18,32)*.

A second DVIU or dilation for early stricture recurrence (at 3 mo) is of limited value in the short term (24 mo) but of no value in the long term (48 mo), whereas a third repeated dilation or urethrotomy is of no value *(11)*. Some authors state that in children a second urethrotomy may provide long-term cure in 71% *(80)*, whereas others feel that if the child fails the initial DVIU, repeat attempts at endoscopic correction should be abandoned in favor of definitive urethroplasty *(31)*. Specific contraindications to DVIU include suspicion of urethral carcinoma, bleeding diathesis, and active infection, that is, cystitis, urethritis or periurethral abscess *(12)*.

Editorial Comment

It is difficult to make any meaningful additional comments after such a comprehensive and well-written chapter as this one by Chris Heyns. Instead, we will make more of a summary statement. Internal urethrotomy encompasses all methods of transurethral incision or ablation to open a stricture. Direct visual urethrotomy by cold knife (after Sachse), with a deep cut at the 12-o'clock position (generally to 22 F) is the traditional method. We prefer not to make deep cuts, but rather multiple small radial incisions, circumferentially, to open up the mucosal scar, without cutting too deep into the corpus spongiosum, which has the potential to bleed profusely (**Table 7.1**). In our recent nationwide survey of U.S. urologists, only 12.1% use the radial cut technique, which suggests that this technique is used by the some "experts" but is not community practice *(105)*.

When available, we prefer to use a pediatric urethrotome for the urethrotomy. As scar revision surgery, the goal of urethrotomy is to have the epithelium regrow before the spongiosal scar recurs; in this way the scar still recurs but creates a larger caliber and diameter lumen/ stricture. Successive urethrotomies or dilations are merely palliative and not curative. Furthermore, single or primary strictures, bulbar location, length <1 cm, and wide caliber are positive predictive factors to long-term urethrotomy success.

Minimally invasive methods for managing urethral strictures, either by urethrotomy or dilation, are commonly performed procedures among U.S. urologists. Because results are not durable, many urologists use adjunctive procedures such as laser urethrotomy or urethral stenting. In contrast, open urethroplasty is not commonly performed despite better long term results.

TABLE 7.1. Urethrotomy technique by U.S. Urologists (From Ref. *[5]*).

Urethrotomy method	Frequency	Percentage
12-o'clock cut	372	86.3
Radial cuts	52	12.1
No response	7	1.6
Total	431	100

Endoscopic methods are thus overly common. Urethral dilation and direct vision urethrotomy with cold knife are popular management techniques for anterior urethral stricture, mainly due to the perception that they are simple procedures that cause little morbidity. Complications can occur, however, in up to 27%.

Another potential reason for urethrotomy popularity is that few urologists have continuing experience with urethroplasty surgery. In our recent nationwide survey of practicing members of the AUA, 60% of urologists surveyed did not perform any urethroplasties in the prior year, and only 0.9% performed >11 urethroplasties in that same year. Most (two-thirds) also believed that the literature supports that urethroplasty should be performed only after repeated failure of urethrotomies or dilations. This adherence to a treatment philosophy of a "reconstructive ladder" where there is a progression from simple to complex surgeries only after successive failures is clearly not supported by the published literature. Also evidenced by our survey, urethral dilation and optical internal urethrotomy are common procedures, performed with periodic frequency by most U.S. urologists, at 93% and 86%, respectively. Other contemporary series have found minimally invasive treatments of stricture to be common in the States, as well as South Africa, and Italy.

For refractory and recurrent strictures, Heyns has nicely summarized and referenced studies herein that show that repeating urethrotomy and dilation is futile, and such patients are usually better served by urethroplasty. However, 81% of surveyed U.S. urologists perform repeat and serial office dilation and approximately 50% recommend either patient self-dilation or patient self-catheterization. This disparity between the literature and common practice appears attributable to a lack of education and surgical experience. The best and most durable results with urethrotomy are for short bulbar strictures, in particular, those less than 1 cm. However, only one in four practicing urologists uses 1 cm as a cut-off to decide on open urethroplasty. What appears to be the U.S. community standard is a cut-off of 2 cm when deciding on a minimally invasive method, with 50% of practicing Urologists using a cut-off >2 cm (**Table 7.2**).

Duration of catheterization after endoscopic incision is variable in prior reports, ranging from 24 h to 6 wk. From our survey, common practice is 1 wk (36%), followed closely by 24 h (35%) and 2 to 5 d (a distant third at 15%; **Table 7.3**). Clearly, duration of catheterization is important to epithelization, as well as helps prevent urinary retention and corpus spongiosum fibrosis (from urine extravasation). Extrapolating from dog experiments on the ureter by Hinman, the urethral epithelium should regenerate and cover the urethrotomy site within one week. Thus, the community practice of leaving an indwelling catheter for one week seems sound. The other issue is if injection of biological modifiers into the stricture sites after urethrotomy improves overall success. Clearly, surveyed U.S. urologists do not believe it does, with only 8% injecting steroids into the urethra. There have been small reports of the use of injecting steroids, interferon, collagenase and more recently botulinum toxin type A (Botox) into the urethra. Such studies are small, not randomized, and not prospective, so few conclusions can be made. Clearly, biological modifiers have been shown to be effective with cutaneous scars after burns. However,

TABLE 7.2. Maximal bulbar urethral stricture length managed by urethrotomy by U.S. Urologists. (From Ref. [97])

Urethral stricture length treated	Frequency	Percentage
<1 cm	99	23
<1.5 cm	91	21.1
<2.0 cm	106	24.6
<2.5 cm	34	7.9
<3.0 cm	67	15.5
>3 cm	13	3
Total	431	100

With permission from Bullock TL, Brandes SB: J Urol 2007,177:685–690.

TABLE 7.3. Time interval from urethrotomy to Foley catheter removal by U.S. Urologists. (From Ref. [97])

Time Foley in place after OIU	Frequency	Percentage
No Foley	7	1.6
24 h	152	35.3
2–5 d	64	14.8
1 wk	157	36.4
2 wk	28	6.5
3 wk	8	1.9
No response	15	3.5
Total	431	100

it remains to be seen if such modifiers improve urethrotomy results.—S.B. Brandes

References

1. Steenkamp JW, Heyns CF, De Kock ML (1997)
Internal urethrotomy versus dilation as treatment for
male urethral strictures: A prospective, randomized
comparison. J Urol 157:98–101
2. Hjortrup A, Sorensen C, Sanders S, Moesgaard F,
Kirkegaard P (1983) Strictures of the male urethra
treated by the Otis method. J Urol 130:903–904
3. Schultheiss D, Truss MC, Jonas U. (1999) History of
direct vision internal urethrotomy. Urology 52:729–
734. Erratum in: Urology 53:456
4. Lipsky H, Hubmer G. (1977) Direct vision urethrotomy in the management of urethral strictures. Br J
Urol 49:725–728
5. Keitzer WA, Cervantes L, Demaculangan A, Cruz B
(1961) Transurethral incision of bladder neck for
contracture. J Urol 86:242–246
6. Sandozi S, Ghazali S. (1988) Sachse optical urethrotomy, a modified technique: 6 years of experience.
J Urol 140:968–969
7. Blandy JP (1976) Urethral stricture and carcinoma.
In: Blandy J, ed. Urology, 1st ed, vol 2. Blackwell,
Oxford, pp 1014–1048
8. Carter HB (2002) Basic instrumentation and cystoscopy. In: Walsh PC, Retik AB, Darracott Vaughan E,
Wein AJ (eds) Campbell's Urology. 8th ed, vol 2.
Saunders, Philadelphia, pp 114–116
9. Jordan GH, Schlossberg SM (2002) Surgery of
the penis and urethra. In: Walsh PC, Retik AB,
Darracott Vaughan E, Wein AJ (eds) Campbell's
Urology. 8th ed, vol 4. Saunders, Philadelphia, pp
3919–3923
10. Stormont TJ, Suman VJ, Oesterling JE (1993) Newly
diagnosed bulbar urethral strictures: etiology and outcome of various treatments. J Urol 150:1725–1728
11. Heyns CF, Steenkamp JW, De Kock ML, Whitaker P
(1998) Treatment of male urethral strictures: is
repeated dilation or internal urethrotomy useful?
J Urol 160 356–358
12. Kinder PW, Rous SN (1979) The treatment of urethral stricture disease by internal urethrotomy: a
clinical review. J Urol 121:45–46
13. Boccon-Gibod L, Le Portz B (1982) Endoscopic
urethrotomy: does it live up to its promises? J Urol
127:433–435
14. Emmett JL, Rous SN, Greene LF, De Weerd JH, Utz
DC (1963) Preliminary internal urethrotomy in 1036
cases to prevent urethral stricture following transurethral resection; caliber of normal adult male urethra.
J Urol 89(6), 829–835
15. Schultz A, Bay-Nielsen H, Bilde T, Christiansen L,
Mikkelsen AM, Steven K (1989) Prevention of
urethral stricture formation after transurethral resection of the prostate: a controlled randomized study
of Otis urethrotomy versus urethral dilation and the
use of the polytetrafluoroethylene coated versus the
uninsulated metal sheath. J Urol 141:73–75
16. Bailey MJ, Shearer RJ (1979) The role of internal
urethrotomy in the prevention of urethral stricture
following transurethral resection of the prostate. Br J
Urol 51:28–31
17. Pain JA, Collier DG (1984) Factors influencing
recurrence of urethral strictures after endoscopic
urethrotomy: The role of infection and peri-operative
antibiotics. Br J Urol 56:217–219
18. Yurkanin JP, Dalkin BL, Cui H (2001) Evaluation of
cold knife urethrotomy for treatment of anastomotic
stricture after radical retropubic prostatectomy. J
Urol 165:1545–1548
19. Al-Ali M, Al-Shukry M (1997) Endoscopic repair
in 154 cases of urethral occlusion: the promise
of guided optical urethral reconstruction. J Urol
157:129–131
20. Gupta NP, Gill IS (1986) Core-through optical
internal urethrotomy in management of impassable traumatic posterior urethral strictures. J Urol
136:1018–1021
21. Matsuoka K, Inoue M, Iida S, Tomiyasu K, Noda
S (2002) Endoscopic antegrade laser incision in the
treatment of urethral stricture. Urology 60:968–72
22. Holm-Nielsen A, Schultz A, Moller-Pedersen V
(1984) Direct vision internal urethrotomy. A critical
review of 365 operations. Br J Urol 56:308–312
23. Netto NR Jr, Lemos GC, Claro JFA (1989) Internal
urethrotomy as a complementary method after urethroplasties for posterior urethral stenosis. J Urol
141:50–51
24. Bødker A, Ostri P, Rye-Andersen J, Edvardsen L,
Struckmann J (1992) Treatment of recurrent urethral
stricture by internal urethrotomy and intermittent
self-catheterization: a controlled study of a new
therapy. J Urol 148:308–310
25. Albers P, Fichtner J, Brühl P, Müller SC (1996)
Long-term results of internal urethrotomy. J Urol
156:1611–1614
26. Pansadoro V, Emiliozzi P (1996) Internal urethrotomy in the management of anterior urethral strictures: Long-term followup. J Urol 156:73–75
27. Chiou RK. (1999) Re: Treatment of male urethral
strictures: Is repeated dilation or internal urethrotomy useful? J Urol 161:1583
28. Djulepa J, Potempa J. (1983) Urethrotomy technique in urethral strictures: 6-year results. J Urol
129:955–957

29. Kreder KJ, Stack R, Thrasher JB, Donatucci CF (1993) Direct vision internal urethrotomy using topical anesthesia. Urology 42:548–550

30. Ye G, Rong-Gui Z (2002) Optical urethrotomy for anterior urethral stricture under a new local anesthesia: intracorpus spongiosum anesthesia. Urology 60:245–247

31. Hsiao KC, Baez-Trinidad L, Lendvay T, Smith EA, Broecker B, Scherz H, Kirsch AJ (2003) Direct vision internal urethrotomy for the treatment of pediatric urethral strictures: analysis of 50 patients. J Urol 170:952–955

32. Dalkin BL. (1996) Endoscopic evaluation and treatment of anastomotic strictures after radical retropubic prostatectomy. J Urol 155:206–208

33. Carr LK, Webster GD. (1996) Endoscopic management of the obliterated anastomosis following radical prostatectomy. J Urol 156:70–72

34. Vaidyanathan S, Hughes PL, Singh G, Soni BM, Watt JW, Darroch J, Oo T. (2005) Location of urethral arteries by colour Doppler ultrasound. Spinal Cord 43:130–132

35. McAninch JW, Laing FC, Jeffrey RB Jr. (1988) Sonourethrography in the evaluation of urethral strictures: A preliminary report. J Urol 139:294–297

36. Merkle W, Wagner W. (1988) Sonography of the distal male urethra – a new diagnostic procedure for urethral strictures: Results of a retrospective study. J Urol 140:1409–1411

37. Kishore TA, Bhat S, John RP (2005) Colour Doppler ultrasonographic location of the bulbourethral artery, and its impact on surgical outcome. BJU Int 96:624–628

38. Geavlete P, Cauni V, Georgescu D. (2005) Value of preoperative urethral ultrasound in optic internal urethrotomy. Eur Urol 47:865–871

39. Turek PJ, Cendron M, Malloy TR, Carpiniello VL, Wein AJ (1992) KTP-532 laser ablation of urethral strictures. Urology 40:330–334

40. Becker HC, Miller J, Noske HD, Klask JP, Weidner W (1995) Transurethral Laser urethrotomy with Argon-Laser—experience with 900 urethrotomies in 450 patients from 1978 to 1993. Urol Int 55:150–153

41. Kamal BA (2001) The use of the diode laser for treating urethral strictures. BJU Int 87:831–833

42. Gurdal M, Tekin A, Yucebas E, Kirecci S, Sengor F (2003) Contact neodymium: YAG laser ablation of recurrent urethral strictures using a side-firing fiber. J Endourol 17:791–794

43. Futao S, Wentong Z, Yan Z, Qingyu D, Aiwu L (2006) Application of endoscopic Ho:YAG laser incision technique treating urethral strictures and urethral atresias in pediatric patients. Pediatr Surg Int 22:514–518

44. Naudé AM, Heyns CF (2005) What is the place of internal urethrotomy in the treatment of urethral stricture disease? Nat Clin Pract Urol 2:538–545

45. Hayashi T, Yoshinaga A, Ohno R, Ishii N, Watanabe T, Yamada T, Kihara K (2005) Successful treatment of recurrent vesicourethral stricture after radical prostatectomy with holmium laser: Report of three cases. Int J Urol 12:414–416

46. Hossain AZ, Khan SA, Hossain S, Salam MA. (2004) Holmium laser urethrotomy for urethral stricture. Bangladesh Med Res Counc Bull 30:78–80

47. Kamp S, Knoll T, Osman MM, Kohrmann KU, Michel MS, Alken P (2006) Low-power holmium: YAG laser urethrotomy for treatment of urethral strictures: Functional outcome and quality of life. J Endourol 20:38–41

48. Gonzalez R, Chiou RK, Hekmat K, Fraley EE. (1983) Endoscopic re-establishment of urethral continuity after traumatic disruption of the membranous urethra. J Urol 130:785–787

49. Chiou RK, Gonzalez R (1985) Endoscopic treatment of complete urethral obstruction using thin trocar. Urology 24:475–478

50. Quint HJ, Stanisic TH (1993) Above and below delayed endoscopic treatment of traumatic posterior urethral disruptions. J Urol 149:484–487

51. Yilmaz U, Gunes A, Soylu A, Balbay MD (2001) Evrim Bougie: a new instrument in the management of urethral strictures. BMC Urol 1:1

52. Chuang C-K, Lai M-K, Chu S-H. (1994) Optic internal urethrotomy under transrectal ultrasonographic guide and suprapubic fiberoscopic aid. J Urol 152:1435–1437

53. Dogra PN, Ansari MS, Gupta NP, Tandon S (2004) Holmium laser core-through urethrotomy for traumatic obliterative strictures of urethra: initial experience. Urology 64:232–236

54. Koraitim MM (2004) Post-traumatic posterior urethral strictures: Preoperative decision making. Urology 64:228–231

55. Kohrmann KU, Henkel TO, Schmidt P, Rassweiler J (1994) Antegrade-retrograde urethrotomy for treatment of severe strictures of the urethra—experience and literature review J Endourol 8:433–438

56. El-Abd SA (1995) Endoscopic treatment of posttraumatic urethral obliteration: Experience in 396 patients. J Urol 153:67–71

57. Dogra PN, Nabi G (2003) Nd-YAG laser core-through urethrotomy in obliterative posttraumatic urethral strictures in children. Pediatr Surg Int 19:652–655

58. Levine J, Wessells H (2001) Comparison of open and endoscopic treatment of posttraumatic posterior urethral strictures. World J Surg 25:1597–1601

59. Pettersson BA, Asklin B, Bratt C (1978) Endourethral urethroplasty: a simple method of treatment of urethral strictures by internal urethrotomy and primary split skin grafting. Br J Urol 50:257–261

60. Naudé JH (1998) Endoscopic skin-graft urethroplasty. World J Urol 16:171–174

61. Chiou RK (1988) Endourethroplasty in the management of complicated posterior urethral stricture. J Urol 140:607–610

62. Le Roux PJ (2005) Endoscopic urethroplasty with unseeded small intestinal submucosa collagen matrix grafts: A pilot study. J Urol 173:140–143

63. Giannakopoulos X, Grammeniatis E, Gartzios A, Tsoumanis P, Kammenos A. (1997) Sachse urethrotomy versus endoscopic urethrotomy plus transurethral resection of the fibrous callus (Guillemin's technique) in the treatment of urethral stricture. Urology 49:243–247

64. Tunc M, Tefekli A, Kadioglu A, Esen T, Uluocak N, Aras N (2002) A prospective, randomized protocol to examine the efficacy of postinternal urethrotomy dilations for recurrent bulbomembranous urethral strictures. Urology 60:239–244

65. Heyns CF, Marais DC (2002) Prospective evaluation of the American Urological Association symptom index and peak urinary flow rate for the followup of men with known urethral stricture disease. J Urol 168:2051–2054

66. Sachse H. (1974) Zur Behandlung der Harnröhrenstriktur: die transurethrale Schlitzung unter Sicht mit shcarfen Schnitt [On the treatment of urethral stricture: transurethral incision under vision using sharp section] [Article in German]. Fortschr Med 92:12–15

67. Hammarsten J, Lindqvist K, Sunzel H. (1989) Urethral strictures following transurethral resection of the prostate. The role of the catheter. Br J Urol 63:397–400

68. Carlton FE, Scardino PL, Quattlebaum RB (1974) Treatment of urethral strictures with internal urethrotomy and 6 weeks of silastic catheter drainage. J Urol 111:191–193

69. Iversen Hansen R, Guldberg O, Moller I (1981) Internal urethrotomy with the Sachse urethrotome. Scand J Urol Nephrol 15:189–191

70. Graversen PH, Rosenkilde P, Colstrup H (1991) Erectile dysfunction following direct vision internal urethrotomy. Scand J Urol Nephrol 25:175–178

71. Schneider T, Sperling H, Lummen G, Rubben H (2001) [Sachse internal urethrotomy. Is erectile dysfuction a possible complication?] [Article in German]. Urologe A 40:38–41

72. Chen GL, Berger RE (1997) Treatment of impotence resulting from internal urethrotomy. J Urol 158:542

73. Bapuraj JR, Sridhar S, Sharma SK, Suri S (1999) Endovascular treatment of a distal urethral-internal pudendal artery fistula complicating internal optical urethrotomy of a post-traumatic urethral stricture. BJU Int 83:353–354

74. Karagiannis AA, Sopilidis OT, Brountzos EN, Staios DN, Kelekis NL, Kelekis DA (2004) High flow priapism secondary to internal urethrotomy treated with embolization. J Urol 171:1631–1632

75. Chilton CP, Shah PJR, Fowler CG, Tiptaft RC, Blandy JP (1983) The impact of optical urethrotomy on the management of urethral strictures. Br J Urol 55:705–710

76. Greenwell TJ, Castle C, Andrich DE, MacDonald JT, Nicol DL, Mundy AR (2004) Repeat urethrotomy and dilation for the treatment of urethral stricture are neither clinically effective nor cost-effective. J Urol 172:275–277

77. Hafez AT, El Assmy A, Dawaba MS, Sarhan O (2005) Bazeed M. Long-term outcome of visual internal urethrotomy for the management of pediatric urethral strictures. J Urol 173:595–597

78. Duel BP, Barthold JS, Gonzalez R (1998) Management of urethral strictures after hypospadias repair. J Urol 160:170–171

79. Pitkämäki KK, Tammela TL, Kontturi MJ (1992) Recurrence of urethral stricture and late results after optical urethrotomy: Comparison of strictures caused by toxic latex catheters and other causes. Scand J Urol Nephrol 26:327–331

80. Koraitim M. (1985) Experience with 170 cases of posterior urethral strictures during 7 years. J Urol 133:408–410

81. Desmond AD, Evans CM, Jameson RM, Woolfenden KA, Gibbon NO (1981) Critical evaluation of direct vision urethrotomy by urine flow measurement. Br J Urol 53:630–633

82. Merkle W, Wagner W (1990) Risk of recurrent stricture following internal urethrotomy. Prospective ultrasound study of distal male urethra. Br J Urol 65:618–620

83. Mandhani A, Chaudhury H, Kapoor R, Srivastava A, Dubey D, Kumar A (2005) Can outcome of internal urethrotomy for short segment bulbar urethral stricture be predicted? J Urol 173:1595–1597

84. Lawrence WT, MacDonagh RP (1988) Treatment of urethral stricture disease by internal urethrotomy followed by intermittent "low-friction" self-catheterization: preliminary communication. J R Soc Med 81:136–139

85. Zambon JV, Delaere KPJ. (1990) Prevention of recurrent urethral strictures by intermittent low-friction self-catheterisation. Eur Urol 18(suppl 1):277, abstract 535

86. Newman LH, Stone NN, Chircus JH, Kramer HC. (1990) Recurrent urethral stricture disease managed by clean intermittent self-catheterization. J Urol 144:1142–1143

87. Kjaergaard B, Walter S, Bartholin J, Andersen JT, Nahr S, Beck H, Jensen BN, Lokdam A, Glavind K. (1994) Prevention of urethral stricture recurrence using clean intermittent self-catheterization. Br J Urol 73:692–695

88. Harriss DR, Beckingham IJ, Lemberger RJ, Lawrence WT (1994) Long-term results of intermittent low-friction self-catheterization in patients with recurrent urethral strictures. Br J Urol 74:790–792

89. Gnanaraj J, Devasia A, Gnanaraj L, Pandey AP (1999) Intermittent self catheterization versus regular outpatient dilatation in urethral stricture: A comparison. Aust N Z J Surg 69:41–43

90. Lin YH, Huang WJ, Chen KK. (2006) Using stainless steel chopstick for self-performing urethral sounding in preventing recurrence of anterior urethral stricture. J Chin Med Assoc 69:189–92

91. Jaidane M, Ali-El-Dein B, Ounaies A, Hafez AT, Mohsen T, Bazeed M (2003) The use of halofuginone in limiting urethral stricture formation and recurrence: an experimental study in rabbits. J Urol 170:2049–2052

92. Khera M, Boone TB, Smith CP (2004) Botulinum toxin type A: a novel approach to the treatment of recurrent urethral strictures. J Urol 172(2):574–575

93. Ayyildiz A, Nuhoglu B, Gulerkaya B, Caydere M, Ustun H, Germiyanoglu C, Erol D (2004) Effect of intraurethral Mitomycin-C on healing and fibrosis in rats with experimentally induced urethral stricture. Int J Urol 11:1122–1126

94. Olschewski T, Kropfl D, Seegenschmiedt MH (2003) Endourethral brachytherapy for prevention of recurrent urethral stricture following internal urethrotomy–first clinical experiences and results. Int J Radiat Oncol Biol Phys 57:1400–1404

95. Sun YH, Xu CL, Gao X, Jin YN, Wang LH, Liao GQ, Wang ZF, Hou JG, Qian SX, Yong-Jiang MA (2001) Intraurethral brachytherapy for prevention of recurrent urethral stricture after internal urethrotomy or transurethral resection of scar. J Endourol 15:859–861

96. Kropfl D, Olschewski T, Seegenschmiedt MH. (2004) [Endourethral brachytherapy for the prevention of recurrent strictures following internal urethrotomy.] [Article in German]. Urologe A 43:1254–61

97. Brandes SB, Smith J, Virgo K, Johnson FE (2001) Adult anterior urethral strictures: a national practice patterns survey. J Urol 165(suppl), abstract 53:13

98. Koraitim MM. (1995) The lessons of 145 post-traumatic posterior urethral strictures treated in 17 years. J Urol 153:63–66

99. Berger B, Sykes Z, Freedman M (1976) Patch graft urethroplasty for stricture disease. J Urol 115:681–684

100. De la Rosette JJ, de Vries JD, Lock MT,Debruyne FM (1991) Urethroplasty using the pedicled island flap technique in complicated urethral strictures. J Urol 146:40–42

101. Roehrborn CG, McConnell JD (1994) Analysis of factors contributing to success or failure of 1-stage urethroplasty for urethral stricture disease. J Urol 151:869–874

102. Martinez-Pineiro JA, Carcamo P, Garcia Matres MJ, Martinez-Pineiro L, Iglesias JR, Rodriguez Ledesma JM (1997) Excision and anastomotic repair for urethral stricture disease: experience with 150 cases. Eur Urol 32:433–441

103. Ziprin P, Wheeler J, Davies G, Stephenson TP (1996) The long-term follow-up of the urethroplasty for non-traumatic urethral strictures. J Urol 155:abstract 762:501A

104. Andrich DE, Dunglison N, Greenwell TJ, Mundy AR (2003) The long-term results of urethroplasty. J Urol 170:90–92

105. Bullock TL, Brandes SB (2000) Adult anterior urethral strictures: A national practice patterns survey of board certified urologists in the United States. J Urol 177:685–690

8
Endourethral Prostheses for Urethral Stricture

Daniel Yachia and Zeljko Markovic

Contents

1. Introduction.. 85
2. Urethral Stricture and Wound Healing.. 86
3. Stents in the Treatment of Recurrent Urethral Strictures.. 86
   3.1. Permanent Stents (Wallstent)... 87
   3.2. Temporary Stents... 89
   3.3. Limitations of Previous Generations of Permanent and Temporary Stents................ 91
   3.4. Allium Bulbar Urethral Stent 91
Editorial Comment... 93
References.. 94

Summary   The gold standard for treating a recurrent urethral stricture in a definitive way remains an open surgical urethroplasty. However, most urologists continue to manage their stricture patients with repeated dilation or urethrotomy, which are typically not curative methods. Since the introduction of urethral stents in the 1980s for the treatment of urethral strictures, two different methods to prevent scarring contraction have been introduced, namely permanent stents versus temporary stents that undergo a staged removal. Examples of permanent urethral stents are the UroLume Wallstent and Memotherm, while that of temporary stents are the UroCoil, Memokath, and Allium. Indications for stent placement are limited and typically for recurrent bulbar urethral strictures. Despite initial enthusiasm, with time, the results obtained with permanent urethral stents have been disappointing. Results with the newer temporary stents are encouraging.

Keywords   Wallstent, temporary urethral stents, Urocoil, Allium, Memokath, hybrid stents

1. Introduction

Urethral stricture is the result of scar tissue development after either traumatic or inflammatory injury of the urethra. Although not a life-threatening condition, the treatment of urethral stricture is one of the most challenging situations for the urologist and a very troublesome condition for the patient *(1,2)*. The treatment of this condition has one main aim: to allow the patient to void with a satisfactory stream and control. This aim can be achieved by creating a urethra with an adequate caliber either by dilation or endoscopic incision of the stricture or preferably by one of the many urethroplasty techniques developed for this purpose. Today, the gold standard for treating a recurrent urethral stricture in a definitive way is to perform an

From: *Current Clinical Urology: Urethral Reconstructive Surgery*
Edited by: S.B. Brandes © Humana Press, Totowa, NJ

urethroplasty. As described in other chapters of this book, if the stricture is short, urethroplasty is performed by excision and reanastomosis or, in longer strictures, by substitution urethroplasty, using tissues from other parts of the body such as skin, bladder or buccal mucosa. However, most urologists manage their stricture patients with repeated dilation or urethrotomy, which are less curative methods.

There is a great variation in reporting recurrence rates after urethral dilations and urethrotomies because of the poor classification of the treated strictures in the reports. Although a 50–60% success rates can be obtained with dilations or urethrotomy in short strictures without spongiofibrosis, in longer strictures and in strictures involving the corpus spongiosum, the recurrence rates is about 80% because of new stenotic scar development. Because of repeated dilations or urethrotomy, local inflammatory reaction can occur and result in more extensive strictures than the treated one.

Conventionally, after an endoscopic manipulation and sometimes after a urethral dilation, a urethral catheter is left indwelling for one or for several days to allow urine drainage during the edematous stage of the dilated urethra and to help in its remodeling. At the time the catheter is removed, the edema disappears, but the tissue-healing process continues to be active. The continuing tissue healing process makes the outcome of the treatment unpredictable which in many cases results in a recurrent stricture.

2. Urethral Stricture and Wound Healing

Wound healing is an integrated series of cellular, physiological, and biochemical events occurring in the tissues. There is a difference between wound repair (scarring) and tissue embryogenesis (tissue regeneration). All wounds seem to heal by the same basic process. However, there are some basic differences between the healing of an acute and a chronic injury wound and between a clean vs an infected wound. During the healing process of a clean wound and under normal conditions, there is equilibrium between collagen synthesis and collagen degradation. Repeated trauma and infection cause disequilibrium in this process. A change in the equilibrium of the healing process causes an increase in collagen synthesis and a decrease in its degradation, creating a

hypertrophic scar tissue development. During the healing process, after the appearance of inflammatory cells, fibroblasts and capillaries invade the fibrin clot to form a contractile granulation tissue. About a week after wounding, the wound clot becomes fully invaded and replaced by activated fibroblasts that are stimulated by growth factors to synthesize and remodel the new collagen-rich matrix (3). This granulation tissue draws the wound margins together, and the epithelial edges migrate forward to cover the wound surface. This is made easier by the underlying contractile connective tissue, which shrinks to bring the wound margins towards one another. In undisturbed tissue healing, programmed cell death occurs in some of the wound fibroblasts, probably the myofibroblasts, after wound contraction has ceased (4), marking the stabilization of the scarring process. The healing of an urethra injured during dilation or urethrotomy also develops under similar conditions as with other injured tissues. Although an incised or dilated urethra may appear to be healed within a few weeks, having a complete epithelial coverage, in most cases the stricture will recur because of the ongoing wound healing/scarring process in the deeper layers of the urethra that continues for several months. In urethral stricture this process results in stricture recurrence. As in other cylindrical organs, when happening in the urethra, this scar usually involves the entire circumference of the injured segment causing the recurrence of the circumferential stricture.

As detailed in Chapter 30 in of this volume by Atala, attempts are being made to stimulate the regeneration of tissues. Some success has been achieved by bridging lesions with artificial or natural biomaterial 'scaffolds' for promoting migration, proliferation and differentiation of cells (5). Until tissue-regenerative technologies become widely available, urethral stents are being used and continually modified as a minimally invasive treatment approach to recurrent urethral strictures.

3. Stents in the Treatment of Recurrent Urethral Strictures

As explained previously, all wounds heal almost by the same basic process. A chronic wound in the urethra usually fails to heal primarily, as would an acute wound. Healing of a chronic wound is unpredictable. A chronic wound heals up to a point and then the healing process turns toward contraction. Attempts to predict this course and to change the direction of the process with pharmaceutical means, such as local injections with biological modifiers, like steroids, is typically ineffective. However, trials to prevent contraction of the wound by mechanical interference showed very encouraging results, especially in urethral strictures. The idea behind the use of large-caliber metallic stents for preventing urethral stricture recurrence is based on mechanical interference to prevent the scarring process from ending in contraction. Since the introduction of stents in the late 1980s for the treatment of urethral strictures, two different concepts have been studied to prevent the scarring contraction, namely stents for permanent implantation versus stents temporarily left indwelling for limited periods of time and then removed.

3.1. Permanent Stents (Wallstent)

The era of self-expanding stents in medicine started with the introduction of the braided Wallstent for vascular disease, as developed by Hans Wallsten (**Fig. 8.1**). This stent became the widely rec-

ognized and used in many medical disciplines, including urology. The design of this stent was based on a wire braiding technology similar to the the "Chinese finger trap"; an old Chinese trick in which one can insert a finger that is trapped when the finger is retracted. This braiding technology is also used widely for the manufacturing of coaxial cables. The concept of using a permanently implanted stent to maintain the patency of a strictured bulbar urethra was first described by Milroy et al. in 1988 (*6*) Urological use was a natural extension of the concept of vascular stenting, where the stent becomes imbedded into the wall of the blood vessel and covered by endothelium. Vascular stents are about 1.2 times the blood vessel diameter to ensure its anchoring, without causing unnecessary pressure to the wall of the vessel. After its release, the entire mesh stent comes in contact with the vessel wall. The constant pressure that the stent struts apply to the wall causes traumatic damage to the endothelium. This damage induces a chain reaction in the tissue until the stent becomes covered with endothelium. In the urethra, these Wallstents were intended to push themselves into the urethral wall and remain permanently as a fixed reinforcement, akin to the reinforcing iron bars (Rebar) of concrete pipes, which help keep the lumen open. Milroy et al. (*6*) first described the use of the UroLume Wallstent (American Medical Systems, Minnetonka, MN) stent after dilating the urethra.

The Urolume Wallstent is made from a biocompatible nonmagnetic superalloy woven into a tubular mesh which is flexible and self-expanding to 42F. Soon after the Urolume Wallstent (**Fig. 8.1A**), another mesh stent (knitted) became available: the thermo-expandable Memotherm (C. R. Bard, Murray Hill, NJ; **Fig. 8.1B**). Both stents were deployed under vision with an endoscopic tool on which the stent comes loaded (**Fig. 8.2**). The large-caliber and the radial expansion force of the stents kept these stents in place until the stent pushes itself into the urethral wall and epithelialization completely buries it.

3.1.1. Urolume Wallstent: Clinical Outcome

Candidates for UroLume Wallstent or Memotherm stent placement are patients with a bulbar urethral

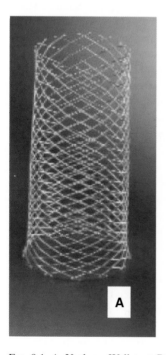
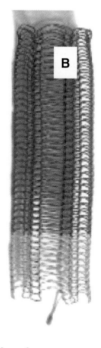

FIG. 8.1. A. Urolume Wallstent. B. Memotherm

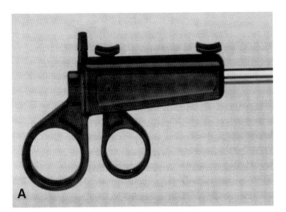

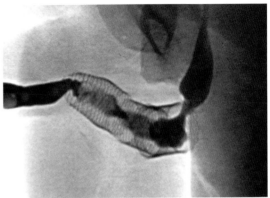

FIG. 8.3. Retrograde urethrogram showing restenosis by hypertrophic tissue within tandem placed Urolume stents in the bulbar urethra

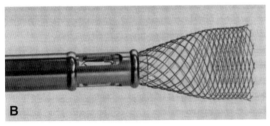

FIG. 8.2. A. The deployment tool for inserting the Urolume stent: B. The Urolume (wire mesh stent) attached to the end of the deployment device. (From Oesterling JE, Kletscher BA: Endourethral stents in urethral stricture management. In Traumatic and Reconstructive Urology, McAnincg JW (ed), WB Saunders, Philadelphia, 1996)

strictures less than 3 cm long and at least an interval of 10 mm of healthy urethra distal to the external sphincter. The stent should be at least 10 mm longer than the stricture, because 5 mm has to be added to each end of the estimated stricture length.

Researchers from The North American UroLume Trial (between March 1989 and April 1996) enrolled 179 patients with recurrent strictures in the bulbar urethra. Most of these patients had been treated for more than 5 years by dilatations or urethrotomies at least 5 times. The initial results of this study were very encouraging. In the short term, insertion of the UroLume stent decreased retreatment rates from 75.3% before insertion to 14.3% after insertion in 105 patients, who were followed for at least 1 year (7). No similar study with large number of patients was performed with the Memotherm. At the 2-year follow-up, narrowing of the Urolume stent lumen was noted in 74 of 179 (41.3%) patients. Narrowing was the result of urethral epithelium overgrowth through the interstices of the stent (**Fig. 8.3**). In 62 (83%) of these cases, the

narrowing was mild, whereas in 12 patients (16%) occlusion was severe enough to require adjunctive procedures, such as transurethral resection of the occluding tissues (7). Other short-term complications (7–28 d) were perineal discomfort (86%) and dribbling (14%). The long-term complications were painful erection (44%), mucous hyperplasia (44%), recurring stricture (29%), and incontinence (14%). Although long-term success of the Urolume stent is generally disappointing, there are some centers which reported higher success rates (8).

The incidence of hyperplastic tissue ingrowth and excessive intrastent tissue proliferation and subsequent urethral stenosis frequently occurred in patients with post-traumatic strictures (9,10). Thus, permanent stents are felt to be contraindicated in traumatic strictures. Furthermore, because of their shape and large caliber, the use of the Urolume Wallstent or other permanent stents are limited to the bulbar urethra. Their use in the mobile parts of the urethra (pendulous) is contraindicated because of the sharp ends of these stents can cause pain, injury or even perforate the urethra, as well as inhibit or preclude urethral extensibility for normal penile tumescence. The permanent stents also had a high failure rate in patients who underwent previous urethroplasty, in particular, prior substitution urethral surgery with skin. Such stents when placed in a prior urethroplasty bed could not become entirely incorporated or covered by urethral epithelium. Such bare wires of the stent were subsequently prone to stone formation, recurrent infection, urethritis and dysuria.

Despite initial optimism, with time, the results obtained with permanent urethral stents are disappointing. Reports started to appear that on longer-term follow up (even at 3 to 6 yr) that the restenosis rates were high. Long-term results with the urethral Urolume wallstent for recurrent bulbar strictures in 60 consecutive men followed for 12 yr showed that 58% had complications, with reoperation required in 45%. The most frequent nonsurgical complications were postmicturition dribble (32%) and recurrent urinary tract infections (27%). The most common surgical interventions required were transurethral resection of obstructing stent hyperplasia (32%), urethral dilatation or urethrotomy for stent obstruction or stricture (25%), and endoscopic litholapaxy for stent encrustation or stone formation (7).

These reports also note difficulties in stent removal that frequently required resection of the entire urethral segment together with the stent and subsequent complex urethroplasty (11–15). (See chapter 24 this volume by Brandes detailing the surgical removal of the Urolume stent.) In some patients who developed an intrastent occlusion, a temporary stent was inserted instead of surgical removal of the permanent stent and a concomitant urethroplasty (**Fig. 8.4**).

The accumulating experience has thus narrowed the indications for use of the self expanding perma-

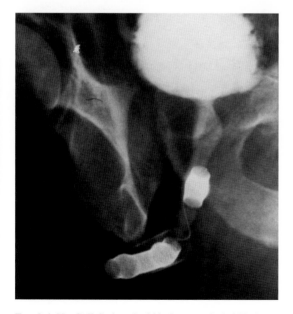

Fig. 8.4. UroCoil-S placed within in an occluded Urolume Wallstent

nent stents (Urolume Wallstent) to the select populace of only frail patients older than 55 years of age or to those refusing surgical treatment (14). The Urolume Wallstent remains the only FDA approved endourethral prosthesis approved by the U.S. Food and Drug Administration for urethral strictures. Such Urolume difficulties and lack of durability have spurred interest in other potential stents, ranging from the retrievable temporary stents to biodegradable stents.

3.2. Temporary Stents

In 1989, the concept of a large-caliber temporary urethral stent was introduced as a reduced profile stent, deployed to self-expand. The concept of using a temporary device instead of a permanent one was based on an entirely different mechanical interference technique. The new concept of a temporary stent was to leave the stent in place only long enough to act as a mold and until stabilization of the scarring process. The presence of the stent in the lumen aimed to prevent scar contraction during the healing process. After up to 12 mo, the stent would be removed, potentially leaving behind a large-caliber urethra, remodeled around the stent. The initial results with a removable temporary stent (UroCoil System, InStent Inc., Minneapolis, MN) in 18 patients was published in 1991 (16). The temporary UroCoil System stents were made of a nickel-titanium alloy (Nitinol) and expanded to 24–30 Fr., with an insertion caliber of 17 Fr. Urocoils came in three different configurations, allowing their use along the entire urethra, from the bladder neck to the external meatus (**Fig. 8.5** [17,18]). Later, the Memokath urethral stent (Engineers & Doctors, Hornbaek, Denmark), which was also made of nitinol was launched in Europe (**Fig. 8.6** [19]). The Memokath is a thermoexpanable stent that softens at >10°C and returns to a preformed shape when warmed to >50°C. Once placed into position, prewarmed saline is flushed through the stent, resulting in stent expansion of the beel shaped ends from 24 Fr. to a final diameter of 44 Fr, anchoring the stent. The main body of the stent remains 24 Fr. This feature makes the stent easy to insert and remove. Furthermore, its tight spiral structure helps prevent urothelial ingrowth

The introduction of these stents opened up a new minimally invasive approach to the treatment of recurrent urethral stricture disease (20). In addition to their use in urethral strictures, they were also

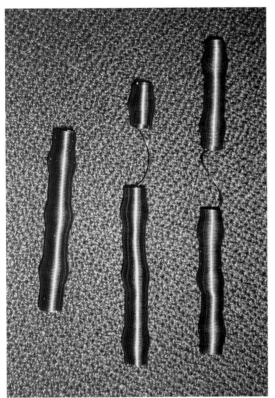

FIG. 8.5. From left to right: The UroCoil for penile urethral strictures, the UroCoil-S, for bulbar strictures and
the UroCoil-Twins for combined posterior urethral and
bulbar strictures

used with varying success in the treatment of
post prostate surgery, urethro-vesical anastomotic
stenoses *(21,22)*. In these cases, a different configuration of the stent (ProstaCoil) was inserted into the
dilated or incised bladder neck and left indwelling
for 1 yr and then removed. In patients with a very
short distance between the external sphincter and
the bladder neck, severe stress incontinence typically
developed while the stent was in place. Patients who
remained continent after stent insertion were advised
to perform Kegel exercises. Those who were continent before stent insertion continued to be continent
shortly after stent removal.

In contrast to permanent stents, temporary stents
showed that they could be used for post-traumatic
strictures or in post urethroplasty strictures, because
such stents rarely become infiltrated by tissue and
did not have to cut through the skin patch to become
imbedded. However, when occlusive hypertrophic scar
did occur in some of the UroCoil or a Memokath stent
patients, it was typically at ends of the stents.

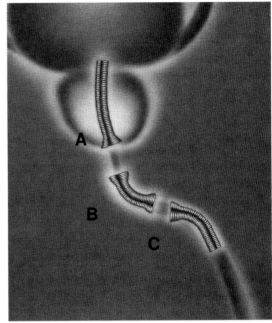

A

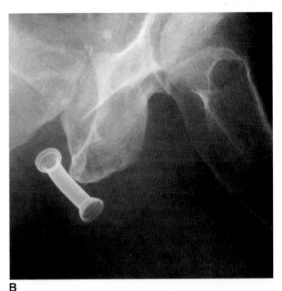

B

FIG. 8.6. A. The 3 configurations of the Memokath urethral stents: a- Memokath 028 for prostatic obstructions;
b- Memokath 044 for bulbar strictures; c- Memokath 045
for post-bulbar strictures. B. Radiograph of Memokath
044 placed in the bulbar urethra

3.2.1. UroCoil System: Clinical Results

From 1990 to 2000, 172 patients with recurrent
urethral strictures have been treated with the three
configurations of the UroCoil-System stents by the

author (**Fig. 8.5**). The strictures were situated all along the urethra, from the urethral meatus up to the posterior urethra *(23)*. All patients had undergone at least three urethral dilatations or two optical urethrotomies during the year preceding the procedure. The average indwelling time of the stent was 12 mo (range, 9–14) and average follow-up after stent removal was 36 months (range, 8–50). At the end of the second year, 83% of the patients had a patent urethra and were voiding with a stream that was found to be within the normal range. The recurrence rate rose to 20% in year 3 but stayed at the same level during year 4.

Although the UroCoil System stents were developed by a U.S.-based company and the results looked promising, they were never approved by the Food and Drug Administration. Regardless, the Urocoil System is no longer commercially available due to fiscal reasons. At this time, there are no temporary urethral for use in the urethral strictures in the United States. However, there is an ongoing multicenter trial in the States with the Memokath urethral stent.

3.3. Limitations of Previous Generations of Permanent and Temporary Stents

Accumulating experience has shown that adopting and then adapting permanent vascular stents for use in the prostatic and bulbar urethra has not been terribly successful. Also the previous generation of temporary urethral stents (UroCoil System, Memokath 044, Memokath 045) also have had their limitations and varied success (**Figs. 8.5 and 8.6**).

One of the problems with the self-expanding metallic permanent and temporary stents is stent for shortening upon release. The deployed Urolume Wallstent is about 30% shorter than its constricted length. Furthermore, the UroCoils shorten by roughly 40–50% upon deployment and the Memokath by about 10%. In inexperienced hands this shortening may cause the stent to not properly overlap the stricture and thus predispose stricture recurrence.

Other common problems seen with both the permanent and temporary stent were:

- development of sphincteric dysfunction when they were deployed near to the the external sphincter;
- tissue proliferation into the stent lumen (mainly seen with the permanent stents, occasionally between the loops of the temporary stents); and

- tissue proliferation at the ends of the stents

The external sphincter, during its contraction, gives a fusiform shape to the urethral lumen at the proximal bulb. Placing a cylindrical stent with a ring shaped end adjacent to the external sphincter often interferes its proper functioning; and thus causes partial or total incontinence in 10–20% *(24)*. Additional problems encountered with the current urethral stents were occasional tissue ingrowth between the loops of the coils or reactive tissue proliferation at their sphincteric end, causing partial or complete obliteration of the stent. The reason for such reactive tissue proliferation is the radial stiffness of the sphincteric end of the stent causes repeated friction to the urethral wall during opening and closure of the sphincter. A similar phenomenon occurs at the ends of vascular stents, and is typically referred to as the "candy-wrap effect."

3.4. Allium Bulbar Urethral Stent

The limitations detailed herein of prior endourethral prostheses (stents) induced us to search for new designs based on the specific needs of proximal bulbar urethra.

3.4.1. Stent Characteristics

The ideal stent for the bulbar urethra needs to accurately fit the dimensions and shape of an adult bulbar urethra (so it can act as a mold), not interfere with the function of the external sphincter, and prevent tissue in-growth into the lumen and tissue proliferation at its ends. Other desirable stent characteristics include the ability to be inserted in reduced caliber, the ability to not shorten upon deployment, and to exhibit a compressibility and recoil ability to make it effective, yet comfortable, to the patient. The Allium Bulbar Stent was engineered to take into consideration all these requirements (**Fig. 8.7A**). An Allium stent for post prostatectomy anastomotic stenoses has also been developed (**Fig. 8.7B**). It has a nitinol wire skeleton that is covered with a biocompatible polymer that is resistant to the urine environment. As an impermeable walled tube, the Allium stent should also prevent tissue in-growth into the lumen. The stent is deployed using a special 24-Fr delivery mechanism for easy endoscopic insertion (**Fig. 8.8**). On deployment, the stent continues to self-expand

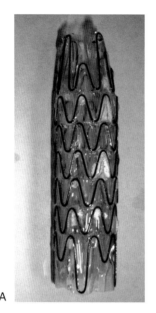

A

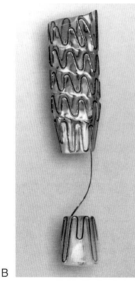

B

FIG. 8.7. A The hybrid (alloy skeleton and polymeric cover) Allium Bulbar Urethral Stent with its slightly conical sphincteric segment and low radial force downstream end. B Allium urethrovesical anastomotic stent for post prostatectomy stenoses

until it reaches its maximum of up to 45 Fr. This self expansion process can take days.

The end segments of the stent exert low radial force and thus reduce mechanical interference to the external sphincter and help reduce the friction between the end of the stent and the urethral wall, and help prevent

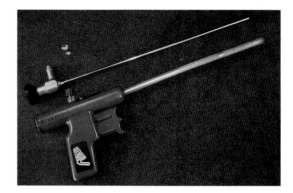

FIG. 8.8. Endoscopic deployment device of the Allium Bulbar Urethral Stent

reactive tissue growth. Having a "sphincter-friendly" segment of dynamic stent with low radial force in a lumen adjacent to a sphincter also allows the stent to be more accurately positioned in the lumen. When the sphincter closes and the diameter of the lumen adjacent to the sphincter decreases, the diameter of the sphincter ends of the stent also decreases into a conical shape while remaining in contact with the lumen wall. When the sphincter opens for voiding, and the diameter of lumen adjacent to the sphincter increases, the diameter of the sphincteric ends of the stent also increases, allowing for unobstructed urination (**Fig. 8.7**). To prevent stent migration, the caliber of the stent is larger than the distal bulbar urethra. The Allium stent is also compressible. Thus, when sitting on a hard surface, the stent is comfortable to the patient. After the compressive force is released, the stent rapidly returns to its original shape and caliber.

3.4.2. Insertion Technique

The entire insertion procedure is performed under direct vision or fluoroscopic guidance. Before insertion of the stent, the stricture needs to be opened up to at least 24 Fr (the size of the delivery device), either by internal urethrotomy, dilation, or progressive dilation. After dilation of the stricture, a Foley-like ruler catheter with centimeter marks is inserted into the bladder. To determine the appropriate length stent to insert, cystoscopic measurements are taken from between the end of the external sphincter and the proximal end of the stricture, and the other measurement being the length of the stricture plus 1 cm. The stent is released under direct vision by pulling the trigger of the device to retract the overtube. After

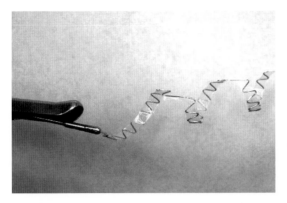

FIG. 8.9. The Allium Bulbar Stent can be removed easily even after 1 year by pulling its downstream end with an endoscopic forceps. If the pulling force is more than 500-600 grams the stent will unravel

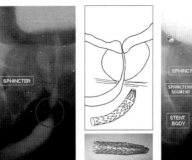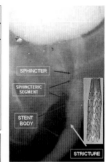

FIG. 8.10. Pre and post-deployment retrograde urography of the Allium Bulbar Urethral Stent within a proximal bulbar stricture

stent release, the radial expansion of the stent opens the stricture to its maximum caliber. Once the release process is started, the stent cannot be retracted back into the delivery device; instead, the stent should be removed and a new one inserted. Under local sedation, the stent can be removed with endoscopic grasping forceps. As a safety feature, if the pulling force during removal exceeds 500–600 g the stent starts to unravel (**Fig. 8.9**).

3.4.3. Clinical Experience With the Allium Bulbar Stent

Since 2003, we have deployed the Allium stent in 24 patients who had recurrent bulbar urethral strictures; 8 of them 1 cm distal to the sphincter. Before stent insertion, the strictures were dilated by a endourethral balloon to 30 F (18 patients) or by urethrotomy (6 patients). Stents were inserted endoscopically (19 patients) or under fluoroscopy (5 patients; **Fig. 8.10**) in ambulatory conditions and under topical anesthesia. Stricture etiology was traumatic in 11 patients and inflammatory in 13. The age of patients ranged from 34 to 72 yrs. During the indwelling period of the stent (≥ 12 mo), the urine was acidified (pH < 6) and encouraged urine outputs of 1500–2000 mL/day, to delay biofilm formation and encrustations. Stents were left indwelling for 8 to 14 mo (mean, 11 mo). Mean follow-up after stent removal has been 20 mo. After stent removal, peak flow rates typically decreased by up to 15% from baseline. In follow-

up, patients with peak flow rates that decreased by >20% were imaged and cystoscoped. In two patients, recurrence was observed after 12 and 18 months. No stent migration was observed. No patients requested stent removal because of discomfort. Patients who were sexually active before stent insertion maintained potency after stent placement. Recently an additional group of patients with anastomotic (bladder neck) strictures after radical prostatectomy are being treated with a slightly different design and larger caliber stent. Initial results of the Allium stent have been encouraging in the short term. However, true stent efficacy and durability are still to be determined.

Editorial Comment

The promise of a successful and durable endourethral prosthesis for urethral stricture has never materialized. The Urolume (American Medical Systems, Minnetonka, MN) stent is approved by the Food and Drug Administration for a very narrow and specific role, and with variable results. Off-label uses of the Urolume stent typically produce high failure rates and complications. For details on the endoscopic and open surgical management of Urolume complications (*see* Chapter 24 by Brandes in this volume).

Initial results with the new Allium stent, however, are very encouraging. Other types of urethral stents that have promise are the biodegradable (nonpermanent) and drug-eluting stents. Drug-eluting stents are a recent innovation to prevent restenosis and intimal hyperplasia in the coronary artery. The principle of drug elution has also been used in the urethra. There are numerous pilot studies with drug elution with such medications as paclitaxel, indomethecin and dexamethasone. Such stents are biocompatible and can be used effectively as a platform for local drug delivery.

Bioabsorable Stents

The concept of a spiral biodegradable stent was introduced in the late 1980s in Finland. The bioabsorbable endourethral stents were made of the high molecular weight polymers of polylactide (PLA) or polyglycolide (PGA; **Fig. 8.11**). A report of the PLA stent noted placement in 22 patients after prior failed urethrotomy (mean 2.5 prior urethrotomies). Bioabsortion time mean was 10 to 12 mo. Stricture recurrence rates were a disappointing 64% at 46 months of follow-up. In many cases, the stent collapsed at the time of bioabsortion, and the fragments of the stent perforated the mucosal lumen and potentially obstructed the lumen.

To emphasize, formal open urethroplasty is clearly the gold standard, with the best long-term success and patency. Urethral stents do occasionally work well and with durability; yet, in the cases in which they fail, the complications can be disastrous and difficult—S.B. Brandes.

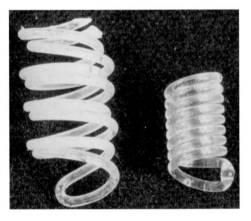

FIG. 8.11. Biodegradable urethral stent showing initial size (on the right), and expanded dimensions after 2 weeks in situ (on the left). (From: Stenting the Urinary System, (2nded), Yachia D, Paterson PJ (eds), MD Martin Dunitz, London)

References

1. Kropp KA (1978) Male urethral strictures. In: Gillenwater JY. Grayhack JT. Howards SS, Duckett JW (eds) Adult and pediatric urology. Year Book Medical, Chicago, 1297–1314
2. McAnnich JW (1992) Disorders of penis and urethra. In: Tanagho AE, McAnnich JW (eds) Smith's general urology, 13th ed. Prentice-Hall International (Lange Medical Books) London, 602–605
3. Martin P (1997) Wound healing—aiming for perfect skin regeneration. Science 276:75–81
4. Desmouliere A, Redard M, Darby I, Gabbiani G (1995) Apoptosis mediates the decrease in cellularity during the transition between granulation tissue and scar. Am J Pathol 146:56–66
5. Stocum DL (1997) Editorial Science 276:156
6. Milroy E, Cooper J, Wallsten H, Chapple C (1989) A new treatment for urethral strictures Lancet 25:1424–1427
7. Badlani G, Press S, Defalco A (1995) Urolume endourethral prosthesis for the treatment of urethral stricture disease: long term results of the North American multicenter Urolume trial. Urology 45:846–856
8. Sertcelik N, Sagnak L, Imamoglu A, et al. (2000) The use of self expanding metallic urethral stents in the treatment of recurrent bulbar urethral strictures: Long term results. BJU Int 86:686–689
9. Sneller Z, Bosch R (1992) Restenosis of the urethra despite indwelling Wallstent. J Urol 148:145–149
10. Verhamme H, Van Poppel H, Wan DeVoorde W (1993) Total fibrotic obliteration of urethral stent. BJU 72:389–390
11. Wilson TS, Lemack GE, Dmochowski RR (2002) Urolume stents: lessons learned. J Urol 167:2477–2480
12. De Vocht TF, Van Venrooij GEPM, Boon TA (2003) Self expanding stent insertion for urethral strictures: a 10-year followup. BJU Int 91:627–630
13. Shah DK, Kapoor R, Badlani GH (2003) Experience with urethral stent explantation. J Urol 169:1398–1400
14. Hussain M, Greenwell TJ, Shah J, Mundy A. (2004) Long-term results of a self-expanding wallstent in the treatment of urethral stricture. BJU Int 94:1037–1039
15. Gupta NP, Ansari MS (2004) Holmium laser core through internal urethrotomy with explantation of Urolume stent. An ideal approach for a complicated posterior urethral stricture. Int J Urol 11:343–344
16. Yachia D, Beyar M (1991) Temporarily implanted urethral coil stent for the treatment of recurrent urethral strictures: a preliminary report. J Urol 146:1001–1004
17. Yachia D (1993) The use of urethral stents for the treatment of urethral strictures Ann Urol 27:245–252

18. Yachia D, Beyar M (1993) New, self-expanding, self-retaining temporary coil stent for recurrent urethral strictures near the external sphincter. Br J Urol 71:317–321

19. Soni BM, Vaidyanathams S. Krishnan KR (1994) Use of Memokath, a second generation urethral stent for relief of urinary retention in male spinal cord injury patients. Paraplegia 32:480–488

20. Sikafi ZH.(1996) A self-expanding, self-retaining temporary urethral stent (UroCoil™) in the treatment of urethral strictures: preliminary results. BJU Int 77:701–704

21. Pizzoccaro M, Catanzaro M, Stubinski R, et al. (2002) The use of temporary stents in the treatment of urethral stenosis. Arch Ital Urol Androl 74:111–112

22. Yachia D (2004) Treatment of recurrent anastomotic stenoses after radical prostatectomy or radical cysto-prostatectomy and orthotopic bladder replacement with temporary stents. In: Yachia D, Paterson PJ (ed) Stenting the urinary system. Martin Dunitz. London, pp 491–493

23. Yachia D (2004) How do temporary urethral stents work in recurrent urethral strictures. In: Yachia D, Paterson PJ (ed) Stenting the urinary system. Martin Dunitz. London, pp 465–474

24. Nordling J, Conort P, Milroy E, Williams G, Yachia DB (1993) Stents: The 2nd International Consultation on Benign Prostatic Hyperplasia (BPH) Scientific Communication International Ltd. Jersey, Channel Islands, pp 468–481

9
Fossa Navicularis and Meatal Reconstruction

Noel A. Armenakas

Contents

1. Introduction 98
2. Etiologic Factors 98
    2.1. Inflammatory 98
    2.2. Iatrogenic 99
3. Patient Evaluation 99
4. Management Considerations 100
5. Minimally Invasive Techniques 100
    5.1. Urethral Dilation 100
    5.2. Direct Visual Internal Urethrotomy 100
    5.3. Meatotomy 101
6. Reconstructive Techniques 101
    6.1. Graft Urethroplasty 101
    6.2. Flap Urethroplasty 102
7. Complications 104
References 104

Summary The correction of strictures involving the fossa navicularis and meatus poses a distinct reconstructive challenge. Unlike surgical repair of strictures involving other urethral segments where the primary concern is restoration of urethral patency, management of fossa navicularis and meatal strictures also requires particular attention to cosmesis. Paramount to the success of any of the described procedures is the careful selection of non-diseased tissue for substitution. If the penile skin is healthy, the preferred urethral substitute is the fasciocutaneous ventral penile transverse island flap. The inherent characteristics of this versatile flap (i.e. well-vascularized predictable pedicle, non-hair bearing, and negligible contraction) provide for an excellent time-tested glanular urethral substitute. In cases where there is a suggestion of penile skin inflammation (especially BXO) or scarring, extragenital tissue transfer techniques should be considered, preferably using buccal mucosa. Equally essential is the need to substitute the entire length of diseased urethra, preferably as an onlay, preserving the dorsal urethral wall. Persistent proximal urethral disease will eventually result in further stricture formation. Finally, the choice of glanuloplasty is particularly important in achieving a cosmetically appealing outcome. A glans-cap repair is preferred because of the limited dissection required with this relatively simple and bloodless technique.

Careful selection of the most appropriate combined urethral substitution and glans reconstruction

From: *Current Clinical Urology: Urethral Reconstructive Surgery*
Edited by: S.B. Brandes © Humana Press, Totowa, NJ

techniques, as well as meticulous attention to surgical details, are mandatory in achieving a satisfactory functional and cosmetic outcome with fossa navicularis and meatal strictures.

Keywords fossa navicularis, meatus, strictures, reconstruction, urethroplasty, glanuloplasty.

1. Introduction

The fossa navicularis and meatus constitute the glanular segment of the anterior urethra. Embryologically, the epithelium of the fossa navicularis develops by the canalization of an ectodermal cord of cells, the glanular plate that extends from the meatus into the glans. Anatomically, the distal portion of the penile urethra dilates, forming the fossa navicularis and then narrows to create a vertical slit, the meatus.

Strictures involving the fossa navicularis and meatus have distinct etiologic characteristics. Moreover, their management is particularly challenging. Reconstruction of these strictures involves creating a functional urethral conduit while maintaining a cosmetically appealing glans penis.

2. Etiologic Factors

A urethral stricture is a scar from tissue injury after local trauma or inflammation. During healing, the scar contracts, compromising the caliber of the urethral lumen and limiting urine and seminal flow. Strictures are classified according to their location and the extent of scarring, with associated spongiofibrosis. Unlike other anterior urethral strictures, which are caused primarily by

TABLE 9.1. Etiology of strictures of the fossa navicularis and meatus.

Inflammatory
Balanitis xerotica obliterans
Vitiligo
Iatrogenic
Endoscopic procedures (cystoscopy, TURP)
Urethral dilation
Urethral fulguration-laser treatment
Circumcision

external trauma, strictures of the fossa navicularis and meatus are usually inflammatory or iatrogenic (**Table 9.1**).

2.1. Inflammatory

2.1.1. Balanitis Xerotica Obliterans

Balanitis xerotica obliterans (BXO) is the most common inflammatory cause of glanular urethral stricture disease. It was first described in 1928 by Stühmer, a dermatologist from Münster, Germany (*1*). He believed that the cause was glans exposure after circumcision; however, this theory has been disproved by the finding of BXO in uncircumcised males.

BXO is the male genital form of lichen sclerosus et atrophicus (*2*). It is a chronic progressive sclerosing process that can involve the glans, prepuce, penile skin, and anterior urethra. Although the exact etiology is uncertain, genetic predisposition, infections and local and autoimmune factors have been implicated in its pathogenesis (*3*). The true incidence of BXO is similarly obscure, but it is has been documented in up to 3.6% of circumcision specimens (*4*). It is more frequently identified in middle-aged men, but incidences in men with ages ranging from 5 to 83 yr have been reported (*5,6*).

The onset of BXO is insidious, evolving over many years. In uncircumcised males, the prepuce is usually involved and can result in phimosis. The lesions appear as diffuse or patchy dry white-colored plaques with well-defined margins, giving the glans a characteristically mottled appearance. Further progression of these sclerotic lesions can include the meatus and fossa navicularis, leading to urethral scarring with proximal meatal migration (**Fig. 9.1**). The disease may involve the penile skin or entire anterior urethra resulting in extensive stricture formation (*7,8*). Besides phimosis, the most common presenting symptom is urinary obstruction, occurring in 47% of patients (*6*). A causal relationship between BXO and squamous cell carcinoma has been suggested but not proven (*9*).

The diagnosis can be suspected clinically, but confirmation by biopsy is necessary. Histologically, BXO is characterized by marked epithelial atrophy with mild hyperkeratosis (*2*). The differential diagnosis includes erythroplasia of Queryat, leukoplakia,

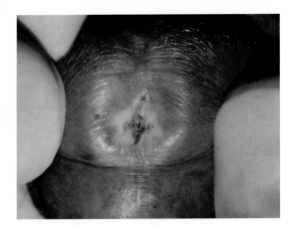

FIG. 9.1. BXO with characteristic patchy white plaques and proximal meatal migration

scleroderma, and cicatricial pemphigoid. Topical therapy using high potency corticosteroids steroids (clobetasol 0.05% ointment) or an immunomodulator (tacrolimus) has been reported with varying efficacy *(10,11)*. Alternatively, intralesional corticosteroid injections have been proposed.

2.1.2. Vitiligo

Vitiligo is an idiopathic pigmentary disorder that can involve the genitalia. Its peak incidence is in the second and third decades, but it can present at any age. Clinically, vitiligo is characterized by pale white macules that enlarge centrifugally over time (**Fig. 9.2** *[12]*). Although they are usually asymptomatic, an inflammatory variant of vitiligo can cause meatal atrophy and stricture.

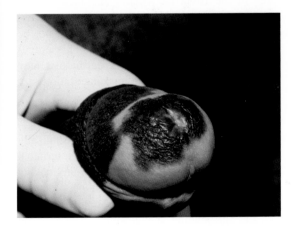

FIG. 9.2. Hypopigmentation caused by vitiligo

Unlike strictures from BXO, those from vitiligo are confined to the meatus. Disorders associated with vitiligo include insulin-dependent diabetes mellitus, pernicious anemia, hypo- and hyperthyroidism, and biliary cirrhosis.

2.2. Iatrogenic

2.2.1. Urethral Instrumentation

Strictures resulting from urethral instrumentation frequently involve the fossa navicularis. They arise from urethral luminal trauma caused by endoscopic procedures, catheterizations,or subsequent infections. These strictures often extend through the urethral mucosa and involve the surrounding spongiosum; consequently, they may not be amenable to cure by minimally invasive techniques.

Diagnostic cystoscopy and urethral dilations are the most common procedure-related causes of fossa navicularis and meatal strictures, but their true incidence is unknown. After transurethral resection of the prostate, a stricture rate of up to 6.3% has been reported, with 41% of these involving the fossa navicularis and meatus *(13)*. Fulgurating or lasing the urethral mucosa, frequently used for the treatment of urethral condylomata acuminata, can similarly result in stricture formation.

2.2.2. Circumcision

Meatal stenosis is the most common significant long-term complication of circumcision. The mechanism is thought to be disruption of the normal preputial-glanular adhesions and excision of the foreskin, resulting in an inflammatory reaction, which causes a meatitis with subsequent scarring.

3. Patient Evaluation

The proper diagnosis and adequate characterization of glanular urethral strictures must be based on data obtained from a combined clinical, radiographic and endoscopic evaluation. The clinical evaluation of a stricture involving the glanular urethra is relatively straightforward. The patient will present with obstructive lower urinary symptoms, including a decreased force of the stream, dribbling or splaying, and prolonged voiding; progression to acute urinary retention may occur. A thorough history should reveal any previous surgery, inflammation, instrumentation, or external trauma to the urethra. On physical examination, a pinpoint opening with permeate scarring is pathognomonic of a meatal stricture. A solitary fossa navicularis stricture may also be diagnosed clinically by direct visualization facilitated by manual meatal retraction; otherwise, a small catheter can be passed through the meatus and advanced to the level of the obstruction. It is very important to inspect the entire glans and penile shaft carefully to identify any coexisting pathology suggesting an inflammatory etiology. The presence of BXO involving the penile skin (better termed penile lichen sclerosus et atrophicus) precludes its use in urethral replacement.

The radiographic evaluation of glanular urethral strictures may be difficult. The introduction of either a small Foley catheter or a catheter-tip syringe in the distal urethra, necessary for retrograde urethrography, will usually obscure the stricture. Sonourethrography, although superior to conventional radiography in defining the degree of spongiofibrosis, is similarly limited by the need for distal urethral instrumentation. If properly performed, a voiding cystourethrogram is the preferred imaging modality for the fossa navicularis and meatus. The bladder should be filled with an enhanced concentration of contrast material (60% solution) and roentgenograms taken while the patient is voiding. The image quality can be optimized by adjusting the contrast resolution to provide opacification of the entire glanular urethra.

Alternatively, if a catheter cannot be passed safely through the narrowing, a voiding cystourethrogram can be performed using contrast material injected intravenously (2 mL/kg body weight). This is more time consuming and the diluted contrast may yield suboptimal images. Urinary flow rates are obtained preoperatively, as a baseline with which postoperative results can be compared. Endoscopic urethral evaluation should be performed to confirm the length of the stricture and to estimate the degree of spongiofibrosis. This can be done at the time of the reconstructive procedure, using a pediatric cystoscope.

4. Management Considerations

Management of fossa navicularis and meatal strictures includes minimally invasive (dilation, urethrotomy) and reconstructive techniques. The selection of the proper procedure is paramount to achieving a successful outcome. Factors affecting this selection should include the age and overall condition of the patient as well as the etiology and specific characteristics of the stricture, glans, and penile skin. Treatment of simple glanular urethral strictures includes dilation and urethrotomy (either direct visual internal or meatotomy). Recurrent or complex glanular urethral strictures are best managed by surgical reconstruction. Dilation and urethrotomy are predominantly palliative procedures with long-term cure limited only to short (<5 mm) mucosal strictures without associated spongiofibrosis. Surgical reconstruction should be regarded as curative.

5. Minimally Invasive Techniques

5.1. Urethral Dilation

Urethral dilation is accomplished by gradual, progressive stretching of the urethra to a maximal diameter of 24 Fr. It must be performed in a manner that will not cause further urethral trauma. Aggressive dilation can lead to excessive urethral stretching and further scarring. Ideally, an acceptable result should limit the interval between dilations to every 6 mos. Select strictures of the fossa navicularis and meatus may respond to dilation; however, long-term success is questionable. Urethral dilation should not be used for the management of BXO. This potentially progressive inflammatory dermatosis may be accelerated by repetitive instrumentation.

5.2. Direct Visual Internal Urethrotomy

Direct visual internal urethrotomy is technically difficult in the fossa navicularis. This terminal urethral segment provides a poor fulcrum, making any cutting motion awkward, with poor manual control. The incision can be inadvertently extended into the surrounding spongiosum, causing undue bleeding.

5.3. Meatotomy

A ventral or dorsal meatotomy can be performed for select meatal and fossa navicularis strictures. The urethra is incised and, where possible, the mucosal edges are sutured. The ventral approach will produce a small degree of hypospadias, which is preferable to a dorsal incision which can result in significant bleeding by cutting into the vascular glans penis.

6. Reconstructive Techniques

Several techniques have been described for reconstructing the fossa navicularis and meatus. Basically, they involve tissue transfer techniques using grafts or flaps. Partial urethral replacement, using an onlay configuration, is preferable to circumferential replacement as the latter has a high restricture rate. For a successful repair, appropriate preoperative urethral and penile skin assessment and adherence to basic surgical principles are mandatory (**Table 9.2**). Penile or urethral biopsies can be helpful in confirming the diagnosis of an inflammatory process.

Most reconstructive procedures can be done safely and effectively in one stage. Two-stage repairs are used for salvage procedures in patients with limited remaining viable tissue from multiple failed operations. The choice of the particular reconstructive technique is dictated by the characteristics of the stricture and proposed tissue to be transferred, as well as the surgeon's familiarity and preference.

6.1. Graft Urethroplasty

Full-thickness, rather than split-thickness, skin grafts should be used to reconstruct the fossa navicularis and meatus. The avoidance of split-thickness grafts is predominantly because of their

TABLE 9.2. Basic surgical principles for reconstructing strictures of the fossa navicularis and meatus.

- Wide exposure of the stricture and surrounding tissue
- Adequate scar excision
- Appropriate choice of healthy tissue for urethral substitution
- Creation of a normal caliber water tight neo-urethra
- Choice of glanuloplasty depending on the physical characteristics of the glans penis
- Maintenance of an uninfected dry suture line

significant and unpredictable contractility, yielding an unacceptably high failure rate.

One of the earliest reconstructive procedures for fossa navicularis strictures is the patch-graft urethroplasty, described by Devine (*14*). It incorporates a full-thickness distal penile skin graft to "re-pave" the fossa navicularis. The rich glanular blood supply can provide an ideal host for successful graft take. More contemporary studies incorporate extragenital tissue, using postauricular and buccal mucosal grafts. Extragenital tissue always should be used in patients with lichen sclerosus et atrophicus involving the penile skin, because urethral substitution using diseased tissue inevitably will lead to recurrent stricture formation.

The use of buccal mucosa was first described by Humby in 1941, but remained relatively dormant until the past decade (*15,16*). Advantages of buccal mucosa over other grafts include its ease in harvesting without any noticeable cosmetic deficit; the tissue's thick epithelium and dense subdermal plexus, providing resilience and improving graft-take; and a normal compliment of dermal collagen limiting contraction. Although buccal mucosal grafts have solidified their place in our armamentarium for reconstruction of urethral strictures, they are best used in the spongiosal-rich bulbar urethra. Indeed, there is limited experience in using buccal mucosal grafts for the reconstruction of fossa navicularis and meatal strictures. Most of the reported series using these grafts in glanular urethral reconstruction are for hypospadias repairs (*16–18*). However, the etiology and tissue characteristics of hypospadias are distinct from those of urethral stricture disease, making direct extrapolation of surgical outcomes potentially inaccurate.

6.1.1. Buccal Urethral Grafting

The buccal graft is harvested using the technique described by Morey and McAninch (*19*). A rectangular full-thickness graft is taken from the inner cheek and the defect closed primarily, grafted with cadaveric fascia or left to heal by secondary intent. A midline longitudinal full-thickness urethrotomy is made incising the entire stricture. The buccal mucosal graft is placed ventrally and sutured to the lateral edges of the native urethra using running absorbable material; interrupted sutures are placed at the proximal anastomosis to limit undue narrowing at this site. Graft immobilization and the appropriate vascular coverage are paramount in ensuring tissue survival.

6.2. Flap Urethroplasty

Penile flap reconstruction for strictures involving both the fossa navicularis and meatus was first described by Cohney in 1963 *(20)*. This technique involves the rotation of a ventrally based penile flap to cover the previously incised glanular urethra. Problems with this repair include glanular torsion and flap necrosis. Several modifications followed, incorporating an inverted U-shaped ventral penile flap to reconstruct the glanular urethra *(21–23)*. These procedures require significant flap mobilization to achieve adequate meatal advancement and can result in a retrusive meatus. In addition, they are limited by their ability to replace only the ventral surface of the glanular urethra; consequently, they cannot be used for circumferential disease requiring tubular urethral substitution.

6.2.1. *Fasciocutaneous Ventral Penile Transverse Island Flap*

A more versatile flap for reconstruction of the fossa navicularis and meatus is the fasciocutaneous ventral penile transverse island flap, initially described by Jordan *(24)*. This is a rectangular broad-based penile skin flap, based on an island of dartos fascia vascularized by the superficial penile vessels. Because of the relative laxity of the penile skin, this flap can easily be used in circumcised patients requiring fossa navicularis and meatal substitution.

The glans reconstruction is an integral part of this procedure. Where possible, avoiding an incision directly on the glans will provide a superior cosmetic result *(25)*. This is of paramount importance to the patient, and can overshadow the functional success of the urethroplasty procedure.

Technique of Repair

Urethral Exposure
The patient is positioned supine on the operating table. Distal urethroscopy can be performed, with a pediatric cystoscope, to evaluate the fossa navicularis as well as the more proximal anterior urethra.

Optical magnification, afforded by surgical loupes, is a valuable aid for the reconstructive procedure.

A subcoronal incision is made on the ventrum of the penis and extended circumferentially around the ventral glanular margin, leaving approximately a 5 mm mucosal cuff (**Fig. 9.3**). The incision is carried down through the dartos and Buck's fascias, exposing the underlying distal anterior urethra.

The appropriate glans reconstruction is chosen, depending on the physical characteristics of the glans. If the glans is conical shaped without undue scarring, inflammation or distortion, a glans-cap glanuloplasty should be used. This has the aesthetic advantage in that it preserves the integrity of the entire glans, limiting unnecessary scarring to this most prominent terminal penile segment. With a severely diseased or flattened glans, glans-wings are preferable because they allow the excision of all fibrotic tissue with anatomic resculpturing of the glans.

Once the choice of glans reconstruction is made, the fossa navicularis can be appropriately exposed. For a glans-cap glanuloplasty, the ventral surface of the glans is dissected off the distal corporal bodies. For a glans-wings glanuloplasty, a full-thickness incision is made in the ventral glanular groove, exposing the underlying urethra. A ventral longitudinal stricturotomy is performed and the incision extended at least 5 mm into normal urethral tissue (**Fig. 9.4**). Usually, the dorsal urethral surface can be preserved unless there is severe circumferential urethral disease necessitating complete urethral excision. Once all the scar tissue is removed, the proximal urethral lumen should be calibrated, with metal bougie-à-boule dilators, ensuring a diameter of at least 24 Fr.

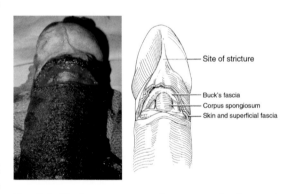

FIG. 9.3. Urethral exposure using a ventral subcoronal incision

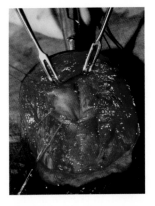
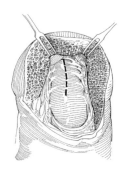

FIG. 9.4. Ventral longitudinal stricturotomy

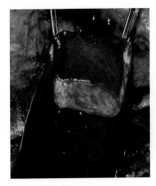
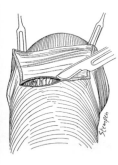

FIG. 9.5. Creation of the fasciocutaneous ventral penile transverse island flap

Creation of a Fasciocutaneous Ventral Penile Transverse Island Flap

The fasciocutaneous ventral penile flap is appropriately marked after measuring the length of the urethral defect. The width of the proposed flap is dependent on the type of urethral substitution required and can be calculated by using the following formula:

$$\text{Circumferential length} = 2\,\pi r,$$

where $\pi = 3.14$ and r = urethral luminal radius.

To create a 24-Fr lumen, necessary for complete urethral substitution, a 2.5-cm flap width is adequate; with an onlay this width can be halved. Because contraction is not a problem with flaps, accurate measurements can limit subsequent sacculation apparent with oversized tissue dimensions.

The flap is developed by superficially incising the previously marked segment of penile skin (**Fig. 9.5**). This is carried through the subdermal fascia, developing a tissue plane between this and Buck's fascia. The dissection is usually continued to the mid-penis, but can be extended proximally, as needed, for adequate flap mobilization (**Fig. 9.6**). Careful preservation of the subdermal fascia is vital in ensuring viability of the remaining penile skin.

Urethral Substitution

The newly created flap is rotated medially, ensuring its unobstructed tension-free interposition in the glanular urethra. The flap is then sutured, preferably as an onlay, using monofilament 6-O. One continuous suture is used, on each side, approxi-

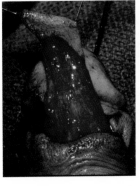
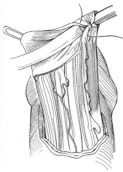

FIG. 9.6. Completed flap mobilization with preservation of thick fascial pedicle

mating the cutaneous side of the flap to the ventral urethral mucosa. In cases were complete urethral substitution is required, the flap is tubularized and sutured over an 18-Fr silicone catheter, creating a watertight seam.

Glanular Reconstruction

Once the urethral reconstruction is complete, attention is directed to the glanuloplasty, the choice of which has been previously decided. With a glans-cap repair, the flap is tunneled under the previously elevated glans (**Fig. 9.7**). A generous core of glanular tissue needs to be taken, ensuring complete removal of all perimeatal fibrosis. With the use of 4-O chromic, the distal flap is then sutured to the tip of the glans, creating an orthotopic, widely patent neo-meatus (**Fig. 9.8**).

With the glans-wings repair, two full thickness glans flaps are elevated laterally, from the ventral

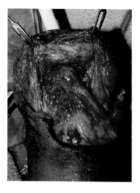
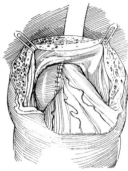

FIG. 9.7. Urethral substitution using an only configuration tunneled below an intact glans

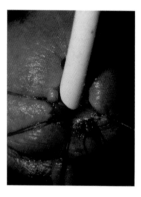
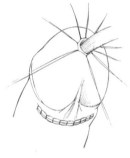

FIG. 9.8. Completed glans-cap repair with the creation of an adequately patent neomeatus

midline, enabling broad neo-urethral coverage. Debridement of any glanular tissue should be limited in order to ensure a tension-free glanular closure. The glans-wings are approximated loosely over the neo-urethra in two layers, using interrupted fine chromic sutures. This gives the glans a physiologic conical shape with a ventrally placed linear suture line.

Penile Skin Closure

Before closing the penile skin, meticulous hemostasis is accomplished with the bipolar cautery forceps. The squared corners of the flap donor site are rounded, to permit reapproximation of the penile skin to the subcoronal mucosa. Burrow triangles can be used to eliminate any dog-ears which can occasionally form at the corners of the closure. Antibiotic ointment is placed on the suture lines and a transparent moisture-permeable dressing is used to cover the penis. The Foley catheter should be taped in a non-dependent position, on the patient's abdomen, decreasing postoperative edema and limiting undue catheter pressure.

Postoperative Management

Postoperative ambulation is started immediately. Perioperative intravenous antibiotics are continued for 24 h. The neo-meatus should be kept lubricated, with antibiotic ointment, to prevent drying. The urethral catheter is removed at 2 wk, at which time a voiding cystourethrogram is obtained. Follow-up is obtained at three and twelve months, using flow rate determinations. Urethrography and urethroscopy can be performed, selectively but, in general, further instrumentation is avoided, in order to limit the risk of additional procedure-induced scarring.

7. Complications

Early complications of fossa navicularis and meatal urethral reconstruction include splaying of the urinary stream and a small degree of glanular torsion. Both of these problems are usually transient, resolving once the initial healing process is complete. Delayed complications include urethral restenosis, skin necrosis, penile torsion, fistula formation, and neourethral prolapse or retrusion. Most recurrent strictures will occur at the proximal urethral anastomosis and are short, making them amenable to treatment by minimally invasive procedures. In cases where a tubular neo-urethral configuration was used, such strictures may require reoperation. Fistulas can be managed by excision and closure, which should be postponed for 6 mo postoperatively.

References

1. Stümer A (1928) Balanitis xerotica obliterans (post operationem) und ihre Beziehungen zur "Kraurosis glandis et praeputii penis." Arch Dertmatol Syphilol 156:613
2. Meffert JJ, Davis BM and Grimwood RE (1995) Lichen sclerosus. J Am Acad Dermatology 32:393
3. Thomas RHM., Ridley CM and Black MM (1983) The association of lichen sclerosus et atrophicus and autoimmune-related disease in males Br J Dermatol 109:661

4. Schinella RA, Miranada D (1974) Posthitis xerotica obliterans in circumcision specimens Urology 3:348

5. Garat JM, Chéchile G, Algaba F, Santaularia JM (1986) Balanitis xerotica obliterans in children. J Urol 136:436

6. Bainbridge DR, Whitaker RH, Chir M, Shepheard BGF. (1971) Balanitis xerotica obliterans and urinary obstruction Br J Urol 43:487

7. Staff WG (1970) Urethral involvement in balanitis xerotica obliterans Br J Urol 47:234

8. Mallo N, Garat JM, Santaularia J and Hernandez J (1978) Urethro-balanitis xerotica obliterans Eur Urol 4:9

9. Pietrzak P, Hadway P, Corbishley CM, Watkin N (2006) Is the association between balanitis xerotica obliterans and penile carcinoma underestimated? BJU 98:74

10. Depaquale I, Park AJ, Bracka A(2000) The treatment of balanitis xerotica obliterans BJU 86:459

11. Pandher BS, Rustin MHA, Kaisary AV (2003) Treatment of balanitis xerotica obliterans with topical tacrolimus J Urol 170:923

12. Gokhale BB, Mehta LN (1983) Histopathology of vitiliginous skin Int J Dermatol 22:477

13. Lentz HC Jr, Mebust WK, Foret JD, Melchior J (1977) Urethral strictures following transurethral prostatectomy: Review of 2,223 resections. J Urol 117:194

14. Devine CJ Jr (1986) Surgery of the urethra. In: Walsh PC, Gittes RF, Perlmutter AD, Stamey TA, (eds) Campbell's urology, 5th ed. WB Saunders, Philadelphia

15. Humby G (1941) A one-stage operation for hypospadias Br J Surg 29:84

16. Bürger RA, Müller SC, El-Damanhoury H, Tschakaloff A, Riedmiller H, Hohenfellner R (1992) The buccal mucosal graft for urethral reconstruction: a preliminary report. J Urol 147:662

17. Caldamone AA, Edstrom LE, Koyle MA, Rabinowitz R, Hulbert WC (1998) Buccal mucosal grafts for urethral reconstruction Urology 51:15

18. Dessanti A, Rigamonti W, Merulla V, Falchetti D, Caccia G (1992) Autologous buccal mucosa graft for hypospadias repair: an initial report. J Urol 147:1081

19. Morey AF, McAninch JW (1996) Technique of harvesting buccal mucosa for urethral reconstruction. J Urol 155:1696

20. Cohney CG (1963) A penile flap procedure for the relief of meatal stricture. Br J Urol 35:182

21. Blandy JP and Tresidder GC (1967) Meatoplasty. Br J Urol 39:633

22. Brannen GE (1976) Meatal reconstruction. J Urol 116:319

23. De Sy WA (1984) Aesthetic repair of meatal stricture. J Urol 132:678

24. Jordan GH (1987) Reconstruction of the fossa navicularis. J Urol 138:102

25. Armenakas NA, Morey AF and McAninch JW (1998) Reconstruction of resistant strictures of the fossa navicularis and meatus. J Urol 160:359

10
Stricture Excision and Primary Anastomosis for Anterior Urethral Strictures

Reynaldo G. Gomez

Contents

1. Stricture Excision and Primary Anastomosis for Anterior Urethral Strictures... 107
2. Etiology.. 108
3. Patient Selection for Excision and Primary Anastomosis... 108
4. Preoperative Evaluation 109
5. Surgical Technique... 109
6. Postoperative Care 114
7. Clinical Outcomes of Excision and Primary Anastomosis 114
8. Summary 115
Editorial Comment.. 116
Appendix... 116
References.. 116

Summary   Stricture excision and primary end to end anastomosis is the best surgical treatment for anterior urethral strictures. After resecting all fibrotic urethral walls, proximal and distal urethral ends are mobilized so they can be approximated without tension to bridge the gap. Natural urethral elasticity is used to elongate the urethra and the distance can be shortened by opening the inter-crural septum. A wide mucosa-to-mucosa tension-free anastomosis is then performed using fine interrupted absorbable sutures. This procedure is ideally suited for bulbar strictures 1–3 cm long, but it can also be successful in some selected cases with proximal bulbar strictures up to 5 cm in length. Because the anterior penile urethra is stretched during erection, this procedure is limited in the pendulous urethra, as it can produce shortening of the urethra and ventral curvature of the penis on erection. Complications are rare, mainly infection or hematoma of the operative wound. Sterile urine at the time of surgery and meticulous hemostasis are required to avoid them. Late failures are related to excessive tension at the anastomosis or incomplete fibrous resection. Complete excision of the fibrotic urethra is essential, and the surgeon must be prepared to perform an alternative form of repair if this resection results in a defect too long for a tension-free end to end reconstruction. When performed properly, excision and primary anastomosis is a well-tolerated, low-morbidity and highly effective procedure, with a long-term cure rate around 95%.

Keywords   Urethra, Urethral stricture, Surgical anastomosis, Urethral reconstruction, Urethroplasty, Bulbar.

1. Stricture Excision and Primary Anastomosis for Anterior Urethral Strictures

When performed properly, excision and primary anastomosis is the best surgical procedure for the treatment of anterior urethral strictures available today.

From: *Current Clinical Urology: Urethral Reconstructive Surgery*
Edited by: S.B. Brandes © Humana Press, Totowa, NJ

The involved principle is simple: a perineal approach with resection of the strictured urethral segment and reconstruction by means of an end-to-end anastomosis. Results are excellent with long-term cure rates at approx 95% in the published experience of major reference centers. Although simple, success with this procedure is related to a number of important clinical and technical details, which are the basis of this chapter.

2. Etiology

Before the antibiotic era, sexually transmitted diseases, mainly gonorrhea, were the main cause of strictures of the urethra. Gonorrhea and other urethritis are still very frequent, but early antibiotic treatment can avoid infectious damage to the urethra so these strictures are less frequent in developed countries nowadays. External trauma and iatrogenic injuries are the etiology of most anterior urethral strictures, although in many cases the etiology is unknown and is reported as "idiopathic." Fenton et al. (1) performed a meta-analysis of the etiology of anterior strictures from 7 series of the literature with a total of 732 patients, founding a 33% idiopathic, 33% iatrogenic, 15% inflammatory, and 19% traumatic etiology.

Traumatic strictures of the bulbar urethra usually are short and, in most cases, result after a straddle injury in which the urethra is crushed against the inferior border of the symphysis pubis. This injury may cause partial damage of the urethra that heals with scar formation, which eventually leads to a stricture. With more severe injuries, the urethra can be transected with total loss of urethral continuity. Some strictures of unknown origin may in fact be the delayed result of an unrecognized childhood perineal trauma, and a stricture appearing many years after one of such injuries has occurred (1,2).

Iatrogenic strictures are related to endoscopic procedures and prolonged urethral catheterization. Although they tend to be longer and located at the penoscrotal junction or pendulous urethra, sometimes they can be short and proximal enough in the bulbar urethra as to be repaired by a primary anastomosis.

Some idiopathic strictures are located in the proximal half of the bulbar urethra, occur in young men, and contain smooth muscle. These strictures are linked with the so-called Cobb's collar and may represent an embryological fusion defect, for which they are referred by some authors as "congenital" (3). These strictures tend to be thin and diaphragmatic, amenable to visual urethrotomy, but some may be candidates for anastomotic repair should the endoscopic treatment fail.

3. Patient Selection for Excision and Primary Anastomosis

Patient selection is essential for success. The objective of this procedure is to obtain a wide mucosa-to-mucosa anastomosis without tension. A 1-cm spatulation of the urethral ends is a useful maneuver to create a wide overlapping oblique anastomosis that reduces the risk of annular retraction and recurrence, which means mobilization of both urethral ends to replace the length of the excised segment plus the urethral spatulation. For this reason, length of the stricture and its location are the limiting factors. The anterior penile urethra is stretched during erection so the length of pendulous urethra than can be excised without causing chordee is very limited. With a 1-cm spatulation on each side, the resection of a 2-cm stricture will cause a 4-cm urethral shortening, which could be unacceptable on many patients and, indeed, some authors stated that excision and primary anastomosis may never be used in the penile urethra, except in previously impotent patients (4). Moreover, strictures of the penile urethra tend to be multiple and long so the number of patients amenable for primary anastomosis in the pendulous urethra is quite small. In some selected cases this technique can be used for strictures up to 1 cm, but in most instances a substitution urethroplasty will be necessary (4–6).

On the contrary, the bulbar urethra does not participate in an erection and can be extensively mobilized proximally to the genitourinary diaphragm and distally to the penoscrotal junction without causing erectile impairment. The bulbar urethra has a very rich blood supply, proximally from the bulbar and urethral arteries and distally by retrograde flow from the glans penis and from perforating arteries, branches of the cavernosal and dorsal arteries. Once mobilized, the natural elasticity of the urethra can be stretched without tension to bridge short defects up to 1–2 cm. If the defect is longer, the natural curve of the bulbar urethra can be straightened to bridge the gap. The curve of the bulbar urethra is produced at the junction of the two crura at the base of the penis, where the urethra bends to penetrate the perineal diaphragm towards the apex of the prostate. Between the crura, there is a virtual space that can be developed by separating the crura to allow the distal urethra to lie between them; this will straighten the urethra gaining additional length to allow a tension-free anastomosis. With these combined maneuvers, up to a 5-cm gap can be bridged without tension in most patients. For this reason, excision and primary anastomosis is suitable for bulbar strictures 1–3 cm long considering a 1-cm spatulation on each end (3–10). Because the elasticity of the bulbar urethra is greater on its distal half than on its proximal half, the more proximal the stricture, the longer the segment that can be removed (6). In a recent paper, Morey and Kizer (11) reported on a series of 11 patients in whom an extended anastomotic repair was performed with strictures 2.6 to 5.0 cm long (average, 3.78 cm). All these patients had proximal bulbar strictures within 1 cm from the membranous urethra and were young sexually active men with healthy and well vascularized tissues. There were no differences in recurrence or sexual dysfunction when compared with a similar group with strictures 2.5 cm or shorter (11). These results suggest that, in some selected cases, proximal strictures longer that 3 cm can also be considered for an anastomotic repair. In the end, the reconstructive surgeon should select the procedure to be used according to the operative findings and be prepared to modify his original plan when required. The patient should be warned that a substitution repair may be necessary if the stricture results to be longer that anticipated.

4. Preoperative Evaluation

Proper selection of patients for primary anastomotic reconstruction requires a thorough clinical and imaging evaluation. Anamnesis should take note of co-morbid conditions that can increase the surgical risk or impair wound healing. Previous surgical management of the stricture may introduce important alterations to the normal anatomy and vascular supply. On physical examination, fibrosis, inflammation, or fistula in the perineal area may be found. Penile and hairless skin, foreskin, and buccal mucosa are evaluated as possible sources of tissue for reconstruction.

Because the feasibility of performing a primary anastomotic repair depends on the stricture's location, its length, and degree of spongiofibrosis, a precise anatomical knowledge of the stricture is essential. Retrograde urethrogram is the standard imaging study for this purpose because it can demonstrate the location and extent of the stricture. In most cases, a voiding cystourethrogram should be also included to best define the proximal urethra and bladder neck. However, it is well known that these radiographic studies often underestimate stricture length because they are preformed in an oblique position with relation to the anteroposterior x-ray beam, resulting in a shorter projected view of the stricture (12,13). Also, in some severe strictures, high voiding pressure will hydrodilate the proximal urethra, masking areas of proximal fibrosis so the stricture may look shorter than it really is. For this reason, when in doubt it may be helpful to allow the urethra to rest for a couple of weeks by means of a temporary suprapubic diversion, to get a more precise estimation of the true length of the stricture (4,5). Because of the limitations of the radiographic studies, sonographic evaluation of the stricture has been advocated to improve preoperative staging. This study has been shown to be highly accurate in predicting the true length of the stricture and may also provide some valuable estimation of the degree of spongiofibrosis and presence of other pathologic conditions like diverticulae, fistulas, urethral calculi, false passages and periurethral abscesses (12–14). Endoscopy, preferably flexible urethroscopy, may be useful to visualize the mucosa at the distal side of the stricture. Pink mucosa means healthy urethra, but a pale–gray mucosal aspect reflects submucosal fibrosis that will need to be removed during surgery. This evaluation may be particularly important in patients with previous urethroplasty or those managed with visual urethrotomy. In patients with complete urethral disruption unable to void, imaging of the proximal urethra may be a problem. These cases will have a suprapubic tube, and flexible cystoscopy through the catheter tract may be very informative.

5. Surgical Technique

The patient is operated under general anesthesia and with broad-spectrum prophylactic antibiotic coverage. It is imperative that the urine be sterile at the time of surgery, which is particularly important in patients with a suprapubic tube, who may be chronically colonized. Failure to operate with sterile urine is the main reason for wound infection and postoperative urinary sepsis.

The patient is placed in the exaggerated lithotomy position. We place a cushion to elevate the pelvis and flexed the patient's hips to make the perineum as horizontal as possible. Slight Trendellenburg tilt of the table can also be useful. Neuroskeletal complications caused by this position have been well documented in the literature, especially severe compartment syndrome *(15–17)*. However, the risk is directly related to the surgical time, especially for surgeries longer than 5 h. Because most primary anastomotic procedures can be completed in less than 3 hours, the incidence of such injuries is negligible. Anyway, care is taken in padding the contacts points to avoid pressure, and Allen type stirrups are used when available to limit flexion at the knee joint and decrease stretch on the peroneal nerve. Thromboembolic prophylaxis is provided by the use of elastic leggings and pneumatic intermittent leg-compression device (**Fig. 10.1**).

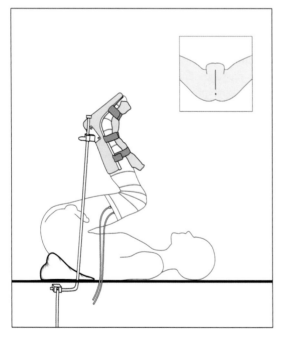

FIG. 10.1. Exaggerated lithotomy position. Note the cushion elevating the pelvis and the horizontal projection of the perineum

Patient's genitalia, perineum, lower abdomen, and thighs are prepared for surgery. Surgical drapes and towels are placed to expose the perineum and hypogastrium. We use a number 1016 adhesive plastic Steri-Drape Irrigation Pouch (3 M Health Care) to keep the anus away from the operative field. Two stitches are placed from the sides of the scrotum to the pubic area to elevate the scrotum and better expose the perineal surgical field. We always use magnification loupes, a head lamp, monopolar, in addition to bipolar electrocautery (for hemostasis around the urethra). Scott's retractor ring is another very useful aid; besides a very effective radial retraction capability, this device also exerts elastic traction of tissues. This traction brings deeper structures to the surface, reducing the depth of the working cavity. The spongiosum is mainly a vascular structure and should be managed as such; consequently we use DeBackey vascular forceps for its dissection. Angled Pott's vascular scissors are very helpful when performing longitudinal urethrotomy incisions. The bougie-a-boule probes are very useful for calibration of the urethral ends and detection of residual spongiofibrosis.

A vertical skin incision is used in most cases extending from the base of the scrotum almost to the anal margin. After incision of Colles' fascia, a 20-F soft rubber catheter is placed in the distal urethra to help with its identification; the urethra is then located by palpation and dissected. The best approach to the urethra is at the distal margin of the bulbospongiosum muscle (**Fig. 10.2**). Buck's fascia is opened on either side of the urethra and a plane is developed between the spongiosum and cavernous bodies. Once the urethra has been separated from the corpus cavernosum, a vascular tape is placed to elevate the urethra and facilitate its proximal and distal dissection. The bulbospongiosum muscle is now opened in the midline with scissors and separated laterally on each side to expose the underlying corpus spongiosum. The muscle is not adhered to the spongiosal tunica albuginea, except in the ventral midline raphe where sharp dissection is necessary to expose the bulb (**Figs. 10.3 and 10.4**).

The location of the stricture is sometimes marked by fibrosis and an hourglass retraction of the spongiosum, especially after traumatic straddle injuries. It can also be determined by gentle retrograde probing of the urethra with the soft rubber catheter; the idea is to locate the stricture site, taking care to

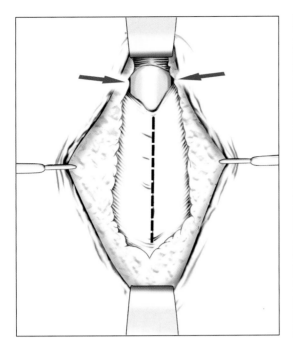

FIG. 10.2. The urethra is best approached at the distal margin of the bulbospongiosum muscle (arrows)

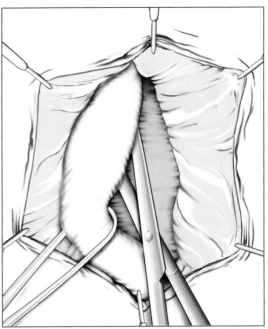

FIG. 10.4. A vascular tape elevates the urethra while it is freed from the corpora

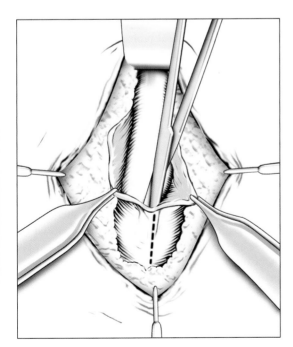

FIG. 10.3. The bulbospongiosum muscle is split along the dotted lines to expose the bulb

avoid urethral perforation or dilation of the stricture with this maneuver. Inadverted perforation of the distal side of the stricture may lead to unnecessary loss of valuable urethral length, whereas dilation of the stricture at this time may make it more difficult to identify the limits of the fibrous process to be resected. Once the urethra has been separated from the corpus cavernosum, it can be transected at the site of maximum stricture. However, if the surgeon is in doubt about the feasibility of performing a primary anastomosis, a longitudinal urethrotomy should be performed through the stricture and extended proximally and distally until healthy urethra is found. If the resulting defect is too long for an end-to-end reconstruction, then a patch graft urethroplasty can be selected. This urethrotomy can be dorsal or ventral and buccal mucosa is the preferred tissue for urethral graft nowadays.

With short strictures amenable to excision and primary anastomosis, the urethra is divided and the strictured portion is excised completely. If too much bleeding occurs after dividing the urethra, soft bulldog-type vascular clamps can be applied to both ends of the urethra to reduce blood loss and improve view, facilitating urethral inspection. All diseased fibrotic urethra is resected until completely healthy urethra is found. This step is crucial, as one main cause of failure is incomplete scar removal. Partially fibrous urethra can look "acceptable," but the mucosa usually has a grayish aspect, clearly distinguishable from the truly healthy pink mucosa. Forceps manipulation should be minimized to avoid attrition damage of this delicate tissue. The bougie-a-boule probes are used to gently calibrate the proximal and distal urethral lumen up to a 28- to 30-F caliber. Failure of bougies to smoothly calibrate the ends indicates residual spongiofibrosis that limits urethral elasticity, which also needs to be removed.

Dissection proceeds now distally separating the urethra from the corpus cavernosum, but not beyond the peno-scrotal angle to avoid penile shortening or chordee during erection. In the impotent patient, this factor is not of concern and the urethra can be completely mobilized distally. The urethra is also dissected proximally, freeing the bulb from the perineal body. At this point the paired bulbar arteries will be found; sometimes they need to be suture-ligated to properly mobilize and advance the bulb. However, with short strictures extensive mobilization of the bulb may not be necessary and these arteries can be preserved. These arteries should be spared whenever possible to ensure good vascular supply of the spongiosum (8,18). Splitting the inter-crural septum in the midline is also very helpful in reducing the distance between both urethral ends. This maneuver will allow the distal portion of the urethra to lie within the inter-crural space, straightening the natural curve of the bulbar urethra and gaining length to relieve tension at the anastomosis.

A 1-cm spatulation is performed on each urethral end to create an oblique anastomotic line, thus reducing the risk of annular retraction recurrence. Typically, the proximal end is spatulated dorsally and the distal end ventrally (**Fig. 10.5**). The anastomosis is performed with six to eight interrupted 5-O poliglecaprone (Monocryl) sutures. In the dorsal half of the urethra, through and through stitches include the urethral wall and the thin spongiosum in one single layer; the knots can be tied from the inside or the outside of the urethra (**Fig. 10.6**). Some surgeons like to anchor these dorsal stitches to the corporal tunica albuginea to stabilize the anastomosis and keep the dorsal plate flat and

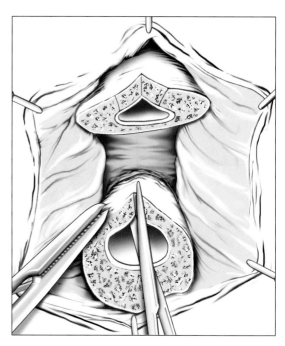

FIG. 10.5. The proximal urethral end is spatulated dorsally and the distal end ventrally

open (8). In the ventral half, the spongiosum is much thicker so the anastomosis can be performed in two layers: the first layer includes only the urethra and the spongiosal tunica is closed separately in a second watertight layer; these knots are tied on the outside (**Figs. 10.7** and **10.8**). In this way, blood is allowed to flow across the anastomosis, ensuring good irrigation. Although some authors use a single layer anastomosis (4,8), most prefer the two layer technique. A 16-F Foley catheter is placed for urinary diversion and secured with tape to the hypogastrium to avoid decubitus at the peno-scrotal angle. All-silicone rubber catheter is used because they cause much less urethral inflammatory reaction than latex rubber catheters. After securing the hemostasis, the incision is closed by layers approximating the bulbospongiosum muscle and Colles' fascia with running absorbable sutures, mainly 3-O poliglactin, and the skin is closed with staples. The wound is permanently irrigated with saline plus Gentamicin throughout the procedure.

The use of drains is a matter of personal preference and case selection. Some leave a quarter-inch Penrose or a small suction drain overnight if there is too much bloody oozing, if a periurethral abscess

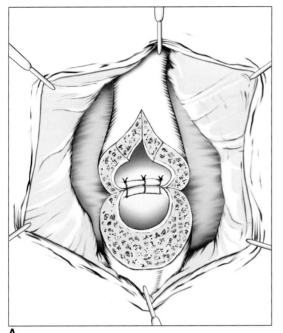

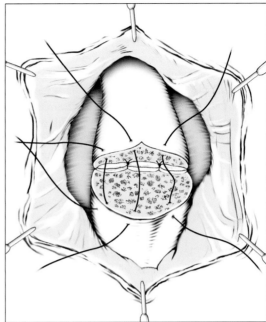

FIG. 10.7. The ventral suture is performed in two layers, a mucosal and a tunical layer

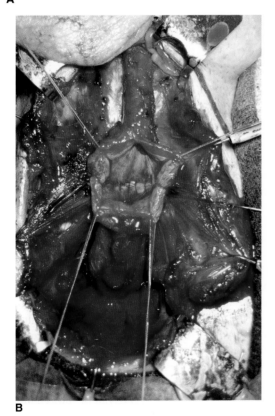

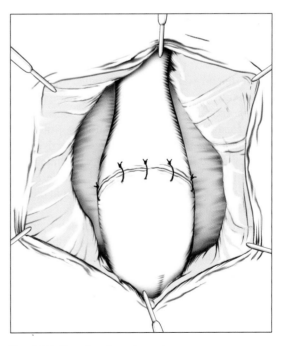

FIG. 10.6 (A) The dorsal suture has been completed in one layer. Knots are in the inside. (B) Mid-bulbar anastomotic urethroplasty. Note wide spatulation

FIG. 10.8. Completed anastomosis

has been drained or if there is a potential space that can collect fluid *(5,8,9)*. Others do not use drains at all, providing careful satisfactory hemostasis has been obtained. Because the spongiosum is a highly vascular structure and wound hematoma is a recognized postoperative complication, it has been our routine to use a closed-suction drain for the first 24 h. This may be particularly useful in young patients who might experience nocturnal erections or patients undergoing extensive inter-crural dissection.

6. Postoperative Care

Oral intake can be resumed 2 h after recovery from anesthesia. Usually patients are kept under bed-rest for 12–24 h and discharged home the day after surgery. However, there is a trend for outpatient surgery in urology just like in most areas of surgery. Anterior urethroplasty and particularly stricture excision and primary anastomosis are well suited for this approach in properly selected cases. According to recent reports, outpatient surgery decreases costs and increases patient satisfaction without compromising the overall surgical outcome *(7,19,20)*. Eligible candidates are well motivated patients, able to understand and follow hospital instructions regarding precautions and postoperative self-care. Patients who are of advanced age or have significant co-morbidities, complex difficult reconstructions, poor reliability, or unsatisfactory social support system are best admitted for hospital management. Nevertheless, even with these restrictions, a considerable percentage of patients can be good candidates for outpatient surgery. Soft elastic compressive perineal dressings, effective oral analgesia, and limited home activity are important. Some patients also use local wound anesthesia and perineal ice-packs. Drains are not used, and precise surgical technique with meticulous hemostasis is very important to avoid hematoma. In our opinion, the decision to perform outpatient urethroplasty should be taken according to the social and cultural status of the particular population under care in each center and, unfortunately, may not be feasible in many parts of the world.

Regarding catheter removal, there is no consensus about the time the catheter is left in place after surgery, and it is mainly an issue of personal preference. Most authors would leave the catheter for 1 to 3 wk and perform a pericatheter urethrogram before its removal to exclude the presence of extravasation *(5,8,9,21)*. However, in the present time of minimal impact surgery some authors have advocated early catheter removal to reduce patient disability. In a recent report, Al-Qudah et al. (15) performed voiding cystourethrogram on day 3 and noted extravasation in only 2 of 12 patients (17%) with anterior anastomotic reconstructions. In the 10 patients without extravasation the catheter was removed immediately while patients with extravasation had their Foley replaced. The voiding cystourethrogram was repeated 1 wk later in these two cases and was normal in both. There were no differences in outcome compared to another group of patients with "late" (8–14 d) catheter removal *(2)*. Although larger series are needed to confirm this approach it seems feasible to individualize the management of each case and each type of reconstruction in order to avoid unnecessary time of catheterization.

7. Clinical Outcomes of Excision and Primary Anastomosis

Excision and primary anastomosis is the procedure that offers the best chance for long-term cure of anterior urethral strictures. **Table 10.1** shows a collection of 10 series from the literature with more than 800 patients and long follow-up; cure rates ranged from 86% to 98.6%, with an average of 93%. Length of follow-up is important because it has been shown that failures may appear many years after surgery. In a cohort of 166 patients Andrich et al published re-stricture rates of 7%, 12%, 13%, and 14% after 1:5, 10, and 15 yr *(23)*. Although late failures can occur after 15 yr, most were diagnosed within the first 5 years *(23,24)*.

As with any open surgery, urethral reconstruction may be associated with significant patient discomfort, and post operative pain. However, in one prospective survey of 25 consecutive patients, Shenfeld et al. *(25)* found that recovery of a normal urinary flow after urethroplasty was linked to a very high degree of patient satisfaction, which clearly overcame the bother and pain associated with the surgery. As it can be anticipated, degree of satisfaction correlated directly with the objective

TABLE 10.1. Results of excision and primary anastomosis for anterior urethal stricture.

Author	No. patients	Avg. length	% Success	Follow-up
Eltahawy et al. *(33)*	213	1.9 cm	98.5	40.5 mo
Santucci et al. *(9)*	168	1.7 cm	95.2	72 mo
Andrich et al. *(23)*	82	-	86	180 mo
Micheli et al. *(6)*	71	0.5–3 cm	93	60 mo
Martinez-Piñeiro et al. *(26)*	69	<3 cm	88	44.4 mo
Jakse et al. *(27)*	60	1–4 cm	93.3	45 mo
Lindell et al. *(35)*	49	<2.5 cm	95.9	12–48 mo
Panagakis et al. *(36)*	42	<2 cm	95.2	3–72 mo
Kessler et al. *(24)*	40	-	86	72 mo
Barbagli et al. *(34)*	20	<2 cm	95	54.5 mo
Total	814		93	

results of surgery, as evaluated by peak urinary flow improvement *(25)*.

Surgical complications of urethroplasty are more frequent and significant with long, time-consuming or complex reconstructions. Excision and primary anastomosis has a low surgical complication rate, ranging from 6% to 10% in different series, most of which were minor *(4,9,26,27)*. Complication rates can be greater when investigated purposefully. In a detailed study of urethroplasty complications, Al-Qudah and Santucci performed a thorough review of their series looking for any possible complication, and also directly questioned the patients for self-reported complaints. Early complications in 24 anterior anastomotic urethroplasty were 25% minor and 0% major. Late complications were 42% minor and 21% major (erectile dysfunction in 4 patients and chordee in 1). All early complications were resolved but some late complications were not *(15)*. However, mean follow-up in this series was only 26 months and some late complications were prone to favorable resolution in time, particularly those related to sexual function.

Impact on sexual function is a well known concern with urethral surgery. Surgery around the bulb can theoretically damage neurovascular structures important for erection. The available information is somewhat limited but in general has shown little lasting deleterious effect on erection. Acute dysfunction as high as 53% after anastomotic urethroplasty has been reported, but it resolved with time in most cases with a definitive erectile failure rate around 5% *(28,29)*. The incidence of sexually related problems may be higher when studied using self-applied questionnaires *(15,30,31)*. In one sur-

vey, questionnaires were mailed to 200 patients who underwent anterior urethroplasty and to 48 patients who underwent circumcision. Overall satisfaction with erection worsened after surgery in 30.9% of patients in the urethroplasty group; however there were no statistical differences in sexual complaints compared with the circumcision group *(30)*. Reported cases with permanent postoperative erectile dysfunction correspond mainly to bulbo-prostatic anastomosis after pelvis fracture injury or tend to have longer strictures and increasing age *(23,29,32)*. Definitive erectile failure after bulbo-bulbar anastomosis is rare and has been reported in large series to go from 0% to 1.8% *(4,9,29,33)*.

Failure of this procedure is usually the result of ischemia or incomplete resection of the fibrous disease. Ischemia occurs because of failure to preserve the bulbar arteries or excessive tension at the anastomosis. Advanced age, previous surgery, heavy smoking and certain co-morbidities are also high risk factors for poor vascular status. Too much tension can also cause suture dehiscence and increased collagen deposit in the healing wound leading to undesired fibrosis. Fortunately, in most cases this fibrosis is mild and failures can be "rescued" with a single optical urethrotomy, taking the final success rate close to 100% *(6,9,24)*.

8. Summary

Stricture excision and primary anastomosis is the simplest and most effective surgical treatment for anterior strictures. After resecting all fibrotic urethra and stenosis, a wide mucosa-to-mucosa tension-free end-to-end anastomosis is performed to restore urethral continuity. This procedure is ideally suited for bulbar strictures 1- to 3-cm long. According to the local anatomy, this technique can also be successful in some selected cases with bulbar strictures up to 5 cm in length. Because the anterior penile urethra is stretched during erection, this procedure is limited in the pendulous urethra, as it can produce excessive shortening of the urethra and ventral curvature of the penis on erection. Complications are rare, mainly infection or hematoma of the operative wound. Sterile urine at the time of surgery and meticulous hemostasis are required to avoid them. Late failures are related to excessive tension at the anastomosis or incomplete stricture resection. Complete excision of the fibrotic urethra is essential, and the surgeon must be prepared to perform an alternative form of repair if this resection results in a defect too long for a tension-free reconstruction. When performed properly, excision and primary anastomosis is a well-tolerated, low-morbidity and highly effective procedure, with a well documented long-term cure rate of up to 95%.

Editorial Comment

Stricture excision and primary anastomosis offers excellent success and durability, with minimal morbidity or complications. Substitution urethroplasty, in contrast, has a lower short term success rate, as well as a recurrence rate that progressively increases with time. Clearly, when ever possible, a tension free, mucosa-to-musosa, end-to-end urethroplasty is the urethral reconstructive method of choice. In order to bridge the gap of excised urethra, either the urethra needs to be lengthened or the distance between the ends of the urethra need to be shortened. To lengthen the urethra, anastomotic urethroplasty takes advantage of the natural elasticity of the mobilized urethra. To shorten the distance between the ends, the corporal bodies can be separated, the inferior pubis can be excised, or the urethra re-routed.

Eltahawy et al. (J Urol 177:1803:2007) recently reported long-term results of the largest cohort of anastomotic (EPA) urethral surgeries in the literature to date. In a series of 260 EPA surgeries, at a mean follow-up of 4 years (50.2 months), strictures recurred in only 2% (3/260). Complications noted were relatively minor, all less then 5%, such as urinary tract infection, self-limited sensory changes in the feet due to positioning, transient ED, scrotalgia, and minor wound problems. Although urethrotomy admittedly has an advantage of shorter operative, catheterization, and recovery time, the near perfect success rates and long-term durability of EPA make it the obvious good standard that all other techniques should be judged.–S.B. Brandes

Appendix

Preferred Instruments and Suture of RG Gomez

Instruments

Although I use pretty much standard surgical instruments for urethroplasty, I also use:

2.5x magnifying loupes
Fiberoptic headlight
Bipolar cautery
DeBakey vascular forceps to handle the spongiosum and urethra
Ball-point curved Potts scissors
A long (6 cm) nasal speculum
A rubber inter-molar retractor (for BM procurement)

I always use the Scott retractor. My favorites are the medium size (blue) hooks and the double (green) hooks.

Suture

As suture material, I almost always use 5/0 and 6/0 Monocryl

References

1. Fenton AS, Morey AF, Aviles R, Garcia CR (2005)Anterior urethral strictures: etiology and characteristics. Urology 65:1055–1058
2. Baskin LS, McAninch JW (1993) Childhood urethral injuries: perspectives on outcome and treatment. Br J Urol 72:241–246
3. Andrich DE and Mundy AR.(2000) Urethral strictures and their surgical management. Br J Urol 86:571–580
4. Jezior JR, Schlossberg SM.(2002)Excision and primary anastomosis for anterior urethral stricture. Urol Clin N Am 29:373–380

5. Rosen MA, McAninch JW.(1996) Stricture excision and primary anastomosis for reconstruction of anterior urethral stricture. In: McAninch JW, Carroll PR, Jordan GH (eds) Traumatic and reconstructive urology. W.B. Saunders, Philadelphia, pp 565–569

6. Micheli E, Ranieri A, Peracchia G and Lembo A (2002) End-to end urethroplasty: long-term results. BJU Int 90:68–71

7. Peterson AC and Webster GD (2004) Management of urethral stricture disease: developing options for surgical intervention. BJU Int 94:971–976

8. Mundy AR (2005) Anastomotic urethroplasty. BJU Int 96:921–944

9. Santucci RA, Mario LA, McAninch JW (2002) Anastomotic urethroplasty for bulbar urethral stricture: analysis of 168 patients. J Urol 167:1715–1719

10. Guralnick ML, Webster GD (2001) The augmented anastomotic urethroplasty: indications and outcome in 29 patients. J Urol 165:1496–1501

11. Morey AF, Kizer WS (2006) Proximal bulbar urethroplasty via extended anastomotic approach— What are the limits? J Urol 175:2145–2149

12. Morey AF, McAninch JW (2000) Sonographic staging of anterior urethral strictures. J Urol 163:1070–1075

13. Gupta N, Dubey D, Mandhani A, Srivastava A, Kapoor R, Kumar A (2006) Urethral stricture assessment: a prospective study evaluating urethral ultrasonography and conventional radiological studies. BJU Int 98:149–153

14. Heidenreich A, Derschum W, Bonfig R, Wilbert DM (1994) Ultrasound in the evaluation of urethral stricture disease: a prospective study in 175 patients. Br J Urol 74:93–98

15. Al-Qudah HS, Santucci RA (2005) Extended complications of urethroplasty. Int Braz J Urol 31:315–325

16. Anema JG, Morey AF, McAninch JW, Mario LA, Wessells H (2000) Complications related to the high lithotomy position during urethral reconstruction. J Urol 164:360–363

17. Angermeier KW, Jordan GH (1994) Complications of the exaggerated lithotomy position: a review of 177 cases. J Urol 151:866

18. Eltahawy EA, Virasoro R, Jordan GH (2006) Vessel sparing excision and primary anastomosis of the urethra. J Urol 175(Suppl):104

19. Lewis JB, Wolgast KA, Ward JA, Morey AF (2002) Outpatient anterior urethroplasty: outcome analysis and patient selection criteria. J Urol 168:1024–1026

20. MacDonald MF, Al-Qudah HS, Santucci RA (2005) Minimal impact urethroplasty allows same-day surgery in most patients. Urology 66:850–853

21. Greenwell TJ, Venn SN, Mundy AR (1999) Changing practice in anterior urethroplasty. BJU Int 83:631–635

22. Al-Qudah HS, Cavalcanti AG, Santucci RA (2005) Early catheter removal after anterior anastomotic (3 days) and ventral buccal mucosa onlay (7days) urethroplasty. Int Braz J Urol 31:459–464

23. Andrich DE, Dunglison N, Greenwell TJ, Mundy AR (2003) The long-term results of urethroplasty. J Urol 170:90–92

24. Kessler TM, Schreiter F, Kralidis G, Heitz M, Olianas R and Fisch M (2003) Long-term results of surgery for urethral stricture: a statistical analysis. J Urol 170:840–844

25. Shenfeld OZ, Goldfarb H, Zvidat S, Gera S, Golan I, Gdor Y, Pode D (2005) A prospective survay of patients' satisfaction with urethral reconstructive surgery. J Urol 173(Suppl.): 35

26. Martinez-Pineiro JA, Carcamo P, Garcia Matres MJ, Martinez-Pineiro L, Iglesias JR, Rodriguez Ledesma JM (1997) Excision and anastomotic repair for urethral stricture disease: experience with 150 cases. Eur Urol 32:433–441

27. Jakse G, Marberger H (1986) Excisional repair of urethral stricture. Follow-up of 90 patients. Urology 27:233

28. Mundy AR (1993) Results and complications of urethroplasty and its future. Br J Urol 71:322

29. Andrich DE, O'Malley K, Holden F, Greenwell TJ, Mundy AR (2005) Erectile dysfunction following urethroplasty. J Urol 173(Suppl):90–91

30. Coursey JW, Morey AF, McAninch JW, Summerton DJ, Secrest C, White P, Miller K, Pieczonka C, Hochberg D, Armenakas N (2001) Erectile function after anterior urethroplasty J Urol 166:2273–2276

31. Erickson BA, Wysock JS, Jang TL, McVary KT, Gonzalez CM (2005) Male sexual function after urethral reconstructive surgery for stricture disease. J Urol 173(Suppl.):36

32. Anger JT, Sherman ND, Webster GD (2005) The effect of bulbar urethroplasty on erectile function. J Urol 173(Suppl):91

33. Eltahawy EA, Schlossberg SM, McCammon KA, Jordan GH (2005) Long term follow up for excision and primary anastomosis in anterior urethral strictures. J Urol 173(Suppl.):87

34. Barbagli G, Palminteri E, Bartoletti R, et al (1997) Long-term results of anterior and posterior urethroplasty with actuarial evaluation of the success rates. J Urol 158:1380–1382

35. Lindell O, Borkowski J, Noll F, Schreiter F (1993) Urethral stricture repair: results in 179 patients. Scand J Urol Nephrol 27:241–245

36. Panagakis A, Smith JC, Williams JL (1978) One-stage excision urethroplasty for stricture. Br J Urol 50:410

11
Buccal Mucosal Graft Urethroplasty

Guido Barbagli

Contents

1. Introduction.. 120
2. Development and Evolution of Dorsal Onlay Graft Urethroplasty 120
3. Significance of Urethral Anatomy and Selection of Surgical Technique 120
4. Preoperative Evaluation 121
5. Surgical Techniques 122
    5.1. Penile One-Stage Dorsal Inlay Buccal Mucosa Graft Urethroplasty......................... 122
    5.2. Preparation of the Bulbar Urethra... 122
    5.3. Ventral Onlay Buccal Mucosal Graft Urethroplasty 124
    5.4. Dorsal Onlay Buccal Mucosal Graft Urethroplasty Using Fibrin Glue...................... 127
6. Postoperative Care and Complications 128
7. Discussion.. 129
    7.1. Penile skin vs Buccal Mucosal Graft 130
    7.2. Flap vs Graft in Penile Urethroplasty 131
    7.3. Ventral vs Dorsal Bulbar Onlay Graft Urethroplasty... 131
    7.4. Excision of the Stricture vs Simple Augmentation of the Stricture............................ 133
Appendix... 133
References.. 133

Summary Buccal mucosa has received increased attention in the field of urological reconstructive surgery because it is readily available, is easily harvested from the cheek or lip and it leaves concealed donor site scar. Surgical treatment of adult penile and bulbar urethral strictures has been a constantly evolving process and considerable changes have recently been introduced. Here we report the development and the evolution of buccal mucosal graft urethroplasty with a detailed surgical techniques. We describe penile one-stage dorsal inlay buccal mucosa graft urethroplasty, ventral onlay buccal mucosal graft urethroplasty and dorsal onlay buccal mucosal graft urethroplasty. As free grafts have been making a comeback, with fewer surgeons using genital flaps we found that short bulbar strictures are amenable using primary anastomosis, with a high success rate. Longer strictures are repaired using ventral or dorsal graft urethroplasty, with the same success rate. New tools such as fibrin glue or engineered material will become a standard in future treatment. In reconstructive urethral surgery, the superiority of one approach over another is not yet clearly defined. The surgeon must be competent in the use of various techniques to deal with any condition of the urethra presented at the time of surgery.

Keywords Buccal mucosa; Graft; Urethroplasty; Urethra; Stricture; Fibrin glue.

From: *Current Clinical Urology: Urethral Reconstructive Surgery*
Edited by: S.B. Brandes © Humana Press, Totowa, NJ

1. Introduction

In an interesting historical overview on the employment of oral mucosa as surgical substitute material, Filipas et al. *(1)* traced its use in other medical areas to its development and application in urology. In 1993, for the first time, El-Kasaby et al. *(2)* reported that a buccal mucosal graft from the lower lip was used for treatment of penile and bulbar urethral strictures in adult patients without hypospadias. In 1996, Morey and McAninch *(3)* reported indications, operative techniques, and outcome in 13 adult patients with complex urethral strictures in which buccal mucosa was used as a non-tubularized ventral onlay graft for bulbar urethra reconstruction. Since that time, buccal mucosa has become an increasingly popular graft tissue for penile or bulbar urethral reconstruction performed in single or multiple stages.

Buccal mucosa has received increased attention in the field of urological reconstructive surgery because it is readily available in all patients and is easily harvested from the cheek or lip with a concealed donor site scar *(4,5)*. Moreover, buccal mucosa is hairless, has a thick elastin-rich epithelium, which makes it tough yet easy to handle, and has a thin and highly vascular lamina propria, which facilitates inosculation and imbibition *(4,5)*. Surgical treatment of adult penile and bulbar urethral strictures has been a constantly evolving process and considerable changes have recently been introduced with the dorsal onlay approach *(6–9)*, also known as the Barbagli procedure *(10)*.

2. Development and Evolution of Dorsal Onlay Graft Urethroplasty

Several experimental studies and clinical experiences have contributed to the development and evolution of dorsal onlay urethroplasty in surgical treatment of penile and bulbar urethral strictures. In 1979, Devine et al. *(11)* popularized the use of free skin graft techniques in anterior urethral reconstruction. In 1980, Monseur *(12)* described a new urethroplasty opening the urethra along its dorsal surface and fixing the opened urethra over the corpora cavernosa. Regeneration of the urethral mucosa is obtained by leaving a catheter

in place for a long period of time *(12)*. In 1995 and 1996, we combined Devine's technique with Monseur's and described the first penile and bulbar dorsal onlay skin graft urethroplasties *(6–9)*. In our technique, the graft is sutured to the corpora cavernosa and the urethra, which is opened along its dorsal surface, is sutured to the lateral margins of the graft. Regeneration of urethral mucosa is facilitated by the graft that works as an epithelial roof strip, thus considerably reducing the time for urethral regeneration. Moreover, according to the results of experimental and clinical studies by Weaver and Schulte *(13,14)* and Moore *(15)*, the dorsal buried strip facilitates urethral regeneration without formation of the scar tissue. Over time, our original technique has been greatly improved *(16–18)* and new changes are continuously being suggested *(19)*. Moreover, the dorsal placement of the graft may be combined with Snodgrass's incision of the urethral plate *(20)*, as suggested by Hayes and Malone for childhood hypospadias surgery *(21)* and by Asopa et al. and Gupta et al. for penile and bulbar urethroplasty in adults *(22,23)*.

3. Significance of Urethral Anatomy and Selection of Surgical Technique

Penile urethroplasty is usually a simple procedure in patients with a normal penis, but it can be a difficult challenge in men with strictures associated to failed hypospadias repair or genital Lichen sclerosus, in which the penis is fully involved in the disease *(24)*. In general, the choice of surgical procedure for repair of penile urethral strictures is based on the etiology of the disease *(24)*. In patients with a normal penis, the penile skin, urethral plate, corpus spongiosum, and dartos fascia are suitable for urethral reconstruction, and one-stage urethroplasty using a dartos fascial flap with a penile skin island or using a free graft is the surgery of choice worldwide. In patients who have experienced failed hypospadias repair or Lichen sclerosus, rendering the penile skin, urethral plate and dartos fascia unsuitable for urethral reconstruction, multistage urethroplasty is generally recommended *(24)*. Selection of a surgical technique for penile urethra reconstruction, in addition to respecting the status of the penile tissue and components, must

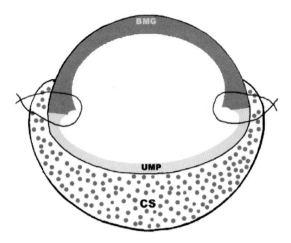

FIG. 11.1. Dorsal onlay graft: the buccal mucosa graft (BMG) is applied on the corpora cavernosa and covered by the urethral mucosal plate (UMP) and by the intact spongiosum tissue (CS)

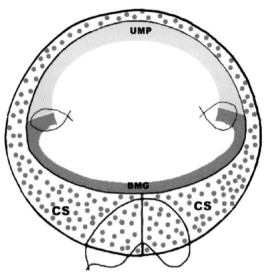

FIG. 11.2. Ventral onlay graft: the buccal mucosal graft (BMG) is applied on the urethral mucosal plate (UMP), and the spongiosum tissue (CS) is closed over the graft

also be based on proper anatomic characteristics of the penile tissues to ensure flap or graft take and survival. Furthermore, sexual function can be placed at risk by any surgery on the genitalia; thus, dissection must avoid interference with neurovascular supply to the penis. Flaps or grafts should not compromise penile length or cause penile chordee and should certainly not untowardly affect penile appearance *(24)*.

In the bulbar urethra, the relationship between the spongiosum tissue and the urethral lumen is different from that noted in the penile urethra. The corpus spongiosum is thicker in its ventral aspect and dorsally thinner *(16,17)*. Furthermore, the urethral lumen is located dorsally and not centrally, thus a dorsal incision may more likely to preserve the residual blood supply to the spongiosum tissue. Adequate neovascularization of the graft is achieved by applying the patch so that it adheres to the corpora cavernosa, and spread fixation may decrease the risk of graft contraction and sacculation. The buccal mucosal graft is covered by the intact overlying urethral mucosal plate and corpus spongiosum (**Fig. 11.1**), and fistula formation or patch necrosis has no yet been reported in the literature following this procedure. In patients who have undergone repeated and deep internal urethrotomies at the 12-o'clock position, the urethral lumen may be adherent and firmly fixed to the tunica albuginea because the longitudinal internal cut involve the urethral mucosa, spongiosum tissue, and tunica

albuginea. Unfortunately, the healing of this kind of urethrotomy, along with the extravasation can cause a scar that fuses the urethral mucosa to the tunica albuginea. In this situation, mobilization of the urethra from the corpora cavernosa may be may be difficult. In patients with an implanted bulbar urethral stent in place, it likewise may by difficult to approach and free the dorsal urethral lumen. In obese patients, exposure of the dorsal aspect of the urethra may also no be optimal. Finally, in patients with previous failed urethroplasty or with bulbar strictures located more proximally to or just at the external distal sphincter, the dorsal approach to the urethra may be particularly difficult. In these situations, the urethra is not mobilized from the corpora cavernosa, but is opened along its ventral surface and the buccal mucosal graft is sutured ventrally to the edges of the mucosal urethral plate and covered by the spongiusum tissue (**Fig. 11.2**). We present here three surgical techniques for one-stage repair of penile or bulbar urethral strictures using buccal mucosal grafts.

4. Preoperative Evaluation

The clinical history and medical charts of the patient requiring penile urethroplasty must be carefully reviewed and the genitalia meticulously inspected taking into consideration glans shape, scars in the penile and scrotal skin, the presence of residual foreskin, or hair in the meatus or stones in the urethra. In addition, the presence of Lichen sclerosus disease must be excluded. Preoperative retrograde urethrography is mandatory to evaluate the urethral plate. Patients selected for a penile one-stage procedure should be informed that early or later complications, such as hematoma, infection, meatal stenosis or fistula may occur with any surgical technique.

In patients undergoing bulbar urethroplasty, clinical history and medical charts are reviewed to evaluate present effects of previous perineal blunt trauma or repeated failed urethrotomy or urethroplasty. Preoperative retrograde urethrography is mandatory to evaluate the site, number and length of stricture and voiding cystourethrography is useful in evaluating continence of the bladder neck and urethral dilation proximally to the stenosis. Sonourethrography and urethroscopy are suggested to collect more detailed information on stricture characteristics. Patients are fully informed that bulbar urethroplasty is a safe procedure as far as sexual function is concerned.

The patient's clinical history, as well as the stricture etiology, location, and length must be carefully examined to better define the characteristics needed in the buccal mucosa graft. Patients who currently had an infectious disease of the mouth (such as Candida, Varicellavirus, or Herpes virus) or who have had previous surgery in the mandibular arch that prevented the mouth from being opened wide, or who play a wind instrument are informed that genital or extra genital skin would be used for the urethroplasty.

Three days before surgery, the patient should begin using clorhexidine mouthwash for oral cleansing and continue using it for three days following surgery. A broad-spectrum antibiotic is administered intravenously during the procedure and for three days afterward.

5. Surgical Techniques

5.1. Penile One-Stage Dorsal Inlay Buccal Mucosa Graft Urethroplasty

A circumcoronal incision is made through the foreskin completely degloving the penis (**Fig. 11.3**). The penile urethra is exposed and

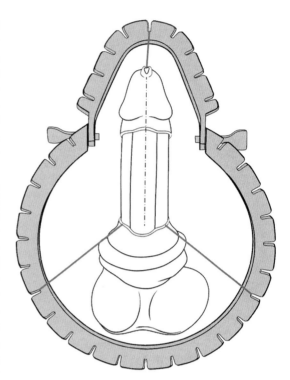

FIG. 11.3. Degloving of the penis with circumcoronal incision. The ventral longitudinal incision on the glans and penile urethra is underlined

the strictured tract is fully opened by a ventral midline incision (**Figs. 11.3 and 11.4**). The urethral mucosal plate is longitudinally incised on the midline down to the tunica albuginea of the corpora cavernosa (**Figs. 11.4 and 11.5**). The wings of the urethral mucosal plate are laterally mobilized to create a bed for the graft (**Fig. 11.5**). The buccal mucosa graft is sutured and quilted onto the bed of the dorsal urethral incision using interrupted 6-O polyglactin sutures, and augmentation of the urethral plate is obtained (**Fig. 11.6**). The urethra is closed and tubularized up to the glans over a Foley 14-French grooved silicone catheter (**Figs. 11.7 and 11.8**), taking advantage of the mobilized wings of the urethral plate. The glans and the penile skin are closed. The catheter is left in place for 2 wk.

5.2. Preparation of the Bulbar Urethra

The patient is placed in simple low lithotomy position. The patient's calves are carefully placed in Allen stirrups with sequential inflatable compression sleeves and the lower extremities are then

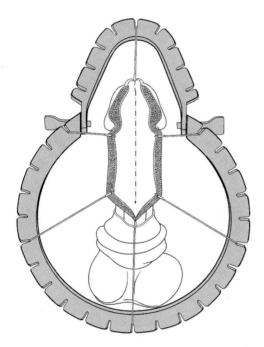

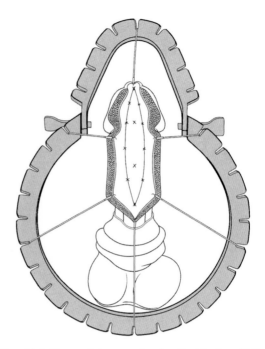

FIG. 11.4. The glans and the penile urethra are fully opened and the midline incision of the mucosal urethral plate is underlined

FIG. 11.6. The graft is sutured and quilted in the middle of the urethral plate

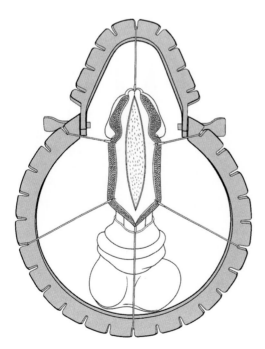

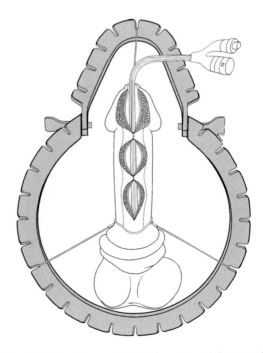

FIG. 11.5. The mucosal urethral plate is incised on the midline

FIG. 11.7. The Foley catheter is inserted and the ventral urethral surface is closed

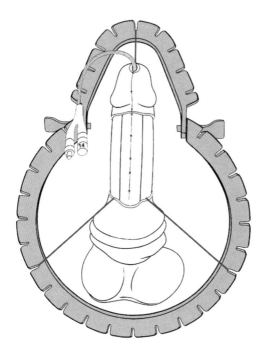

FIG. 11.8. The glans and the urethra are closed

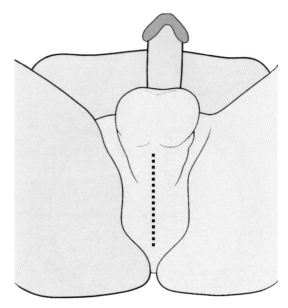

FIG. 11.9. The midline perineal incision is underlined

suspended by the patient's feet within the boots of
the stirrups. Proper positioning ensures that there is
no pressure on any aspect of the calf muscles and
no inward boot rotation to avoid peroneal nerve
injury. The skin of the suprapubic region, scrotum
and perineum is shaved and the region is prepared
and draped appropriately.

Methylene blue is injected into the urethra
to better define the urethral mucosa involved in
the disease, and a midline perineal incision is
made (**Fig. 11.9**). The bulbocavernous muscles
are separated in the midline and a self-retractor
with atraumatic plastic hooks is positioned (**Fig.
11.10**). In patients with a proximal urethral stricture the central tendon of the perineum is dissected (**Fig. 11.11**). The bulbar urethra is freed
for its entire length (**Fig. 11.12**) and the ventral
or dorsal onlay graft urethroplasty is performed.

5.3. Ventral Onlay Buccal Mucosal Graft Urethroplasty

The distal extent of the stenosis is identified by
gently inserting a 16-French catheter with a soft
round tip until it meets resistance (**Fig. 11.13**).
The corpus spongiosum is incised in the ventral

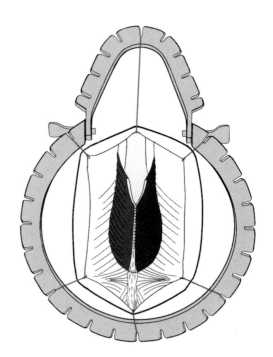

FIG. 11.10. The muscles are separated, and the self-
retractor is placed

midline until the catheter tip and urethral lumen
are exposed. The stricture is then incised along its
entire length by extending the urethrotomy distally
and proximally (**Fig. 11.14**). Once the entire stric-

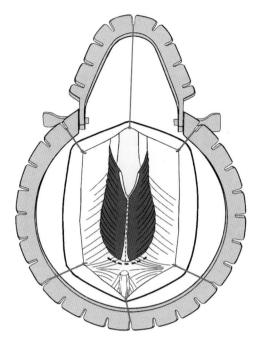

FIG. 11.11. The section of the central tendon of perineum is underlined

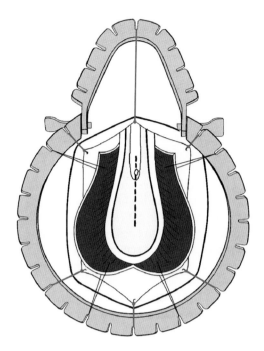

FIG. 11.13. The distal extent of stricture is identified and the incision on the ventral urethral surface is underlined

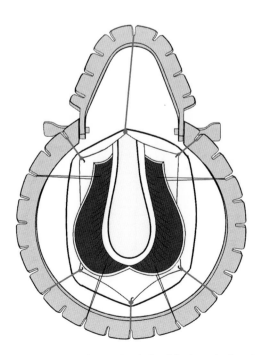

FIG. 11.12. The bulbar urethra is freed for its entire length

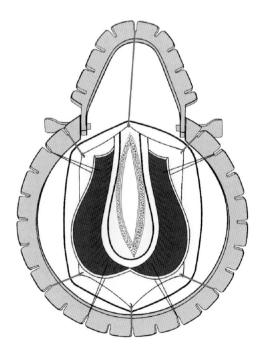

FIG. 11.14. The bulbar urethra is fully opened along its ventral surface

ture has been incised, the length and width of the remaining urethral plate are measured. Proximal and distal calibration of the urethra with a special modified nasal speculum is critical for identifying any residual narrowing. The buccal mucosal graft is trimmed to its appropriate size, according to the length and width of the urethrotomy. The two ends of the graft are sutured to the proximal and distal apices of the urethrotomy and running 6-O polyglactin suture is used to complete a watertight anastomosis between the left margin of the graft and the left margin of the urethral mucosal plate (**Fig. 11.15**). A Foley 16-Fr grooved silicone catheter is inserted. The graft is rotated over the catheter and running 6-O polyglactin suture is used to complete a watertight anastomosis between the right margin of the graft and the right margin of the mucosal urethral plate (**Fig. 11.16**). After completion of graft suturing the corpus spongiosum is closed over the graft with 4-O polyglactin interrupted suture (**Fig. 11.7**). The bulbocavernous muscle is re-approximated over the spongiosum tissue (**Fig. 11.18**) and Colles' fascia, the perineal fat and the skin are closed with interrupted absorbable sutures (**Fig. 11.19**). The catheter is left in place for 3 wk.

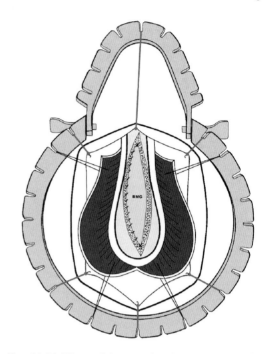

FIG. 11.16. The graft is rotated and sutured to the right margin of the mucosal urethral plate

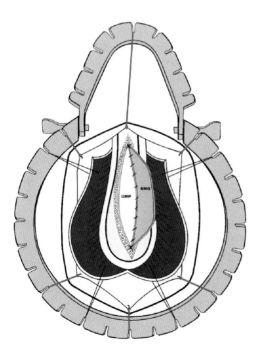

FIG. 11.15. The margin of the graft is sutured to the left margin of the mucosal urethral plate

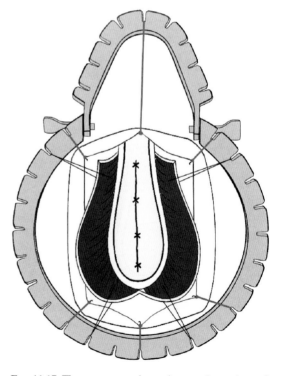

FIG. 11.17. The corpus spongiosum is sutured over the graft

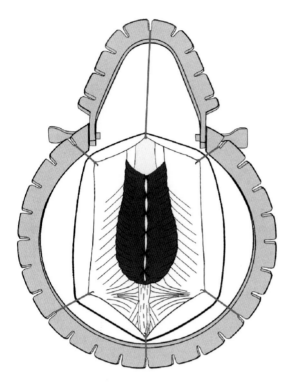

FIG. 11.18. The bulbocavernous muscles are sutured on the midline

5.4. Dorsal Onlay Buccal Mucosal Graft Urethroplasty Using Fibrin Glue

The bulbar urethra is dissected from the corpora cavernosa (**Fig. 11.20**). The urethra is rotated 180 degrees and the distal extent of the stenosis is identified by gently inserting a 16-Fr catheter with a soft round tip until it meets resistance (**Fig. 11.21**). The dorsal urethral surface is incised in the midline until the catheter tip and urethral lumen are exposed. The stricture is then incised along its entire length by extending the urethrotomy distally and proximally (**Fig. 11.22**). Once the entire stricture has been incised, the length and width of the remaining urethral plate is measured. Proximal and distal calibration of the urethra with a specially modified nasal speculum is critical for identifying any residual narrowing. The buccal mucosal graft is trimmed to an appropriate size according to the length and width of the urethrotomy. The bulbar urethra is moved to the right side and 2 ml of fibrin glue are injected over the albuginea of the corpora cavernosa (**Fig. 11.22**). The buccal mucosal graft is spread fixed over the fibrin glue bed (**Fig. 11.23**). The two apices of the graft are sutured to the

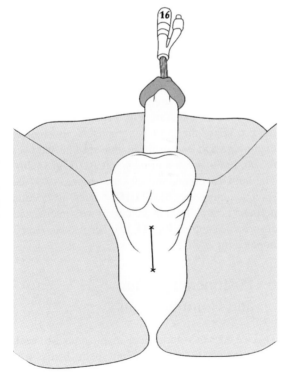

FIG. 11.19. The Foley catheter is in place and the perineal incision is closed

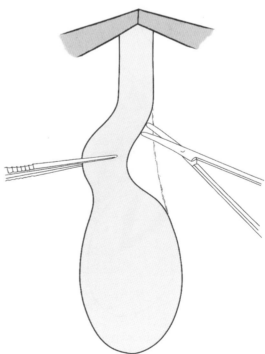

FIG. 11.20. The urethra is freed from the corpora cavernosa

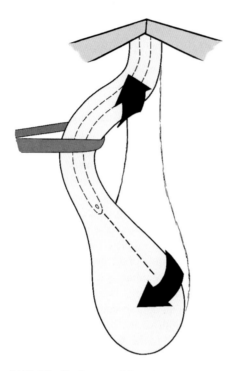

FIG. 11.21. The distal extent of the stricture is identified and the incision on the dorsal urethral surface is underlined

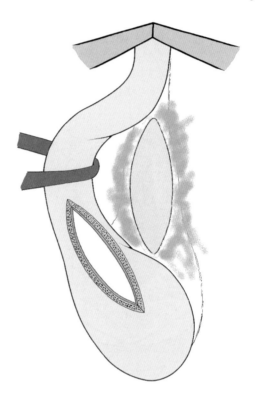

FIG. 11.23. The graft is applied over the fibrin glue bed

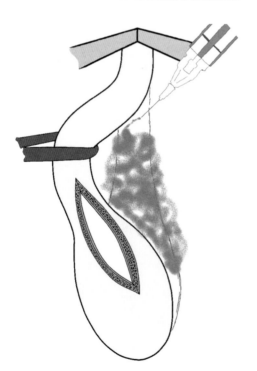

FIG. 11.22. The bulbar urethra is fully opened along its dorsal surface and fibrin glue is injected over the albuginea of the corpora cavernosa

proximal and distal apices of the urethrotomy (**Fig. 11.24**). A Foley 16-Fr grooved silicone catheter is inserted. The bulbar urethra is rotated to its original position over the graft (**Fig. 11.25**). Three interrupted 4-zero polyglactin sutures for each side are used to stabilize the urethral margins to the corpora cavernosa over the graft (**Fig. 11.26**). At the end of the procedure the graft is completely covered by the urethra and 2 ml of fibrin glue are injected over the urethra to prevent urinary leakage (**Fig. 11.26**). The bulbocavernous muscles are sutured over the spongiosum tissue (**Fig. 11.18**). Colles' fascia, the perineal fat and the skin are closed with interrupted absorbable sutures (**Fig. 11.19**). The catheter is left in place for 2 wk.

6. Postoperative Care and Complications

Two ice bags are immediately applied on the cheek and genitalia to reduce edema, pain, hematoma, and nocturnal erections. The patient initially consumes a clear liquid diet and ice cream before

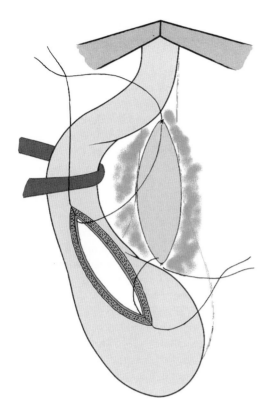

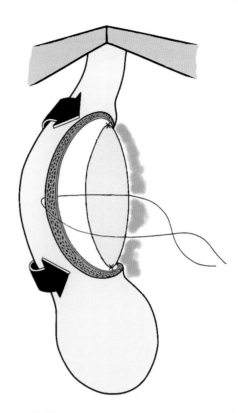

FIG. 11.24. The apices of the graft are sutured to the apices of urethrotomy

FIG. 11.25. The urethra is moved to its original position to completely cover the graft

advancing to a soft, then regular diet. The patient is discharged from the hospital three days after surgery. Two or three weeks after surgery, the catheter is removed and voiding cystourethrography is at that time obtained. All patients are maintained on oral antibiotics until the catheter is removed.

In patients who have undergone penile urethroplasty, early complications include edema, hematoma, and infection. If infection is present and pus discharges from the urethral meatus, the catheter should be immediately removed and a suprapubic urinary drain left in place. In addition, the patient should be instructed to void through the new urethra twice daily to wash the pus from it. Unfortunately, patients who have early complications such as hematoma and infection, frequently develop major complications such as suture dehiscence, tissue necrosis and fistulas. Additional late complications include fistulas, meatal stenosis, meatal retraction, cosmetic defects, and penile skin necrosis.

Spontaneous fistula closure has rarely been observed. In such cases, a new surgical approach may be necessary to open the fistulous tract or a wide meatotomy may be required for meatal stenosis. In patients who have undergone ventral or dorsal bulbar urethroplasty, a possible early minor complication is urethrorrhagia due to nocturnal erections. Possible later minor complications are temporary numbness, dysesthesia to the perineum, and scrotal swelling.

7. Discussion

The surgical treatment of adult anterior urethral strictures is continually evolving, and renewed controversy exists over the best means of reconstructing the anterior urethra, since the superiority of one approach over another is not yet clearly defined. The reconstructive urologist must be fully familiar with the use of both flaps and grafts to deal with any condition of the urethra at the time of surgery.

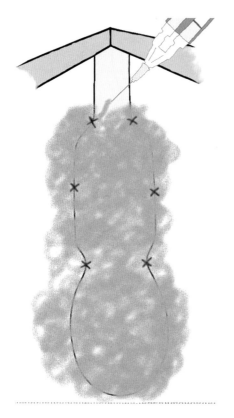

Fig. 11.26. The urethra is fixed to the corpora and fibrin glue is injected over the urethra

7.1. Penile skin vs Buccal Mucosal Graft

Buccal mucosa has become the most popular substitute material in the treatment of urethral stricture disease and its success is well documented in numerous series of patients having undergone anterior urethral reconstruction. Before the use of buccal mucosa as a substitute material, penile skin was the substitute material suggested for anterior urethroplasty. However, is buccal mucosa really superior to penile skin? Alsikafi et al. *(25)* compared the outcome of 95 buccal urethroplasty and 24 penile skin graft urethroplasties in an effort to answer whether buccal mucosa is really best. The overall success rate of penile skin urethroplasty was 84%, with a mean follow-up of 201 months, whereas the success rate of buccal urethroplasty was 87% with a mean follow-up of 48 months and no statistically significant difference was found between the two groups (**Table 10.11** *[25]*). Alsikafi et al. *(25)* concluded that penile skin and

buccal mucosa are excellent materials for substitution urethroplasty with a comparable success rate, though penile skin appears to have a longer follow-up. Gozzi et al. *(26)* reported the outcome of 194 patients with penile, bulbar and posterior urethral strictures treated using genital and extragenital free skin grafts and concluded that the skin grafts provide excellent results with an average follow-up of 31 months (**Table 11.1**).

At our Center, 95 consecutive patients, average age 44 yy (range 17 to 79 yr), underwent bulbar urethra reconstruction between January 1994 and December 2004 for urethral strictures *(27,28)*. In 45 patients the stricture was treated using penile skin as a substitute material *(27)* and in 50 patients buccal mucosa was used as a substitute material *(28)*. Thirty-three of the 45 penile skin urethroplasties were successful (73%) and 12 (27%) were failures *(27)*. Forty-two of the 50 buccal mucosa urethroplasty were successful (84%) and 8 (16%) were failures *(28)*. Thus, the skin graft urethroplasty showed a higher failure rate (27%) compared to buccal mucosa (16%; **Table 11.1**). The penile skin group of patients did have a longer follow-up (mean, 71 mo) compared with the buccal mucosa group of patients (mean, 42 mo; **Table 11.1**). Yet, the penile skin group showed a higher number of failures involving the entire graft area (17% vs 6%), requiring surgical revision using a multi-stage procedure *(28)*.

Finally, in patients requiring anterior urethroplasty, the use of buccal mucosa avoids cosmetic disadvantages and consequences caused by the use of genital skin, as it is readily available in all

Table 11.1. Penile skin vs buccal mucosal (BM) onlay grafts.

Authors	Journal, year	No. patients	Substitute material	Success rate (%)	Mean follow-up (months)
Alsikafi et al. *(25)*	J Urol, 2005	119	Skin 24 BM 95	84% 87%	201 48
Barbagli et al. *(27,28)*	J Urol, 2004–2005	95	Skin 45BM 50	73% 84%	71 42
Gozzi et al. *(26)*	J Urol, 2006	194	Skin	Excellent	31

patients with a concealed donor site scar *(4,5)*. Moreover, the elasticity and easy handling of the buccal mucosa is superior to penile skin promoting the use of graft in original techniques *(16–18)*.

7.2. Flap vs Graft in Penile Urethroplasty

The controversy over the best mean of reconstructing the penile urethra has been renewed and in recent years free grafts have been making a comeback, with fewer surgeons using genital flaps *(18,29,30)*. The current literature, however, does not clearly support the use of one technique over the other. Rarely has a prospective study compared the graft with the flap, making it hard to declare a clear favorite *(29)*. That being said, however, the use of free grafts does not require extensive training in tissue-transfer procedures, as is required with the use of penile flaps *(18)*.

At present, we do not know which patients undergoing one-stage penile urethroplasty with a buccal mucosa graft will have a successful outcome *(18)*. Nor are we certain about the proper anatomic characteristics the penis should have to ensure that the grafts take *(18)*. The penile spongiosum tissue and dartos fascia do not ensure good vascular and mechanical support to the graft in all patients *(18,29)*. This leads to a number of questions *(18,29–31)*. What type of vascular support can be used? In which patients will the use of a pedicled flap have better chances of success than a free graft? What is the role of urethral plate salvage in the reconstructive armamentarium? Morey *(31)* suggests that urethral plate replacement may be necessary in patients with complex, long, severe strictures, and he describes a new penile urethroplasty that uses a combined graft-flap procedure. Identification and use of criteria to more carefully select the appropriate procedure for the patient should help answer all of these questions, and might clarify whether the use of a buccal mucosa graft is preferable to the use of a penile flap.

7.3. Ventral vs Dorsal Bulbar Onlay Graft Urethroplasty

Buccal mucosa graft onlay urethroplasty represents the most widespread method used for the repair of strictures in the bulbar urethra because of its thick and highly vascular spongiosum tissue

(24). Location of the patch has recently become a contentious issue *(10,32,33)*. Wessells suggests that the technical advantages of ventral onlay urethroplasty are considerable: complete circumferential mobilization of the bulbar urethra is not necessary, thus preserving arterial and venous connections to the corpora cavernosa; the stricture is easily visualized; the lumen is clearly delineated with urethrotomy, allowing the surgeon to identify mucosal edges, measure the size of the plate, carry out a watertight anastomosis, and , if necessary, excise portions of the stricture and perform dorsal reanastomosis *(34)*. Moreover, Armenakas *(35)* emphasizes that ventral graft placement, requiring less urethral dissection and mobilization, is technically easier.

Success with buccal mucosa grafts for repairing bulbar urethral strictures has generally been high with dorsal *(7,10,26,27,36–39)* or ventral onlay grafts *(3,29,34,35,40–42)*, and the different graft positions have shown no difference in success rate (**Table 11.2** *[28,43]*). We retrospectively reviewed the outcome analysis of 50 patients who underwent three types of urethroplasty with the buccal mucosal graft placed on the ventral, dorsal or lateral surface of the bulbar urethra *(28)*. Of 50 cases, 42 (84%) were successful and 8 (16%) failed. The 17 ventral grafts were successful in 14 cases (83%) and failed in 3 (17%); the 27 dorsal grafts were successful in 23 cases (85%) and failed in 4 (15%); the 6 lateral grafts were successful in 5 cases (83%) and failed in 1 (17%) (**Table 11.2**). Failures involved the anastomotic site (distal in two and proximal in three) and the entire grafted area in three cases. In our experience, the placement of the buccal mucosa grafts onto the ventral, dorsal or lateral surface of the bulbar urethra showed the same success rates (83% to 85%), outcome was not affected by the surgical technique and stricture recurrence was uniformly distributed in all patients (**Table 11.2** *[28]*). Others authors have found that these rings cause stricture recurrence after substitution bulbar urethroplasty *(36,41–43)*.

Recently, we retrospectively reviewed the patterns of failure after bulbar substitution urethroplasty *(44)*. In particular, we investigated the prevalence and location of anastomotic fibrous ring strictures occurring at the apical anastomoses between the graft and urethral plate after using the above three types of onlay graft techniques (**Table 11.3**).

TABLE 11.2. Ventral vs. dorsal buccal mucosal (BM) onlay grafts.

Authors	Journal, year	Sub-stitute material	Graft location	No. patients	Success rate (%)	Fail-ures (%)
Barbagli et al. *(28)*	J Urol, 2005	BM	Ventral	17	83	17
			Dorsal	27	85	15
			Lateral	6	83	17
Abouassaly et al. *(43)*	J Urol, 2005	BM	Ventral	100	92	8
			Dorsal			
			Combined			

TABLE 11.3. Prevalence of anastomotic fibrous rings in 107 substitution bulbar onlay graft urethroplasty.

				Type of failure		
Urethroplasty (substitute material)	No. patients	Success rate, no. (%)	Failure rate, no. (%)	Entire grafted area, no. (%)	Anastomotic ring stricture, no. (%)	Site of ring (no.)
Dorsal onlay skin graft urethroplasty (skin)	45	33 (73)	12 (27)	8 (17)	4 (8)	distal (2); proximal (2)
Buccal mucosal onlay graft urethroplasty (buccal mucosa)	50	42 (84)	8 (16)	3 (6)	5 (10)	distal (2); proximal (3)
Augmented end-to-end urethroplasty (buccal mucosa)	12	10 (84)	2 (16)	1 (8)	1 (8)	proximal (1)
Total	107	85 (80)	22 (20)	12 (11)	10 (9)	distal (5); proximal (5)

A review of 107 patients undergoing bulbar urethroplasty between 1994 and 2004 was performed ***(44)***. The mean patient age was 44 yr old. Forty-five patients underwent dorsal onlay skin graft urethroplasty, 50 patients underwent buccal mucosa onlay graft urethroplasty, and 12 patients underwent augmented end-to-end urethroplasty. Clinical outcome was considered either a success or a failure depending on whether any postoperative procedure was needed, including dilation. The mean follow-up was 74 months (range, 12–130). Out of 107 patients, 85 (80%) were successful and 22 (20%) failures. Failure in 12 patients (11%) involved the entire grafted area and in 10 patients (9%) involved the anastomotic site (five distal, five proximal; **Table 11.3**). Urethrography, sonourethrography, and urethroscopy were fundamental to see the difference between full-length or focal extension of restricture. The prevalence and location of anastomotic ring strictures after bulbar urethroplasty were uniformly distributed in the three different surgical techniques using skin or buccal mucosa (**Table 11.3** *[44]*). Further studies are necessary to clarify the etiology of these fibrous ring strictures.

We recently developed a new and interesting step in the use of our dorsal onlay graft urethroplasty, using fibrin glue to fix the graft to the albuginea of the corpora cavernosa ***(19)***. The use of fibrin glue avoids the necessity of numerous interrupted stitches to fix the graft: this is a tedious and time-consuming step in onlay urethroplasty. Moreover, the apposition of the graft and its adhesion to the corpora cavernosa can be simplified by the use of fibrin glue, which allows ideal fixation of the graft to its vascular bed and therefore better revascularization of the transplanted tissue. Tenacious adhesion of the graft keeps it wide open reducing the risk of sacculation and shrinkage, thus allowing the surgeon to perform an easier anastomosis between the graft and the urethral margins. Fibrin glue shortens graft revascularization time, because a fibrin clot represents the first link in a chain of events, which rules the process of revascularization of any free graft (followed by imbibition and inosculation). Experimental studies done in the rat documented better healing and smaller shrinkage of the free skin graft when fibrin glue was utilized *(45)*.

7.4. Excision of the Stricture vs Simple Augmentation of the Stricture

In 2004, Delvecchio et al. *(46)* suggested that the use of augmented roof-strip anastomotic urethroplasty using incorporation of the graft onlay into the receiving urethral plate is less successful, either because of the inherent deterioration of transferred tissues exposed to urine or to the fact that the onlay is performed in a densely spongiofibrotic area, generally at the site the stricture disease originated, that is unsuitable for simple onlay grafting. These authors propose always excising this area, followed by direct reanastomosis of the floor strip and onlay of the adjacent "better" stricture, whatever its length *(46)*. The authors show that this technique had only a 5.2% failure rate in 38 patients, compared with 9% failure rate in 11 patients who underwent a simple augmented graft urethroplasty without excision of the strictured tract, and conclude that excision of the worst stricture segment (up to 2 cm) avoids a long onlay in a poor urethral bed where failure often occurs at the location of even the smallest stricture caliber *(46)*. Recently, Al-Qudah and Santucci *(47)* reported 47 short urethral strictures treated with end-to-end anastomosis or buccal mucosal onlay grafts and compared early and intermediate outcome to determine which is the best technique. Buccal mucosal urethroplasty had superior success rates and fewer complications than anastomotic urethroplasty and it is suggested as the operation of choice even for short bulbar strictures *(47)*. In 2006, Abouassaly and Angermeier *(48)* recommended the complete excision of the stricture and the use of an augmented anastomotic repair in patients undergoing substitution urethroplasty for strictures that contain a particularly narrow or dense area of 1–2 cm in length.

Recently, we retrospectively reviewed 107 patients who underwent surgical reconstruction for bulbar urethral strictures between 1994 and 2004 *(44)*. The mean patient age was 44 yr. Ninety-five patients underwent simple augmentation of the stricture with the onlay graft and 12 patients underwent excision of the stricture with anastomotic graft urethroplasty. Out of 107 patients, 85 (80%)

treatments were considered successful and 22 (20%) failures. Seventy-five of 95 augmented graft urethroplasties were successful (79%), and 20 (21%) were failures. Ten out of 12 anastomotic graft urethroplasties were successful (84%) and 2 (16%) were failures *(44)*.

Appendix

Preferred Instruments of G Barbagli

Allen stirrups (Allen Medical System, The Org Group, Anton, MA, USA)
Sequential Compression Sleeves (Tyco Healthcare Group LP, Mansfield, MA, USA)
Mouth self-retractor with its own light (Ce.Di.Sa. Srl, Sesto Fiorentino, Italy)
Plastic ring retractor with atraumatic plastic hooks (Lone Star, Medical Products, Huston, TX, USA)
Modified nasal speculum with atraumatic thin round tip (Ce.Di.Sa. Srl, Sesto Fiorentino, Italy)
Silicone board (Ce.Di.Sa. Srl, Sesto Fiorentino, Italy)
Turner-Warwick needle holder (Lawton G.m.b.H and Company, Fridingen, Germany)
Super-light titanium needle holder (Lawton G.m.b.H and Company, Fridingen, Germany)
Microsurgical needle holder (Lawton G.m.b.H and Company, Fridingen, Germany)
Microsurgical scissors (Lawton G.m.b.H and Company, Fridingen, Germany)
Black porcelain scissors (Lawton G.m.b.H and Company, Fridingen, Germany)
Methylene blue
Foley grooved silicone catheter (Rush GMBH, Kernen, Germany)
Polyglactin suture (Vicryl) (Ethicon, Johnson & Johnson Intl., St-Stevens-Woluwe, Belgium)

References

1. Filipas D, Wahlmann U, Hohenfellner R (1998) History of oral mucosa. Eur Urol 34:165–168
2. El-Kasaby AW, Fath-Alla M, Noweir AM, El-Halaby MR, Zakaria W, El-Beialy MH. (1993) The use of buccal mucosa patch graft in the management of anterior urethral strictures. J Urol 149:276–278
3. Morey AF, McAninch J W (1996) When and how to use buccal mucosal grafts in adult bulbar urethroplasty. Urology 48:194–198
4. Wood DN, Allen SE, Andrich DE, Greenwell TJ, Mundy AR (2004) The morbidity of buccal mucosal

graft harvest for urethroplasty and the effect of non-closure of the graft harvest site on postoperative pain. J Urol 172:580–583

5. Barbagli G, Palminteri E, De Stefani S, Lazzeri M (2006) Harvesting buccal mucosal grafts. Keys to successs. Contemp Urol 18:16–24

6. Barbagli G, Menghetti I, Azzaro F (1995) A new urethroplasty for bulbous urethral strictures. Acta Urol Ital 9:313–317

7. Barbagli G, Selli C, Tosto A, Palminteri E (1996) Dorsal free graft urethroplasty. J Urol 155:123–126

8. Barbagli G, Selli C, Di Cello V, Mottola A (1996) A one-stage dorsal free-graft urethroplasty for bulbar urethral strictures. Br J Urol 78:929–932

9. Barbagli G, Azzaro F, Lombardi G, Palminteri E (1996) A new one-stage free skin patch graft urethroplasty for anterior urethral strictures. Afr J Urol 2:103–108

10. Andrich DE, Leach CJ, Mundy AR (2001) The Barbagli procedure gives the best results for patch urethroplasty of the bulbar urethra. BJU Int 88:385–389

11. Devine PC, Wendelken JR, Devine CJ (1979) Free full thickness skin graft urethroplasty: current technique. J Urol 121:282–285

12. Monseur J. (1980) L'elargissement de l'urètre au moyen du plan sus urètral. J Urol 86:439–449

13. Weaver RG, Schulte JW (1962) Experimental and clinical studies of urethral regeneration Surg Gynecol Obstet 115:729–736

14. Weaver RG, Schulte JW (1965) Clinical aspects of urethral regeneration. J Urol 93:247–254.

15. Moore CA. (1963) One-stage repair of stricture of bulbous urethra. J Urol 90:203–207

16. Barbagli G, Palminteri E, Lazzeri M. (2002) Dorsal onlay techniques for urethroplasty. Urol Clin N Am 29:389–395

17. Barbagli G, Palminteri E, Lazzeri M, Bracka A (2003) Penile and bulbar urethroplasty using dorsal onlay techniques. Atlas Urol Clin 11:29–41.

18. Barbagli G, Palminteri E, De Stefani S, Lazzeri M (2006) Penile urethroplasty. Techniques and outcomes using buccal mucosa grafts. Contemp Urol 18:25–33

19. Barbagli G, De Stefani S, Sighinolfi C, Annino F, Micali S, Bianchi G (2006) Dorsal buccal mucosa onlay graft bulbar urethroplasty using fibrin glue. J Urol 175:160–161.

20. Snodgrass W (1994) Tubularized, incised plate urethroplasty for distal hypospadias. J Urol 151:464–465

21. Hayes MC, Malone PS (1999) The use of a dorsal buccal mucosal graft with urethral plate incision (Snodgrass) for hypospadias salvage. BJU Int 83:508–509

22. Asopa HS, Garg M, Singhal GG, Singh L, Asopa J, Nischal A (2001) Dorsal free graft urethroplasty for urethral stricture by ventral sagittal urethrotomy approach. Urology 58:657–659

23. Gupta NP, Ansari MS, Dogra PN, Tandon S (2004) Dorsal buccal mucosal graft urethroplasty by a ventral sagittal urethrotomy and minimal-access perineal approach for anterior urethral stricture. BJU Intl 93:1287–1290

24. Barbagli G, Palminteri E, Lazzeri M, Guazzoni G (2003) Anterior urethral strictures. BJU Int 92:497–505

25. Alsikafi NF, Eisenberg M, McAninch JW (2005) Long-term outcomes of penile skin graft versus buccal mucosal graft for substitution urethroplasty of the anterior urethra. J Urol 173:87

26. Gozzi C, Pelzer AE, Bartsch G, Rehder P (2006) Genital free skin graft as dorsal onlay for urethral reconstruction. J Urol 175:38

27. Barbagli G, Palminteri E, Lazzeri M, Turini D. Interim outcomes of dorsal skin graft bulbar urethroplasty. J Urol 172:1365–1367

28. Barbagli G, Palminteri E, Guazzoni G, Montorsi F, Turini D, Lazzeri M (2005) Bulbar urethroplasty using buccal mucosa grafts placed on the ventral, dorsal or lateral surface of the urethra: are the results affected by the surgical technique? J Urol 174:955–958

29. Wessells H, McAninch JW (1998) Current controversies in anterior urethral stricture repair: free-graft versus pedicled skin-flap reconstruction. Word J Urol 16:175–180

30. Wessells H, McAninch JW (1996) Use of free grafts in urethral stricture reconstruction. J Urol 155:1912–1915

31. Morey AF. (2001) Urethral plate salvage with dorsal graft promotes successful penile flap onlay reconstruction of severe pendulous strictures. J Urol 166:1376–1378

32. Bhandari M, Dubey D, Verma BS (2001) Dorsal or ventral placement of the preputial/penile skin onlay flap for anterior urethral strictures: does it make a difference? BJU Int 88:39–43

33. Dubey D, Kumar A, Bansal P, Srivastava A, Kapoor R, Mandhani A, Bhandari M (2003) Substitution urethroplasty for anterior urethral strictures: a critical appraisal of various techniques. BJU Int 91:215–218

34. Wessells H (2002) Ventral onlay graft techniques for urethroplasty. Urol Clin N Am 29:381–387

35. Armenakas NA (2004) Long-term outcome of ventral buccal mucosal grafts for anterior urethral strictures. AUANews 9:17–18.

36. Iselin CE, Webster GD (1999) Dorsal onlay graft urethroplasty for repair of bulbar urethral stricture. J Urol 161:815–818

37. Barbagli G, Palminteri E, Rizzo M (1998) Dorsal onlay graft urethroplasty using penile skin or buccal

mucosa in adult bulbourethral strictures. J Urol 160:1307–1309

38. Rosestein DI, Jordan GH (2002) Dorsal onlay graft urethroplasty using buccal mucosa graft in bulbous urethral reconstruction. J Urol 167:16

39. Dubey D, Kumar A, Mandhani A, Kapoor R, Srivastava A (2006) Dorsal onlay buccal mucosa versus penile skin flap urethroplasty for anterior urethral strictures: results for a randomized prospective trials. J Urol 175:151

40. Kane CJ, Tarman GJ, Summerton DJ, Buchmann CE, Ward JF, O'Reilly KJ, Ruiz H, Thrascher JB, Zorn B, Smith C, Morey AF (2002) Multi-institutional experience with buccal mucosa onlay urethroplasty for bulbar urethral reconstruction. J Urol 167:1314–1317.

41. Elliot SP, Metro MJ, McAninch JW (2003) Long-term followup of the ventrally placed buccal mucosa onlay graft in bulbar urethral reconstruction. J Urol 169:1754–1757.

42. Kellner DS, Fracchia JA, Armenakas NA (2004) Ventral onlay buccal mucosal grafts for anterior urethral strictures: long-term followup. J Urol 171:726–729

43. Abouassaly R, Angermeier KW (2005) Cleveland clinic experience with buccal mucosa graft urethroplasty: intermediate-term results. J Urol 173:33.

44. Barbagli G, Palminteri E, Guazzoni G, Turini D, Lazzeri M (2006) Anastomotic fibrous rings as cause of stricture recurrence after bulbar onlay graft urethroplasty: an open issue. J Urol 175:104

45. Bach AD, Bannasch H, Galla TJ, et al (2001) Fibrin glue as matrix for cultured autologous urothelial cells in urethral reconstruction. Tissue Eng 7:45–53

46. Delvecchio FC, Anger JT, Webster GD (2004) A proposal that whenever possible stricture excision be a part of all bulbar urethroplasties: a progressive approach to patient selection. J Urol 171:17

47. Al-Qudah HS, Santucci RA (2006) Buccal mucosal onlay urethroplasty versus anastomotic urethroplasty (AU) for short urethral strictures: which is better? J Urol 175:103

48. Abouassaly R, Angermeier KW. Augmented anastomotic urethroplasty (AAR) in patients with dense urethral stricture disease. J Urol 175:38

12
Lingual Mucosa and Posterior Auricular Skin Grafts

Steven B. Brandes

Contents

1. Introduction.. 137
2. Lingual Mucosal Grafts 137
    2.1. Technique 138
    2.2. Posterior Auricular Grafts... 139
References... 139

Summary Patients who lack suitable skin or buccal graft for substitution urethroplasty, can be successfully reconstructed with the alternative extragenital sources of lingual mucosa and posterior auricular skin. Both alternative grafts are easy to harvest, readily available, and have a high degree of take.

Keywords lingual mucosa, grafts, auricular skin, substitution urethroplasty

1. Introduction

For patients who lack suitable substitution skin or buccal graft or failed prior buccal graft urethroplasty, reasonable alternative extragenital sources for urethral reconstruction are the posterior auricular skin or the lingual mucosa. Grafting entails tissue transfer without preservation of its blood supply. Instead, it relies on the host bed for graft survival by inosculation and imbibition. Characteristics of the host bed that maximize graft success are: 1) host bed viability: the host bed must be débrided first of all nonliving tissue and have a reliable blood supply; 2) hemostasis: after debridement

of the host bed, control of bleeding is important to prevent a hematoma from separating the graft from bed; 3) bacterial equilibrium: all granulating surfaces need to be débrided first because they are all contaminated; and 4) systemic equilibrium: diabetes, venous stasis, previous radiation, and exogenous steroids are comorbid conditions that compromise graft take. Characteristics of a good graft are as follows 1) ease of harvest, 2) readily available, 3) excellent graft take, and 4) small degree of contracture. Both lingual and posterior auricular grafts fulfill all four qualities.

2. Lingual Mucosal Grafts

The lingual mucosal graft has been recently described *(1)*. In the short term, it appears to have little harvest morbidity and good success as a urethral reconstructive material. The advantage of harvesting a lingual graft is that it is readily available, easy to harvest, resistant to infection, and has tissue characteristics similar to a buccal graft (namely a thick epithelium, thin lamina propria, rich vascularization, and elastic). Thus, the lingual graft is an ideal graft for rapid and predictable inosculation and imbibition.

From: *Current Clinical Urology: Urethral Reconstructive Surgery*
Edited by: S.B. Brandes © Humana Press, Totowa, NJ

2.1. Technique

A 2-O Prolene suture is placed at the apex of
the tongue for traction. A segment 1.5 to 2 cm
wide and as long as the tongue (range 3 to 8 cm,
mean 3.3 cm) is marked out on a lateral posterior aspect, between the papilla on the dorsum
(anterior two-thirds) and the midline frenulum of
the sublingual mucosa (**Fig. 12.1**) The margins
of the dissection are clear in that the dorsum is
visibly rough as the result of numerous papillae (taste buds). The smooth mucosal aspects of
the lateral and posterior tongue have no papillae.
A submucosal wheel of lidocaine and epinephrine
(1:100,000) is injected submucosally to facilitate
graft elevation and decrease bleeding. A full-thickness graft, superficial to the genioglossus muscle,
is harvested sharply with a scalpel and Stevens
tenotomy scissors. (**Fig 12.2a–d**) If needed, grafts
can be harvested from both sides of the tongue. The
lingual artery and nerve run deep and posterior,
and are safe during mucosal dissection. Avoid the
middle frenulum, at the tongue base, for this is
where wharton's duct lies. The graft is then defatted on the back table with Metzenbaum scissors
in the same manner as a buccal graft. The donor
site is then closed with interrupted 3-O absorbable
sutures, after hemostasis with bipolar electrocautery. In small case series reports and in our own
anecdotal experience, oral discomfort in the donor
lasts for roughly 3 days. No esthetic or functional
side effects on chewing, taste, swallowing, or

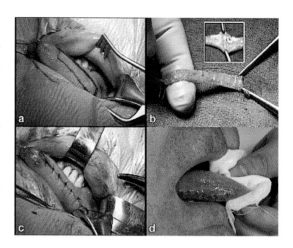

FIG. 12.2. Lingual graft dissection. (A) Graft margins.
(B) Full-thickness graft harvested and defatted. (C)
Donor site closure. (D) Excellent healing of donor site.
(Reprinted from Simonta et al. *[1]*)

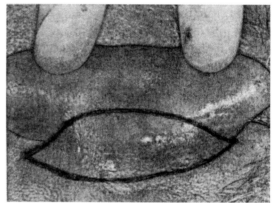

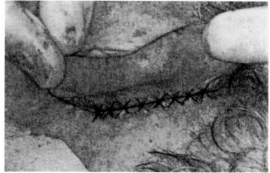

FIG. 12.3. Posterior auricular full-thickness graft harvest.
(A) Ear is folded forward and an oval shaped piece of
skin marked out (B) Primary closure after graft harvest.
(Reprinted from Rudolph et al. *[2]*)

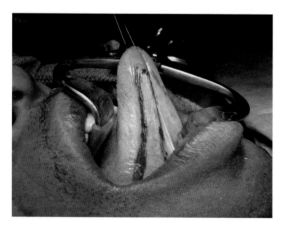

FIG. 12.1. Lingual mucosal graft. Stay suture at tongue
apex, as traction. Margins for graft dissection marked out
(Courtesy of Allen F. Morey)

salivatory/oral cleansing ability have been noted or reported from the donor site harvest. However, there are anecdotal reports of slight speech slurring, but these all resolved by 3 months. To date, reported success rates for lingual graft urethroplasty at 18 months follow-up approach 87%, which is very similar to other grafts like buccal mucosa (1).

2.2. Posterior Auricular Grafts

Posterior auricular-free, full-thickness skin grafting (PAG) was first described in 1875 by Wolfe. To date, the main use of PAG has been for plastics eyelid reconstruction. As an additional extragenital graft site, use of the PAG is a useful graft for reconstruction to have in the surgical armamentarium. Posterior auricular skin is selected because it is hairless and, aside from the eyelid, it is the thinnest extragenital skin on the body. A full-thickness skin graft that is thin, is unique in its high rate of "take" and small degree of contracture after application.

Because the posterior auricular skin overlies the firm bone and cartilage, the graft can be harvested easily and free from the underlying fat.) The donor site is injected with lidocaine and epinephrine (1:100,000) to facilitate tissue separation and hemostasis. The ear is folded forward and an oval shaped piece of skin, centered over the posterior auricular groove is harvested, in the size needed. (**Fig. 12.3A**) The limits of graft size that can be harvested is roughly 2 × 5 cm. If needed, both posterior auricular grooves can be used for harvest. The graft is then prepared by defatting it with Metzenbaum scissors. Tacking the graft to a pin board and scrapping it with the belly of a 15 blade is another method to defat the graft. The donor site is sutured closed primarily and typically heals as a linear and cosmetic scar (**Fig. 12.3B**). Although it is our practice to suture the harvest site closed, others report stapling the harvest site closed with acceptable cosmetic results.

References

1. Simonta A, Gregori A, Lissiani A, Galli S, et al (2006) The tongue as an alternative donor site for graft urethroplasty: a pilot study. J Urol 175:589–592
2. Rudolph R, Fisher JC, Ninnemann JL (1980) Skin grafting. Boston, Little, Brown.

13
Augmented Anastomotic Urethroplasty

Neil D. Sherman and George D. Webster

Contents

1. Introduction 142
2. The Rational for Using the Augmented Anastomotic Repair 142
3. Stricture Factors Important in Procedure Selection 144
4. A Graded Approach for the Management of Bulbar Urethral Stricture Disease ... 144
    4.1. Graft Location 144
    4.2. Preoperative Evaluation 145
5. Surgical Technique 146
    5.1. Exposing the Urethra 146
    5.2. Obtaining The Graft 148
    5.3. Placing the Graft 148
    5.4. Postsurgical Follow-Up 149
6. Results 150
7. Postoperative Complications 150
    7.1. Stricture Recurrence 150
    7.2. Donor-Site Complications 150
    7.3. Sexual Function 150
Appendix 150
References 151

Summary Primary anastomotic urethroplasty with complete stricture excision provides for the most successful outcome in bulbar urethral reconstruction. For strictures too long to allow for a tension free anastomosis a substitution urethroplasty is often used.

The augmented anastomotic urethroplasty is a combination repair that incorporates the principles of excision and substitution urethroplasty and is primarily used for those bulbar strictures deemed too long for straight forward primary anastomosis. In this repair, up to two centimeters of afflicted urethra is excised, and the ventral urethra is reapproximated and a buccal graft is applied dorsally, thus augmenting the anastomosis and addressing any adjacent wide-caliber stricture.

An evolution in graft use has led to our current exclusive use of buccal mucosa placed in a dorsal location. We also spread fix the graft to the overlying corporal bodies which securely applies the graft to its bed and reduces graft shrinkage and sacculation.

When the entire stricture cannot be excised we advocate removing the worst portion (up to two centimeters) a technique we term the 'complex' augmented anastomotic urethroplasty. We do still use pure onlay repairs but in less common scenarios.

In this chapter we discuss our graded approach to the management of bulbar strictures as well as our rationale for utilizing the augmented anastomotic repair. In addition our surgical technique is described.

From: *Current Clinical Urology: Urethral Reconstructive Surgery*
Edited by: S.B. Brandes © Humana Press, Totowa, NJ

We believe that by incorporating the benefits of primary anastomosis with dorsal buccal graft augmentation, the augmented anastomotic urethroplasty provides patients with a durable repair.

Keywords urethra, urethral stricture, urethroplasty, surgical grafts

1. Introduction

A number of urethroplasty techniques may be appropriate for the repair of a bulbar urethral stricture but, ultimately, it is stricture length that will be most important in determining the procedure chosen. The most successful procedure is one that requires only complete stricture excision and a spatulated, circumferential reanastomosis of normal urethra to normal urethra (**Fig. 13.1**). Although a primary anastomosis is appropriate for the majority of bulbar strictures encountered in current practice its use is limited by the risk of causing penile chordee or shortening when used too aggressively. When stricture length or adjacent wider-caliber stricture disease preclude the safe use of primary anastomosis, a combination of stricture excision and graft augmentation may be useful, a procedure termed the augmented anastomotic repair. It is in less common circumstances nowa-

days that graft or flap onlay alone or multistaged repairs are used for bulbar urethroplasty.

The term substitution urethroplasty is used when the urethral lumen is augmented by use of a graft or a flap. Invariably, the substitute is fashioned into an appropriately sized and shaped patch that is applied to the strictured portion of the urethra in either a dorsal or a ventral location. Full circumference replacement by either graft or flap is rarely used because it has a poor success rate. In the past, flaps constructed as pedicle islands of penile (and less commonly scrotal) skin were favored to repair bulbar strictures; however, their difficulty of construction and ultimately their long-term results have lessened enthusiasm for their use. Mundy et al. (*1*) reported a steady annual attrition rate of about 5% for all types of pedicle reconstruction, and this, combined with the poor cosmetic results using flaps has tilted the pendulum in favor of grafts.

There has also been a continuing evolution in the use of grafts for urethral reconstruction. Although the use of split- and full-thickness extragenital skin is somewhat historic, the move from full-thickness penile (or preputial) skin to the now widely used buccal mucosa is current. Whereas it is suggested that buccal grafts are particularly resistant to infection and skin diseases, such as lichen sclerosus, and are easier to work with, there is currently no hard data favoring buccal mucosa over full-thickness penile grafts in terms of urethroplasty outcomes. However, we are personally biased as to the advantages of this "wet" epithelium and have adopted it as our substitute of choice since 1998.

2. The Rational for Using the Augmented Anastomotic Repair

An augmented anastomotic procedure is a combination repair and embodies the principles of both excision and substitution urethroplasty. The term was first coined by Turner-Warwick (*2*), who described the technique as a means by which an "anastomotic" repair could still be performed when the stricture was marginally longer than could be safely repaired by a spatulated end to end reanastomosis. He described excision of the stricture and reanastomosis of the roof strip of the urethra alone. The urethra was spatulated ventrally on both ends, and a small flap or graft placed to augment the size of the anastomosis.

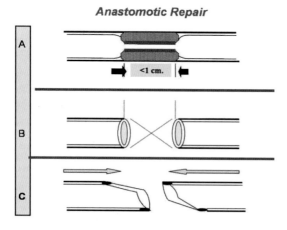

FIG. 13.1. Primary anastomotic repair. When bulbar urethral stricture disease is approximately 1 cm in length (line A), the entire stricture can be excised (line B) and then the urethra is spatulated into healthy tissue (line C) to allow for a direct anastomosis of healthy urethra mucosa

In essence, it was a technique that saved the 1 cm or so required for a standard end to end anastomosis hence allowing for the advantage of excisional urethroplasty for slightly longer strictures **(Fig. 13.2)**.

This ability to extend the indications for anastomotic urethroplasty is valuable but, interestingly, the length of bulbar stricture repaired by excision and anastomosis alone has increased in recent reports, and in our practice. Certainly, one cannot give a numeric value as to just how much bulbar stricture can be excised and yet still safely perform a spatulated tension free reconnection that will apply in all cases. Variables will include genital length, urethral elasticity, the extent of proximal and distal urethral mobilization, and such maneuvers as release of the midline perineal tendon or separation of the corporal bodies at the crus. Ultimately the patient's acceptance of some penile shortening or chordee make the decision easier.

The augmented anastomotic technique finds even greater value in its ability to address wide caliber spongiofibrosis adjacent to a stricture that otherwise would easily fit the criteria for a simple excisional repair *(3)*. In this circumstance, the main body of the stricture (up to the allowable limits of the individual patient based on the variables we have discussed previously) is excised, and the urethra then spatulated dorsally through all remaining spongiofibrotic urethra for whatever length. The graft is then fashioned to a length to allow for augmentation of the floor strip anastomosis as well as onlay over the spatulated proximal and distal spongiofibrosis.

We have elaborated our use of this technique one step further in recent years to address many strictures that, because of length, would otherwise be candidates only for pure onlay repair. We suggest that many long strictures have their origins somewhere in the midst of the stricture at a location where the lumen will be its smallest and the spongiofibrosis at its worst. Onlay of a graft or flap to this location carries poor results as the urethral "foundation" is so poor. We prefer to identify this location and excise it and then proceed as in the manner described in the scenario above. For example, if a stricture 6 cm in length contains a 2-cm tight stricture and a less tight but still-structured 4-cm area, the tight 2-cm stricture is completely excised and the remaining urethral ends are anastomosed as a floor strip. On the dorsal aspect, the urethra is opened through the remaining stricture and for an additional 1 cm into healthy urethra proximally and distally. A 6-cm onlay is then placed on the urethral wall opposite the anastomosis and the resultant urethral shortening is only 2 cm **(Fig. 13.3)**.

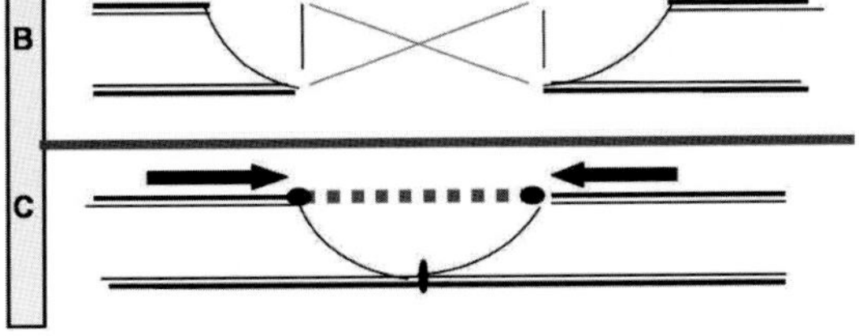

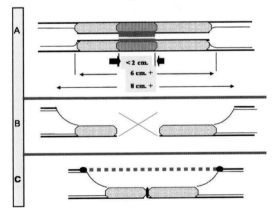

The 'Complex' Augmented Anastomotic Repair

FIG. 13.3. "Complex" augmented anastomotic repair. With longer stricture disease, there is frequently an area of stricture that is more diseased than the remainder of the stricture **(line A)**. Up to two centimeters of the most afflicted urethra is excised and the remainder of the diseased urethra is spatulated dorsally **(line B)**. The ventral urethra is primarily anastomosed and a graft (dashed line) that is long enough to extend into the spatulated healthy urethra is placed dorsally **(line C)**

Augmented Anastomotic Repair

FIG. 13.2. Augmented anastomotic repair. When bulbar stricture disease is greater than about 1 cm and usually less than 2 cm **(line A)**, the diseased urethra is completely excised and the dorsal urethra is spatulated for 1 cm proximally and distally **(line B)**. The ventral native urethra is then re-approximated and a graft (dashed line) is placed across the dorsal defect

This chapter will explain our graded approach to the surgical management of bulbar urethral stricture disease as well as the intraoperative technique and postoperative management for the augmented anastomotic urethroplasty using buccal mucosa.

3. Stricture Factors Important in Procedure Selection

A variety of factors influence the management of bulbar urethral stricture disease. Variables that must be taken into account include stricture location, length, and etiology. In addition, local adverse events such as inflammation, scarring from previous treatments (spongiofibrosis), radiation effects, and surgeon preference all dictate the course of repair.

Stricture length is typically the most important variable in determining an appropriate repair. One must realize that at least 1 cm of healthy urethra must be spatulated in both the proximal and distal direction prior to anastomosis. Thus for strictures 1 cm in length, one will create a gap of 2 cm that must be traversed. The elasticity of the mobilized bulbar urethra can accommodate this gap without causing tension or penile chordee (2). Although others have reported extended anastomotic repairs (4), it is important not to take this as license to perform, but rather to recognize the possibility and consider the necessary patient and technical variations as we discussed earlier.

Stricture location will dictate how much urethral mobilization is safe before urethral shortening and penile chordee may develop. For the pendulous urethra, any amount of mobilization may lead to chordee unless extensive proximal urethral mobilization is performed to "gain length." In contrast, the bulbar urethra typically allows for up to 2 cm of excision without creating adverse outcomes. For posterior urethral injury after pelvic fracture, i.e., pelvic fracture urethral distraction defect, gaps of any length may be bridged. If after urethral mobilization to the region of the suspensory ligament of the penis the defect cannot be bridged without tension then other maneuvers such as separation of the corporal bodies, inferior pubectomy and supracorporal rerouting of the urethra will generally allow for safe bulboprostatic anastomosis (5).

Stricture etiology is variable and often times the exact cause is not known. Although stricture etiology and previous therapies may complicate procedure selection and adversely affect outcome, most strictures are surgically correctable. Exceptions to this predictability are those associated with balantis xerotica obliterans (6), radiation therapy and local inflammatory changes from multiple fistulae.

4. A Graded Approach for the Management of Bulbar Urethral Stricture Disease

We approach repair of bulbar urethral stricture, guided by the retrograde urethrogram, but recognizing that intraoperative findings sometimes dictate a need to elaborate the repair. Our goal is always to repair by primary anastomotic urethroplasty if possible, as these provide the most durable outcomes for urethral stricture disease.

If the stricture is marginally too long (**Fig. 13.4**) but there is no associated adjacent spongiofibrosis, we elaborate to a dorsal buccal graft onlay augmented anastomotic procedure. This saves 1 cm of urethral shortening, as described above (**Fig. 13.2**). When the bulbar stricture is long but there is a central location of bad urethra (**Fig. 13.5**), this bad segment is excised and the dorsal urethrotomy is extended into the adjacent spongiofibrosis. The graft length is increased accordingly and the dorsal onlay performed customarily. We term this technique the 'complex' augmented anastomotic repair (**Fig. 13.3**). The final step in our progression is to simply onlay the graft dorsally, particularly if the stricture is long and uniform with no particularly bad area that requires excision (**Fig. 13.6**).

4.1. Graft Location

Through the years, substitution urethroplasty has used various locations for graft and flap placement. Each of these location has its' pros and cons. In 1996, Barbagli (7) proposed a dorsal application of the graft (dorsal stricturotomy and patch technique) securing the graft to the corporal bodies. Since that time, we too have used a dorsal graft location, believing in its perceived benefits. These benefits include the fact that dorsal graft placement allows

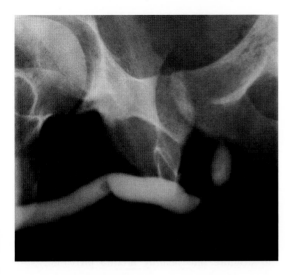

FIG. 13.4. Retrograde urethrogram: A tight 2-cm bulbar urethral stricture amenable to an augmented anastomotic urethroplasty

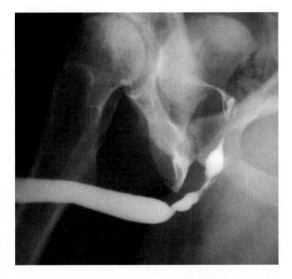

FIG. 13.5. Retrograde urethrogram: Long bulbar urethral stricture with tight proximal segment and an adjacent, distal portion of affected urethra. The proximal segment was excised and a dorsal stricturotomy performed on the distal portion. The floor strip was primarily anastomosed and a buccal graft was placed dorsally as a "complex" augmented anastomotic repair

the graft to be spread and anchored (spread fixed) to the undersurface of the corporal bodies and thus offers a secure bed for neovascularization. This spread fixation probably reduces the chances of

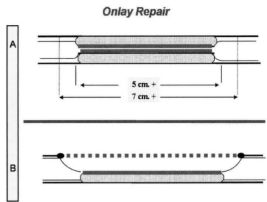

Onlay Repair

FIG. 13.6. Dorsal onlay repair. In some long strictures, disease is uniform and a discrete area is unable to be identified (**line A**). In these cases a segment of stricture is not excised and the entire stricture in onlayed with graft (dashed line) extending 1 cm into healthy urethra proximally and distally (**line B**)

graft shrinkage and graft sacculation *(8)*. Finally, it is possible that limiting incision of the thicker ventral spongiosum may help to preserve its' residual blood supply *(9)*. Despite these advantages, our rationale for utilizing dorsal graft placement is not universally acclaimed *(10,11)*.

4.2. Preoperative Evaluation

Attention to factors that may complicate surgery or mitigate against success are important. These include previous managements, radiation therapy to the area, co-morbidities such as obesity and diabetes, the presence of lichen sclerosus, and other skin problems in the genital area. If buccal graft is too be used, the mouth should be examined and oral hygiene improved as necessary.

A recent retrograde urethrogram delineating all features of the stricture should be available, and if necessary a voiding cystourethrogram performed. Cystourethroscopy is performed for correlation if necessary.

Before surgical exploration, it is ideal for there to be no recent incisions or dilations of the stricture. This ensures that the maximum extent of diseased urethra can be identified at the time of urethroplasty. Timing between the last endoscopic intervention and repair is unique to each patient and based on the time interval of prior dilations and the patient's voiding symptoms. If necessary, a suprapubic cystostomy tube may be inserted during the time leading up to surgical repair.

5. Surgical Technique

5.1. Exposing the Urethra

The augmented anastomotic urethroplasty is performed with the patient in dorsal lithotomy position with the thighs just cephalad of vertical. We prefer padded Allen stirrups and all patients wear sequential compression devices on the lower extremities. A table-fixed Bookwalter retractor, a surgeon's headlight and 2.5 x magnification loupes are advantageous (**Fig. 13.7**).

Before perineal incision, undiluted methylene blue is instilled per urethra to differentially stain normal from scarred mucosa. It also assists in the accurate placement of closure sutures. A 22-French red-rubber catheter is passed down the urethra to the stricture (but NOT through) to identify its distal limit and to guide location of the incision.

For a midbulbar urethral stricture, the incision is midline perineal with posterior bilateral bifurcation. The bulbospongiosus muscle is incised in the midline and dissected off the urethra. Buck's

fascia on the ventral corporal body is opened bilaterally at the level of the bifurcation of the crura, creating "windows" in the fascia that allow for safe circumferential mobilization of the urethra. The strictured urethra, as well as 2 cm of proximal and distal healthy urethra, is circumferentially mobilized. Ventral dissection is taken proximally through the central perineal tendon. This maneuver allows one to take advantage of the elasticity of the bulbar urethra and increases its length.

With guidance from the red rubber catheter, the urethra is transected at the distal level of the obstruction. The severed urethral ends are stabilized with 4-O silk suture tags, and the strictured urethra is then opened dorsally (12-o'clock position) through the stricture into healthy urethra proximally. As the urethra is spatulated 4-O silk suture tags are placed on the bulbospongiosus to assist with traction and exposure (**Fig. 13.8**). A change in color of the previously injected methylene blue, and appearance of the spongy tissue, help clarify when the proximal limit of stricture is reached. Bougie a boule calibration to 26 French ensures that the proximal limit of the diseased urethra has been reached. When clinically indicated, cystoscopy can now be performed. At this point, the length of the diseased urethra is measured and factors, such as urethral length and elasticity, are assessed to

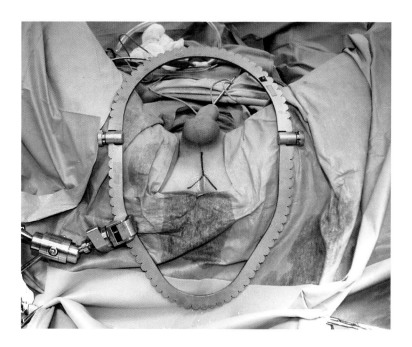

FIG. 13.7. Patient in lithotomy position with table fixed Bookwalter retractor in place. Note the marking for a midline perineal incision with posterior bifurcation

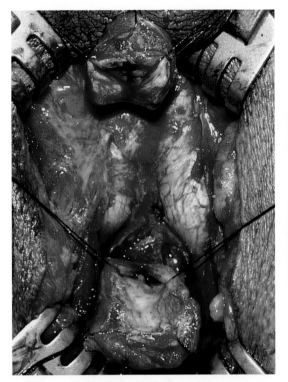

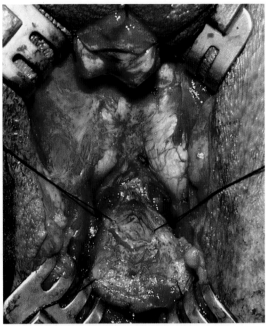

FIG. 13.9. The proximal, ventral urethral stump is on traction ,and 2 cm of strictured urethra has been excised. The residual "raw," healthy spongiosum is a posteriorly based flap that will be used to cover the ventral urethral anastomosis

FIG. 13.8. The proximal urethra is placed on traction and dorsal stricturotomy is performed into healthy proximal urethra. Two centimeters of afflicted urethral tissue in the foreground will be excised

determine the most appropriate repair to perform (see previous paragraph). Although preoperative retrograde urethrography provides some guidance, the final determination for type of repair is based predominantly on the intraoperative findings of stricture length as well as the appearance of the mucosa and spongy tissue.

When stricture length suggests that a simple anastomotic repair cannot be performed but the retrograde urethrogram (RUG) characteristics and operative findings imply the worst stricture can be excised and still allow the floor of the urethra to be approximated tension free, such is done. In most cases, the scarred mucosa and spongy tissue is excised leaving the "raw" healthy underlying bulb as a posteriorly based flap to ultimately cover the anastomosis ventrally (**Fig. 13.9**). The important considerations at this juncture are whether one can approximate healthy urethra to healthy urethra and whether the dorsal urethrotomy has gone sufficiently far

into the healthy urethra such that all adjacent spongiofibrosis will be encompassed by the dorsal graft. If tension free re-approximation is not possible, further distal urethral mobilization or proximal urethral release of the central perineal tendon is performed.

After preparation is complete, one must determine the length of graft to obtain. The proximal and distal stumps are brought together and the urethrotomy length on the dorsal urethra is measured to determine the length of graft required. Measurement includes one centimeter into the healthy proximal and distal dorsal urethra.

The major variation on the above described approach is the circumstance in which the initial RUG suggests that a 'complex' approach is required (**Fig. 13.5**). This is exemplified by the very long stricture with a central tight area needing excision. In this situation, the urethra is circumferentially mobilized and then the long dorsal urethrotomy is performed. We then assess the urethra for excision of a segment or perhaps elect to simply perform a long dorsal onlay.

5.2. Obtaining The Graft

The inner cheek is preferred over the lower lip as the harvest site. The endotracheal tube is secured off to the contralateral side of the mouth and gauze is used to pack away the tongue and to prevent pooling of blood and irrigation in the pharynx. Stenson's duct is identified and marked at the level of the second upper molar. An ellipse of predetermined length is then marked on the cheek, making sure to avoid Stenson's duct nor to encroach too close to the alveolar margin nor to the labial angle of the mouth. A graft width of 1.5 cm, at its' wide point, is customary.

The submucosa beneath the graft harvest site is infiltrated with normal saline and 4-O silk traction sutures are placed at the anterior apex of the future graft. Army-Navy retractors placed inside the cheek and lower lip help in providing adequate exposure and we do not use purpose made mouth retractors. The marked outlines for the graft are incised with a no. 15 blade knife and then sharply dissected off of the underlying buccinator muscle (**Fig. 13.10**). We prefer to close the graft donor site with a 5-O running, interlocking polyglycolic acid suture (**Fig. 13.11**).

The harvested graft is fixed to a foam block with radial 25-gauge needles, thinned with metzenbaum scissors, shaped as needed and fenestrated with a no. 15 blade knife (**Fig. 13.12**). The graft is now ready for placement.

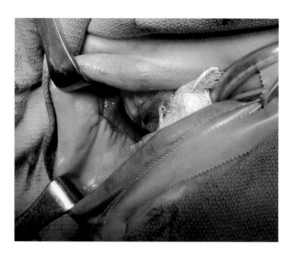

FIG. 13.11. A running, interlocking 5–O polyglycolic acid suture is used to close the buccal graft donor site

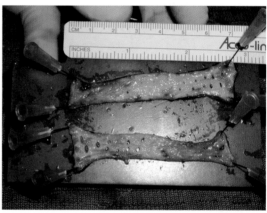

FIG. 13.12. The graft is spread fixed to a paraffin block with 25-gage needles and then fenestrated with the tip of an 11 blade knife

5.3. Placing the Graft

The graft is placed dorsally and spread fixed over the corporal bodies as originally described by Barbagli (*12*). A number techniques have been used to affix the graft to the corporal bodies and to the margins of the dorsally spatulated urethra. Some spread fix the graft and then apply the edges of the urethra to the graft perimeter. We prefer to commence graft placement with the proximal, apical suture. A small portion of the intercrural fascia is incorporated into the suture with knot placement inside the future urethral lumen. Particularly when this apical suture is at the

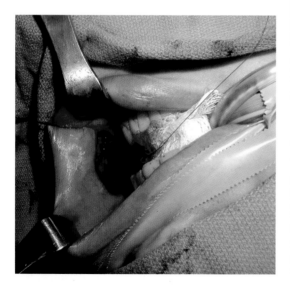

FIG. 13.10. Army-Navy retractors expose the donor graft site of the inner cheek. Gauze is packed between the teeth and the endotracheal tube is secured to the contralateral side

bulbo-membranous region, this and the adjacent sutures also are hemostatic as they tamponade the midline veins exposed and opened by the dorsal mobilization of the urethra. We use diathermy rarely in this intercrural space as there is risk to the nearby, laterally lying cavernous nerves. Graft handling is made easier by temporarily tacking the distal apex to the corporal bodies. Proximal graft suturing then continues with 5-O polyglycolic acid suture in an interrupted fashion around the dorsal spatulation, each suture picking up the urethral margin then a small bite of the corporal tunica and then the graft. Most, but not all, sutures are tied within the urethral lumen. Incorporation of the underlying corporal body helps secure the graft in position (**Fig. 13.13**).

After securing the proximal aspect of the spatulated urethra to the spread fixed graft, the distal graft is anastomosed to the spatulated distal urethra in a similar fashion. Quilting sutures securing the graft to overlying corporal body are placed centrally on the graft to minimize central detachment. At this point only a few lateral sutures and the urethral floor strip reconnection sutures remain to be placed. After the anastomosis is completed, the proximal

bulbospongiosus flap from the previously excised stricture is utilized as a second closure layer.

A 12-French fenestrated, silicone catheter is inserted. A suprapubic catheter is rarely placed. The bulbospongiousus muscle is then re-approximated as is Colle's fascia. The skin is closed with interrupted absorbable suture. Drainage of the operative space is not typically required. The incision is dressed with xeroform gauze and a scrotal support. Patients are discharged on the day of surgery *(13)*. Postoperative erections are limited during the first week by prn use of inhaled amyl nitrite ampules.

5.4. Postsurgical Follow-Up

We do not restrict ambulation or reasonable activity in the early postoperative course despite use of a graft. We believe the secure spread fixation of the graft in a dorsal location protects it from dislodging from its bed. If, at 3 weeks, a pericatheter urethrogram confirms complete healing, the Foley catheter is removed (**Fig. 13.14**). A repeat urethrogram is performed at 3 months, by which time future durability of the repair is likely to be evident. At 12 months postoperatively, a uroflow study is performed and a retrograde urethrogram is repeated as indicated. Cystoscopy is also invaluable to evaluate abnormal RVG findings and indeed some prefer it to RVG. Follow-up thereafter is then dictated by patient symptomatology.

All patients are instructed to manually compress the perineum at the conclusion of voiding. This procedure helps to evacuate the few urine drops that may be sequestered at the graft lumen and thus avoid the problem of terminal dribbling that may accompany substitution urethroplasty. The cause of this dribbling is typically attributed to a redundant

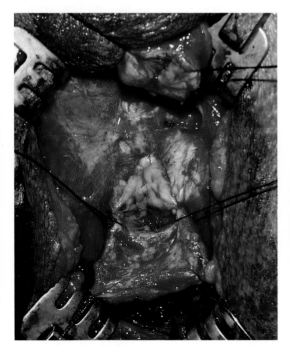

FIG. 13.13. The buccal graft is spread fixed to the corporal body and anastomosed to the dorsal, proximal urethra

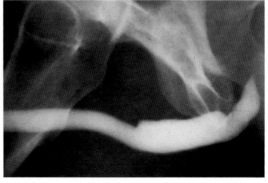

FIG. 13.14. Postoperative urethrogram with patent bulbar urethra after an augmented anastomotic urethroplasty.

ventral graft but in reality it may also be seen with dorsal graft placement. The true etiology is probably a disruption of the natural closing mechanism of the spongy tissue and surrounding musculature that occurs with dissection of the anterior urethra at the time of urethroplasty *(2)*.

6. Results

In 2001, we reported a series of patients in which the augmented anastomotic technique was used *(14)*. At a mean follow-up of 28 months, 93% of patients were free of stricture. Those cases that recurred did so at the ends of the repair, while most of the grafted urethra remained patent. The most likely explanation for this finding is that the repair did not extend far enough into healthy urethra.

The original patients reported on in 2001 were incorporated into a larger cohort of patients presented in 2004 *(15)*. In these 47 patients, there was 100% success for augmented anastomotic repairs and a 95% success for 'complex' augmented anastomotic repairs. To date, there have not been any other series that critically assessed those patients that have undergone an augmented anastomotic repair.

Our philosophy in choosing buccal mucosa is confirmed by our transition from other tissues to using buccal mucosa for all substitution urethroplasties *(16)*. Early data has indicated that stricture excision with the more appropriate buccal mucosa graft provides for durable success when indicated.

7. Postoperative Complications

Generally, complications are infrequent and minor. The most common complaint is postvoid dribbling. This may be due to the disruption of the natural closing mechanism of the bulbar spongy tissue and its surrounding muscle. It is best managed by having the patient manually milk the urethra from the perineum to the meatus after each void *(14)*.

7.1. Stricture Recurrence

As previously discussed, when a postoperative stricture occurs it is frequently at one of the anastomotic suture lines although it is possible for the entire graft to obstruct *(17)*. When failures do

occur, a variety of management options are available. Initial treatment with internal optic urethrotomy or dilations is frequently all that is necessary. Strictures that encompass the entire graft area are typically treated with redo-urethroplasty *(18)*.

7.2. Donor-Site Complications

Sensory changes at the donor site may occur with buccal mucosa graft use. Other potential problems related to graft harvest include persistent pain, neurologic changes, changes to salivary flow and contracture. These appear to be a greater problem with grafts taken from the lower lip versus the inner cheek *(19)*. The associated increases in post-operative discomfort with grafts taken from the lower lip are also associated with a decrease in patient satisfaction *(20)*.

7.3. Sexual Function

One must always be conscientious of the rare complication of altering erectile function during anterior urethroplasty *(21)*, and concerns about sexual function remain a major component of our preoperative counseling. Although the neurovascular bundles are not visualized from the perineal approach, dissection does occur in proximity to the corporal bodies and the erectile neurovascular structures. It has been our experience that erectile function is related to patient age and pre-operative erectile status rather than with the type of bulbar urethroplasty repair *(22)*.

Appendix

Preferred Instruments and Suture of GD Webster

Instruments

Jordan retractor system (C&S Surgical, Slidell, LA) for Bookwalter retractor system (Codman, Raynam, MA)
Wagenstein forceps
Flexible self-retaining retractor
Turner-Warwick needle driver

Suture

5-0 polyglycolic acid suture for donor site closure
5-0 polyglycolic acid suture for anastomosis

References

1. Mundy AR (1995) The long-term results of skin inlay urethroplasty. Br J Urol 75:59–61
2. Turner-Warwick R (1993) Principles of urethral reconstruction, in Webster G, Kirby R, King L, et al (eds) Reconstructive urology, vol. 2. Boston, Blackwell Scientific, pp 609–642
3. Guralnick ML, Webster GD (2003) The augmented anastomotic urethroplasty. Atlas Urol Clin 11:43–49
4. Morey AF, Kizer WS (2006) Proximal bulbar urethroplasty via an extended anastamotic approach: what are the limits? J Urol 175:2145–2149
5. Mark SD, Webster GD (1996) Reconstruction of the failed repair of posterior urethral rupture, in McAninch JW (ed) Traumatic and reconstructive urology. Philadelphia W.B. Saunders, pp 439–451
6. Peterson AC, Palminteri E, Lazzeri M, Guazzoni G, Barbagli G, Webster GD (2003) Heroic measures may not always be justified in extensive urethral stricture due to lichen sclerosis (balanitis xerotica obliterans). J Urol 169(S4):178, Abstract 688
7. Barbagli G, Selli C, di Cello V, Mottola A (1996) A one-stage dorsal free-graft urethroplasty for bulbar urethral strictures. Br J Urol 78:929–932
8. Barbagli G, Palminteri E, Rizzo M (1998) Dorsal onlay graft urethroplasty using penile skin or buccal mucosa in adult bulbourethral strictures. J Urol 160:1307–1309
9. Pansadoro V, Emiliozzi P, Gaffi M. Scarpone P.(1999) Buccal mucosa urethroplasty for the treatment of bulbar urethral strictures. J Urol 161:1501–1503
10. Barbagli G, Palminteri E, Guazzoni G, Montorsi F, Turini D, Lazzeri M (2005) Bulbar urethroplasty using buccal mucosa grafts placed on the ventral, dorsal or lateral surface of the urethra: are results affected by the surgical technique? J Urol 174:955–958
11. Kane CJ, Tarman GJ, Summerton DJ, Buchmann CE, Ward JF, O'Reilly KJ, et al (2002) Multi-institutional experience with buccal mucosa onlay urethroplasty for bulbar urethral reconstruction. J Urol 167:1314–1317
12. Barbagli G, Selli C, Tosto A, Palminteri E (1996) Dorsal free graft urethroplasty. J Urol 155:123–126
13. MacDonald MF, Al-Qudah HS, Santucci RA (2005) Minimal impact urethroplasty allows same day surgery in most patients. J Urol 66:850–853
14. Guralnick ML, Webster GD (2001) The augmented anastomotic urethroplasty: indications and outcome in 29 patients. J Urol 165:1496–1501
15 Delvecchio FC, Anger JT, Webster GD (2004) A proposal that whenever possible stricture excision be a part of all bulbar urethroplasties: a progressive approach to patient selection. J Urol 171(S4):17, Abstract 66.
16. Peterson AC, Delvecchio FC, Flynn BJ, Webster GD (2003) Evolving urethroplasty options for bulbar urethral stricture: a current rationale for procedure selection. J Urol 169(S4):97, Abstract 377.
17. Barbagli G, Guazzoni G, Palminteri E, Lazzeri M (2006) Anastamotic fibrous ring as cause of stricture recurrent after bulbar onlay graft urethroplasty. J Urol 176:614–619
18. Peterson AC, Delvecchio FC, Palminteri E, Lazzeri M, Guazzoni G, Barbagli G, Webster GD (2003) Dorsal onlay urethroplasty using penile skin: a multi-institutional review of long term results. J Urol 169(S4):19, Abstract 72.
19. Jang TL, Erickson B, Medendorp A, Gonzalez CM (2005) Comparison of donor site intraoral morbidity after mucosal graft harvensting for urethral reconstruction. Urology 66:716–720
20. Kamp S, Knoll T, Osman M, Hacker A, Michel MS, Alken P (2005) Donor-site morbidity in buccal mucosa urethroplasty: lower lip or inner cheek? BJU Int 96:619–623
21. Mundy AR (1993) Results of complications of urethroplasty and its future. Br J Urol 71:322–325
22. Tash JT, Sherman ND, Webster GD (2007) The effect of bulbar urethroplasty on erectile function. J Urol 178:1009–1111.

14
Penile Skin Flaps for Urethral Reconstruction

Sean P. Elliott and Jack W. McAninch

Contents

1. Introduction.. 154
2. Patient Selection... 154
3. Desirable Flap Characteristics 154
4. Fascial and Vascular Anatomy of the Penis 155
5. Types of Flaps 155
    5.1. Longitudinal vs Transverse 156
    5.2. Proximal vs Distal Penile Skin.. 157
    5.3. Dorsal vs Ventral vs Lateral Pedicle 157
    5.4. Ventral Onlay vs Tube Flap vs Combined Tissue Transfer................. 158
6. Technique.. 158
    6.1. Preoperative Preparation 158
    6.2. Patient Positioning 158
    6.3. Flap Harvest 158
    6.4. Urethral Closure With Ventral Onlay Island Skin Flap 161
    6.5. Urethral Closure in Combined Tissue Transfer 162
7. Results... 163
    7.1. Success Rates 163
    7.2. Complications 163
Editorial Comment.. 163
Appendix 164
References.. 164

Summary The penile skin flap is a versatile tool in the reconstruction of anterior urethral stricture disease. When adequate non-diseased skin exists and when the arterial supply is dependable, a flap may be used for single stage reconstruction of strictures from the bulbar urethra to the urethral meatus. The surgical technique is challenging; a thorough understanding of the penile anatomy, particularly the vascular anatomy and fascial layers, is necessary to successful flap harvest. While based on similar principles, the various penile skin flaps described in this chapter have distinct differences in their technique of harvest as well as their appropriateness for strictures of the bulbar and penile urethra. All share a common blood supply in the external pudendal arteries. All involve the isolation of an island of skin dependent on this vascular pedicle. The differences in technique center on whether the island is isolated transversely or longitudinally, to what degree the pedicle is developed proximally and whether the pedicle is primarily ventrally-based or dorsally-based. With a proper understanding of each of these techniques a surgeon is well-prepared to approach the difficult task of anterior urethral reconstruction.

Keywords Island flap, anterior urethral stricture, lichen sclerosus, single-stage reconstruction, combined tissue transfer

1. Introduction

The ultimate goal of anterior urethral reconstruction should be unobstructed micturition from a glanular meatus with excellent cosmesis. At times, it is appropriate to compromise meatal location or cosmesis to better achieve unobstructed micturition. Ideally, anterior urethral reconstruction should be achieved in a single stage; however, two-stage repairs are acceptable when they lead to optimum results. The penile skin flap provides a versatile mechanism for achieving excellent results in the single-stage repair of complex anterior urethral strictures.

The penile skin flap is generally used as a ventral-onlay, but it can be tubularized or used in combination with a dorsal graft. With appropriate modifications in technique, the penile skin flap can be used for strictures of nearly any length, occurring in any location throughout the anterior urethra. Given the good cosmetic and long-term outcome results with anastomotic urethroplasty for bulbar strictures <2 cm and with patch graft urethroplasty for longer bulbar strictures, the primary role of the penile skin flap has become in the reconstruction of penile urethral strictures. Success rates are approximately 80% with long-term follow-up.

This chapter will focus on the penile skin flap in anterior urethral reconstruction. We will discuss the anatomy of the skin flap. We will review the technical aspects and success rates of each technique. The various types of penile skin flaps can often lead to confusion on the part of the reader and the young reconstructive surgeon. We will attempt to arrive at a more intuitive classification scheme based on descriptive terminology rather than eponyms or acronyms.

2. Patient Selection

Complex urethral strictures may benefit from reconstruction with a penile skin flap; however, certain patient characteristics should be considered when counseling such patients. First, advanced

patient age may make one more strongly consider periodic urethral dilation or a permanent first-stage urethroplasty; whereas the younger patient may prefer complex urethral reconstruction. Second, other patient factors such as adverse wound characteristics (caused by concomitant periurethral abscess or fistula) or poor wound healing (caused by peripheral vascular disease, diabetes or previous radiation therapy) should cause one to reconsider proceeding with a complex single stage urethral reconstruction. Specifically, there has been much debate about the use of the penile skin flap for reconstruction of urethral stricture disease as the result of lichen sclerosus et atrophicans (LSA *[1]*). Although no one would advocate using skin afflicted with LSA, we have documented good long-term results in patients with LSA when the penile skin used in the flap is not clinically involved by the LSA *(2)*. Others believe a two-stage repair utilizing extragenital skin is preferable *(3)*. Third, the length and location of the stricture are paramount to the choice of urethral reconstruction technique. The penile skin flap serves best in the reconstruction of penile urethral strictures from the urethral meatus to the distal bulbar urethra. The excellent success rates with anastomotic urethroplasty and buccal mucosa graft in the bulbar urethra argue for avoiding using the penile skin flap in these cases, although there are exceptions.

3. Desirable Flap Characteristics

The ideal penile skin flap should be hairless, perform well in an aqueous environment, be adaptable, and leave the patient with an excellent cosmetic outcome. The distal penile shaft and prepuce are hairless whereas the proximal and mid penile shaft contain variable amounts of hair, especially ventrally. Hair in the urethra leads to chronic bacterial colonization, inflammation, and stone formation. The inner preputial skin is particularly well-suited to use in urethral reconstruction as it is accustomed to functioning in a moist environment.

Flap adaptability depends on flap mobility and the ability to harvest flaps of various lengths using the same technique. Flap mobility allows one to use the same flap for reconstruction anywhere from the meatus to the bulbar urethra and depends on the degree of pedicle dissection. Good mobility can be obtained with most of the described flap techniques. Regarding length, the transverse island flap techniques allow the surgeon to harvest a flap of up to 15 cm. Although longitudinal flaps are shorter, they can be lengthened with a "hockey-stick" extension.

Cosmetic outcomes are best when the skin incision and resultant wound are created along already present skin lines. Longitudinal flaps attain this by making an incision along the median raphe whereas transverse flaps use a circumcision incision.

4. Fascial and Vascular Anatomy of the Penis

The anatomy of the penis is described in detail chapters one and two in this volume. The aspects of the anatomy that are relevant to a discussion of penile skin flaps are reviewed herein. The confusion about the various types of penile skin flaps is attributable, at least in part, to inconsistent anatomical terminology. In the interest of clarity we will relate our terminology with that of Dr. Quartey's.

The dermis of the penile and scrotal skin is composed of dartos muscle (**Fig. 14.1**). This muscle contracts in response to stimuli such as cold temperature. This muscle is distinct from the dartos fascia. Deep to the dartos muscle is a subdermal vascular plexus. Beneath this is the dartos/Colle's fascia, which is continuous with Scarpas's fascia on the anterior abdominal wall. Deep to Colle's fascia is a loose subcutaneous areolar tissue containing the axial arteries of the penis. This layer is often termed the tunica dartos. Below this is Buck's fascia, a multilamellar fascia that surrounds the neurovascular bundle of the erectile bodies dorsally and splits ventrally to wrap around the corpus spongiosum.

The penile skin derives its blood supply from the superior (superficial) and inferior (deep) external pudendal arteries, branches of the femoral artery. Venous drainage parallels the arterial supply (**Fig. 14.2** *[5]*). All the various penile skin flaps are developed based on this blood supply. At the base of the penis, the external pudendal arteries split into ventrolateral and dorsolateral axial penile arteries. These then give off delicate superficial branches to the subdermal plexus. It is incorrect to say that the vessels run in a particu-

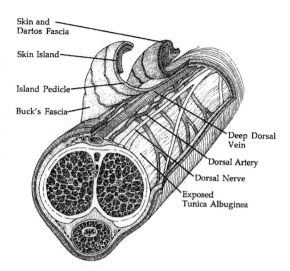

FIG. 14.1. The fascial anatomy of the penis

lar fascia, as fascia is by definition avascular. In fact, the subdermal plexus runs superficial to the dartos/Colle's fascia but deep to the dartos muscle (dermis) whereas the subcutaneous plexus runs deep to the dartos/Colle's fascia but superficial to Buck's fascia.

Although there is no fascia in the vascular pedicle, the pedicle is certainly developed with a fascial layer supporting the subcutaneous plexus. When one examines a well-developed penile skin flap, it is undoubtedly supported by a layer of fascia; otherwise, it would just be a loose network of vessels and areolar fat, just which fascial layer supports the flap is unclear. McAninch and others have described that layer as being the superficial layer of Buck's fascia (which lies just deep to the pedicle *[4,5]*), whereas others have described it being supported by the dartos fascia (which lies just superficial to the pedicle *[6]*). Likely, the surgical techniques used by the reconstructive surgeons are similar, what differs is their interpretation of the anatomy.

5. Types of Flaps

There are numerous, often confusing terms used to describe the various penile skin flaps. In fact, it would lead you to believe that no two flaps are the same. Actually, as alluded to previously, the flaps

Fig. 14.2. Arterial supply and
venous drainage of the penis

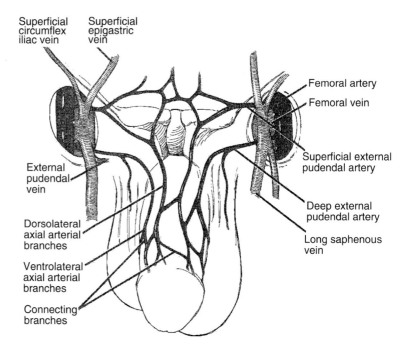

are more similar than they are different. As opposed to a graft, a flap carries with it its own blood supply. An axial flap is based on a defined vascular pedicle, whereas a random flap is based on a blood supply that is not as well defined. Penile skin flaps are an example of an axial flap based on the subcutaneous plexus of vessels traveling in the tunica dartos. An axial flap can be a peninsular flap in which the skin of the flap remains in continuity with the skin body. Alternatively, an axial flap may be created as an island flap in which the skin of the flap is separated from the skin of the body, its only remaining connection with the body being its vascular pedicle. Peninsular skin flaps are not applicable to urethral reconstruction, as they do not allow for urethral closure. Peninsular skin flaps do have a role in genital reconstruction when used as an advancement skin flap for the reconstruction of genital skin defects. All penile skin flaps used in urethral reconstruction are island flaps. After the island flap is raised and the pedicle is dissected from the underlying skin, one has in essence created a second flap, that is, the remaining shaft skin has now been separated from its underlying subcutaneous plexus of vessels and becomes dependent upon the subdermal plexus alone, which communicates with the axial vessels at the base of the penis.

To avoid confusing nomenclature we will now review the different types of penile skin island flaps based on an intuitive anatomical classification. Flaps should be characterized as longitudinal vs transverse penile skin island, proximal penile skin vs distal penile skin/preputial skin, dorsal vs ventral vs lateral pedicle and ventral onlay vs tube flap vs combined tissue transfer.

5.1. Longitudinal vs Transverse

The most intuitive direction in which to develop a flap is longitudinal. This creates a flap that parallels the urethra and can easily be tailored to the appropriate length and width and rolled onto the area of the urethrotomy. Obviously, such a flap is best harvested from the ventral penile skin to minimize the amount of dissection needed to bring it to the urethra. Such a ventral skin incision is well-hidden in the median raphe during wound closure. A major disadvantage of this type of flap is that in longer strictures, hair-bearing skin from the proximal penis is used in the reconstruction. This, combined with the length of the penis, limits the length of flap.

The transverse penile flap is less intuitive and requires a greater degree of dissection of the pedicle to allow the flap to be rotated 90 degrees such that it parallels the urethra. In this case, the width of the onlay is determined by the width of the ring of penile skin harvested. The length of the flap can be varied from quite short if just a ventral patch of skin is used in the island or as long as 15 cm if a completely circular ring of skin is used. A "hockey stick" extension of the circular penile skin flap has been described (7), but we have not found this to be necessary, with extensive proximal mobilization of the flap a long, mobile flap is achieved. Like the longitudinal flap, the transverse flap scar is cosmetically excellent in that the appearance is no different than if the patient had been circumcised. The major critique of the transverse flap is that the dissection is more difficult; however, the more extensive dissection of the pedicle may have a distinct advantage in blood supply to the skin island. The pedicle of the longitudinal flap must be divided on one side of the flap to roll that side of the skin onto the urethrotomy. In contrast, the transverse island flap, particularly when it is harvested as a circular penile skin flap demands circumferential dissection of the tunica dartos pedicle ensuring a more broad-based blood supply.

5.2. Proximal vs Distal Penile Skin

The quality of the distal penile is skin is better suited to urethral reconstruction than is the proximal penile skin. First, the proximal penile skin can be hair-bearing leading to inflammation, infection, stone formation and restricture. In contrast, the distal penile skin has only a fine lanugo and the inner prepuce is completely devoid of hair follicles. Likewise, the distal penile skin and, in particular, the inner prepuce is better-accustomed to a moist environment than is the proximal penile skin which can become soggy and inflamed when continuously exposed to urine. When designing a transverse island flap one should harvest the skin flap as distally as possible.

5.3. Dorsal vs Ventral vs Lateral Pedicle

As reviewed previously, the source of the blood supply in the pedicle of the penile skin flap is the same regardless of the type of skin flap, always from the superficial and deep external pudendal arteries. The only difference is whether the ventrolateral or dorsolateral branches of the external

pudendal arteries contribute to the flap. A dorsally based flap theoretically maximizes blood supply from the left and right dorsolateral branches, at the risk of compromising the ventrolateral branches. The opposite is true for a ventrally based flap. A laterally based flap derives the majority of its blood supply from the ipsilateral ventrolateral branch with some collateral supply from the ipsilateral dorsolateral branch.

The type of flap, in part, dictates the direction of dissection of the pedicle. A longitudinal skin flap harvested from ventral penile skin could not, obviously, be supplied by a dorsally-based pedicle. It can, however, be based on a ventral or lateral pedicle. When developing a ventral pedicle a plane is developed over the urethra at the distal end of the flap and dissection of the pedicle continues proximally. As the dissection continues proximally the direction of dissection is carried out laterally to ensure a broad-based ventral flap. This is the technique described by Turner-Warwick (8).

An alternative approach is to dissect the skin island off the urethra from medial to lateral and continue the dissection out laterally along the corporal body, creating a laterally-based pedicle. This is the technique described by Ornadi (5). When constructing a transverse island onlay flap, the pedicle a segment of distal penile skin is outlined and the flap dissected off the shaft of the penis proximally. If only a small island of skin is used, then this is generally taken from the ventral aspect of the penis and the pedicle is, thus, ventrally based. This technique is described in detail elsewhere in this book by Dr. Armenakas. If a longer segment of urethra is to be reconstructed then a circular flap of distal penile skin is harvested.

To maximize blood supply to this long flap, it is essential to circumferentially dissect the tunica dartos off of the shaft. The skin island and flap can then be divided longitudinally either ventrally or dorsally, creating a rectangular skin flap and a dorsal or ventral pedicle, respectively. Although the blood supply to the edges of the island flap is relatively compromised compared with the center of the skin flap, blood supply to the edges is maximized by the initial complete degloving of the penile shaft such that the contribution of the ventrolateral branches is maximized as much as possible in a dorsally based flap and vice-a-versa. This is the technique described by McAninch (9).

5.4. Ventral Onlay vs Tube Flap vs Combined Tissue Transfer

After a ventral urethrotomy is made and the flap is isolated and tapered to the appropriate length, the flap is then sewn as an augment to the cut edges of the ventral urethrotomy. The dorsal onlay technique has been described for use in graft reconstruction of the anterior urethra but it is not used in flap reconstruction techniques.

Because the ventral onlay flap acts as an augment, it relies on an intact dorsal urethral plate; therefore, it is not appropriate in completely obliterative strictures. Short (<2 cm) obliterative strictures may be treated with excision and anastomotic urethroplasty but longer obliterative strictures require recreation of a dorsal urethral plate. One way to accomplish this is to perform a two-stage repair in which the first stage serves to recreate the dorsal plate with local skin flaps or a graft and the second stage to tubularize the urethral opening. For more detail on two-stage techniques, (see Chapter 18 by Dr. Coburn in this volume). For strictures slightly longer than 2 cm, an augmented anastomotic urethroplasty may be possible (see Chapter 13 by Sherman and Webster in this volume). One-stage solutions to the repair of obliterative strictures that are too long for an augmented anastomotic urethroplasty are a tube flap or a dorsal graft followed by a ventral penile skin island flap.

As with any obliterative stricture, the first step involves complete excision of the diseased urethra, leaving only the bare corporal bodies. A tube flap involves forming a cylinder of the island skin flap, sewing it into a tube longitudinally with open edges at both ends, and then anastomosing the open edges to the cut ends of the urethra. The tube flap has been used in complete urethral replacement for the treatment of long obliterative strictures; however, results have been poor (4), and this technique has been largely replaced by combined tissue transfer techniques or two-stage repairs. The tube flap will not be discussed further.

Combined tissue transfer refers to combining two or more techniques and/or tissue in urethral reconstruction. The most common example of this technique is a graft in one part of the urethra and a flap in another. However, for the case of long-segment urethral obliteration, combined tissue transfer can be used as a dorsal graft used to recreate the urethral plate followed by a ventral onlay flap. This technique will be described further below.

6. Technique

6.1. Preoperative Preparation

Preoperative delineation of stricture length and character is essential for careful selection of the type of reconstruction and patient positioning. The techniques of retrograde urethrogram, voiding cystourethrogram and sonourethrogram are described in detail by Dr. Siegel in chapter 4 of this book.

6.2. Patient Positioning

Urethral reconstruction requires meticulous technique. As such, the operative times can be long. Ensuring proper positioning before beginning the procedure will improve technical efficiency and will minimize positioning-related complications. For a discussion of positioning related complication, see Chapter 19 by *Al-Qudah* and Santucci in this volume. The length and location of the stricture will dictate whether the procedure is performed with the patient in the supine, low lithotomy, or high lithotomy position. Every effort should be made to keep the patient in the supine position as much as possible in order to minimize positioning-related complications. For pendulous urethral strictures the entire case can be performed in the supine position. When exposure of a more proximal stricture requires the lithotomy position and a flap repair is planned, it is essential that the flap be harvested with the patient in the supine position in order to minimize time in lithotomy.

6.3. Flap Harvest

We place a 2-O silk stay suture in the midsagittal plane of the glans penis to be used as traction suture. We do not shave the penile shaft preoperatively because this allows us to design a flap that does not incorporate hair-bearing skin. Careful tissue handling is essential in flap harvest and urethral reconstruction so as to minimize tissue necrosis and flap loss. One must move carefully so as to remain in the proper tissue plane at all times as failure to do so will compromise the vascular supply of the flap. Similarly, the use of bipolar electrocautery to control bleeding vessels is essential: poor vascular control leads to hematoma formation, which can compromise the flap.

A flap should be designed to match the length and width of the urethral defect. An estimation of length and width can be made based on preoperative imaging but the final measurements should be made after complete stricturotomy. The measurement of length is intuitive. Flap width, however, should equal the expected circumference of the normal urethra in the affected area minus the width of the urethral plate as measured after stricturotomy. As an example, if the expected circumference of the native urethra is 24 mm and the width of the urethral plate after stricturotomy is 4 mm then a 20 mm wide flap is selected. The circumference of the native urethra correlates with the size in "French," can vary from 30 mm in the bulbar urethra to 18 mm near the meatus and is also dependent on age. All this should be taken into consideration.

The remainder of the flap harvest technique varies by the type of flap, so each type of flap will be reviewed separately below. Although a particular flap might be harvested in a variety of ways, in the interest of clarity and brevity we will describe the technique of one expert surgeon for each type of flap. Again, we have taken the liberty of slightly modifying the terminology of fascial layers described by each of these expert surgeons so that all of the terminology is congruent. For instance, we will avoid describing whether the deep incision extends below or above the superficial layer of Buck's fascia and whether the superficial incision extends below or above the dartos fascia. Rather, we will describe the superficial and deep incisions only as such, superficial or deep to the pedicle.

6.3.1. *Longitudinal Ventral Penile Skin Flap With a Lateral Pedicle (Technique of Orandi [5])*

With the penis on stretch, a ventral vertical penile shaft incision is made over the area of stricture, approximating the length of the stricture. This incision, which will serve as the deep incision, is deepened to the lateral border of the corpus spongiosum. The plane is developed medially over the urethra. A lateral urethrotomy is made contralateral to the side of the initial skin incision and extended proximally and distally until normal urethra is encountered. The lateral urethrotomy helps minimize the amount of flap dissection necessary to obtain a tension-free anastamosis in this flap based on a lateral pedicle. The length and width urethral defect are then measured and the flap is marked out in an elongated hexagonal shape (**Fig. 14.3**). The deep longitudinal incision serves as one of the two long segments of the hexagon with the second long hexagonal segment becoming the superficial incision. This superficial incision is carried down to but not through the pedicle and developed laterally until the flap can be rotated over onto the urethrotomy in a tension-free manner (**Fig. 14.4**).

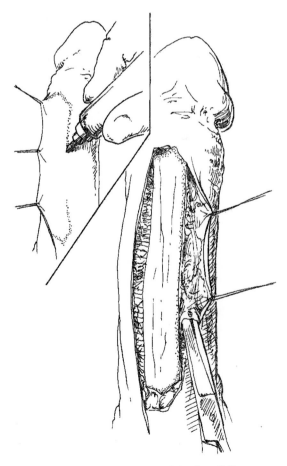

FIG. 14.3. Technique of harvest of the Orandi flap

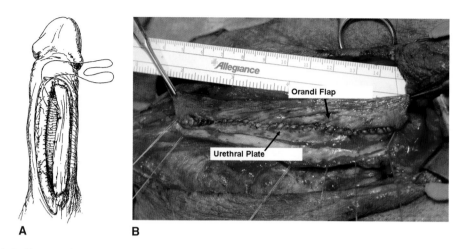

A   **B**

FIG. 14.4. A. Cartoon of rotation and onlay anastomosis of the Orandi flap. B. Orandi skin flap sewn to urethral plate. Foley catheter then placed and contralateral side of flap anastomosed

6.3.2. Longitudinal Ventral Penile Skin Flap With a Ventral Pedicle (Technique of Turner-Warwick [8])

Mr. Turner-Warwick described this flap as a bilaterally pedicled island penile skin flap (or BiPIPS). This is to differentiate it from the unilaterally pedicled island penile skin flap. Both flaps are based on a ventral pedicle. The broad bilateral pedicle (i.e. right and left ventrolateral branches of the external pudendal artery) ensures a more robust blood supply than the unilateral pedicle he described previously. Like the Orandi flap, this flap uses an elongated hexagonal patch of ventral penile skin. The skin island may be marked out preoperatively based on imaging of the stricture; if the flap is being used for bulbar urethral reconstruction, the skin island can be marked out after the bulbar urethra has been exposed via a separate perineal incision and the stricture measured. A deep plane is developed below the level of the pedicle around the distal apex of the island and a superficial layer is developed around the proximal apex of the island (**Fig. 14.5**) The island and its pedicle are thus elevated off the underlying penile urethra and overlying proximal penile shaft skin and scrotal skin. Development of the pedicle continues down into the scrotum. Because of the direction of development of the pedicle, Turner-Warwick described this flap to be most useful in bulbar urethral reconstruction where the flap is retrogradely inverted through a scrotal tunnel and brought out through a separate perineal incision and sewn to the bulbar urethrotomy.

6.3.3. Transverse Circular Penile Skin Flap With a Primarily Dorsal Pedicle (Technique of McAninch [9])

The penis is placed on stretch and the flap is marked out with calipers and brilliant green dye. The width of the flap varies between 2.0 and 2.5 cm, depending on the caliber of the stricture. If the penis is uncircumcised then the inner prepuce is chosen for the flap whereas if the penis is circumcised then the distal penile skin is used, for reasons described earlier. The distal incision is carried down through the pedicle, leaving the pedicle with the proximal penile skin. Once a satisfactory plane is established, the dissection is continued proximally, degloving the entire penile shaft. The proximal/superficial incision is then made and the pedicle dissected off the proximal penile skin, circumferentially all the way to the base of the penis. This leaves a very mobile circular ring of penile skin supported by a circumferential pedicle (**Fig. 14.6**). The flap and pedicle are generally divided ventrally as we feel the dorsal branches of the pedicle are more robust. (**Fig. 14.7**) The flap is then rotated 90 degrees and brought around ventrally (**Fig. 14.8** and **14.9**). The skin island is trimmed to meet the length of the stricturotomy and sutured to the urethral edge (**Fig. 14.10**).

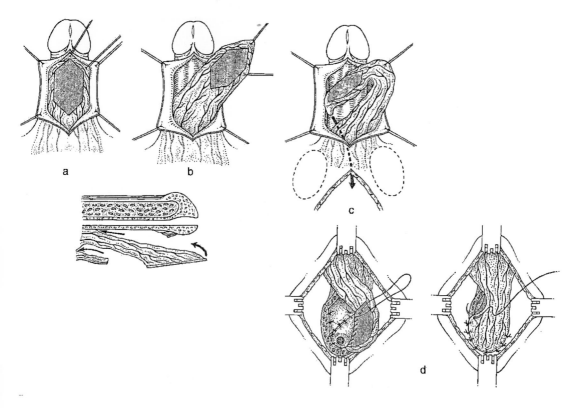

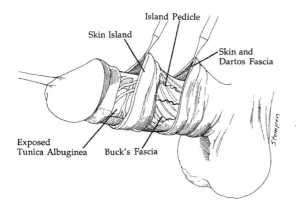

Fig. 14.5. Technique of harvest of the Turner-Warwick flap

Island Pedicle

Skin Island

Skin and
Dartos Fascia

Exposed
Tunica Albuginea   Buck's Fascia

Fig. 14.6. Technique of harvest of the McAninch flap

6.4. Urethral Closure With Ventral Onlay Island Skin Flap

Regardless of the technique of flap harvest, the principles of urethral closure using a ventral onlay of a penile skin island flap are the same. First, the stricture should be completely opened, extending into

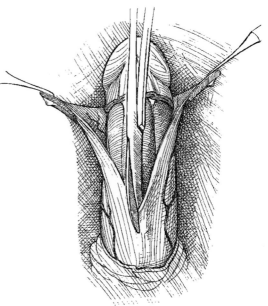

Fig. 14.7. Ventral splitting of the McAninch flap

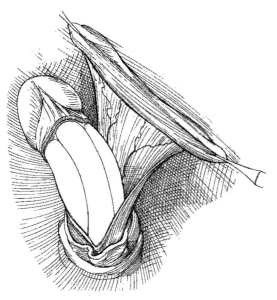

FIG. 14.8. Rotation of the McAninch flap

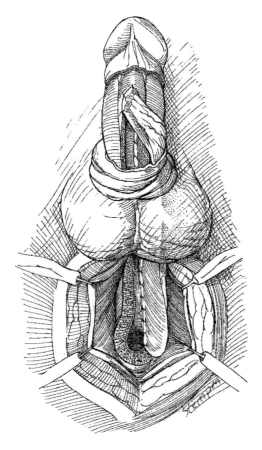

FIG. 14.9. Onlay anastomosis of the McAninch flap

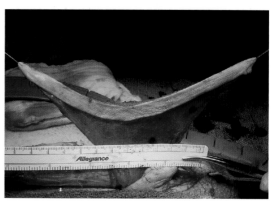

FIG. 14.10. Mobilized circular (McAninch) skin flap demonstrating versatility and long length

normal urethra. Second, the skin island should be tapered and fashioned to the length and width necessary for urethral reconstruction, as described above. Third, a meticulous epithelium to urethral edge anastomosis should be done. This is best accomplished with loupe magnification, fine suture and delicate instruments. Neither running nor interrupted suture has ever been proven to be superior to the other; the surgeon should follow whatever technique he feels gives him the best control. The urethral closure is done over a 14- to 18-French catheter. Too small a catheter does not optimally drain the bladder, especially when clots may be present, while too large a catheter may induce pressure ischemia of the flap. The catheter is left indwelling for 1–3 wk depending on the length and location of the flap.

6.5. Urethral Closure in Combined Tissue Transfer

As described previously, combined tissue transfer techniques are useful as one-stage solutions to obliterative long anterior urethral strictures. The most common scenario in which a pedicled island penile skin flap is used in combined tissue transfer is as a ventral onlay in combination with a dorsally placed buccal mucosa graft. After the stricture is completely excised down to the bare corporal bodies, the buccal mucosa graft is fixed in place at the apices by stitches that pass through the buccal graft, the dorsal aspect of the native urethral lumen and the tunica albuginea.

It is then helpful to place the graft on stretch with four to six additional stitches between only the tunica and the graft along the lateral edges of the graft. The remainder of the graft fixation can be incorporated into the stitches used to lay in the ventral flap as described below. First, taper the flap to the appropriate length and width. Second, suture the proximal and distal apices of the flap to the ventral aspect of the proximal and distal cut ends of the native urethra. Third, place enough interrupted sutures at the apices to complete the anastomosis of the flap to the native urethral lumen. These are difficult sutures and it is easy to get confused, which is why we prefer to place these sutures in an interrupted fashion. Finally, a running suture is used to anastomose the flap to the lateral edges of the buccal graft and concomitantly anchor both the flap and the graft to the tunica albuginea. After one side is completed, a urethral catheter is inserted and the second side is closed in the same running fashion.

7. Results

7.1. Success Rates

For several reasons, it is difficult to compare success rates with the different techniques of penile skin flap urethroplasty. Most surgeons perform only one type of flap urethroplasty meaning that any comparison of one technique against another must be done across several institutions in many countries. Etiology of stricture disease, length and location of stricture, mechanisms of patient referral, indications for surgery, surgical technique, quality of follow-up, and the definition of failure may differ at each of these institutions. Finally, most studies are retrospective reviews of case series. These all contribute to multiple forms of selection bias and observation bias. Given these shortcomings in the data, it appears that the success rates of at least the Orandi and McAninch flaps, and likely the Turner-Warwick flap as well, are similar: 5% failure at 1 yr and 20% at 3–5 yr *(4,10)*. Results are better with onlay flap (10–15% failure long-term) than tubularized flaps (30–60% failure long-term).

7.2. Complications

Restenosis can occur from flap failure, inadequate stricturotomy, imprecise suturing of the flap to the urethral edges, or progression of the original disease. Flap failure occurs early and results from a compro-

mised pedicle due to improper dissection at the time of flap harvest, hematoma or infection. This results in a long restricture. Inadequate stricturotomy also occurs early but results in a short segment re-stenosis at one of the ends of the flap. Errors in suturing of the flap to the urethral edges occur most commonly at the apices, resulting in early restenosis at one of the ends of the flap. Finally, progression of the original disease also results in re-stenosis at one of the ends of the flap or distant from the flap, but this generally occurs later in follow-up.

Urethrocutaneous fistula may result from hematoma, infection, catheter obstruction, or errors in surgical technique. It is believed that interposing additional layers between the urethral anastomosis and the skin or avoiding overlapping suture lines will minimize the risk of fistula formation.

Penile skin necrosis may result from dissecting in the wrong plane when raising the flap, resulting in compromising the collateral blood supply to the skin. A complete discussion of complications may be found in Chapter 19 by Al-Qudah and Santucci in this volume.

Editorial Comment

Penile flaps are the mainstay of urethral reconstruction. Penile skin flaps rely on the rich vascular collaterals within the tunica Dartos for its blood supply. The anterior lamella of Buck's fascia is elevated to ensure taking the entire Dartos. The correct planes are relatively avascular. Island flaps are versatile and can be mobilized to all areas of the anterior urethra. For on-lay flaps where the urethral plate remains intact, failure rates are progressive and increase over the long-term. Tubularized flaps fail roughly one-half the time.

Depending on the location and the length of the stricture, flaps can be ventral–longitudinal (Orandi, for pendulous urethra), ventral–transverse (Jordan/Devine, for fossa strictures), or transverse–circumferential (Quartey, McAninch, or Q-type, for anterior urethra) and rotated to reach the defect. Proper mobilization and are easier to construct, will not put the flap on tension or cause penile torsion. The advantages of transverse–circumferential flaps are they are hairless, can be mobilized to any area of the anterior urethra and are long (10–15 cm). Ventral flaps require less mobilization and are easier to construct, but hair is often present at the proximal aspect. Although we have been generally been moving away from the use of flaps to buccal graft urethroplasty over the last few years, they still have an important role in the armamentarium. Flaps are particularly useful for reconstructing a prior graft failure, long (near panurethral) strictures, or as a combination flap of both dorsal graft (replacing the urethral plate) and a ventral onlay flap, instead of the typically unsuccessful tubularized flap or graft. In general, we try to mobilize flaps with the patient in the supine position, and if the stricture extends into the bulbar urethra, we subsequently redrape and prep the patient in the lithotomy position. In this way, the morbidity of excessive time in the lithotomy position can be avoided. From a technical view point, when dissecting out the pedicle of the flap, we will typically err on the skin side in our attempt to make the Dartos pedicle as thick as possible. Our feeling is that if we make it a little thin on the skin side, the skin may slough in a small area, but this is something that with dressing changes will granulate in nicely with time and leave little long-term morbidity. If we skimp on the pedicle side out of fear of devascularizing a small segment of skin, we potentially compromise the success of the urethroplasty (which is a much bigger problem to deal with). For this reason, we typically first start with the distal skin incision that extends deep, to mobilize the sub-Dartos plane, and then make the more proximal skin incision (usually 2 cm proximal) that extends only into the subepithelial avascular plane. When dissecting out the subepithelial plane we typically keep an index finger under the Dartos pedicle (and periodically palpate with a thumb) to insure that we are keeping the pedicle as thick as possible.—S.B. Brandes.

Appendix

Preferred Instruments and Suture of JW McAninch

a) Castroviejo Caliper
b) Bayonet bipolar cautery forceps
c) Bougie-a-Boule
d) Forceps
   i) Gerald forceps with teeth
   ii) DeBakey forceps
   iii) Bishop-Harmon forceps
   iv) McAninch blue titanium forceps (Sontec #2600-582)
e) Scissors
   i) Supercut curved endarterectomy Scissors, 6¾ inches (Jarit #102-315)
   ii) Supercut straight Mayo Scissors, 5 ½ inches (Jarit #102-100)
   iii) Supercut curved Jamison Scissors, 5½ inches (Jarit #102-300)
f) Needle Holders:
   i) Euphrates-Pasque (2300-661)
g) Suture
   i) 2-0 silk pop-off (glans stitch)
   ii) 5-0 chromic (to repair holes in the corpus spongiosum)
   iii) 4-0 Dexon RB-1 (for holding stitches and wound closure)
   iv) 5-0 or 6-0 Maxon, RB-1 (for urethral anastomosis)

References

1. Barbagli G, Palminteri E, Balo S, Vallasciani S, Mearini E, Constantini E, Mearini L, Zucchi A, Vivacqua C, Porena M (2004) Lichen sclerosis of the male genitalia ans urethral stricture disease. Urol Int 73:1–5
2. Garcia M, Elliott SP, McAninch JW (2006) Single-stage fasciocutaneous flap urethral reconstruction of strictures involving the fossa navicularis and meatus Abstract presented at the national Meeting of the American urological Association, Atlanta, GA
3. Venn SN, Mundy AR (1998) Urethroplasty for balanitis xerotica obliterans. Br J Urol 81:735–737
4. Carney KJ, McAninch JW (2002) Penile circular fasciocutaneous flaps to reconstruct complex anterior urethral strictures. Urol Clin N Am 29:97–409
5. Kodama RT, Ordorica RC (1996) Ornadi flap for urethral stricture management, in McAninch JW (ed) Traumatic and reconstructive urology. Philadelphia, Saunders, pp 595–600
6. Jordan GH, Schlossberg SM. Surgery of the penis and urethra, in Walsh PC, Retik AB, Vaughan, Jr, Wein AJ (ed) Campbell's urology, vol. 4. Philadelphia, Saunders, pp 3886–3954
7. Quartey JKM (1996) Quartey flap reconstruction of urethral stricture, in McAninch JW (ed) Traumatic and reconstructive urology. Philadelphia, Saunders, pp 601–608
8. Chapple C, Turner-Warwick R (1996) Substitution urethroplasty and the pedicled island penile skin procedure, in McAninch JW (ed) Traumatic and reconstructive urology. Philadelphia, Saunders, pp 571–594
9. Mcaninch JW (1993) Reconstruction of extensive urethral strictures: circular fasciocutaneous penile flap. J Urol 149:488–491
10. Greenwell TJ, Venn SN, Mundy AR (1999) Changing practice in anterior urethroplasty. BJU Int 83, 631–635

15
Panurethral Strictures

Steven B. Brandes

Contents

1. Introduction... 165
2. Evaluation 166
3. Patient Positioning 166
4. Surgical Reconstruction 166
    4.1. Bilateral Buccal Mucosal Grafts.. 166
    4.2. Circular Fasciocutaneous Onlay flaps, "Q flap" 166
    4.3. Flap Combined With Graft... 168
    4.4. Proximal Buccal Graft and Distal Staged Urethroplasty 169
    4.5. LSA-Induced Panurethral Stricture... 169
    4.6. Panurethral Stricture With Areas of Complete Lumen Obliteration............................ 170
References... 170

Summary Panurethral strictures are complex and long strictures that involve both the pendulous and bulbar urethra. Such strictures are among the most difficult to successfully reconstruct, and require the use of the entire surgical armamentarium. Surgical methods for reconstructing such long and diffuse strictures are: bilateral buccal mucosal grafts, "Q" penile skin flaps, McAninch (circular penile skin) flaps, Orandi (vertical penile skin) flap, or a combination of such onlay flaps and grafts. In these combination cases, the graft is typically placed proximally to benefit from spongiosal blood supply, and the flap placed on the distal bulb or pendulous urethra. Bilateral buccal grafts will allow repair in strictures up to 12 cm, while the mean penile lengths from flaps are roughly: Q flap (17 cm), Ornadi flap (9 cm), McAninch (15 cm). For refractory panurethral strictures, a staged urethroplasty using skin grafting is usually needed.

Keywords penile skin flap, fasciocutaneous flap, buccal mucosal graft, staged urethroplasty, lichen sclerosus

1. Introduction

Panurethral strictures are complex and long strictures that involve both the pendulous and bulbar urethra. Such strictures are difficult to reconstruct and require the use of the entire surgical armamentarium for successful urethral reconstruction. The anterior urethra length is on average from 15 to 20 cm. Thus, to bridge a pan urethral stricture, a combination of grafts and/or flaps is needed for reconstruction. The initial surgical steps include exposure of the entire anterior urethra and then opening up the stricture longitudinally for visual inspection of the epithelium and spongiofibrosis, followed by intraoperative bougienage of the

From: *Current Clinical Urology: Urethral Reconstructive Surgery*
Edited by: S.B. Brandes © Humana Press, Totowa, NJ

spatulated urethra and repeat cystoscopy to assess for residual stenosis and disease.

2. Evaluation

The first common pitfall is to not properly diagnose the stricture as being panurethral. On urethrography, the narrowing of the lumen can be fairly uniform, with short areas of more severe stenosis. Such a panurethral stricture can be misread as just a short stricture and the other less-narrow areas underestimated as being a "normal" caliber. Some of the ways to avoid this error in diagnosis is that, no matter how uniform the urethra may look, if it does not expand to ≥8 mm in diameter on imaging, then it is probably stenosed. In addition, full evaluation of the urethra requires both urethroscopy and bougienage. If the preoperative image is confusing, endoscopy and bougienage will help clarify the extent of stricture. If it is still confusing, then we typically take such patients for an "examination under anesthesia" (EUA) and repeat all the studies. Oftentimes, it is only by a liberal use of EUA and endoscopy that a proper and timely surgical plan can be made. Moreover, it is our feeling that for successful reconstruction of long and complex strictures, it is best to determine the length and full extent of the stricture preoperatively, with a well thought out plan for reconstruction, rather then attempting to "figure it out" during the surgery.

3. Patient Positioning

In general, we start with the patient in the supine position and open and repair the pendulous urethral stricture. We then reposition the patient lithotomy and work on the more proximal strictures that involve the bulb. By following this order of positioning, the morbidity of lithotomy positioning is minimized, by limiting the time in lithotomy. We typically place our patients with pan urethral strictures in adjustable "Allen" or "Yellowfin" stirrups, initially in the low lithotomy position, almost supine, with the patient's buttock at the edge of the bed. Thus, when the pendulous aspects of the urethral stricture are completed, the legs can be easily placed into lithotomy without repositioning or redraping.

4. Surgical Reconstruction Methods

4.1. Bilateral Buccal Mucosal Grafts

Bilateral buccal mucosal graft harvest from the cheeks typically will give grafts of 6 cm each (depending on oral anatomy), and thus can be used to repair strictures of up to 12 cm. When phallic length is short, two buccal grafts alone may be able to bridge the whole gap. Otherwise, a combination of flap and graft or a two-stage reconstruction method is needed. For pendulous and distal bulbar strictures, we prefer to place the grafts dorsally (quilted to the corpus cavernosum) because there is typically insufficient distal spongiosum to properly cover a ventrally placed graft. Unsupported and inadequate "spongioplasty" to ventral grafts, are prone to ischemic failure and sacculation.

4.2. Circular Fasciocutaneous Onlay flaps, "Q flap"

Another option for reconstructing the panurethral stricture is the "Q-flap." The Q-flap is a modification of a circular penile fasciocutaneous skin flap procedure (McAninch flap) (1). It is so-called because it incorporates an additional midline ventral longitudinal penile extension, thus resembling the letter Q. Similar "hockey-stick" flap configurations have also been described by Quartey and Jordan (2).

Morey et al. (1) reported their experience with 15 men undergoing single-stage urethral reconstruction with a distal circumferential penile skin flap incorporating a ventral midline extension (i.e., Q-flap [1]). None had undergone previous urethroplasty and all still had a prepuce. Mean stricture length was 15.5 cm (range, 12–21 cm). The Q-flap provided a pedicled strip of penile skin with a mean length of 17 cm (range, 15–24 cm). Operative times averaged 5 h. The Q-flap provides an abundant hairless penile skin flap that enables single-stage panurethral reconstruction while eliminating the additional time and morbidity of harvesting further grafts. No proximal grafts were necessary for stricture repair. Excellent results were obtained in 10 of 15 (67%) of patients.

Complications were fairly common at one-third, which included recurrent stricture (in two) and (in one patient each), urethrocutaneous fistula, meatal stenosis, femoral neuropathy, and prolonged catheterization for focal extravasation. Of the 15 patients, 13 were followed for a mean of 42.6 mo (range, 12–102 mo) and the remaining two for only 6 mo. Of the former, 11 void standing and have excellent cosmetic results. Focal failure occurred in one at 5 yr. Moderate penile skin edema and ecchymosis occurred routinely for days to weeks after surgery.

To minimize the complications of lithotomy positioning, the Q-flap flap is dissected with the patient initially in the supine position. The flap is outlined with the penis on stretch and the penis degloved, carefully preserving the vascular pedicle of tunica dartos (**Fig. 15.1**). A ventral urethrotomy is then made into the stricture. In the uncircumcised patient, the outer sleeve of the prepuce is then mobilized carefully from the tunica dartos skin flap pedicle. The Q-flap is typically 2-cm wide, depending on the width of the urethral "plate," to create a urethra of normal caliber (typically, 24 French). The ventral and longitudinal extension typically adds an additional 3–6 cm. Hair-bearing skin from the proximal penile shaft is avoided whenever possible. Once the pedicle is dissected back to the penoscrotal junction, the flap pedicle is divided ventrally along the edge of the Q-extension and then further, to the penoscrotal area. Relaxing incisions can be useful along the lateral margins of the flap to allow a

tension-free transfer to the perineum and prevent penile torsion. The Q-flap in sewn into place after ventral urethrotomy as an onlay flap (Fig. 15.2). The fossa navicularis typically is reconstructed with the use of either a glans-wings or a glans-preserving technique. Anastomosis of the flap to the urethral plate is typically performed with running 4–O polyglactin or polydioxanone sutures. It is important to keep the flap on stretch while it is sewn into place to prevent redundancy and sacculations (which can cause bothersome post void dribbling). Redundant pedicle should also be loosely advanced over the contralateral suture line to help prevent fistula formation.

Once the pendulous aspects of the onlay flap were sewn in, the patient is repositioned into the lithotomy position. To transfer the flap to the

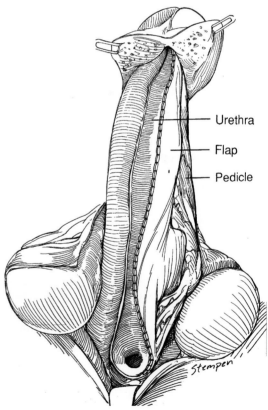

FIG. 15.2. Circular fasciocutaneous flap rotated vertically and sewn into place as an onlay to the urethral plate. (From Quartey JKM (1996). Quartey flap reconstruction of urethral strictures, in McAninch JW (ed) Traumatic and reconstructive urology. Philadelphia, WB Saunders)

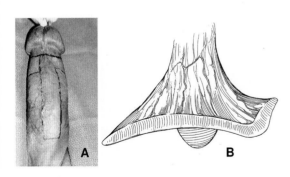

FIG. 15.1. Q FLAP. (A) Circular fasciocutaneous skin flap with ventral longitudinal extension, as outlined on the penis. (B) Illustration of a fully mobilized hockey stick-shaped flap (i.e., Q-flap). (A is courtesy Allen F Morey B. From Quartey JKM (1996). Quartey flap reconstruction of urethral strictures, in McAninch JW (ed) Traumatic and reconstructive urology. Philadelphia, WB Saunders)

perineum with no tension, a scrotal tunnel roughly 4 cm wide in diameter is made. Redundant distal prepuce, if present, is excised at the end of the reconstruction. Most patients are kept in hospital for 1 to 2 d postoperatively. A 16-F silicone urethral catheter is typically maintained for 3 to 4 wk, followed by a voiding cystourethrogram. For comfort and to prevent inadvertent pulling on the urethral catheter, we typically also place a suprapubic catheter and cap the urethral Foley catheter after 48 h. The major advantage of the Q-flap is offers one-stage reconstruction of difficult and long strictures; and it eliminates the need for additional, potentially morbid and time-consuming tissue-transfer techniques, which otherwise would be necessary for panurethral reconstruction.

4.3. Flap Combined With Graft

We prefer to first develop a subcoronal, circular fasciocutaneous onlay flap in the supine position. The circular pedicle island skin (McAninch) flap will typically be roughly 15 cm in length and 2 cm in width (**Fig. 15.3**) Others have used an Orandi flap in combination with a proximal graft *(3)*; however, the Orandi flap is typically limited by shaft hair, and thus typically only 8–9 cm in length (depending on penile size). If the pedicle of Dartos and anterior lamella of Buck's fascia is adequately mobilized, the flap can be transposed even to the proximal bulbar urethra, through a window underneath the scrotum. By adequate mobilization, we mean that when the penis is placed on full stretch, there is redundancy and no tension on the vascular pedicle (**Fig. 15.4**).

Inadequate pedicle mobilization will result in a tethering of the penis and cause the penis to rotate with erection (the direction of the "torsion" is clockwise when the pedicle is developed on the left and counterclockwise when the pedicle comes from the right).

The onlay flap is used to cover the pendulous and distal bulbar urethras. A ventral urethrotomy is made until the urethral can be bougied to at least 24 Fr. The edges of the cut spongiosum are sewn to the urethral plate with a running suture for hemostasis. For the distal margin of the circular skin flap, the incision is deep to the Dartos of the penis and includes the anterior lamella of Buck's fascia. Such a depth is avascular. For the proximal margin of the skin flap, the skin is incised sharply with a scalpel, until the skin easily separates from

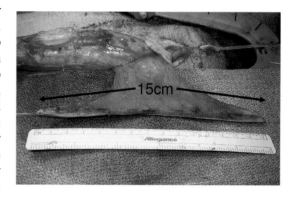

FIG. 15.3. Another circular fasciocutaneous onlay flap, fully mobilized and rotated vertically for use as an onlay flap. Note near panurethral length at 15 cm

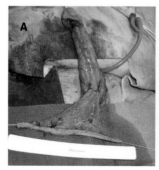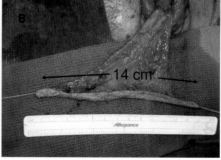

FIG. 15.4. (A) and (B) Circular fasciocutaneous onlay flap fully mobilized till the penoscrotal junction. Note the length of the skin flap (14 cm) and versatility of its long vascular pedicle of Dartos, for reconstruction of any aspect of the anterior urethra

its underlying Dartos tissue. The skin can then be mobilized away from the Dartos vascular pedicle in an avascular, areolar like layer.

For the remaining proximal bulbar stricture, a buccal graft if placed ventrally and the covered by spongioplasty. The reason the buccal graft and not the flap is placed proximally is because the spongiosum is thickest in the proximal bulb and will provide the most vascularity to a ventrally placed graft; thus, maximizing success. In order to continuously bridge the entire stricture, we prefer to suture the distal end of the graft to the proximal end of the flap with interrupted sutures. Berlund and Angermeier *(3)* noted that, in 18 patients, they were able to reconstruct near pan urethral strictures with a combined graft and flap. Mean stricture lengths were 15.1 cm (range, 9.5–22 cm). Such strictures could have been reconstructed with a circular onlay flap or Q-flap alone. Regardless, they used a combination of buccal graft (mean, 6.3 cm) and Orandi flap (ventral-longitudinal flap; mean, 8.5 cm). Etiology of their panurethral strictures were hypospadias repair failures (22%), instrumentation (22%), pelvic trauma (17%), lichen sclerosus et atrophicus (LSA; 17%), and unknown in 22%.

4.4. Proximal Buccal Graft and Distal Staged Urethroplasty

When the patient has a pendulous urethral stricture that has failed multiple prior urethroplasty, hypospadias surgery, or LSA surgery, and there is an associated bulbar urethral stricture, then such patients can often be successfully managed with a staged urethroplasty to the pendulous urethra and a buccal graft to the more proximal bulbar stricture.

For the bulbar stricture, we start out in the lithotomy position with a perineal incision and repair the stricture with a buccal mucosal graft placed either ventrally or dorsally, based on surgeon preference. The patient is then repositioned supine or low lithotomy. The ventral midline penile incision is made to expose the spongiosum, followed by a ventral urethrotomy, extending up to the glandular stenosis, and glans wings are developed. The tunica Dartos of the penis is then quilted to the side of the urethral plate, to act as a host bed for the subsequent graft. For recurrent meatal and fossa strictures, where the tissues are often very scarred, we favor excision of the

glandular and fossa urethral plate, followed by complete grafting. Stay sutures are placed at the corners of each of the glans wings. The rest of the pendulous urethral plate is preserved. Depending on the length of the stricture, a split thickness skin graft of a buccal mucosal graft is fenestrated with a no. 11 blade and then quilted to the corpora with multiple 4-O chromic sutures. For strictures longer then 3 cm, bilateral buccal grafts are often needed to recreate a wide enough plate for staged tubularization. The buccal graft should be oversized by 20% and a split-thickness skin graft oversized by 50% to allow for graft contracture as it matures. A neomeatus is then made at the proximal aspect of the pendulous urethral stricture. A 16-French silicone Foley is placed and a typical bolster dressing of Xeroform, cotton batting soaked in mineral oil, and fluff bolster tied into place with purple dyed 2-O Vicryl sutures placed at the edges of the graft. The dressing and bolster are taken down after 3 to 5 d. After the grafts have matured and the tissue is supple (typically 6 or more mo) the second stage is performed. At the time of tubularization, we prefer to interpose an onlay flap of tunical vaginalis, to act as a second layer to prevent fistulization.

4.5. LSA-Induced Panurethral Stricture

Panurethral strictures that are LSA induced typically start as meatal stenosis and meatitis. The high pressure voiding and infected urine, lead to secondary Littritis, which then results in corresponding annular (band-like) strictures at the level of each of the glands. The stenotic bands that develop are typically multiple and throughout the bulb and pendulous urethra. LSA is a good example of how untreated and ignored meatal stenosis can progress to the complex and difficult to repair paraurethral stricture. Because the epithelium is infected with LSA, in our experience, over prolonged follow-up, such onlay flap or grafts eventually become infected and re-stenose.

Although it was our prior common practice to reconstruct the LSA stricture with an onlay flap of penile skin, such flaps typically progressively failed, in our hands. Avoiding the use of local skin makes sense because the LSA often affects all genital skin fairly diffusely and, thus, the nonvisible, subclinical disease will often just manifest later. Therefore, to achieve durable results, we favor that panurethral strictures from LSA be reconstructed by a staged method of grafting followed by tubularization of the graft, months later. Details for staged grafting techniques are detailed above (in section 4.4), as well as Chapter 18 by Coburn in this volume.

4.6. Panurethral Stricture With Areas of Complete Lumen Obliteration

As detailed previously in this chapter, the initial surgical steps include exposure of the anterior urethra and ventral urethrotomy, followed by reconstruction with augmentation of the stenotic urethral plate by a graft or flap. In general, if we assume the residual plate will be roughly 1 cm, then a graft or flap 2 cm wide will create a tubular structure 3 cm in circumference (which translates to a lumen >24 French) For strictures where there is barely a residual plate or an obliterated lumen to augment, then either a two stage reconstruction is required, or a one stage method (after Morey) is performed *(4)*. (**Fig. 15.5**) In general, tubularized flap reconstruction of the urethra has a high (over 50%) failure rate. An alternative and more successful one-stage method of reconstructing the obliterated urethra is to place a buccal graft ventrally, quilted to the corpora, combined with a dorsal onlay skin flap. The combination of ventral graft and dorsal flap creates a tubular structure that has more durable success then a tubularized flap *(3)*.

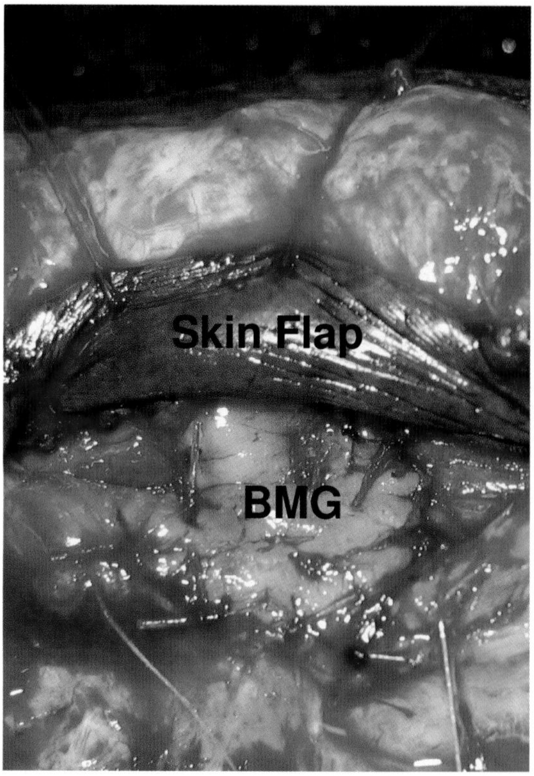

FIG. 15.5. Obliterated urethral segment reconstructed with ventral skin island flap (Orandi) and dorsal buccal graft

References

1. Morey AF, Tran LK, Zinman LM (2000) Q flap reconstruction of panurethral strictures. BJU Int 86: 1039–1042.
2. Quartey JKM (1996) Quartey flap reconstruction of urethral strictures. In McAninch JW (ed). Traumatic and Reconstructive Urology, Philadelphia, WB Saunders
3. Berglund RK, Angermeier KW (2006) Combined buccal mucosa graft and genital skin flap for reconstruction of extensive anterior urethral strictures. Urology 68:707–710
4. Morey AF (2001) Urethral plate salvage with dorsal graft promotes successful penile flap onlay reconstruction of severe pendulous strictures. J Urol 166:1376–1378

16

The Combined Use of Fasciocutaneous, Muscular and Myocutaneous Flaps and Graft Onlays in Urethral Reconstruction

Leonard N. Zinman

Contents

1. Introduction 171
2. Muscle Assisted Full-Thickness Skin and Buccal Graft Urethroplasty 172
3. Gracilis Flap: Anatomy and Retrieval for Urethral Stricture Disease 172
    3.1. Technique of Buccal Mucosal Graft Onlay With Gracilis Support 173
    3.2. Short Gracilis Flap 173
    3.3. Dorsal Placement of Buccal Graft and Gracilis Muscle 174
    3.4. Prefabricated Combined Skin and Gracilis Flap Reconstruction 175
    3.5. The Gracilis Myofasciocutaneous Flap 176
    3.6. Operative Technique for Transfer of the Gracilis Myofasciocutaneous Flap 178
4. Perineal Artery Fasciocutaneous Flap (Singapore) 180
    4.1. Flap Design and Technique of Elevation for Onlay Patch Urethroplasty 180
5. Gluteus Maximus Muscle Flap 182
    5.1. Gluteal Flaps for Bulbomembranous Urethral Reconstruction 182
    5.2. Gluteal Anatomy and Clinical Applications 183
    5.3. Techniques of Gluteal Maximus Repair of a Perineal-Urethral Strictures (and Fistulas) 183
6. Conclusion 186
Editorial Comment 187
References 187

Summary For refractory urethral strictures and fistulas with compromised vascularity and multiple failed previous procedures, salvage methods for successful reconstruction require tissue transfer of muscle-assisted skin and buccal graft composites, such as with the gracilis muscle flap, the perineal artery - medial thigh - fasciocutaneous flap, and the inferior gluteus maximus muscle flap. Such extragenital axial flaps are reliable and suitable for local genital skin substitution. These muscle flap composites are relatively simple in design, easy to harvest and transfer, possess reliable vascular and cutaneous landmarks, and can be mobilized to the perineum without tension or significant donor site morbidity.

Keywords gracilis muscle flap, buccal graft, myocutaneous flap, Singapore flap, gluteus maximus muscle flap

1. Introduction

The ability to achieve a long-term, stable, stricture-free, and hairless urethral lumen in patients with complex anterior strictures and posterior urethral separation defects in the presence of adverse wound settings, is one of the ongoing challenges of reconstructive urologic surgery. Genital fasciocutaneous flaps, buccal mucosal grafts, or some combination of the two in a one-stage or multistage

From: *Current Clinical Urology: Urethral Reconstructive Surgery*
Edited by: S.B. Brandes © Humana Press, Totowa, NJ

fashion is presently the standard of surgical care for strictures not suitable for anastomotic repair. There is, however, a unique subset of patients with complex urethral pathology and refractory fistulas that have undergone multiple failed previous procedures, previous radiation therapy, skin loss from trauma or decubiti, and impaired wound healing that will require transfer of an extragenital flap for successful resolution. With the advent of the axial flap and an understanding of the vascular anatomy of muscular, myocutaneous, and fasciocutaneous flaps and their ability to cover and enhance the healing ability of a compromised wound, an alternative armamentarium of reliable flaps are presently available as critical adjuncts for this challenging pathology. They can be transferred as islands, hinges (peninsular) and free forms with minimal donor site morbidity. A group of extragenital flaps used in the trunk and lower-extremity defects are the most suitable for salvage of high-risk urethral disorders (1,2).

2. Muscle Assisted Full-Thickness Skin and Buccal Graft Urethroplasty

The expectations of full-thickness skin grafts have not been consistently achieved, but their advantages for the repair of anterior urethral stricture are hard to overlook (3). The advantages of buccal mucosa or skin grafts include ease of application, wide versatility, multiple hairless donor source, and the ability to construct a conduit that most closely resembles a normal functioning urethra with rare sacculation. The addition of the buccal mucosa graft, a major change in the reconstructive paradigm, has proven to be an invaluable addition as a one- or two-stage procedure for the complex posthypospadiac, the patient with BXO or radiated, or reoperated patient. Buccal graft's unique anatomy includes a thin and highly vascular lamina propria (4,5). It has extended the ability of free graft material to resolve a longer stricture or a large, fixed refractory fistula with an early impressive record of success but still remains at risk of partial or complete graft loss in the presence of an adverse fibrotic hypovascular periurethral tissue bed. This clinical setting requires a change in graft recipient site vascularity

to ensure reliable inosculation, a concern that can be managed by transferring a number of trunk or thigh muscle flaps adjacent to the graft subdermal or lamina propria surface.

Skeletal muscles have an established role in resolving complex wounds, osteomyelitis, prosthetic graft sepsis, and repair of tissue defects and fistulas that develop under unfavorable condition (6). They can provide coverage, obliterate dead space, separate suture lines, and improve vascularity and enhanced white cell function in chronically fibrotic and impaired wounds with minimal morbidity (7). The use of a skeletal muscle surface intimately secured to the dermal side of a skin graft or buccal mucosal undersurface with proper immobilization will promote more predictable and rapid inosculation and prevent seroma formation and contracture.

The optimal muscle flaps available for urethral and perineal reconstruction include gracilis muscle utilizing four different techniques, the rectus abdominis, gluteus maximus, rectus femoris, semitendinosis and the free latissimus dorsi. The most versatile and readily retrieved muscle is the gracilis, which can be transferred simply as a support for a skin or buccal graft in either a dorsal or ventral position. Three additional variations of transfer of the gracilis muscle include a short version of the gracilis, which offers more muscle volume for preventing dead space, the myocutaneous technique, which is the incorporation of a potential skin paddle for defect coverage in an island or peninsular form, or the prefabrication of a skin graft and subsequent transfer of the muscle, which carries with it an established neovascularized skin graft island.

3. Gracilis Flap: Anatomy and Retrieval for Urethral Stricture Disease

The gracilis muscle remains the reconstructive workhorse of the perineum, groin, genitalia, and anal musculature. As a free flap, it has widespread application in coverage of the head, neck, and extremities, as well as a functional muscle in facial reanimation, and can play a major role in the salvage of high-risk urethral pathology burdened

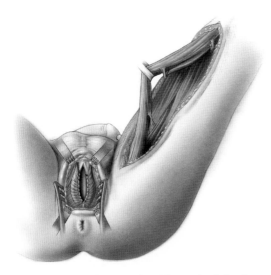

FIG. 16.1. The gracilis muscle with proximal dominant pedicle and two distant minor pedicles

by wound healing adversities. Its anatomy has been reliably defined by numerous studies that have identified its blood supply (**Fig. 16.1**), innervation, and functional characteristics *(8,9)*. *See* Chapter 22 by Brandes in this volume for more details about the gracilis muscle anatomy and its mobilization.

3.1. Technique of Buccal Mucosal Graft Onlay With Gracilis Support

The proper sequence for this procedure is to 1) prepare the urethra, 2) mobilize the muscle, and 3) harvest the buccal graft after a suprapubic diverting cystotomy is established. The urethra is prepared ventrally with exposure through a midline perineal incision extending into the midscrotal raphe. The bulbocavernosis muscle is divided and carefully preserved because it will be sutured to the edges of the applied gracilis. A urethrotomy is started distally and extended for 2 to 3 cm beyond both ends of the stricture. Hemostasis from spongiosal edge is achieved with locked running 5-O chromic catgut sutures along the urethrotomy margin. Extensive, severely fibrotic, or radiated corpus spongiosa should not be excised unless there are obliterated segments since the traditional expected elasticity is often absent in the presence of severe spongiosis so that ventral penile tethering may develop.

A buccal graft is preferably obtained from the inner cheek, where a 6- to 10-cm × 2- to 2.5-cm strip of mucosa can be harvested with minimal morbidity, depending on the contour and shape of the mouth. The length and width of the urethral defect should be measured over a 28-French template. The head and neck are hyperextended, and the face and jaw are draped without antiseptic preparation. A side bite (Jensen) retractor or a small Weitlaner is placed in the lateral edge of the mouth opposite the site of retrieval, after a transoral endotracheal tube has been inserted. Two short, right angle retractors are placed under the lips and a rectangle of mucosa measuring 2- to 2.5 × 6 to 10 cm just inferior to Stensen's duct is retrieved after submucosal infiltration with adrenalin 1:100,000 dilution (**Fig. 16.2**). The graft is transected at the level of the anterior tonsilar pillar and placed in a saline-soaked sponge while the donor site is closed. If a lower lip retrieval donor site is used, it should be left open. A lower lip donor site is best avoided if possible because the complication of contraction of the lip and perioral numbness is not an uncommon complication of this donor site. The graft is meticulously defatted on the surgeon's forefinger until a thin, white surface is obtained. The measured graft is fixed into the urethrostomy with three stabilizing apical sutures of 5–O Monocryl at each end followed by a running suture along the margins. Excess graft length is managed by extending the urethrotomy distally until there is a proper fit (**Fig. 16.3**).

The gracilis muscle is transferred into the perineum through a capacious tunnel to prevent compression ischemia. The muscle surface is placed over the graft and anchored firmly to periurethral tissues. The bulobocavernosis muscle is sutured to the lateral surface of the gracilis (**Fig. 16.4**). If there is residual dead space or a larger perineal defect than expected is created by the repair, then both gracilis muscles are transferred for muscle bulk.

3.2. Short Gracilis Flap

The long traditional gracilis muscle may not always be suitable for some patients when the morbidity is limited by the location of the vascular pedicle and the defect is not adequately covered. The short version of the muscle offers a very useful alterative with more morbidity, a larger bulk of muscle mass

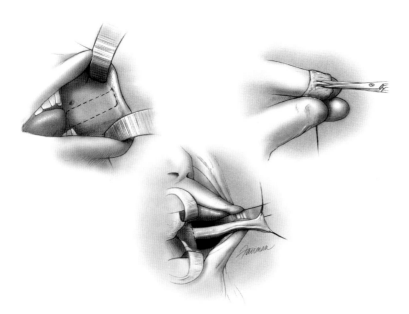

FIG. 16.2. Buccal mucosa graft can be retrieved from one or both cheeks. The opening to Stenson's duct is identified opposite the second Molar. The lower lip should be avoided as a donor. A 2.5 × 6- to 10-cm graft can be potentially harvested if the dissection is extended from tonsilar pillar to the lip edge. The graft is carefully cleaned and thinned by placing it on the forefinger under tension, removing the fibro-fatty surface until a white, shiny surface is obtained

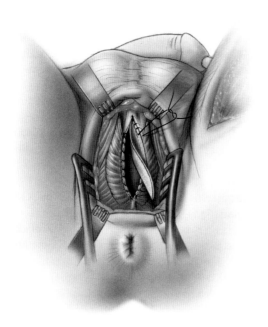

FIG. 16.3. A full-thickness buccal mucosa graft is sutured into the urethrotomy over a no. 24 catheter

proximal vascular pedicle is first occluded with a vascular clamp and an intact axial circulation confirmed by a Doppler probe (**Fig. 16.5**). It is then divided and the muscle dissected proximally to its origin on the inferior pubic ramus dividing the fascia and rotating it through a previously created wide tunnel. This fully mobilized muscle with cutaneous component will also consistently survive on circulation from the terminal branches of the obturator artery, which enters the muscle at its origin (*10,11*).

3.3. Dorsal Placement of Buccal Graft and Gracilis Muscle

In the paraplegic patient with a bulb stricture, a traumatic fistula secondary to erosion of the dorsal surface of the urethra from pressure against the pubic arch or a central decubitis, a dorsal approach to the urethra with a muscular buttress on either surface may be the optimal reconstructive procedure (Fig. 16.6).The bulbar urethra is widely mobilizedand a dorsal urethrotomy is created by rotating the spongiosa to gain access for a 12-o'clock urethrotomy in a relatively avascular site. The graft onlay is completed with interrupted 5–O Monocryl sutures and the muscle is transferred to the perineum in the long form and placed between the dorsal graft bearing surface and

to fill a large defect, and prevents a bulky appearing deformed upper medial thigh, which can easily abduct without tension (*10*). To achieve this kind of morbidity for more extended coverage, the main

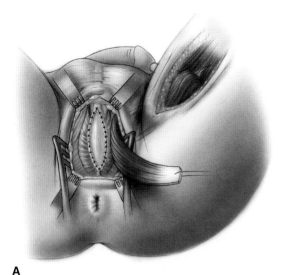

A

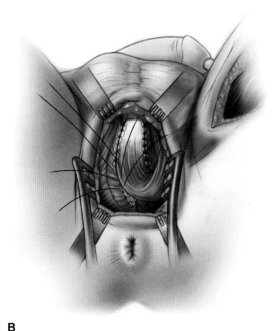

B

Fig. 16.4. The gracilis muscle is detached distally, and the muscle flap is transferred through a capacious subcutaneous medial thigh tunnel. It is applied securely to the dermal surface or lamina propria undersurface of the buccal graft by suturing its margin to the periurethral fascia

corpora cavernosa. The muscle edges are sutured to the spongiosa and a perineal artery or posterior thigh fasciocutaneous flap can be transferred for a perineal cover (**Fig. 16.4**).

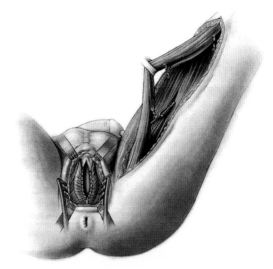

Fig. 16.5. The use of a "short" gracilis muscle with the proximal dominant medial circumflex femoral vascular pedicle divided permits a larger mass of muscle for transfer is more extensive coverage is needed

3.4. Prefabricated Combined Skin and Gracilis Flap Reconstruction

The concept of establishing a vascularized skin graft by initially securing its vascular support before tissue transfer offers an entirely new dimension in the management of strictures with periurethral beds compromised by extensive avascular fibrosis, fistulas, and radiation by prefabricating a skin or buccal graft at a distant site in the medial thigh to establish a reliable circulation and transferring it to the urethra as an onlay. The uncertainty of precarious, unpredictable inosculation can thus be avoided. This permits a skin component without excessive bulk in a more distal site on the muscle flap. The gracilis muscle is first exteriorized through a 10- to 12- cm incision over its distal third, suturing it to the dermis at skin's edge (**Fig. 16.7A**). A graft is sutured to the edges of the exposed anterior muscle surface, pie crusted and quilted to the muscle with 5–O Monocryl sutures. It is then supported with a large stent-like compression bolster dressing. These grafts develop new vascular patterns that have been observed experimentally to appear in a stable manner at a 3- to 4-wk interval and offer the advantages of a custom-created neovascularized skin flap (*14*). This type of flap then avoids the use of a large, bulky myocutaneous skin paddle. When

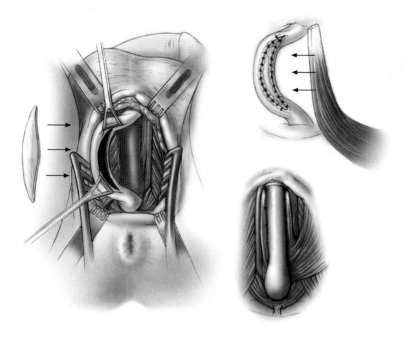

FIG. 16.6. Dorsal wall injuries can be repaired by making a dorsal urethrotomy and fixing a buccal onlay at both apices followed by a muscle flap interrupted between the graft and the ventral corpora

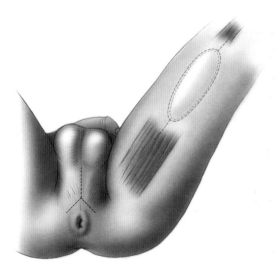

FIG. 16.7. The muscle is exteriorized through a 12-cm incision over its distal third suturing it to the dermis at the skin's edge. The full-thickness skin graft is sutured to the edge with interrupted 4–O Monocryl sutures completely covering the exposed muscle surface. The graft is pie crusted and quilted against the muscle

the graft maturity is established (4 to 6 wk) and the maximum contracture is noted, the muscle and skin are retrieved with a circumferential incision around the graft including a 3-mm margin of thigh

skin. The skin graft, which is now a flap by definition, is tailored to fit the urethral defect, including a redundant margin (**Fig. 16.8**). The distal gracilis tendon is transected and the long muscle flap with the adherent skin graft composite is transferred on its proximal pedicle into the perineum for a proximal urethral repair (**Fig. 16.9**).

3.5. The Gracilis Myofasciocutaneous Flap

The gracilis muscle with a cutaneous component has a more limited application in urologic reconstruction, but can be an invaluable adjunct when a supportive muscle and a skin cover are required. The perineal decubitis with a urethral or prostatic defect, the radiated prostatoperineal fistula following abdominoperineal rectal excision, inflammatory bowel disease with multiple urethrocutaneous fistulas and the genital and perineal defect following debridement for necrotizing fasciitis are some indications for this flap combination (**Fig. 16.10**). Because partial and total necrosis of the cutaneous portion of the flap occurs in 13% and 6.8% of this combined tissue transfer (*15*) using the classic flap, a modified harvesting technique has been described by Whetzel and Lechman (*16*) in attempt to overcome and avoid the hazards of retrieving an

FIG. 16.8. When the graft take is secure, the muscle is explored through a circumferential incision around the graft margin extending distally and proximally to expose the entire flap

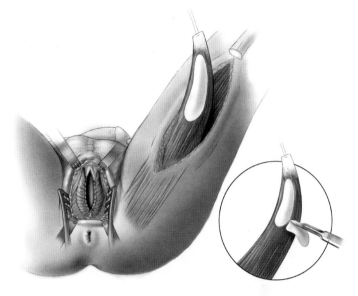

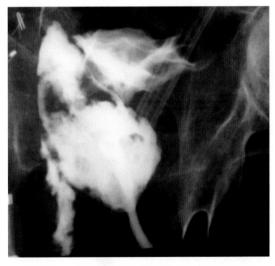

FIG. 16.10. Retrograde urethrogram in a 67-yr-old patient with a radiation prostatocutaneous fistula eleven years after rectal excision

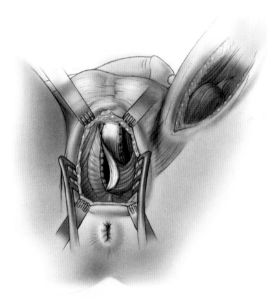

FIG. 16.9. The urethral stricture is first exposed and the appropriate stricturotomy is performed. The thigh incision is extended proximally and distally, dividing the gracilis tendon near its insertion. The urethroplasty is completed by transferring the gracilis muscle with its newly added skin component through a generous medial thigh and perineal tunnel. The skin patch is sutured to the urethral edge

overlying skin segment that has an absent cutaneous vasculariztion derived directly from the muscle surface. During elevation of the muscle, the deep investing perigracilis septal fascia, including fascia of the adductor longus, vastus medialis, adductor magnus, semitendinosis, and sartorius, is included so that no gracilis muscle fibers are seen. The proximal end of the greater saphenous vein can be left in situ and mobilized with the flap. The approach is based on the observation that blood supply to this skin over the gracilis muscle comes primarily from vessels traveling around it, rather than through the muscle. The anterior border is the predominant route for blood vessels on their way to the skin, so the flap is designed with its center based on the anterior edge of the muscle rather than on the midline. This concept is in opposition to the original description where the blood supply was consistently and directly through the muscle by the perforators to the surface *(17)*. This vascular pattern accounts for both muscular and fasciocutaneous vascular concepts in the gracilis environment. The fasciocutaneous component needs to be integrated into the planning of a viable musculocutaneous flap, because the vascular basis is primarily by means of the septocutaneous vessels within the septum between the gracilis and the adductor longus muscles most of which originate from the main gracilis pedicle and travel around the muscle rather than through it to the overlying skin. This anatomic approach to the vascular anatomy of the cutaneous paddle has been validated by Chuang et al. *(18)* in head and neck reconstruction, where the gracilis has been transferred as a free flap.

3.6. Operative Technique for Transfer of the Gracilis Myofasciocutaneous Flap

The patient is placed in the lithotomy position for flap transfer to the perineum, vagina, or the inguinal location with the legs in adjustable and flexible multijoined yellow-fin stirrups. This position permits the patient's knees and thighs to be flexed or straightened for the transfer after flap dissection. Cutaneous flap size is determined by measurement of the defect to be covered or the size of the space that will require the appropriate volume of muscle and deepithelialized skin for replacement and fistula closure (**Fig. 16.11**). Cutaneous vascular perfusion is more reliable when the size of the skin paddle is reduced to an 8 × 20-cm measurement along with excision of the distal gracilis muscle when a "short" gracilis flap is used after ligating the medial circumflex femoral pedicle. A guideline is drawn initially on the unflexed thigh from the pubic tubercle to the medial femoral condyle. A large oval vertical skin island is outlined with its center over the anterior edge of the muscle in its proximal two-thirds (**Fig. 16.12**). The distal tendon is then mobilized anterior to the semitendinosis muscle tendon. A larger flap tends to be more secure

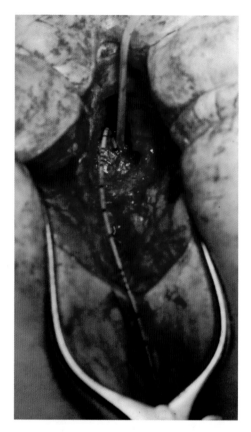

FIG. 16.11. Exposure of prostatic radiation fistula and excision of radionecrotic intergluteal skin surface in prone position

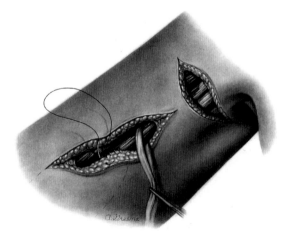

FIG. 16.12. Gracilis myofasciocutaneous flap with skin paddle centered over borders of the proximal two-thirds of the muscle

with regard to blood supply since the critical perforators have a more likely chance of being included in the flap (**Fig. 16.13**). The anterior flap margin is dissected deep into the subcutaneous tissue to the fascia (**Fig. 16.14**). The medial fascia of adductor longus and vastus medialis, adductor brevis, and semitendinosis is included with the gracilis along with all of the sartorius and all the gracilis fascia so that no gracilis muscle should be seen. This includes all the tissue between the adductor longus and the gracilis. The saphenous vein segment is included to attain the maximal rotation for vaginal and any deep perineal spaces. The skin margin is sutured to the fascia underside to avoid disruption of the muscular septocutaneous perforating vessels by shearing of the skin off the muscles during further elevation of the proximal incision. The distal tendon is divided and the flap elevated with the attached skin island proximally (**Fig. 16.15**). The distal two minor pedicles from superficial artery are ligated and divided. The relation of the skin to the muscle is again confirmed as it is elevated and changed if not correctly centered over the muscle. The dominant pedicle will be seen by retracting the adductor longus medially as it passes over the deeper adductor magnus. The flap is rotated on its pedicle to the defect by making a wide suprafascial subcutaneous tunnel to accommodate the flap without tension or compression.

If compression potential exists, then the skin bridge is divided. If further skin paddle rotation or advancement is required at the recipient site, the legs are then brought down with some adduction

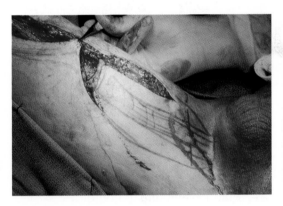

FIG. 16.13. The skin margin of the flap is sutured to the fascial underside of the muscle to avoid shearing disruption of the muscular and septocutaneous perforators during elevation

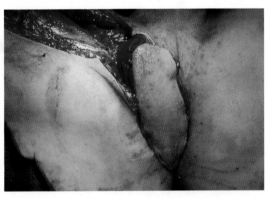

FIG. 16.15. The flap is rotated on its pedicle with tension in the defect after dividing the groin skin bridge

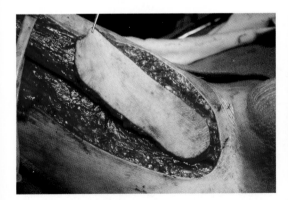

FIG. 16.14. The distal tendon medial to the semitendinosis is divided and the flap is elevated after the skin flap is prepared

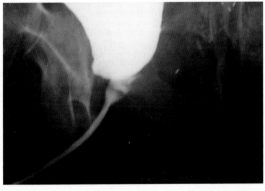

FIG. 16.16. The postoperative urethrogram reveals fistula closure under an effective perineal skin cover

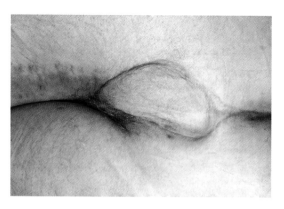

FIG. 16.17. The perigracilis septocutaneous perforators that come around the muscle result in a well perfused viable myocutaneous axial flap

and muscle shortening which provides an additional 3 to 6 cm in length. The thigh and perineal incisions are closed with a suction drain (Blake) that is left in for 72 h. The leg is firmly wrapped and the patient is immobilized for 72 h, and subcutaneous heparin is administered for 7 d. If any of the surface demonstrates necrosis then early debridement with a stented skin graft is instituted.

The anatomical approach to the harvest of the myofasciocutaneous flap with aggressive inclusion of the perigracilis fascia creates the most reliable vascular inflow to the middle third of the skin island (**Fig. 16.17**). All the cases have been retrieved by preseptic debridement and a stented split thickness skin graft cover.

4. Perineal Artery Fasciocutaneous Flap (Singapore)

The perineal artery medial thigh fasciocutaneous flap is another concept in tissue transfer that has the potential of salvaging the complex proximal prostato-membranous and bulb stricture. It is particularly suited for the repair of radiation prostato-membranous strictures, recurrent failed post anastomotic urethral distraction defects and the rare rectourethral fistula associated with a proximal stricture. The flap can be a valuable adjunct in the initial perineal and thigh coverage of defects following necrotizing fasciitis. The radiation vesicovaginal fistula has also been successfuly closed by using the skin cover to replace the ischemic vaginal

wall. Its robust blood supply, predictable measurements, minimal donor site morbidity, and prior reported success in vaginoplasty make this flap an ideal alternative option for complex proximal urethral reconstruction. The proximal portion of the medially rotated flap increases the safety and security of the perineal cover in patients with overlying perineal skin loss, prior surgery, or radiation injury in conjunction with the urethral replacement. It belongs to the class of axial fasciocutaneous flap constructs consisting of skin, subcutaneous tissue, and a well-developed fascial undersurface.

The flap has a defined skin territory supported by an identifiable vascular pedicle, the perineal artery which is a distal branch of the internal pudendal. The perineal artery penetrates the fascia at its base and develops a suprafascial plexus, which arborizes with the subdermal plexus and reliably perfuses the skin (*19*). The flap has the advantages of a simple dissection, minimal bleeding, no loss of function and minimal bulk, making it more suitable for a smaller defect such as those seen in urethral, vaginal and scrotal reconstructions. It can be transferred to the urethra using three different techniques of flap rotation. The onlay patch is the most commonly used for urethral repair and best designed in a transverse direction (*20,21*).

4.1. Flap Design and Technique of Elevation for Onlay Patch Urethroplasty

The perineal artery, or Singapore Flap, is a vertically oriented composite of skin with an underlying deep fascia and adductor epimysium measuring 6 × 15 cm with its proximal base located at the level of the mid perineum 3 cm distal to the anal margin (**Fig. 16.18**). The perineal artery arises just medial to the groin crease with branches to the scrotum and medial thigh skin. This circulation is richly enhanced by its arborization with the deep external pudendal, medial circumflex femoral from the profunda femoris and the anterior branch of the obturator artery. This is a partially sensate flap innervated by the pudendal and the posterior cutaneous nerve of the thigh with good sensory perception in the mid perineal portions of the transferred flap. The urethral stricture is exposed by a thorough ventral urethrotomy,

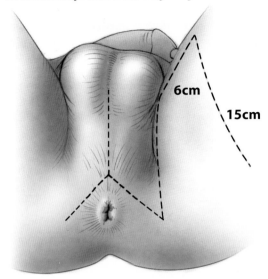

FIG. 16.18. Perineal artery medial thigh flap measurements are consistently 15 × 6 cm with its proximal base located at the level of the mid perineum. The medial border is the groin crease lateral to the edge of the scrotum

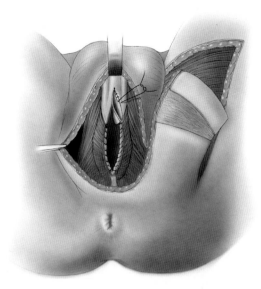

FIG. 16.19. A proximal urethrotomy is performed from the distal bulbous urethra across the trans-sphincter segment to the prostatic apex. A buccal mucosal graft can be utilized to repair the distal portion of the bulbar stricture if the suture is longer than 6–8 cm. A distal transverse island is outlined at the distal margin of the flap and a 3-cm wide strip of skin is deepithelialized just proximal to the island leaving a thin layer of dermis

which is started distally with an indwelling 5-French Fogarty vascular balloon catheter as an intraluminal guide and carried proximally to a point 2 cm beyond the balloon to establish a 30-French proximal lumen and a 26-French distal lumen. This flap is outlined initially with a skin marker defining the measurements with the skin on stretch and extending it, if needed, an extra 2 cm into the femoral triangle, where random circulation based skin extension occurs.

The incisions are started in parallel vertical lines down to the fascia on both sides, raising the epimysium with the fascia and suturing it to the dermis to prevent shearing injury to the segmental vessels. The flap is then lifted back to its proximal transverse margin after completing the distal transverse incision. Effective blood flow is confirmed by de-epithelializing a 2- to 3-mm area at the distal margin to identify a bleeding dermis. The tissue bridge between the base of the flap and the urethral exposure is divided to prevent tunnel pressure effect and the potential compromise of flap circulation. This procedure permits ease of transfer to the deep proximal urethra and a lateral rotation of the scrotal and perineal tissues to help close the donor site.

A 6- to 8-cm transverse island is outlined at the distal edge of the flap by de-epithelializing a 3- to 4-cm strip of skin just proximal to the island onlay segment, leaving a thin layer of dermis to prevent ischemic injury to the transverse island (**Fig. 16.19**). If the urethrotomy is greater than 6 cm in length, it will require an additional segment of buccal mucosa in a combined composite to repair the entire stricture. The buccal mucosa graft is always placed in the more distal portion to avoid the trans-sphincteric site where flaps are more likely to succeed than grafts. The flap is then rotated medially and inferiorly and the island patch is sutured by initially placing the apical sutures at each end to establish a good fit without folds or bunching. If the proximal apex is in the prostatic floor then six 4–O Monocryl sutures are initially placed at the site, rearmed and inserted into the inferior edge of the flap (**Fig. 16.20**). The donor site is closed by advancing the thigh incision toward the scrotum and transferring the scrotal bridge laterally (**Fig. 16.21**). A small suction drain exiting through

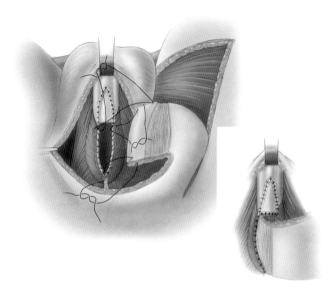

FIG. 16.20. A transverse island is rotated medially and inferiorly, and the island of skin is applied to the urethrotomy defect and sutured with running 4–O Monocryl sutures. The distal edge of the island flap is approximated to the proximal margin of the buccal graft completing the combined reconstruction

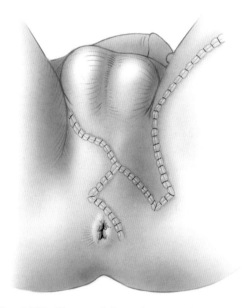

FIG. 16.21. Closure of the perineum and donor site is accomplished by rotating the inguinal and scrotal bridge laterally into the thigh defect and advancing the inferior margin of the thigh incision toward the groin. No donor site morbidity has been noted

the thigh incision is removed in three days. The urethral catheter and suprapubic cystotomy are left in for three weeks pending a normal voiding cystourethrogram.

5. Gluteus Maximus Muscle Flap

5.1. Gluteal Flaps for Bulbomembranous Urethral Reconstruction

Prostatocutaneous and proximal bulbomembranous urethral fistulas and strictures may occur from surgical trauma after abdominoperineal resection of rectum for cancer and inflammatory disease, as a delayed phenomena associated with adjunctive radiation therapy, or the result of a pressure induced decubitis with associated perineal skin loss. This recalcitrant problem requires a large, reliable muscle flap that will buttress the repair, fill in the noncollapsible retrovesical dead space and tissue loss surrounding the fistulas and offer a good blood supply to a rigid fibrotic tract and a buccal graft onlay.

There needs to be a sufficient tissue bulk for covering the perineum and intergluteal space and a well vascularized surface to assist the closure of the defect in the face of impaired wound healing. This can be accomplished by a number of muscle flaps including transabdominal transfer of the rectus abdominus bilateral coapted gracilis muscle flaps combined with a semitendinosis, a gracilis myofasciocutaneous flap or a free latissimus dorsi flap. Our use of unilateral or bilateral inferior gluteus maximus has been the most effective for this pathology. The anatomical insights gained over the past decade have resulted in the development of a number of gluteus maximus muscle flap designs which permit preservation of function and the ability to transfer a large muscle bulk to the deep perineum and presacral space *(22)*. The inferior gluteus maximus or lower segment of this muscle based on the inferior gluteal artery vascular pedicle permits rotation of the muscle into an intergluteal, subcoccygeal and perineal space without incurring impaired motor function or contour deformity of the buttocks *(23)*.

5.2. Gluteal Anatomy and Clinical Applications

The gluteus maximus is a large, quadrilateral muscle that forms the prominence of the buttocks. It measures 24 × 24 cm on average and arises from the posterior gluteal line of the ileum and the sacrum, the side of the coccyx, the aponeurosis of the sacrospinalis, the sacrotuberous ligament and the fascia over the gluteus medius muscle. The fibers from a diffuse origin course laterally and inferiorly to insert into the ileotibial tract and the gluteal tuberosity of the femur. The muscle is nourished by the superior and inferior gluteal arteries, which are branches of the internal iliac arteries. There are two minor vascular pedicles, which anastomose freely with the gluteal vessels. These are the first perforators of the profunda femoris artery and vein and the intra-muscular branches of the lateral circumflex femoral artery from the profunda. The first perforator enters the muscle adjacent to its insertion and the two or three intramuscular branches enter beneath the inferior gluteal muscle insertion. The superior and inferior gluteal arteries pass above and below the piriformis muscle and are located 4 cm medial to the midline (**Fig. 16.22**). The inferior gluteal nerve (L5–S1) courses through the sciatic foreman, accompanies the inferior gluteal artery medial to the sciatic nerve, and enters the gluteus maximus muscle on its deep surface at the level of the piriformis muscle, where it supplies motor innervation to the entire muscle.

Loss of muscle function does not become evident in casual activities such as easy walking or standing because other muscles will compensate for its loss. The gluteus maximus extends and rotates the thigh laterally and is important for more forceful activities such as running, climbing and jumping. The superior or inferior half of the muscle may be elevated as a flap without loss of function if the other half is intact. The muscle segment can be rotated to cover the sacrum where the dominant pedicles enter the muscle very close to the fibers of origin from the sacral edge. The muscle is split into two segments and the inferior portion is used primarily for perineal and vaginal reconstruction. The lower distal portion is adjacent to the intergluteal and perineal space, making it an optimal skeletal muscle flap for repair of this portion of the urethra and for obliteration of the pelvic space.

5.3. Techniques of Gluteal Maximus Repair of a Perineal-Urethral Strictures (and Fistulas)

The patient is initially cystoscoped in the lithotomy position, at which time any fistulous tracts are cannulated with a ureteral catheter and the bladder drained with a urethral catheter. The patient is the placed in the prone position with the waist flexed and the legs separated. Protective padding is then used for the legs and feet and chest rolls are placed to prevent pelvic and breast compression. The lateral edge of the sacrum and greater trocanter are initially identified and marked as respective origin and insertion of the gluteus maximus muscle. The fistula tract is excised by making a circumferential incision and extending in cephalas and caudal along the perineal midline in the intergluteal groove. The intergluteal midline cleft is incised from the scrotum to the coccyx deep to the ventral urethral and prostatic surface. The incision is extended horizontally along the inferior gluteal crease to expose the superficial surface of the muscle. The dissection proceeds cephalas under the coccyx and laterally down the pelvic sidewall. More exposure can be achieved by extending the incision parasacrally. The urethra is identified and the lateral fibrous and radiated tissues are excised. The overlying skin on the gluteus muscle is retracted upward and laterally. The coccyx is resected and the prostatic surface exposed. More sacral bone is removed if there is poor exposure or obvious radionecrotic bone involvement. A prostatic fistula is closed with a buccal mucosa graft following exposure and lateral

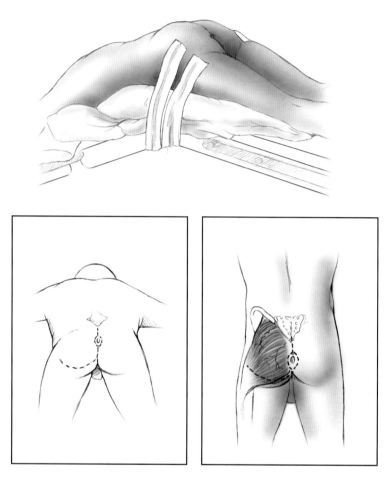

FIG. 16.22. The patient is placed in the prone position with the waist and pelvis flexed. The legs and feet are protectively padded and chest rolls are placed under the chest and pelvis to prevent pressure point injury. The fistulous tract is excised with the indwelling stent. The incision is extended in the mid perineal line in both directions and laterally to expose the surface of the inferior gluteus maximus. The inferior segment of the muscle is identified after the horizontal component of the incision is made

retraction of the levator ani muscle. A proximal urethral stricture can also be repaired with a buccal mucosal onlay in a ventral position followed by support to both grafts with a muscle surface. This well-vascularized muscle will overcome completely the adversity of the radiated pelvis.

To elevate the inferior half of the gluteus maximus after exposure of its superficial surface, the muscle is split at its midportion. The inferior half of the fibers of insertion are divided and separated from the ileotibial tract and the gluteal tuberosity and the muscle is mobilized from lateral to medial, identifying the inferior vascular pedicle. The origin can be completely detached from the sacrum

without endangering the blood supply, if needed. The piriformis muscle is the key reference point in locating the sciatic nerve deep to the gluteus maximus. With the sciatic nerve carefully preserved and the location of the gluteal vessels confirmed, the muscle can be split to the level of the sacrum in preparation for transfer (**Fig. 16.23**). A 10 × 20-cm flap can be retrieved based on the inferior gluteal artery. Gradual detachment of the inserting fibers of the muscle on the ileotibial tract, intermuscular septum, and the lesser trochanter of femur can be readily performed once the underlying structures are identified. Partial release of the gluteus origin from the sacrum will facilitate further flap trans-

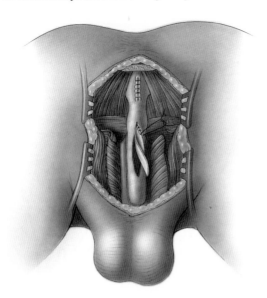

FIG. 16.23. The prostate and proximal urethra are exposed through an intergluteal dissection following excision of the fistula tract. A buccal mucosa patch onlay is placed ventrally to repair a proximal stricture and prostatic fistula

position, which can be easily moved an additional 5 to 9 cm.

The distal flap surface is then advanced into the perineal defect from the buttock and fixed to the periurethral fascia, completing the buttress effect over the urethral and prostatic graft and fistula (**Fig. 16.24**). With adequate mobility, the muscle can also be placed under the sacral roof to completely obliterate the entire retroprostatic and urethral compartment (**Fig. 16.25**). The donor site can be closed by mobilizing the contralateral skin edge and turning the skin and subcutaneous tissue over in a medial direction and suturing it to the contralateral skin edge. It is rarely necessary to place a skin graft for exposed muscle because lateral buttock and inferior subcutaneous thigh skin dissection will allow closure without tension *(23)*. If the muscle does not reach the buccal graft surface, a gracilis or semitendinosis muscle can be retrieved in the prone position and transferred in the space under the inferior gluteus maximus. The gluteus maximus muscle

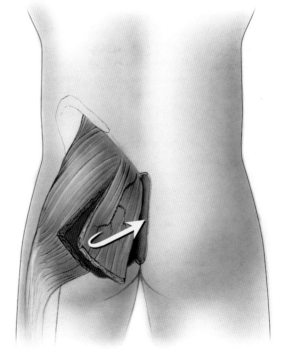

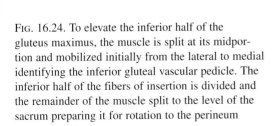

FIG. 16.24. To elevate the inferior half of the gluteus maximus, the muscle is split at its midportion and mobilized initially from the lateral to medial identifying the inferior gluteal vascular pedicle. The inferior half of the fibers of insertion is divided and the remainder of the muscle split to the level of the sacrum preparing it for rotation to the perineum

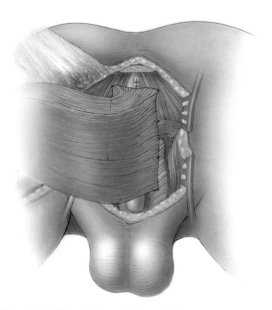

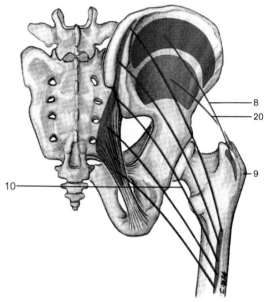

FIG. 16.25. The distal muscle flap edge is advanced medially into the perineal defect obliterating the rectourethral and prostatic space from the sacrum to the perineal skin edge where it is fixed to the periprostatic and periurethral fascia

FIG. 16.26. Course of gluteal muscles as to origin and insertion. 8 = Gluteus medius, 9 = Greater trochanter, 10 = Gluteus maximus, 20 = Gluteus minimus. (From Rohen JW (1983) Yokochi: Color Atlas of Anatomy. New York, Igaku Shoin)

or musculocutaneous flap provides reliable support and buttressing of recalcitrant prostatic and urethrocutaneous fistulas and urethral strictures in patients who have undergone a prior procto-colectomy. The technique advances a large bulk of well-vascularized muscle, which permits complete obliteration of perineal and intergluteal spaces that have been injured by prior radiation or tissue loss. This is not an expendable muscle but proper mobilization of the inferior gluteal segment with preservation of the superior segment, loss of strength in extension and abduction of the hip can be prevented permitting the use of a local muscle flap with minimal donor site morbidity (Fig. 16.26).

6. Conclusion

For refractory urethral strictures and fistulas, skin and buccal graft muscle flap composites, such as with the gracilis muscle, the Singapore medial thigh flap, and the inferior gluteus maximus muscle flap are reliable and successful techniques for reconstruction. These flaps are all particularly valuable resources in the management of recalcitrant pathology or the presence of wound healing impairment such as radiation or other adverse conditions that would jeopardize genital skin graft and flap survival. These expendable muscle-and-tissue covering flaps will not result in impaired motor function if careful attention is paid to the details of their retrieval. Other axial flaps that are available as an enhancing support system include the posterior thigh fasciocutaneous, rectus abdominis, rectus femoris, semimembranosis, semitendinosis and latissimus dorsi free flap, all of which require more complex retrieval techniques. The only consistent option for repair of the complex urethral stricture pathology in patients who have undergone numerous failed prior procedures in the proximal and posterior urethra is the combined use of a ventral buccal mucosal, posterior auricular Wolfe or penile skin graft supported by a transferred skeletal muscle surface.

Editorial Comment

The methods detailed above by Lenny Zinman are not out of realm of the reconstructive urologist. Although such tissue-transfer techniques for urethral reconstruction often are used for the most complex or reoperative cases, we feel strongly that all urologists can learn to harvest such fasciocutaneous, muscular and myocutaneous flaps and graft onlays. They should be part of the surgical armamentarium of all urologists who choose to perform urethroplasty surgery. Furthermore, the plastic surgery surgical principles detailed in the above chapter are familiar to us all as urologists. The harvest of such flaps and muscles can be easily learned and mastered, and should not be relegated or deferred to the Plastic surgeon. This is a well-detailed chapter that will serve you well as a surgical atlas.—S.B. Brandes

References

1. Zinman L (1996) Muscle-assisted full thickness skin graft urethroplasty, in McAninch JW (ed) Traumatic and reconstructive urology. Philadelphia, W.B. Saunders, pp 623–630
2. Zinman L (2002) Myocutaneous and faciocutaneous flaps in complex urethral reconstruction. Urol Clin North Am 29:443–446
3. Roehrborn CG, McConnell JD (1994) Analysis for factors contributing to the success or failure of 1-stage urethroplasty for urethral stricture disease. J Urol 1518:69–74
4. Morey AF, McAninch JW (1996) When and how to use buccal mucosal grafts in adult bulbar urethroplasty. Br J Urol 48:194–198
5. Venn SN, Mundy AR (1998) Early experience with the use of buccal mucosal grafts in adult bulbar urethroplasty. Br J Urol 81:738–40
6. Meland NB, Arnold PG, Weiss HC (1991) Management of the recalcitrant total hip arthroplasty. Wound Plast Reconstr Surg 88:681–685
7. Asaadi M, Murray KA, Russell RC, et al (1986) Experimental evaluation of free-tissue transfer to promote healing of infected wounds in dogs. Ann Plast Surg 17:6–12
8. Giordano PA, Abbes M, Pequignot JB. (1990) Gracilis blood supply: anatomical and clinical re-evaluation. Br J Plast Surg 43:266–72
9. Morris SF, Yang D (1999) Gracilis muscle: aerial and neural basis for subdivision. Ann Plast Surg 42:630–633
10. Chen SH.T., Hentz V, Wei F, Chen Y (1995) Short gracilis myocutaneous flaps for vulvoperineal and inguinal reconstruction. Plast Reconstr Surg 95:372
11. Soper JT, Larson D, Hunter VJ, Berchusk A, Clark-Person DP (1989) Short gracilis myocutaneous flaps for vulvovaginal reconstruction after radical pelvic surgery. Obstet Gynecol 74:823
12. Erol OO (1976) The transformation of a free skin graft into a vascularized pedicle flap. Plast Reconstr Surg 58:470–477
13. Zinman L (1987) Muscle and myocutaneous grafts in urologic surgery, in Libertino JA (ed) Pediatric and adult reconstructive urologic surgery. Baltimore, Williams and Wilkins, pp 567–97
14. Hallock GG (1991) Skin recycling following neovascularization using the rat musculocutenous flap model. Plast Reconstr Surg 88:673–680
15. Woods JE, Beart RW (1983) Reconstruction of non-healing perineal wounds with gracilis muscle flaps. Ann Plast Surg 11:513–516
16. Whetzel T, Lechman AN (1997) The gracilis myofasciocutaneous flap: vascular anatomy and clinical application. Plast Reconstr Surg 99:1642
17. Reddy VR, Stevenson TR, Whetzel TP (2006) 10 year experience with gracilis myofasciocutaneous flap. Plast Reconstr Surg 117:635
18. Chuang DC, Mardini S, Lin SH, Chen HC. (2004) Free proximal gracilis muscle and its skin paddle compound flap transplantation for complex fascial paralysis. Plast Reconstr Surg 113:126
19. Wee JT, Joseph VT (1989) A new technique of vaginal reconstruction using neurovascular pudendal-thigh flaps. A preliminary report. Plast Reconstr Surg 83:701–709
20. Zinman L (1997) Perineal artery axial fasciocutaneous flap in urethral reconstruction. Atlas Urol Clin N Am 5:91–107
21. Tzarnas CD, Raezer DM, Castillo OA. (1994) A unique faciocutaneous flap for posterior urethral repair. Urology 43:379–381
22. Ramirez OM, Swartz WM, Futrell JW (1987) The gluteus maximus muscle: experimental and clinical considerations relevant to reconstruction in ambulatory patients. Br J Plast Surg 40:1–10
23. Stevenson TR, Pollack RA, Rohrich RJ, Vanderkolk CA (1987) The gluteus maximus musculocutaneous island flap; refinements in design and application. Plast Reconstr Surg 79:761–768

17
Posterior Urethral Strictures

Daniela E. Andrich and Anthony R. Mundy

Contents

1. Introduction 189
2. Assessment 190
3. Preparation 191
4. Principles 192
5. Procedure 192
    5.1. Postoperative Follow-Up 196
6. Complications 197
References 200

Summary Posterior urethral strictures are not common and in the context of this chapter they are not really strictures – they are best called pelvic fracture-related urethral injuries. They are generally repaired transperineally with very satisfactory results but some injuries can be technically very challenging and the consequences of inadequate or inexpert surgery of even straightforward cases can be devastating. This is not an area for amateurs.

Keywords Pelvic fracture, urethra, injury, urethroplasty, technique

1. Introduction

The male urethra is traditionally divided into the anterior urethra, which is surrounded by the corpus spongiosum, and the posterior urethra, which is surrounded by the sphincter mechanisms and the prostate. The posterior urethra is subdivided into the bladder neck (or preprostatic urethra),

the prostatic urethra, and the membranous urethra. Bladder neck strictures and strictures of the prostatic urethra are largely a consequence of the treatment of carcinoma of the prostate and of benign prostatic hyperplasia with the use of the "new technology" and are considered elsewhere in this volume. Posterior urethral strictures affecting the membranous segment are most commonly caused by instrumentation of the urethra and by transurethral resection of the prostate. As a consequence of this, not only are the epithelium and the subepithelial vascular tissue strictured, probably as a result of ischemia, but the same fibrotic process infiltrates the urethral sphincter mechanism. Treatment is largely directed toward the preservation of urethral sphincter mechanism, and these so-called "sphincter strictures" are best treated by urethral dilation for this reason. Relatively common as they are, these will not be considered further in this chapter. Posterior urethral strictures otherwise are uncommon and are most commonly caused by pelvic fracture-related urethral injury. It is these "strictures" that are the subject of this chapter.

From: *Current Clinical Urology: Urethral Reconstructive Surgery*
Edited by: S.B. Brandes © Humana Press, Totowa, NJ

As a result of the (well-justified) pronounced influence of Richard Turner-Warwick on the assessment and management of these "strictures," they have come to be termed pelvic fracture urethral distraction defects rather than strictures proper. Such thinking is largely based on the concept that injury leads to a shearing force that plucks the prostatic urethra from the membranous urethra or, more probably, the membranous urethra from the bulbar urethra, and that this is more commonly a complete injury rather than a partial injury, leading to distraction of the two ends. Recent evidence suggests otherwise on both counts.

Recent evidence (1) suggests that most pelvic fracture-related injuries are partial injuries rather than complete injuries. It also suggests that although "switchblade" transection of the urethra, partial or complete, by a bone fragment can occur, most commonly urethral injury depends on what happens to the soft tissues of the pelvis rather than the bones, and particularly on what happens to the perineal membrane and puboprostatic ligaments. Most commonly, it is argued, the injury that causes disruption of the pelvic ring causes a rupture of the perineal membrane and the other supporting ligaments of the lower urinary tract "midsubstance," that is to say at a point between the bony attachments laterally and the visceral attachments medially, and as a result of this the urinary tract is preserved unless it is damaged by a switchblade mechanism as described above. It is only when the injury causes the perineal membrane to avulse a part or the whole of the urethral circumference, rather than to rupture midsubstance, that urethral injury results. Because it is the perineal membrane that "does the damage" when this happens, it is the bulbomembranous junction that is the most common site of urethral injury. This most commonly occurs with disruptions of the pelvic ring that are both vertically and rotationally unstable but even then urethral injury is not particularly common. It is in this same category of pelvic ring injuries that bladder neck injuries and other more complicated injuries to the lower urinary tract occur. Switchblade injuries more commonly injure the proximal bulbar urethra, sometimes extensively.

The incidence of pelvic fracture has been estimated at 20 per 100,000 population. The male to female incidence ratio is about 1.8 to 1, although this varies considerably with age. The mortality of such trauma is about 10% and the incidence of urethral injury is variably reported at about 5–10%, which means that the annual incidence of pelvic fracture-related urethral injuries per million population is approx. 5–10. Not all of these urethral injuries require surgical treatment, and some may respond just to a simple occasional urethral dilation. Thus, the number of those coming for urethroplasty are few. In the United Kingdom, this is approx. 1 per million population as compared with about 12 per million population requiring urethroplasty for anterior urethral stricture disease. This frequency is lower than it might be if some surgeons with no experience of urethroplasty did not persist with dilatation or urethrotomy rather than refer a patient on to a surgeon with such expertise. The incidence, of course, depends on how well the original injury is handled as well and the current standard of care is suprapubic catheterization followed by urethroplasty 3 mo or so later when the patient has recovered from his other injuries (2).

2. Assessment

If a patient has a partial or a complete obstruction to the urethra 3 mo or so after their injury, the investigations of choice are a flow rate study, if the patient is able to void, together with an ascending urethrogram (retrograde urethrogram) and micturating cystogram to define both the upper and lower limits of the stricture (**Fig. 17.1**). A retrograde urethrogram alone may show the distal limit of the obstruction with great clarity but not the proximal limit. The deformity in most instances is characteristic: the posterior urethra is displaced posteriorly, and there is a characteristic S-bend deformity at the site of injury.

It is common to see an apparently long gap between the distal limit of a complete obliteration on ascending (retrograde) urethrogram and the bladder neck on a cystogram (through a suprapubic catheter). This doesn't mean that the stricture extends all the way up to the bladder neck, only that the detrusor is unable to contract and open the bladder neck and so allow contrast down to the upper end of the obliteration (3).

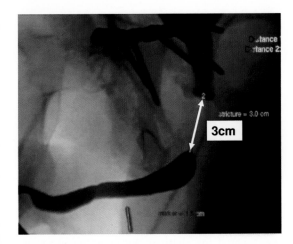

FIG. 17.1. Combined ascending urethrogram and micturating cystogram helps to define the proximal and distal limits of the stricture

It is also quite common to see an apparently incompetent bladder neck in association with a complete obstruction but this is usually misleading. The reason for this appearance (of a so-called "beaked" bladder neck) is not clear, but the vast majority of such patients have a perfectly competent bladder neck postoperatively. When the bladder neck has been damaged, it produces an altogether different appearance; indeed, it looks as thought it has been damaged rather than simply being beaked open.

A flexible cystoscopy may be helpful in determining the nature of an apparently obstructed or incompetent bladder neck and indeed might be helpful in the overall assessment of the urethra on either side of the obstruction. Clinically, it is important to document clearly, objectively, and subjectively whether the patient has normal erections or erectile dysfunction, for obvious medicolegal reasons and also because those patients with complete erectile dysfunction, particularly if associated with a cold numb penis, are likely to have a more profound disruption of the local blood supply and may therefore be more prone to recurrent stricturing after urethroplasty. Assessment of the pelvic and perineal vasculature may be advisable and in some instances revascularisation of the pudendal and penile blood supply might be considered both for the erectile dysfunction and to improve the chances of a successful urethroplasty by improving the local blood supply (4).

It is also important to check that the patient can abduct his hips to allow access to the perineum. Without easy perineal access, urethroplasty may be extremely difficult. Other investigations might be helpful in certain circumstances and some surgeons seem to recommend them almost routinely, most notably magnetic resonance imaging. We have often found the use of magnetic resonance imaging interesting, but we have rarely found it to be helpful. Where it has been helpful has been in circumstances in which patients have had more than usually severe injuries, causing more than usually severe anatomical distortion, or when they have had previous surgery creating complications such as fistulae or false passages. Even then, good-quality contrast radiography of the bladder and urethra is usually more helpful. In those who have sustained rectal injuries the patient will usually have a covering colostomy in which case a barium enema study will be important.

3. Preparation

The patient is admitted on the day of surgery and requires no special preparation. It is sensible to know the patient's blood group, although blood transfusion is rarely necessary except in complicated cases. It is also sensible to have an up to date urine culture, although prophylactic antibiotics will almost always be given with the pre-medication or with the anaesthesia.

Urethroplasty for posterior urethral strictures requires a lithotomy position to give access to the perineum. There should also be access to the suprapubic area. Most patients have an indwelling suprapubic catheter because they have complete obstruction. This provides a channel for passing a urethral dilator through the track and into the bladder neck to demonstrate the upper level of the obstruction by palpitation during the course of the procedure. When this is not available it may be necessary to do a suprapubic cystostomy through a short vertical stab incision just above the pubic symphysis to allow this manoeuvre. In a few patients, most notably those with complex injuries, an abdominoperineal approach may be necessary, in which case the whole abdomen will need to be prepared for a long anterior midline incision.

Some experts like to use the so-called exaggerated lithotomy position to give access to the perineum *(5)*. We find this unnecessary and more prone to complications and use what is call "social lithotomy," which speaks for itself. Articulated leg supports are necessary in either case. It is also useful to have inflatable leggings to provide intermittent compression of venous thromboembolism and of the legs during the course of the procedure to reduce the risk of compartment syndromes. These are rare but can be a devastating complication when they occur. With social lithotomy this is in any case less likely.

4. Principles

The general principles of urethroplasty for posterior urethral strictures were worked out many years ago. Those principles are that it is almost always possible to define the healthy urethra above and below the site of the injury of the surrounding fibrosis and perform a spatulated end-to-end anastomosis. Indeed, substitution urethroplasty should never be performed, except in very exceptional circumstances, usually as a consequence of previous surgery or of neglect. Second, it is almost always necessary to reduce tension of the anastomosis to reduce the risk of recurrent stricturing. In some instances, tension is relieved simply by a full mobilization of the bulbar urethra depending on the retrograde blood flow down the bulbar urethra to maintain its vascularity. When mobilization of the urethra alone is insufficient to reduce tension of the anastomosis, tension can be further reduced by straightening out the natural curved course of the bulbar urethral from the penoscrotal junction to the apex of the prostate. This curve may be as much as a half or five-eighths of a circle and the curve is produced by the fusion of the corpora cavernosa over the inferior aspect of the pubic symphysis. Thus, the urethra can be straightened out by separating the crura of the penis, as far as this is possible, and by performing a wedge resection of the inferior pubic arch. Unfortunately, the degree to which the crura can be separated is variable and it may not be possible to completely straighten out the urethra by crural separation alone, in which case the urethra must be re-routed in some patients around the shaft of the penis rather than between the two component

parts of the shaft of the penis *(6)*. This point is controversial and some surgeons believe that re-routing of the urethra is never necessary *(7)*. Those against re-routing argue that they are always able to get a tension free anastomosis without it *(8)*. To me this suggests that there is a finite limit to the gap between the two ends of the trausmatised urethra which seems to me nonsensical. I suppose it all depends on how a surgeon assesses tension and what his or her casemix is.

This sequence of mobilization proceeding to crural separation when necessary, proceeding to inferior wedge pubectomy when necessary, proceeding ultimately to re-routing of the urethra around the shaft of the penis when necessary, is known as the "transperineal progression approach" and was first referred to as such by Webster. The various component parts of the progression approach had been described decades beforehand by Marion, Waterhouse, and Turner-Warwick amongst others. Webster's particular contribution was to rationalise their innovations in one approach *(8)*.

Occasionally, the proximal urinary tract—the bladder and prostatic urethra—is displaced anteriorly rather than posteriorly and stuck on to the back of the pubis is inaccessible from below. Occasionally there is bladder neck injury, or simultaneous rectal injury, or a false passage. These all require an adominoperineal approach rather then a purely perineal approach. This is more common in children in whom the corpus spongiosum is less well developed and therefore is less elastic.

5. Procedure

The urethra is exposed by a midline perineal incision, about 10 cm long, along the line of the raphe from the posterior aspect of the scrotum to just short of the anal margin. Some surgeons prefer to use a curved or S-shaped incision or to extend the incision on one or other or both sides of the anal margin but we find this unnecessary.

The incision is deepened through the subcutaneous tissue down on to the bulbo-spongiosus muscle (**Fig. 17.2**). At the anterior margin of the bulbospongiosus, there is a layer of fascia called Gallaudet's fascia. Incising Gallaudet's fascia puts you into a plane between that fascia

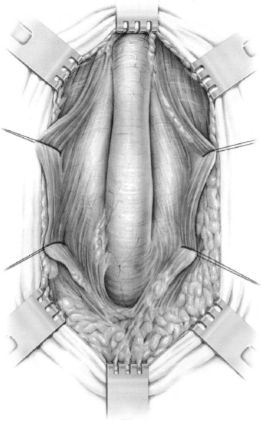

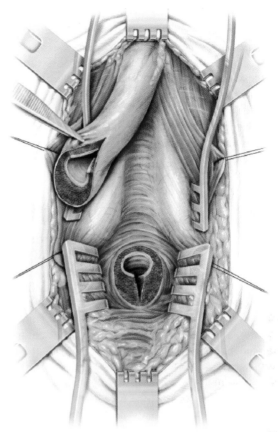

Fig. 17.2. Exposure and mobilization of the bulbar urethra from within the bulbospongiosus muscle

Fig. 17.3. The urethra is then transected through the site of obliteration to free it. It is then trimmed back to healthy tissue and spatulated on its dorsal aspect, then lightly clamped with an atraumatic vascular clamp and retracted out of the way

and Buck's fascia as you dissect distally and allows you to get into the plane between bulbospongiosus and Buck's fascia more proximally *(9)*. The bulbo spongiosus muscle can be divided along the line of its raphe all the way back to the perineal body and can then be reflected off the surface of the corpus spongiosum on both sides. Buck's fascia is then divided on both sides where the corpus spongiosus lies against the ipsilateral corpus cavernosum. By dividing Buck's fascia and deepening this towards the midline on each side the corpus spongiosum can be freed up from the corpora cavernosa as far distally as necessary and as far proximally as the site of the obliteration. Posterolaterally, at the site of obliteration or thereabouts, are the short stout arteries to the bulb which may bleed impressively if they are divided. They are often thrombosed by the original injury

but should be looked for and suture-ligated if they can be identified. Anteriorly on the surface of the urethra as the bulbar segment becomes the membranous segment there is a urethral artery on each side at 11 o'clock and 1 o'clock, which may bleed irritatingly if it is not secured by diathermy first. In the midline there are commonly venous sinuses that may ooze a little but are rarely troublesome. These are best dealt with by suture-ligation if necessary.

The site of the obliteration of the urethra is easily defined by passing a Foley catheter up the urethra until it can pass no further and at this site the urethra is transacted (**Fig. 17.3**). If the bulb of the urethra has not been fully mobilized, then this transection will be through the remaining stump of the bulb and instead of dividing the arteries to the bulb as described above, their branches will be divided in the substance of the spongy tissue and bleeding can be profuse. A bit of pressure for a couple of minutes with a swab will reduce this to the level where the bleeding is easily secured with diathermy or a stitch.

Having mobilized and divided the bulbar urethra, the fibrosis around the margins of the transection can be trimmed back to healthy tissues and the urethra itself spatulated. The corpus spongiosum can then be retracted out of the operative field by means of a lightly applied vascular clamp.

Occasionally, there is still a lumen through the site of the transection to the healthy posterior urethra above but this is rare. More commonly the posterior urethra above the site of the fibrosis and obliteration is best defined by passing a metal sound such as a Van Buren in the United States, a Clutton's sound in the UK or a Benique sound in Europe, through the suprapubic catheter track, if there is one, or through a suprapubic cystostomy if there is not (**Fig. 17.4**). This allows the tip of the sound to be palpated in the upper end of the wound usually posterior to the point at which the bulbar urethra was mobilised and transected. It is then usually just a simple matter to cut down onto the posterior urethra, trim away sufficient fibrosis to expose the upper end and then spatulate it open. Surgeons vary in the degree in which they profess to excise fibrotic tissue from the apex of the proximal urethra but all will be careful anterior-laterally on either side of the proximal urethra where the neurovascular structures to the corpora cavernosa responsible for erection will be vulnerable. At this point the verumontanum should be clearly visible within the posterior urethra – a useful point for distinguishing the urethra proper from a false passage. It is very unusual for the verumontanum to have been damaged by the injury.

If the proximal urethra is not identifiable by palpation in this way an abdomino- perineal approach may be necessary as described to follow.

Having cleared the two ends of the urethra of fibrosis and spatulated them back into healthy tissue it is a simple matter to see whether they will come together without tension or not. If so, they can be sutured together with six or eight 5-O absorbable

sutures **Figs. 17.5** and **17.6**). Again, opinions vary as to which suture material is best but this probably means that it makes not the slightest difference what you choose. We prefer Vicryl (for no very good reason). It is important to approximate the epithelium with each stitch and to take an adequate bit of the surrounding tissue to make sure the sutures hold. It is obviously important that this should be healthy epithelium. This is not always easy to discern with the naked eye and magnification may be helpful.

Working in a confined space in the posterior urethra it is often easier to place sutures if the needle is bent into a J-shape then held in the needle holder so that it emerges end on. Rotation of the wrist then manoeuvres the needle through a significantly smaller axis of rotation rather than when the needle is held in the traditional way at right-angles to

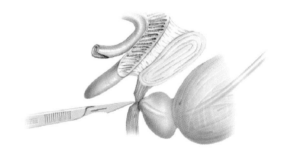

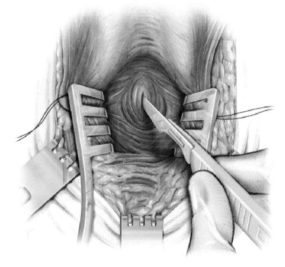

FIG. 17.4. Identification of the proximal urethra when the lumen is obliterated, and incision onto a sound passed antegrade

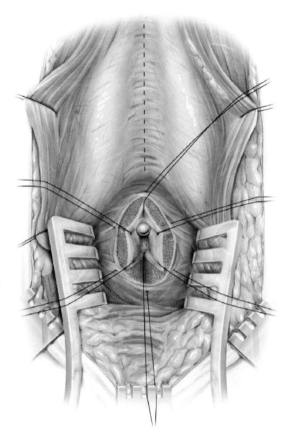

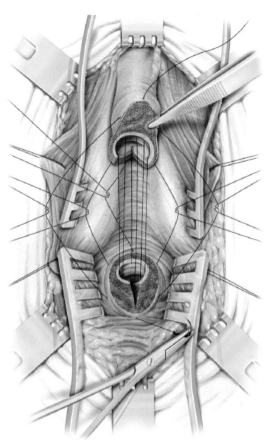

FIG. 17.5. Six 5-O polyglactin sutures can then be placed through the full thickness of the proximal urethra at 2:4-, 6:8-, 10-, and 12-o'clock positions as a preliminary move to the anastomosis, and to spatulate open the posterior urethra to make sure that this is clearly visible and healthy

FIG. 17.6. The sutures are then passed through the distal end of the urethra and tied "parachute" style

the jaws of the needle holder. A gorget facilitates suture placement and also protects the inside of the urethra (**Fig. 17.7**).

If there is tension of the anastomosis, which there usually is after urethral mobilisation alone, then the natural curve of the urethra can be straightened out, as alluded to above, in stages: firstly by incising the tunica albuginea that binds the two crura of the copora cavernosa together in the anterior midline (**Figs. 17.8** and **17.9**). Opening this inter-crural plane allows the urethra to lie between the crura rather than on the surface of the crura and reduces tension quite considerably. Indeed, in more than 50% of patients this will be sufficient to allow a tension-free anastomosis. If

it is not it may be seen that the urethra is being curved over the inferior pubic arch on its way to the anastomosis in which case a wedge pubectomy of the inferior pubic arch can be performed (**Figs. 17.10** and **17.11**). Having fully opened the intercrural plane, and taking great care not to damage the dorsal arteries and nerves of the penis on either side of the inner aspects of the separated crura (as well as the nerves of the corpora cavernosa on either side apex of the prostate and the membranous urethra) the pubic periostium can be incised with diathermy down to bone and the bone can then be removed either using a Capener's gouge, or a bone punch, or some similar instrument. In about another 10% or 15% this

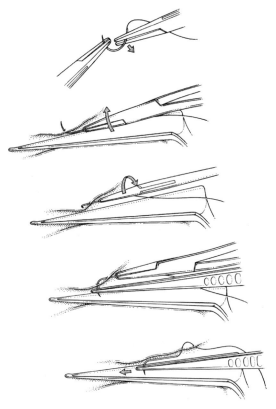

FIG. 17.7. The needle and gorget are useful to facilitate suture placement

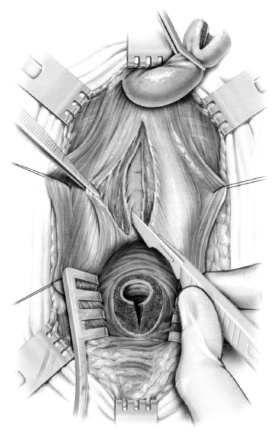

FIG. 17.8. If the ventral midline between the corpora is carefully incised to open the plane between them then

will allow a tension-free anastomosis. For some surgeons, there will still be a group of patients for whom there is still unacceptable tension at the anastomosis despite both a crural separation and an inferior wedge pubectomy. In such patients those surgeons will mobilize the urethra further distally off the corpora cavernosa beyond the point where possible. Then, by exposure of the anterior aspect of the pubic symphysis at the anterior limit of the skin incision a bony channel can be created through to the wedge pubectomy already created and the urethra can be passed through this channel for anastomosis to the proximal urethra (**Figs. 17.12–17.14**). It is obviously important during this to make sure that there is an adequate bony channel and that there are no sharp bony spikes to damage the urethra.

Having completed the anastomosis, a 14- or 16-French silicone Foley urethral catheter is passed up into the bladder, and if there was a pre-existing suprapubic catheter, then this is replaced as well. The wound is then closed in layers taking care to obliterate all the dead space as far as possible to reduce the risk of haematoma formation. If there is a space left behind that cannot be obliterated by suture, then a wound drain should be left in place but this is usually only necessary in those patients who have had a wedge pubectomy or re-routing of the urethra.

5.1. Postoperative Follow-Up

The wound is usually healed and the urethra intact after 2 wk. We arrange for our patients to have a pericatheter urethrogram at this point

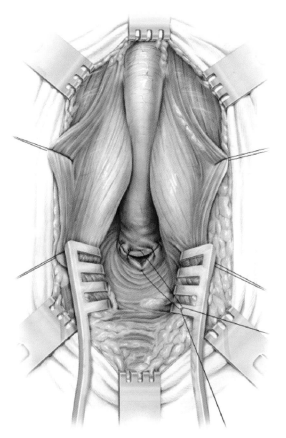

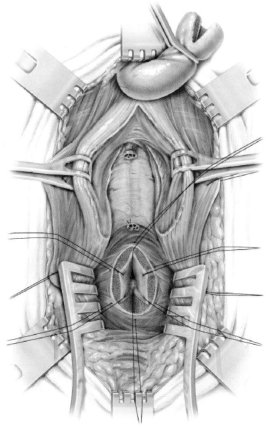

FIG. 17.9. The reconstructed urethra can lie within the inter-crural plane and tension on the anastomosis is relieved

FIG. 17.10. Maximum separation of the crura to expose the inferior pubic symphysis

to make sure that there is no extravasation in which case the catheter can be removed and the patient can start normal voiding. If there is any irregularity we leave the catheter in for a further week and then repeat the x-ray, by which time it is almost always satisfactory. We get a baseline flow rate study at this stage. We then see the patient 6 mo or so later and repeat the flow rate study and the ascending urethrogram and micturating cystogram. Although there are occasional instances of patients who deteriorate with time we have yet to see a patient with a widely patent urethra on urethrography and a normal flow rate 6 mo postoperatively who shows signs of deterioration thereafter. We therefore don't follow-up such patients unless there is some other reason. If the urethrogram is unsatisfactory, for whatever

reason, then however good the flow rate might be, we will follow those patients up with an annual ascending urethrogram and micturating cystogram and flowrate study as it in this group of patients that the occasional long term recurrent stricture occurs.

6. Complications

However, much the most common presentation of a recurrent stricture is that the patient runs into trouble within hours or days of having their postoperative catheter removed. This is because such problems are as a result of ischaemia of the anastomosis because the blood supply is insufficient to sustain adequate vascularity of the

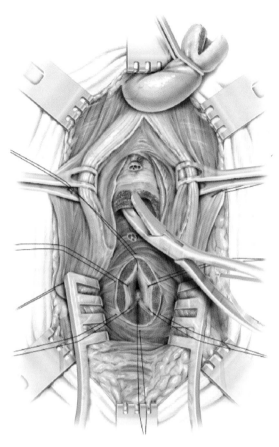

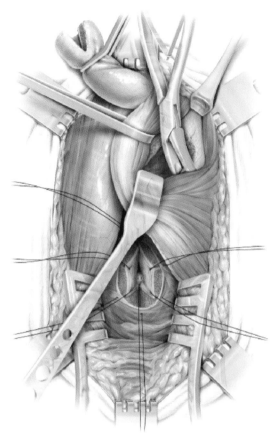

Fig. 17.11. Wedge resection of the inferior part of the pubic symphysis

Fig. 17.12. Medial retraction of the left crus of the penis and resection of a bony channel.

anastomosis, or because fibrotic tissue was left behind, or more commonly, because there was tension at the anastomosis. If the procedure was performed technically competently then almost always the patients who show this early failure also have complete erectile dysfunction support-ing the concept that this recurrent stricture is vas-culogenic and ischaemic in origin. In such cases the suprapubic catheter must be replaced (if it has been removed) and the patient must wait another three months and the procedure is repeated. This is usually successful because the length of the ischaemic segment is usually short.

When the proximal urethra cannot be identified by a sound in the apex of the prostate and mem-branous urethra, or if there is some other indica-

tion that requires it, then an abdomino-perineal approach is necessary (10). Through a long lower midline incision the apex of the prostate is exposed by dividing the haematoma-fibrosis that plasters the bladder, bladder neck and prostatic urethra to the pubic bone and symphysis. This is easier said than done and will often require a wedge resection of the posterior aspect of the pubic symphysis to allow the apex of the prostate to be exposed. Once it has been exposed a chan-nel is created through to the perineal incision and the procedure continues as described previ-ously (Fig. 17.15). When rerouting the urethra is necessary during an abdomino-perineal repair, it is usually easier to reroute it through a superior wedge pubectomy rather than an inferior wedge

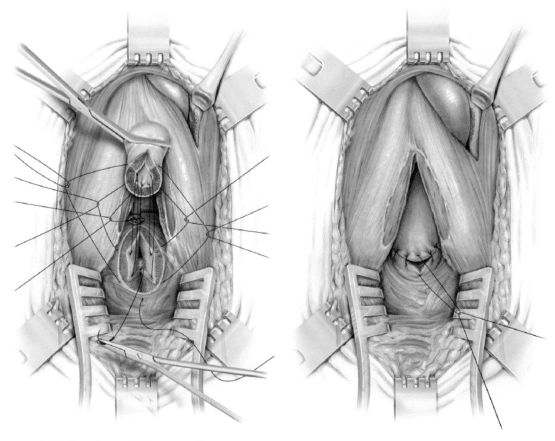

FIG. 17.13. "Parachute-style" anastomosis

FIG. 17.14. The completed anastomosis

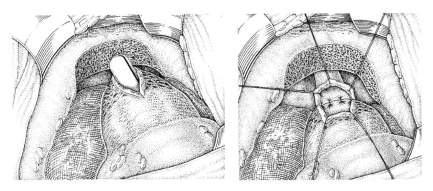

FIG. 17.15. Abdomino-perineal approach. (A) Exposed prostate apex after pubis wedge resection and incision onto sound passed antegrade. (B) Completing the primary anastomosis

pubectomy, particularly in children and teenagers (**Fig. 17.16**).

Bladder neck injuries are a particular problem. They never heal spontaneously, they are always associated with more severe injuries to the urinary tract, they are almost always associated with injury to the bulbomembranous urethra as well, and they are commonly associated with

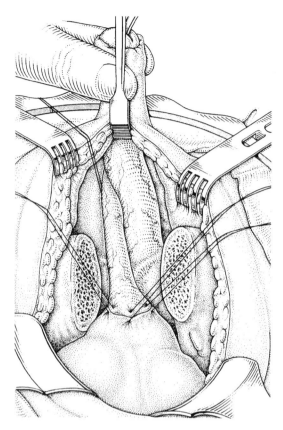

FIG. 17.16. Abdominoperineal approach. Pubectomy and primary anastomosis

infected cavities and fistulation of those cavities through to the perineum or into the adductor compartment to the leg. When a bladder neck injury is identified, it should be repaired as early as possible to reduce the risk of the latter complications. More minor bladder neck injuries may appear to heal in the first instance but they always give rise to problems later on: incontinence, persistent or recurrent bleeding, or recurrent cavitation and infection. The longer they are left, the more difficult they are to repair. Fortunately, most ruptures are in the anterior or anterolateral midline and they can be carefully

identified and reconstructed with reconstruction of the urethra as well, although such repairs may be difficult, lengthy and tedious.

After abdominoperineal reconstruction of the urethra, with our without bladder neck reconstruction, mobilization of the omentum to fill the dead space, line the raw bony areas, and wrap around the reconstruction seems sensible. Postoperatively such patients are managed in exactly the same way as after transperineal bulbo prostatic anastomotic urethroplasty.

References

1. Andrich DE, Day AC, Mundy AR (2007) Proposed mechanisms of lower urinary tract injury in fractures of the pelvic ring. BJU Int 100:567–573
2. Chapple CR (2000) Urethral injury. BJU Int 86: 318–326
3. Jordan GH, Secrest CL (1992) Arteriography in select patients with posterior urethral distraction injuries (abstract). J Urol 147:289 A.
4. Marion G, Pérard J (1942) Technique des operations plastiques sue la vessie et sur l'urètre. Paris, Masson et Cie, pp 113–122, 158–183
5. Mundy AR (1997) Reconstruction of posterior urethral distraction defects. Atlas Urol Clin North Am 5:139–174.
6. Mundy AR (2005) Anastomotic urethroplasty. BJU Int 96:921–944
7. Kizer WS, Armenakas NA, Brandes SB, Cavalcanti AG, Santucci RA, Morey AF (2007) Simplified reconstruction of posterior urethral disruption defects: limited role of supracrural rerouting. J Urol 177:1378–1381
8. Turner-Warwick R (1988) Urethral stricture surgery, in Mundy AR (ed) Current operative surgery. London, Balliere Tindall, pp 160–218
9. Waterhouse K, Abrahams JI, Gruber H, et al (1973) The transpubic approach to the lower urinary tract. J Urol 109:486–490
10. Webster GD, Ramon J (1991) Repair of pelvic fracture posterior urethral defects using an elaborated perineal approach: experience with 74 cases. J Urol 145:744–748

18
Staged Urethroplasty

Michael Coburn

Contents

1. Introduction.. 202
2. History and Rationale 202
3. Staged Procedures for Posterior Urethral Distraction Injuries 203
    3.1. Indications.. 203
4. Technical Approach to Staged Urethroplasty for Posterior Urethral Distraction Injuries.............. 204
5. Staged Procedures for Anterior Urethral Stricture Disease 205
    5.1. Indications.. 205
6. Technical Approaches for Staged Urethroplasty for Anterior Urethral Stricture Disease.............. 208
Editorial Comment... 210
References... 211

Summary Staged urethroplasty is an important element in the armamentarium of the urethral reconstructive surgeon. While the vast majority of urethral injuries and strictures may be addressed with single stage reconstructive techniques, there are various situations in which a staged approach may be preferable or essential. The underlying disease process, the condition of the local tissues, or the history of prior surgical interventions may create situations in which a single stage procedure is ill-advised. The presence of local infection or inflammation or the problem of an obliterated urethral segment with an inhospitable graft bed may necessitate the temporary creation of a proximal urethrostomy with replacement or augmentation of the strictured urethral segment. Previous penile skin mobilization from prior flaps or hypospadias procedures may prevent repeat single stage flap procedures, requiring a staged approach. Classic descriptions of staged urethroplasty techniques by Blandy, Turner-Warwick and Johanson are still applicable today, and have provided an important set of alternatives in the management of complex stricture disease and urethral trauma. Staged approaches generally involve two discrete steps: the surgical opening, augmentation or replacement of the diseased urethral segment with creation of a proximal urethrostomy, followed, after 6 months or more, by a tubularization of the neourethra to recreate intact urethral structure and function. At times, additional intervening stages are required prior to tubularization to correct interval stenosis or partial graft loss or contracture. Current applicability and technical aspects of staged urethral reconstruction.

Keywords Blandy, Turner-Warwick, Johanson, Schreiter, staged urethroplasty, urethral tubularization

From: *Current Clinical Urology: Urethral Reconstructive Surgery*
Edited by: S.B. Brandes © Humana Press, Totowa, NJ

1. Introduction

Most cases of urethral reconstruction may be managed with single-stage surgery. There are, however, certain situations in which a staged approach is preferable. It is important that the surgeon pursuing an interest in urethral reconstructive surgery have a clear sense of when a staged approach offers advantages over single-stage procedures, as well as thorough familiarity with the technical aspects of performing staged surgery to increase the likelihood of a successful outcome. Both in stricture surgery and in the setting of acute trauma, staged repairs may offer significant advantages over single-stage procedures. The term "staged urethroplasty" is applied and in this discussion rather than "two-stage" surgery to reflect the fact that when one decides to pursue one of the staged options, the process is not necessarily limited to two procedures; at times more than two interventions are necessary.

2. History and Rationale

Historically, staged procedures were the norm for many settings of urethral reconstruction. Early descriptions of staged procedures for correction of urethral stricture disease by notable urethral surgery luminaries such as Johanson, Turner-Warwick, Blandy, and others addressed the merits and technical details of staged surgery (1–4). In the area of urethral trauma, various authors also addressed the merits of staged approaches to the reestablishment of urethral continuity. As a general principle, the concept of the staged approach involved an effort to bring vascularized tissue into the bed of a urethral stricture with the use of either a graft or a flap and either complete substitution for the full urethral circumference or augmentation of existing tissue, as a first stage. At the conclusion of the first stage, the patient would void through a urethrostomy at some level: penile shaft, scrotal, or perineal. A period of approximately 3–6 mo to 1 yr or more

is allowed to elapse after the first stage. In so doing, the transferred tissue can gain a stable blood supply and allow the tissues to become mature: supple and manageable for staged surgical manipulation.

The next stage focused on assuring adequate caliber and tissue quality at the proximal, distal, and central portions of the urethrostomy site. At times, the urethrostomy has strictured and thus requires further tissue augmentation, dilation, incision, or plastic reconfiguration (i.e., Y-V plasty). When the initial surgical site is of adequate quality and caliber, the final stage could be pursued directly. The final stage of the planned staged procedures involved tubularizing the transferred tissue over a sound or catheter to achieve a specific caliber, along with soft tissue and skin coverage of the tubularized urethra, to close the urethrostomy and redirect the urinary stream distally, hopefully to the urethral meatus or at least to the distal shaft level depending on the state of the most distal penile urethra.

The rationale for proposing staged urethral surgery for stricture was a reflection of both the nature of stricture disease at the time much of the relevant literature was written, as well as existing biases and the state of the art of grafting materials and tissue transfer techniques during those periods. Before the modern era of antibacterial therapy and because of the limited access to health care for large populations in the 19th and first half of the 20th centuries, presentation with highly complex stricture disease was commonplace. Severe strictures involving loss of or near-obliteration of long segments of urethra, complex fistulae, chronic infection, and abscess or stone formation greatly challenged stricture surgeons and created extraordinarily hostile local environments to support reconstructive efforts.

The "watering pot" perineum, with multiple fistula sites coursing through an indurated and severely diseased perineum, was not uncommon. The tissue transfer materials of choice for graft placement in urethral reconstruction consisted mainly of genital skin or skin from relatively hairless areas such as the inner arm or hip region. Such skin grafts were prone to scarring and contracture due to the inflammatory effects of urine contact and local infection, such that interval procedures to "touch up" the first stage were often necessary prior to tubularization at the final stage. The use of local flap techniques, especially in the scrotum and perineum, often resulted in hair-bearing skin being placed within the neourethra, which created the risk of stone formation, restenosis and obstructive uropathy. Single-stage procedures were often not feasible in such settings because of the potential for graft loss caused by ischemia from placement into a suboptimal bed and the need for the development of new blood supply to transferred tissue before late tubularization.

In the trauma setting, catheter-realignment techniques for posterior urethral distraction injuries were crude and traumatic and resulted in high rates of functional impairment and restricturing. The placement of scrotal and perineal flaps into a urethral defect for creation of temporary perineal urethrostomies, with delayed closure, represented appealing ways out of very difficult situations. The merits of suprapubic diversion with delayed anastomotic repair for both posterior injuries and bulbar straddle injuries were under debate, with strong proponents of various approaches pursuing markedly differing strategies.

The modern era of urethral trauma management and urethral stricture surgery has altered the concept of the indications for staged urethroplasty. Modern tissue-transfer techniques, and especially the advent of the use of buccal mucosal grafts, has impacted on the evolving approaches. Combined tissue transfer techniques such as dorsal buccal grafting plus ventral fasciocutaneous flap placement, as proposed by McAninch and others, have offered expanded applicability of single stage surgery for obliterated strictures involving loss of significant lengths of complete urethral circumference, which in the past would have required staged approaches. The use of minimally invasive catheter realignment techniques to avoid marked lateral and coronal displacement after pelvic fracture urethral disruption injuries, along with careful monitoring and management of suprapubic cystostomies and prevention of related complications while awaiting definitive reconstruction, has also impacted on the role of staged repairs.

3. Staged Procedures for Posterior Urethral Distraction Injuries

3.1. Indications

3.1.1. Length of Urethral Defect

With the valuable descriptions of single stage repairs for posterior urethral injuries which have been published in recent years, even relatively long defects may be managed without using a staged approach. Webster's description of the progressive approach to gaining urethral length, which involves anterior urethral mobilization, midline separation of the corpora cavernosa at the root of the penis, inferior pubectomy and when necessary, urethral rerouting above the corpus cavernosum, for significant length deficiencies, has facilitated single stage anastomotic urethroplasty in the vast majority of cases.

There are, however, exceptions to this generalization and, at times, staged approaches may be necessary because of an exceptionally long defect between the obliterated ends of the urethra. Such significant tissue loss may be observed when there is concomitant injury to the membranous urethral along with loss of the bulbar urethra caused by penetrating injuries or ischemic loss of bulbar urethral tissue, when the bladder and prostate are markedly displaced into the upper pelvis and do not descend with resolution of the pelvic hematoma, or when there is obliteration of the prostatic urethra due to laceration, crush injury or extensive bladder neck trauma. In such cases, transpubic urethroplasty may be considered with the anterior urethra being routed alongside the corpora and brought directly to the prostate or bladder neck anteriorly. It may, however, simply be impossible to bring the anterior urethra to an appropriate location with extensive displacement and tissue loss, necessitating a staged repair.

3.1.2. Vascular Insufficiency of Anterior Urethra

Depending on the magnitude and specific anatomy of the original pelvic trauma, penile vascular insufficiency may result. One should be suspicious of this complication of pelvic fracture if the patient lacks erectile function and does not respond with appropriate arterial dilatation with intracavernosal injection of vasodilatory agents as demonstrated by Duplex Doppler assessment. Such findings should prompt pelvic arteriography or other vascular imaging (magnetic resonance angiography or computed tomography angiography); if bilateral pudendal artery or significant branch arterial occlusion is noted, the anterior urethra may not tolerate significant mobilization, placing the patient at risk for ischemic stricture and failure of an anastomotic repair. For such cases, Jordan has advised preemptive penile revascularization prior to urethroplasty. If revascularization if not feasible or is unsuccessful, staged urethroplasty with tissue transfer techniques, rather than a high-risk anastomotic repair, may be necessary.

3.1.3. Condition of Local Tissues

Ongoing infection, abscess formation, calculus formation, severe pubic bone deformity, or concomitant original rectal injury may cause alteration in the local environment so as to make primary anastomotic repair very difficult or potentially ill-advised. A hostile local environment should be corrected by providing appropriate diversion and bladder drainage, local incision and drainage with adequate time allowed for healing and resolution of cellulities before urethroplasty. If such adverse findings are encountered unexpectedly at the time of planned urethroplasty, conversion to a staged approach may be a preferable strategy.

4. Technical Approach to Staged Urethroplasty for Posterior Urethral Distraction Injuries

A variety of procedures have been described to pursue a staged approach to posterior urethroplasty. Among the best recognized are the techniques described by Blandy and that described by Turner-Warwick (1,4). The "Blandy flap" staged urethroplasty involves rotating an inverted V-shaped perineal flap into the proximal urethral segment and performing a local skin closure which amounts to partly tubularizing the perineal skin flap to create a perineal urethrostomy (**Fig. 18.1, A–D**). The

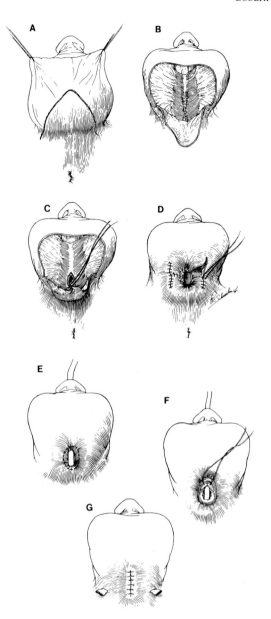

FIG. 18.1. **Blandy two-stage urethroplasty with posteriorly based scrotal inlay flap** A, inverted V incision is marked, extending sufficiently onto the scrotal wall to allow adequate reach to the prostatic apex. B, The scrotal flap is developed, exposing the perineum and the area of the opened urethral margin proximal to the stricture. D, The first–stage procedure is completed by suturing the posterior scrotal skin to the flap. E-G, The second-stage closure, with skin incision around the marsupialized urethra and closure of the tubularized segment in layers. (Modified after Coburn M. Two stage reconstruction of posterior urethral rupture defects. In Traumatic and Reconstructive Urology ed McAninch JW WB Saunders, 1996)

final stage of this procedure, which typically would occur at least 6 mo after the initial stage, involves incision of the perineal skin to produce a continuous tubularized neourethra from the proximal to the anterior urethra, with lateral mobilization of the adjacent skin to provide coverage of the neourethra (**Fig 18.1, E–G**). Meticulous care should be taken when performing the final closure procedure to avoid excessively undermining the neourethral skin which may produce devascularization and subsequent stenosis. Sufficient mobilization of the skin and underlying supporting tissue must be performed to allow tubularization without suture line tension; whenever possible, an intervening layer of local soft tissue between the neourethral suture line and the covering skin is highly desirable to avoid immediately overlapping suture lines and minimize the risk of fistula formation.

The final closure stage should await full maturation of the perineal urethrostomy, with the local tissues becoming maximally soft and pliable and the stoma being stable for sufficient time to minimize the risk of late stenosis. In our experience, 6 mo is usually adequate to reach this level of stability. This procedure does typically result in the inclusion of some hair-bearing skin in the neourethra which can be problematic in some cases. Epilation of the skin before the final tubularization stage with the use of laser fulguration or electrocautery fulguration of visible hair roots, and subsequent endoscopic examination of the internalized flap to assess adequacy of epilation is desirable before the final closure stage. In a moderate percentage of cases, an intermediate stage to modify the first stage anatomy may be necessary if the first stage flap placement results in stenosis with a significantly reduced caliber; Y-V-plasty or additional tissue transfer to widen the proximal neourethra may be necessary to avoid unacceptable stenosis with final tubularization. Endoscopic assessment and calibration of the first stage result should be performed before final tubularization to be certain that an intermediate procedure is not necessary.

The Turner-Warwick urethroplasty (*4*) is similar to the Blandy flap in principle but simply involves displacement of local skin into the opened urethra, rather than creation of the V-shaped flap. The relevance of epilation, the potential need for an intermediate procedure depending on the result of the first stage, and the approach to the final closure stage are similar for the two types of staged procedures. Depending on the depth of the proximal urethra, either of these approaches may be most suitable and the surgeon planning a staged repair should be comfortable with both techniques (**Fig. 18.2**).

An alternative to local perineal or scrotal skin transposition into the proximal urethral to create the perineal urethrostomy is to apply graft techniques using split-thickness skin (meshed or unmeshed) or buccal mucosal grafts to place sufficient tissue into the region of the proximal urethral end to allow anticipated late tubularization for a final closure stage (*5–7*) (**Fig. 18.3, A–C**). The advantage of these approaches are the avoidance of the placement of hair-bearing skin into the proximal urethral region, and the opportunity to utilize tissue from a remote location when the local skin is abnormal or not sufficiently mobile to place into the proximal urethral region. In this author's view, placement of paired parallel strips of buccal mucosa is the preferred approach in such cases, due to its lower likelihood of contracture and longstanding durability in a moist environment.

Some patients will choose to remain with the perineal urethrostomy as a permanent or long-term approach to voiding. This personal decision, based on the patient's individual goals, cosmetic, and functional concerns, should be supported by the urologist in a well-informed patient. A permanent perineal urethrostomy is also an option for the refractory pendulous urethral stricture that has failed prior reconstructions (**Fig. 18.4, A** and **B**). The long-term consequences of the perineal urethrostomy are generally favorable, though monitoring for stomal stenosis with resultant obstructive uropathy, or stone formation especially when hair-bearing skin is present within the proximal segment are important maintenance considerations.

5. Staged Procedures for Anterior Urethral Stricture Disease

5.1. Indications

In the setting of anterior urethral stricture surgery, staged urethroplasty may be advisable or unavoidable in several types of circumstances. In most cases, these settings relate to the challenge of dealing with

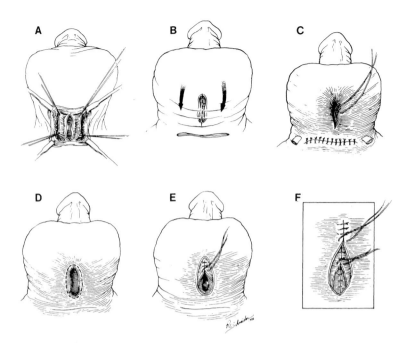

FIG. 18.2. **Turner-Warwick two-stage scrotal inlay procedure.** A, Incision through bulbomembranous stricture via perineal incision. B, Transposition of posterior scrotum over urethrotomy to determine the appropriate level for secondary scrotal incision. C, Completion of the fist stage of repair with the secondary scrotal incision sutured to the urethral edges. D, Marking of incision for second-stage closure. E and F, after elevation of skin and subcutaneous tissue borders, closure of the neourethra is performed, followed by closure of the periurethral tissues (bulbocavernosus muscle), subcutaneous tissue, and skin. (From Coburn M. Two stage reconstruction of posterior urethral rupture defects. In Traumatic and Reconstructive Urology ed McAninch JW WB Saunders, 1996)

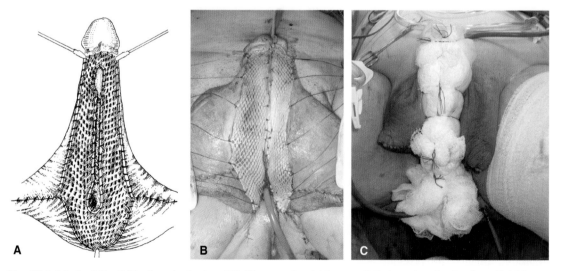

FIG. 18.3. **Meshed Graft Urethroplasty.** A and B, The completed 1st stage. C. Bolster dressing for the spli thickness skin-graft. (Images courtesy SB Brandes)

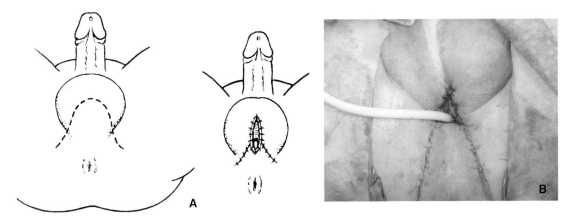

FIG. 18.4. **Perineal urethrostomy with inverted "U" flap, after Blandy.** A. Cartoon B. Completed urethrostomy for a pendulous urethral stricture that has failed multiple surgical reconstructions (Images courtesy of SB Brandes)

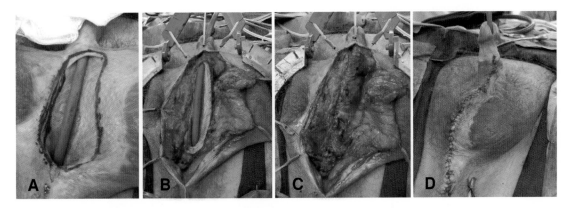

FIG. 18.5. **2nd Stage Urethroplasty, after Schreiter.** 62 year old patient with LSA who had failed two prior one stage urethroplasties. Figures A-D. 2nd stage Schreiter urethroplasty with tubularization of matured (>6months) grafted skin over a 24F Robnel catheter. (Images courtesy SB Brandes)

long strictures, before surgery, or management of meatal, submeatal or fossa navicularis strictures. Strictures caused by the inflammatory, atrophic and obliterative effects of lichen sclerosus et atrophicus (formerly termed "balanitis xerotica obliterans") may be best managed with staged urethroplasty with tissue transfer techniques being applied to bring tissue into the region which may be less likely to become affected by the same process than occurs when local tissue is utilized for reconstruction (**Fig 18.5, A–D**).

5.1.1. Obliterated Anterior Urethra, Inadequate Anterior Urethral Graft Bed

When there is significant luminal obliteration of the anterior urethra and anastomotic or augmented anastomotic repair is not feasible, options include tubularized pedicle skin flaps for creation of a neourethra, combination techniques such as dorsal buccal graft plus ventral skin island placement to create a neourethra, and staged urethroplasty with excision/replacement or augmentation of the dorsal urethral plate with transferred graft tissue, followed by late tubularization and closure. Tubularized skin flaps have a significant late stenosis rate and have been largely replaced by the combination techniques, such as those noted already. When such single-stage reconstructions are not feasible, the staged urethroplasty provides an appealing solution. Failed prior urethroplasty or severe inflammatory disease may result in extensive scarring of the ventral corpora cavernosa such that Dartos or other local tissue must be rotated into position to support a dorsal graft. This need may obviate the option of creating a vascularized skin pedicle for ventral placement, such that a staged approach may be preferable.

5.1.2. Meatal, Submeatal, Fossa Navicularis, Lichen Sclerosus et Atrophicus-Related Distal Urethral Strictures

The entity is addressed elsewhere in this text, but its discussion in the context of staged urethroplasty is important. For surgical reconstruction of distal urethral stenoses some patients may prefer to simply have a more proximal meatus created to void upstream from the stenotic segment. This is often the simplest approach, and many times may constitute an acceptable solution to distal urethral stricture disease, especially when other reconstructive options have failed. When dilation programs or meatal advancement procedures are not successful or acceptable, a variety of local skin flap techniques have been described. The failure rate for such approaches is significant, however, especially when lichen sclerosus is present based on histological analysis or clinical impression. When local skin flap reconstruction is unsuccessful or ill-advised, a staged approach is an excellent alternative.

6. Technical Approaches for Staged Urethroplasty for Anterior Urethral Structure Disease

The essential concept in this group of procedures involves two stages. The first is the creation of an anterior urethral meatus or anterior urethrostomy. This is performed either by the marsupialization of

the anterior urethra to the ventral penile skin via a longitudinal incision and suturing of the urethral wall bilaterally to the adjacent incised ventral penile skin, or by the replacement or augmentation of the anterior urethral by placement of longitudinally-oriented grafts or flaps (**Fig. 18.6**). The stenotic or obliterated urethra may be excised at the time of this tissue transfer procedure, or it may simply be incised longitudinally, with the transferred tissue being placed on one, or more typically both sides of the created dorsal urethral plate to augment the urethral already present. Whether to excise or augment the stenotic urethra depends upon its condition: if the lumen is obliterated or the appearance of the dorsal strip after incision appears inappropriate for use in the reconstruction becaues of extremely narrow-caliber or fibrotic or inflammatory changes, excision of the full urethral circumference with replacement using transferred tissue is preferable.

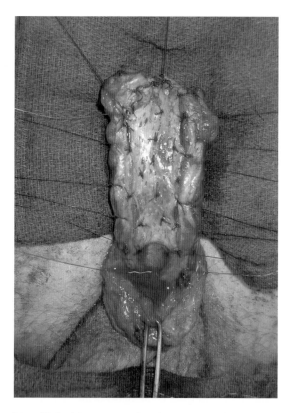

FIG. 18.6. 1st stage urethroplasty with skin graft to pendulous urethra, in a hypospadias "cripple" who had failed 7 prior one stage reconstructions. (Image courtesy SB Brandes)

The final stage, which is performed after an adequate period of maturation after the first stage, is tubularization of the neourethral plate over an appropriately sized catheter with skin coverage and closure. As in the case for the posterior urethra discussion above, an intermediate stage (or stages) may be necessary to deal with proximal meatal stenosis or contracture of the transferred tissue; careful endoscopic assessment of the first stage reconstruction result with calibration and determination of the tissue's readiness for further mobilization and tubularization is critical.

The traditional approach of the Johansen procedure involves marsupialization of the anterior urethra to the adjacent penile skin following full thickness longitudinal ventral incision as the first stage *(3)* (**Fig. 18.7**). The second stage involves tubularization of the neourethra, which consists of the dorsal urethral plate, in addition to a variable width of the adjacent penile skin which is incised longitudinally and included with the tissue tubularized into the neourethra. Sufficient skin is turned inwards to create the neourethra to allow predictable contracture (variably reported but possibly 30% or more) with late maintenance of an acceptable lumen (**Fig. 18.8**). It is desirable to create an intervening layer of viable tissue when possible over the neourethral suture line and

under the covering skin; local dartos is adequate in some cases, although it may be deficient for this purpose; when necessary, dartos flaps from the scrotum or scrotal tunica vaginalis flaps may be created for the purpose of tissue interposition to minimize the risk of fistula formation. If inadequate skin is present to close over the neourethra, it is possible to make a longitudinal relaxing incision on the dorsum of the penis to bring native penile skin together over the neourethral reconstruction, and graft the dorsum of the penis on a healthy dartos or Buck's fascial bed.

A more contemporary approach involves the use of longitudinally placed buccal mucosal grafts (either paired or single, depending on the width of neourethra needed) on the ventral surface of the penis (refs). These grafts appear to be quite durable and less prone to contracture than skin grafts or skin flaps. They can be left in place to form a long-term anterior urethrostomy, or can be mobilized and tubularized as a final stage to create a neourethra, with skin coverage as described previously. If the urethral plate is excised and is to be completely replaced by buccal graft tissue, paired grafts, longitudinally placed and sutured in the midline are generally necessary to allow for an adequate lumen at the time of final stage closure. When the healed graft tissues are ready for final

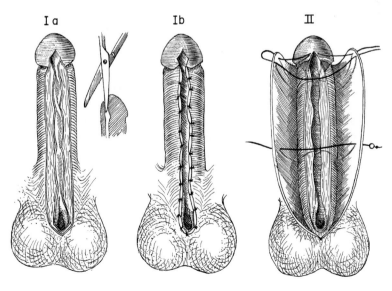

FIG. 18.7. Johanson's original staged urethral reconstruction. (From Glenn JF, Boyce WH: Urologic Surgery, Harper & Row, Pub., New York, 1969)

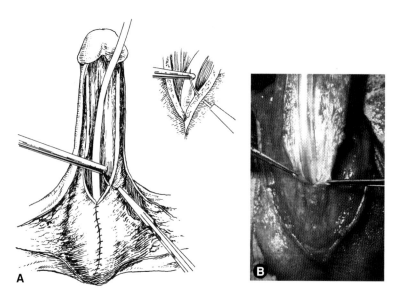

FIG. 18.8. **Second stage Schreiter-type Urethroplasty A.** Forming the neourethra over a 24F catheter. B. Neourethral reconstruction by inverting sutures. (From Coburn M. Two stage reconstruction of posterior urethral rupture defects. In Traumatic and Reconstructive Urology ed McAninch JW WB Saunders, 1996)

stage tubularization and closure, it is important to incise the underlying tissues which will support the neourethra such that the underlying tissues extend a few millimeters beyond the epithelial incision to avoid ischemia at the neourethral suture line. We try to create a second layer suture line with the neourethral closure using these subepithelial tissues to support the vascularization of the neourethra.

Suture material selection for these various approaches to staged urethroplasty generally involves the use of fine absorbable suture, of either gut, braided or monofilament types. Depending on the tissue quality, a 4-O to 6-O suture is usually selected; finest gauge that is adequate for the tissues is preferred. A catheter is generally left in place after the first-stage procedures, and also after any intermediate-stage intervention necessary, to allow initial healing without the patient needing to handle the surgical site or allow urinary extravasation until grafts are stable. Soft bulky gauze dressings are advisable to allow complete early graft or flap immobilization following the first stage reconstructions to minimize the risk of graft loss. We cover the grafts with petrolatum gauze augmented with antibiotic ointment to avoid desiccation and adherence of gauze to the reconstruction site.

Editorial Comment

Johanson's surgical principles that he introduced in the 1950 are still in use today, directly and indirectly. His original article is one of the seminal articles in the field of urology because he introduced a novel method for reconstructing the urethra that was simple, straightforward, and successful. In today's setting, for relatively uncomplicated urethral strictures, there are many safe, effective and durable one stage reconstructions, as an alternative to a staged Johanson. However, when the ideal tissue (local or distant) for urethral reconstruction is deficient or not available (either from prior failed urethral surgery, hypospadias, infection or trauma), then it is best to fall back on the technique of staged urethroplasty. The technique by Schreiter, a modification of the original two-stage urethroplasty by Johanson, uses a ventral urethrotomy to marsupialize the urethra and a meshed skin graft to the Dartos and urethral edges. After 6 to 12 mo (the longer the better) of graft maturation, the urethra is tubularized in a standard Thiersch-Duplay fashion. The key to a successful staged repair is waiting long enough after the first stage until the skin is supple. The typical error here is to perform the second stage too early. After 6 mo, we typically reevaluate the patient every 3 mo until, on physical exam, the skin graft has matured enough to be supple and thus more easily mobilized for a delayed reconstruction.—S.B. Brandes

References

1. Blandy JP, Singh M, Tressider GL (1968) Urethroplasty by scrotal flap fo long urethral strictures. Br J Urol 40:261
2. Blandy JP, Singh M, Notley RG, Tresidder GC (1971) The results and complications of scrotal flap urethroplasty for stricture. Br J Urol 43:52
3. Johanson B (1953) Reconstruction of the male urethra in strictures. Application of the buried intact epithelium tube. Acta Chir Scand 176(Suppl):1
4. Turner-Warwick RT (1960) A technique for posterior urethroplasty. J Urol 83:416
5. Carr LK, MacDiarmid SA, Webster GD (1997) Treatment of complex anterior urethral stricture disease with mesh graft urethroplasty. J Urol 157:104–108
6. Lindell O, Borkowski J, Noll F, Schreiter F (1993) Urethral stricture repair: results in 179 patients. Scand J Urol Nephrol 27:241
7. Schreiter F, Noll F (1989) Mesh graft urethroplasty using split thickness skin graft or foreskin. J Urol 142:1223

19
Complications of Urethroplasty

Hosam S. Al-Qudah, Osama Al-Omar, and Richard A. Santucci

Contents

1. Introduction..214
2. Buccal Mucosal Urethroplasty (BMU) Complications..214
    2.1. Urine Leak..214
    2.2. Fistula..214
    2.3. Recurrence..215
    2.4. Urinary Tract Infection (UTI)..216
    2.5. Erectile Dysfunction (ED)...216
    2.6. Postvoid Dribbling..216
    2.7. Urethral Sacculation..216
    2.8. Other Uncommon Complications...217
    2.9. Oral Complications..217
3. Fasciocutaneous Urethroplasty Complications..217
    3.1. Recurrent Stricture..217
    3.2. Urethral Diverticulum..218
    3.3. Postvoid Dribbling..218
    3.4. Ejaculatory Dysfunction..218
    3.5. Urinary Extravasation..219
    3.6. Urethrocutaneous Fistula...219
    3.7. Erectile Dysfunction/Diminished Penile Sensation....................................219
    3.8. Penile Skin Necrosis..219
4. Anterior Anastomotic Urethroplasty Complications..219
    4.1. Acute Urinary Extravasation..219
    4.2. Postvoid Dribbling..219
    4.3. Erectile Dysfunction..220
    4.4. Chordee...220
    4.5. Recurrence..220
    4.6. Urinary Tract Infection..221
5. Posterior Urethroplasty Complications...221
    5.1. Failure of Repair..221
    5.2. Erectile Dysfunction..222
    5.3. Incontinence..223
    5.4. Positioning-Related Complications...223
Appendix..224
References...224

From: *Current Clinical Urology: Urethral Reconstructive Surgery*
Edited by: S.B. Brandes © Humana Press, Totowa, NJ

Summary Urethroplasty has excellent success rates against urethral stricture that far exceed that found with direct visual internal urethrotomy (DVIU) and dilation. Different forms of urethroplasty were employed including, buccal mucosal (BM), fasciocutaneous and anastomotic urethroplasty. Complications of urethroplasty are directly related to location of stricture, surgical technique, type of substitution tissue, and length of stricture. These complications range from mild and temporary to severe and complicated ones, which result in failure of urethroplasty. We present in this chapter an extensive review of the literature for complications of urethroplasty. Limitations in current published papers are the lack of a universally accepted definition of treatment failure and that reports are mixed complications for heterogeneous groups of strictures, treated by different modalities and surgeons.

Keywords Urethroplasty, buccal, graft, fistula, stricture, fasciocutaneous, flap

1. Introduction

Urethroplasty has excellent success rates against urethral stricture that far exceed that found with direct visual internal urethrotomy (DVIU) and dilation *(1–10)*. The total impact of urethroplasty on the patient is unknown, however, because only one extensive study of complications after urethroplasty has been published *(1)*. In this chapter, we have collected all the published data, to our knowledge, on urethroplasty complications.

There are two major problems that faced us when reviewing this material. The first is that most of the urethroplasty published papers contains heterogeneous groups of strictures treated by different modalities and surgeons. Usually, these reports concentrate on the description of the procedures and often only report raw success rates. Complications, if they are mentioned, are mixed for all the procedures. The second pitfall is in comparing success rates in different series that have variable definitions of treatment failure. We think establishing a unified definition is one of the important targets of any reconstructive urology consensus in the future.

Mild postoperative complications may happen after any urethral surgery. These include wound infection and dehiscence, skin ecchymosis, wound hematoma, wound tightness and numbness, and irritative lower urinary tract symptoms *(1,3,11–15)*. These mild complaints seem to be unimportant to the reconstructive urologist, and are rarely reported in papers. However, they are important to the patient and should be understood and discussed when the patient is being counseled for surgery *(1)*.

2. Buccal Mucosal Urethroplasty (BMU) Complications

Buccal mucosal grafts are now considered the standard substitution material for urethral stricture disease. Buccal mucosal onlay has greaer success rates and less morbidity compared with fasciocutaneous grafts or flaps. (**Tables 19.1** and **19.2** *[1,6,16,17]*) Because it is a relatively newer substitution material, most pertinent reports concentrate on success rates and include only brief description of complications. In general, greater rates of complications are reported with long urethral strictures, especially pendulous urethral strictures, and pan-urethral strictures that require two stage repairs *(18)*.

2.1. Urine Leak

Many centers do not consider urine leak at the time of urethrogram as a complication, whereas others reported it as a (temporary) fistula *(19–21)*. We tend to remove Foley catheters early (1 wk), and our series showed leak in 3 of 19 patients (16%). All were cured by Foley reinsertions for 7 d *(1)*. Others report urine leak in 0–25% of patients which, also were cured with 1–6 additional weeks of Foley catheter placement *(5,19–22)*.

2.2. Fistula

Persistent urine leak caused by breakdown of the urethral suture line leads to fistula formation. This complication is rare after bulbar urethroplasty, and is reported in only one patient (after ventral onlay repair) in published series to date *(23)*.The complications has not yet been reported after dorsal onlay grafts.

TABLE 19.1. Complication rate after buccal mucosal urethroplasty.

Reference	n	Approach	Mean followup (months)	Early complications (%)	Late complications (%)	Recurrence rate (%)
Kellner et al. *(32)*	23	Ventral	50	9		13
Kane et al. *(31)*	53	Ventral	25	6		6
Pansadoro et al. *(5)*	65	Ventral and dorsal	41	6	8	3
Elliott et al. *(4)*	60	Ventral	47	0		10
Andrich et al. *(6)*	29	Ventral	60		21	14
Andrich et al. *(6)*	42	Dorsal	60		17	5
Fichtner et al. *(23)*	32	Ventral	>60		13	13
Al-Qudah and Santucci *(1)*	19	Ventral	19	42	37	0

TABLE 19.2. Complication rate after fasciocutaneous urethroplasty.

Reference	n	Type of urethroplasty	Mean follow up (months)	Early complications (%)	Late complications (%)	Recurrence rate (%)	All complications (%)
Andrich et al. *(30)*	84	fasciocutaneous	120			31	33
Andrich et al. *(30)*	84	fasciocutaneous	60			21	
McAninch and Morey *(56)*	54	fasciocutaneous	41			13	
El-Kasaby et al. *(90)*	29	fasciocutaneous (for stricture and complex hypospadias)	19				17
Morey et al. *(58)*	15	fasciocutaneous (Q flap)	43 (in 13)			13	33
Lindell et al. *(91)*	18	Quartey	48			6	67
Al-Qudah and Santucci *(1)*	10	fasciocutaneous	26	60	60	40	60

Fistulas after one- or two-stage buccal urethroplasty of penile strictures is reported in 3% of patients *(18)*. Fistulae are treated by surgical excision and multilayer closure, with or without a small patch of additional buccal graft *(18)*. Increased fistulae in penile strictures compared to bulbar strictures reflects a general tendency for increased complications in 1) longer strictures and 2) penile urethral strictures.

2.3. Recurrence

One of the most troublesome and significant complications after urethral stricture surgery is recurrence of stricture. Recurrence after BMU for bulbar urethral stricture is reported in 0–20% of cases (**Table 19.3** *[4,21–26]*) Unlike the fasciocutaneous urethroplasty where recurrence is reported in a rate of 5% per year, most of the BMU recurrences occur

TABLE 19.3. Specific complications of fasciocutaneous urethroplasty.

Complication	Andrich et al. *(30)* (%)	Al-Qudah and Santucci *(1)* (%)
Erectile dysfunction	2	0
Post void dribbling	28	50
Diverticulum	12	0
UTI	5	0
Fistula	3	20
Chordee	3	20
Recurrence	21 (at 5 years)	40

in the first 2 yr after surgery *(4,5,21–24,27–31)*. The most frequent site of recurrence is the proximal or distal anastomotic end. It is less common in the mid-portion *(4,16,23,26,29,32)*.

We believe that proximal recurrence might be due to undertreating of the stricture and that modifications in operative technique may decrease the incidence of failure. We extend the urethral incision 5 mm into the normal urethra, and suture the proximal and distal anastomotic ends of the buccal graft with six or so simple interrupted sutures to "tack open" the distal and proximal graft ends in the hopes of decreasing the rate of recurrence *(33)*. Strictures at the proximal or distal graft sites are called "ring recurrences" by Barbagli and are usually easily treated with a single DVIU. Their successful treatment increases the success rates of BMU in most series to 94–100% *(5,26,31,32)*. Recent report by Barbagli et al. *(16)* reported suggest that 70 % (7/10 patients) of these ring recurrences are successfully treated with DVIU, and that the remainder of patients require surgical revision.

There is great controversy as to whether a dorsal or ventral BMU technique affects recurrence rates. Although several authors reported higher success rates with dorsal onlay urethroplasty *(6,34)*, multiple other studies show that ventral techniques have equal failure rates *(1,4,23,32,31)*. Barbagli himself compared the success of ventral grafts versus dorsal grafts and found no effect on graft position on success rates. The best technique in his opinion is the one the surgeon is most comfortable in performing *(33)*.

As always, long strictures and penile strictures have greaer failure rates. Recurrence rates after pan urethral and penile strictures have been reported as high as 10–45% after single-stage repair *(21,35)*. Recurrence rates after complex urethral strictures repaired by two-stage buccal mucosal grafts are 7–45% *(18,20)*. Lichen sclerosus patients also are thought to have worse results than patients with strictures from other causes *(27)*.

2.4. Urinary Tract Infection (UTI)

Acute UTI after BMU is reported in several series, with rates from 0% to 6% *(5,6,31)*. It is usually treated with antibiotics *(5,31)*, although we and others keep the patient on antibiotics during the entire period he is catheterized after surgery and we seldom see this complication. Prolonged Foley catheter drainage will increase the rate of this complication, and this is one of the many reasons we try to remove the Foley 7 d after BMU *(36)*. In our series, we had one patient representing 5% of the series, who developed urosepsis immediately after surgery, and required admission to the hospital for intravenous antibiotics *(1)*.

2.5. Erectile Dysfunction (ED)

This is not a commonly reported complication after ventral BMU for bulbar urethral strictures. Its absence is one of the major advantages of the ventral buccal mucosal technique *(1)*. The exception to this finding was published by Coursey et al., who reported in a questionnaire based evaluation of ED that 19% and 27% of patients reported worse erection after BMU and AU, respectively. The significance of this is unclear, because 27% of patients after a control operation (circumcision) reported worse erections too *(37)*.

2.6. Postvoid Dribbling

Minimal dribbling of a small amount of postvoid urine is the most common patient complaint after buccal mucosal urethroplasty. Although notable to the patient, it is not considered a "complication" per se and many centers do not report it as such. When reported, it is present in 8–21% *(24)*.

Andrich et al. *(6)* reported a rate of 69% of dribbling after two-stage urethroplasty, but the symptom was bothersome in 8% of patients. When comparing ventral onlay to dorsal onlay, Andrich noted dribbling in 100% of the patients, but it was bothersome in only 21% of ventral onlay patients and 17% of dorsal onlay patients.

Although the true cause of post void dribbling in urethral stricture patients is unknown *(38)*, we believe that it is a result of decreased urethral elasticity, either due to the original stricture or its surgical repair. During voiding, the normal urethra balloons outward, and at the end of voiding the elastic fibers in the urethra cause it to collapse down and naturally empty itself of urine. This process is disrupted by the urethral scarring present in all urethral stricture patients. Further, injury to periurethral nerve fibers supplying the bulbospongiosus muscle may also play a role in this symptom *(39)*. These same mechanism may also result in semen sequestration *(6,40)*.

2.7. Urethral Sacculation

Urethral sacculation is sometimes present after BMU, but only rarely is associating with complications such a bothersome post void dribbling, or is large enough to be named a urethrocele or diverticuli *(4,26,31)*. It is less common after dorsally placed BMU *(33)*. Elliot et al. emphasized the importance of proper tailoring of ventrally-placed buccal graft in avoiding this complication. Further, proper closure of the adventitia of the corpora spongiosum over the graft will provide backing and further decrease this complication *(4)*.

2.8. Other Uncommon Complications

Sporadic complications have been reported, usually in patients with long penile or pan-urethral strictures. They include: graft loss *(27)*, anastomotic breakdown *(27)*, penile skin necrosis *(15,41)* and penile cordee or deformity. Of note, these complications are usually much less frequent after BMU than fasciocutaneous urethroplasty *(21,27)*.

2.9. Oral Complications

Buccal mucosal grafts are most commonly harvested from the inner cheek. Cheek harvest is reported to have less early and late complications than lip harvesting *(34)*. Early complications include pain and discomfort, which usually disappears or decrease to mild in 90% of cases in 5–7 d, self-limited oral numbness (30–65%), and mouth tightness (50–75%) which usually disappears by 6 months *(42,43)*.

Late complications include persistent oral numbness (2–26%) or persistent oral tightness in (9–32%) after 6–20 mo of surgery *(5,21)*. Change in salivation occurred in 1–11% *(1,21,44)*. Several authors reported no donor site complications *(20,45,46)*. Others reported only mild temporary complications such as mouth dryness, parasthesia and pain which all resolved with time *(21,23,28,31,47,48)*. Rare complications include intraoral bleeding, hematoma, infection, cheek granuloma and Stensen's duct damage *(1,5,49)*.

Lip contracture is a devastating complication reported in 3–5 % of patients after lip graft harvest *(23,44,50)*. It is avoided, of course, by avoiding the harvest of graft material from the lip. In expert hands, it can be rare, as Barbagli reported only two cases among 650 BMU done at his center (0.3%). We avoid using lip grafts and Barbagli reports using them only in extreme circumstances, such as inability to open the mouth sufficiently to harvest a cheek graft, or previous bilateral cheek grafts *(49)*.

Some have reported that leaving the cheek wound open and allowing it to heal by secondary intention decreases pain and tightness postoperatively *(44)*. However, others have not found pain and tightness to be problematic after closure of the buccal graft site, and we have had troublesome bleeding in patients that were left open, so we tend to close our buccal wounds primarily with 3–O chromic gut suture.

3. Fasciocutaneous Urethroplasty Complications

A major advance in treatment of anterior urethral stricture came in 1953, when Pressman and Greenfield described the use of full thickness skin graft as an onlay patch *(51,51)*. Fasciocutaneous flaps are a reliable urethral substitute and are particularly useful in long, recurrent, or poorly vascularized strictures. They have been reported to have comparable long term results to BMU *(41)*. The best fasciocutaneous onlay flaps are hairless, flexible, and well vascularized as in the distal penile skin or preputial skin *(52)*. Some authors advocate the use of scrotal skin but we avoid it due to the potential for complications from intraurethral hair growth after surgery.

The complications of fasciocutaneous patch are variable (**Tables 19.2** and **19.3**) and depend on several factors, including but not limited to position of patch (dorsal vs. ventral *[38]*), shape of patch (tubularized vs. onlay *[53]*), length of patch *(53)*, and donor site (preputial/penile skin vs. scrotal skin *[53]*).

The complications rate of fasciocutaneous onlay urethroplasty is reported between 3% and 56% *(19)*. Most published papers are not explicit about the details of complications, so it is difficult to understand the details of this wide range of reported complications. Further, reported complications are not stratified according to factors such as stricture length or patient age, and most of these studies were based on nonhomogeneous series of cases that may include strictures of different etiologies and locations, that were treated by more than one surgeon using different techniques with relatively short follow up, and using varying criteria for success and failure *(54)*.

3.1. Recurrent Stricture

Recurrent stricture after initial fasciocutaneous urethroplasty is the most common complication for this type of surgery, and it is reported in 5–56% of cases *(38)*. Failure occurs more often in cases where the vascular supply of the flap is compromised, or extensive fibrosis surrounds the graft *(52,55)*. It usually presents at the proximal or distal anastomosis *(16,56)*. Generally, tube flaps like tube grafts have higher re-stricture rate than onlay patch *(55)*. We avoid tube grafts whenever possible.

Recurrent strictures can be treated with dilation, DVIU, or repeat urethroplasty (including anastomotic urethroplasty for short segments, primary buccal mucosa graft if adequate graft bed is present, or two-stage Johanson urethroplasty with or without buccal grafts placed in the first stage *[16,56]*). Our preferred treatment of recurrent stricture after any urethroplasty is an initial DVIU, followed by open urethroplasty only if the patient recurs after salvage DVIU.

Few authors have reported their long-term results with fasciocutaneous urethroplasty *(53)*. Mundy in 1995 reported an annual restricture rate of 5% in 73 patients with 10 years' follow-up. Restricture after onlay patch was 40% (preputial/penile vs. scrotal skin patch was 31% and 62%, respectively), and in tube urethroplasty was 56% (preputial/penile vs. scrotal skin was 38%, and 89%, respectively). Mundy attributed the difference in restricture rate among these subgroups to several factors including patient's age/health, length of compromised urethra and previous surgeries *(53)*. In 2003 Andrich et al. reported restructure in 58% of 84 patients after 15 years' follow-up *(30)*.

McAninch and Morey in 1998 reported a 21% (14/66 patients) recurrence rate with mean follow up of 41 mo, after using penile circular fasciocutaneous flap in one stage for reconstruction of anterior urethral stricture. The average stricture length was 9 cm. All of these patients but two have been treated successfully with repeat urethroplasty for long stricture, and a single DVIU or dilation for shorter one *(56)*. Dubey et al. compared the restricture rate between dorsal fasciocutaneous flaps (17%) and ventral fasciocutaneous flaps (23%), with follow up times of 22 and 38 months respectively *(41)*. Barbagli et al. initially reported a 5% restricture rate in 20 patients with dorsally positioned fasciocutaneous grafts after an intermediate follow up time of 46 months, but this number ballooned to 27% after 71 months of follow-up *(16)*.

3.2. Urethral Diverticulum

Urethral diverticuli are reported between 2% and 15% of the time after fasciocutaneous onlay urethroplasty *(30,56)* and usually occur either because of redundancy in the patch or poor surrounding tissue support in ventrally positioned patches. Initial ballooning of the tissue can lead to progressive weakening of the patch, sacculation and diverticulum formation *(57)*. Urethral diverticuli often require manual perineal expression to expel residual urine and may result in recurrent urinary tract infections if urinary stasis and pooling is extreme *(57)*. Urethrocele formation has not been reported in dorsal fasciocutaneous graft but Bhandari et al. *(57)* reported it 28.5% of patients who got ventrally placed flaps. McAninch and Morey *(56)* suggest that this complication can be largely avoided by careful tailoring of the flap, and report an incidence closer to 2% in their patients.

3.3. Postvoid Dribbling

Postvoid dribbling is likely underreported in the literature, as many authors do not consider it as a real complication, or even attempt to question their patients about it. The reported rate is 10–50% *(30,38)* It is possible that urethral sacculations increase the incidence of dribbling, especially after ventral onlay *(30,57)*. We advocate that all patients should be warned about this complication before surgery, as surgery seems to cause or unmask it clinically in a certain percentage. It is significantly less common with dorsal patching *(19,41)*. We reported a 50% incidence of post-void dribbling in 10 patients treated with fasciocutaneous onlay ventral flaps *(1)*.

3.4. Ejaculatory Dysfunction

Ejaculatory failure after augmented urethroplasty can be a direct consequence of urethrocele formation *(57)*, or neuromuscular injury to the ejaculatory apparatus (particularly the bulbospongiosus muscle, which is often divided during urethroplasty). Bhandari et al. in 2001 reported 19% ejaculation dysfunction in 21 ventrally placed flaps, 3 patients had scanty ejaculation, and 1 patient had anejaculation. However, no such complication has been reported in series reporting dorsal onlay flaps *(19,57)*.

3.5. Urinary Extravasation

Temporary urinary extravasation is a common complication, which can lead to formation of urethrocutaneous fistula if it does not resolve with prolonged urethral catheter drainage. It is reported at rates from 10% to 20%, and of course the rate will vary depending on when the urethral catheter is removed *(57)*. It usually resolves after leaving a Foley catheter for further drainage *(58)*.

3.6. Urethrocutaneous Fistula

Fistula can happen in up to 20% of cases of fasciocutaneous onlay urethroplasty *(1,30)*. Fistula formation is thought to be less common if extra layers of tissue can be interposed over the suture line, such as dartos or tunica vaginalis fascia, and is thought to be resultant from necrosis of the skin, the graft, or the intervening tissue *(55)*. It is significantly less common in dorsal compared to ventral patch urethroplasty *(57)*. Treatment is excision and multilayer fistula closure, usually after 3 to 6 mo. Strictures distal to the fistula must be aggressively looked-for and treated.

3.7. Erectile Dysfunction/Diminished Penile Sensation

This complication is not commonly reported or is under-reported in the literature probably due to not questioning the patient specifically about erectile function *(41)*. Few authors addressed this complication specifically *(30,41,59)*. Although the specific causes are unknown, extensive dissection of the penis and the urethra is thought to injures the fine distal branches of the penile nerves that run along the dorsal corpora cavernosa, then diverge and fan out all along the penis *(60)*. This leads to diminished penile sensation and/or dysfunctional erection. Dubey et al. *(41)* reported 14% diminished penile sensation after flap fasciocutaneous urethroplasty. However, Coursey et al. used a validated male sexual performance questionnaire in 174 patients who underwent anterior urethroplasty, of whom 44 patients had flap fasciocutaneous urethroplasty, and compared them to other group of patients who underwent circumcision. In their report, the patients who underwent anterior urethro-plasty including penile skin one didn't have more impaired sexual function than those undergone circumcision, and the alterations in penile appearance (length and/or angle) and sexual performance were transient *(37)*. Mundy reported temporary ED after fasciocutaneous urethroplasty in 33% of patients, while persistent ED was reported in only 1% of patients *(59)*.

3.8. Penile Skin Necrosis

This complication has been reported in 0–15% of patients after fasciocutaneous urethroplasty using penile skin *(56)*. Penile skin necrosis usually occurs in the penile skin proximal to the flap because during harvest of the flap, the skin vascular supply via the subdermal plexus was disturbed *(56)*. Although this complication usually heals spontaneously in most cases *(41)*, it can result in a temporarily alarming appearance of the penis for both patient and doctor.

4. Anterior Anastomotic Urethroplasty Complications

Anastomotic urethroplasty is still the gold standard technique for short urethral stricture (although we and others tend to perform BMU for increasingly short strictures because it works better and has less complications). Anastomotic urethroplasty is usually a safe, short procedure with minimal morbidity (**Tables 19.4** and **19.5**). In reviewing the anterior anastomotic literature, we found that most series has combined anterior and posterior anastomotic urethroplasty this made it difficult to differentiate where did the reported complications occur.

4.1. Acute Urinary Extravasation

Urinary extravasation after anastomotic urethroplasty is reported in 1–4% of patients *(1,3)*. It is usually successfully treated with 1–2 weeks of Foley catheter insertion *(1,3)*.

4.2. Postvoid Dribbling

Postvoid dribbling of (usually) a minor amount of urine is reported in 17% of cases, and has similar

TABLE 19.4. Complication rate after anterior anastomotic urethroplasty.

Reference	n	Mean follow up (months)	Early compli- cations (%)	Late compli- cations (%)	Recur- rence rate (%)	All compli- cations (%)
Lindell et al. (91)	49	48	-	10	4	-
Schlossberg (15)	130	45	-	-	2	8
Santucci et al. (3)	168	70	6	-	5	-
Al-Qudah and Santucci (1)	24	26	25	54	8	-

TABLE 19.5. Specific complications of anterior anastomotic urethroplasty.

Complication	Santucci et al. (3) (%)	Al-Qudah and Santucci (1) (%)
Thigh numbness	2	0
Small wound dehiscence	1	0
Scrotal hematoma	<1	0
Erectile dysfunction	<1	17
Catheter dislodgment	<1	9
Wound infection	<1	0

etiology to postvoid dribbling after buccal or fasciocutaneous urethroplasty (discussed previously in the chapter). It is usually a minor symptom with minimal bother to the patient (1).

4.3. Erectile Dysfunction

ED is found between 1–17% of patients (1). Kessler et al. evaluated patient satisfaction with outcomes of urethral stricture surgery in 333 patients by a questionnaire. He reported that overall satisfaction with sexual function post operatively was 74%, 72%, and 97% for anastomotic, fasciocutaneous, and graft urethroplasty, respectively (61).

4.4. Chordee

This complication is usually reported when a urethral stricture longer than 2–3 cm is treated with anastomotic urethroplasty (1,62). It is seen in <5 % of patients (1). It is less common now with the trend to use BMU for strictures longer than 1.5 cm. Kessler et al. (61) evaluated patient satisfaction with outcomes of urethral stricture surgery in 333 patients by a questionnaire. He reported penile shortening post operatively in 30%, 11%, and 0% for anastomotic, fasciocutaneous, and graft urethroplasty, respectively.

4.5. Recurrence

Recurrence after anastomotic urethroplasty is less than 10% in most recent series (3,11,62). Andrich et al. reported long-term follow up after anastomotic urethroplasty, including posterior urethral stricture caused by pelvic fractures. They report a recurrence rate of 12% after 5 yr of follow-up, which stabilize and increase only to 14% after 15 yr of follow up (30). Most of these recurrences (50–100%) seem to be successfully treated with a single DVIU (1,62); however, longitudinal long-term follow-up on the fate of these patients has not yet been published.

In our review of 168 anastomotic urethroplasty patients, recurrence occurred in 8 (5%) patients. Five of eight were treated with DVIU, and three required repeated urethroplasty. However, all the patients who required repeated urethroplasty had complicating factors (one with catheter dislodgment post operatively, the second had preoperative urethrocutaneous fistula and the third had radiation therapy [3]).

Martinez-Pineiro et al. (13) reported in a review of 150 anastomotic urethroplasty patients (including 56 posterior urethral distraction injuries) that recurrence rates are dependant on: primary versus secondary repair, etiology, length, and location of the stricture. Several other reports emphasized the importance of these factors (12,63–65).

Recently, Morey and Kizer presented a cohort of 22 proximal bulbar urethral strictures treated by anastomotic urethroplasty, and compared those patients with short strictures (<2.5 cm) to those with longer strictures (2.6–5.0 cm). Success rates in both groups were 92% without any difference in sexual outcomes. Surprisingly chordee was reported in 44% of the short stricture group and 0 % of the long stricture group (66). However, we as many others prefer to treat these patients with

BMU, and its difficult to know what to make of these data since they so strongly diverge from the expected outcome.

4.6. Urinary Tract Infection

UTI is reported in 2–4% of patients after urethroplasty. It may include simple UTI or febrile UTI (complicated by epididymitis, pyelonephritis or sepsis *[1,11]*). We emphasize the importance of removing Foley catheters as early as possible to decrease these rates, and tend to keep patients on antibiotics during the entire catheterization period *(1,36)*.

5. Posterior Urethroplasty Complications

Posterior urethral strictures most commonly result from urethral distraction injury associated with pelvic fractures. However, rarely they can be caused by perineal straddle injury which involves the bulbomembranous junction, iatrogenic injuries (TURP, radical prostatectomy, radiation therapy *[67,68]*), and gonococcal urethritis *(67)*. Traumatic disruption of the posterior urethra occurs in 3–25% of patients with pelvic fractures *(68)*. The most common site of distraction injury is the bulbomembranous junction (70%) and less commonly the prostatomembranous junction (30% *[69]*).

Surgical repair of distraction urethral injury remains one of the most technically difficult problems in urology *(70)*. Immediate surgical repair

of posterior urethral injury has been abandoned because of high rates of postoperative ED and incontinence, at 56% and 21% respectively *(71)*. Delayed primary urethral repair, usually at least 3 months after the trauma using one stage perineal approach, remains the recommended approach. 68 Only a minority of cases requires the combined abdominoperineal approach *(69)*. The lifelong success rate of delayed repair is more than 90%, without the need for complementary urethrotomy or urethral dilation *(72)*. Treatment of posterior urethral injuries can be complicated by recurrent stricture formation *(68)*, stress urinary incontinence *(73,74)*, ED *(75)*, and position related injuries (**Table 19.6 *[76]***).

5.1. Failure of Repair

The current approach for posterior urethral distraction injury relies on early catheter realignment of the urethra or, failing that, insertion of a suprapubic tube followed by delayed urethroplasty at least 3 mo later. Stricture formation after early urethral realignment over a catheter is reported in 38–69%, which means that a significant portion of these patients never develop a urethral stricture *(68)*. Koraitim, in a personal series of 100 patients combined with review of 771 patients from previous reports, found that early realignment is associated with only a 53% stricture rate *(77)*. Mouraviev et al. *(73)* reported a mean stricture rate of 47% in a review of personal series of 57 patients and 7 other previous published reports encompassing hundreds

TABLE 19.6. Complications after posterior urethroplasty for posterior urethral distraction injury

Reference	n	Approach	Mean follow up (months)	Early complications (%)	Late complications (%)	Recurrence rate (%)
Mundy *(74)*	82	Perineal[a]	60	Urgency 66 Stress Incontinence 37 Impotence 26	Impotence 7[b]	12
Morey and McAninch *(70)*	52	Perineal and transpubic	>12 mo	-	-	11
Flynn *(2)*	109	Perineal	64	-	-	5
Al-Qudah and Santucci *(1)*	9	Perineal	26	56	44	0

[a] Procedures including inferior pubectomy and supra-corporal re-routing of urethra.
[b] Permanent erectile dysfunction.

more other patients. Failure to perform early cath-eter realignment results in stricture with a reported rate of 98–100% *(68,73)*. Once stricture has devel-oped, delayed anastomotic urethroplasty is highly successful, with a reported failure rate of less than 13% at experienced centers *(54,74)*.

Several authors looked into the reasons for failure repair after anastomotic urethroplasty. Koraitim *(54)*, in an interesting paper addressed the subject of failed posterior urethroplasty, found a restric-ture rate of 8% after anastomotic urethroplasty in 130 patients who undergone 145 procedures. He suggested three factors contributing to the failed repair, including inadequate lateral fixation of prostatic mucosa (six patients), failure to achieve a tension free anastomosis (two patients), and incomplete excision of the surrounding scar tissue (three patients). Morey and McAninch stressed that careful and complete excision of scar tissue is the single most important factor for achieving successful repair after posterior urethral recon-struction *(70)*. Mundy *(74)* suggested a tendency to restricture with advancing of age, presumably the result of deterioration of retrograde blood flow in the urethra with age, which is critical for ure-thral healing. Berger et al. *(78)* found that 27% of restrictures occurred due to non-tension free anas-tomosis, which in his opinion lead to ischemia, scar formation, and restricture.

Endoscopic treatment of recurrent stricture by DVIU appears to be highly successful as the under-lining surrounding scar tissue is already excised during urethroplasty *(54)*. Morey and McAninch *(70)* reported 88% success rate with DVIU. Netto et al. *(79)* reported 72% success rate with DVIU for recurrent strictures after anastomotic prostatomem-branous urethroplasty, which confirms the validity of this approach.

5.2. Erectile Dysfunction

Impairment of male sexual function after distrac-tion urethral injury is well known. The reported incidence varies from 3% to 50% *(80)*. Mouraviev et al. *(73)* analyzed 8 papers and combining them with their own series of 96 patients, they found a mean ED rate of 24% (range 14–42%) after (suc-cessful) early realignment, and mean 46% (range 42–50%) after delayed anastomotic urethroplasty. These differences are likely due to the fact that

patients who are cured by early realignment alone likely have less serious urethral distraction injuries than those who ultimately require open urethro-plasty. Koraitim, in a review of personal series of 100 patients combined with 771 patients from previous reports, found a 36% ED rate after early realignment and 19% after delayed repair *(68)*. ED is usually related to the original pelvic fracture urethral injury and rarely to the urethroplasty itself *(75)*. The proposed mechanism appears to be direct damage of penile vasculature and/or nerve supply at the original injury *(80)*. ED as a direct conse-quence of surgery still a possibility and has been reported in about 3% *(81)*. Only one report showed a greater incidence of ED (21%) as a direct result of anastomotic urethroplasty, but it was attributable to a learning curve in the surgeon experience because of unnecessary extensive retropubic dissection *(75)*. However, delayed recovery of sexual func-tion after anastomotic urethroplasty is a described phenomenon, and some authors observed recovery of erectile function after urethroplasty surgery *(72)*. Koraitim reported 66% (29/44 patients) regaining of potency after successful anastomotic urethro-plasty *(72)*. A similar finding reported by Morey and McAninch *(70)* as potency increased from 46% to 62% in their patients after anastomotic ure-throplasty. Dhabuwala et al. *(80)* noted that potency increased from 28% before urethroplasty to 44% after anastomotic urethroplasty. This phenomenon may be partly attributed to the delayed recovery of potency *(70,72)* and perhaps partly attributable to the improvement of patient morale after resump-tion of urethral voiding, after being dependent on a suprapubic catheter for several months, as suggested by Koraitim *(72)*. It is important in evaluating these patients to know whether the ED is caused by psychological, vascular, or neurogenic dysfunction. All patients may benefit from PDE5 inhibitors; however, the patients with a psycho-genic etiology will fare best with this therapy. Patients who do not respond should be evaluated with color Duplex ultrasound with intracavernosal injection, and nocturnal penile tumescence studies. Patients with normal vascular function with Duplex are diagnosed with neurogenic ED and have the choice of intracavernosal injection of prostaglandin E1, vacuum device, or penile prosthesis as treat-ment options, if oral agents fail. Patients who have abnormal vascular duplex will need arteriography to identify the extent and location of vascular damage. Revascularization is an additional option in this group *(82–84)*.

5.3. Incontinence

Stress urinary incontinence as a direct result of urethral injury itself has been reported in 0–37% depending on the initial management after urethral injury *(73)*. Koraitim reports a 5% incidence of incontinence after early realignment and 4% after delayed repair *(68)*. Mouraviev et al. reviewed seven papers in addition to their own patients and found a mean incontinence rate of 4% (range 0–18%) after early urethral realignment, and a mean of 18% (range 10–25%) after delayed repair (the delayed repair numbers were obtained by including 1 previous paper in addition to their own series *[73]*). Elliott and Barrett in a series of 57 patients who had undergone primary endoscopic urethral realignment with mean follow up of 10.5 yr, found a 4% rate of mild stress incontinence. 68 Mundy reported a 37% of stress urinary incontinence at 5 yr of follow-up with delayed anastomotic urethroplasty *(74)*. However Morey and McAninch had a low incontinence rate of 5% in 82 patients treated by delayed transperineal urethroplasty *(70)*. Many experts believe that urinary incontinence after distraction urethral injury is exclusively a result of primary injury rather than the anastomotic urethral repair *(73,74)*. Moreover, incontinence as a direct result of anastomotic urethroplasty has not often been reported as a complication of this type of surgery *(72)*. Many authors reported 0% incontinence rate as a direct result of the transperineal or perineo-abdominal anastomotic urethroplasty itself *(72)*. Koraitim in a series of 155 patients who underwent transperineal urethroplasty (115 patients) and perineo-abdominal repair (40 patients) has not had any case of urinary incontinence as a direct result of anastomotic urethroplasty *(72)*. Pratap et al. *(75)* had the same observation, as none of their patients had urinary incontinence as a direct result of perineo-abdominal anastomotic urethroplasty.

The proposed mechanism of injury in posterior urethral distraction injury has the potential to involve the urethral sphincter mechanism in addition to the bladder neck mechanism *(72)*. However, perhaps 8–10 of these injuries occur distal to the sphincter *(73)* and of the ones that

don't, some experts suggest that continence is primarily dependent on the competence of the bladder neck *(72)*. Concomitant injury to the bladder neck should worsen the continence status of these patients, and accordingly, Pratap et al. *(75)* found 19% (2/21 patients) urinary incontinence in patients with severe bladder neck injury at the time of primary injury. Repair of the injured bladder neck might help. Koraitim reported 80% (4/5 patients) achieved satisfactory continence after being previously completely incontinent after with bladder neck injury, after he repaired the bladder neck *(72)*. Finally, many authors *(67,85)* believe that even if the urethral sphincteric mechanism is partially compromised by trauma, nerve damage, or subsequent surgery, it may still function satisfactorily to achieve satisfactory continence.

5.4. Positioning-Related Complications

Positioning-related complications, usually but not exclusively involving the extremities, of the lower extremities can jeopardize the outcome of procedures requiring high lithotomy position, especially after reconstruction of complex urethral injuries *(76)* The most common complications are superficial peroneal nerve neuropraxia, rhabdomyolysis, and the lower extremity compartmental syndrome *(76)*. Other less-reported complications are temporary upper-extremity neuropathy *(1,32)* lower- extremity neuropathy (sciatic, femoral, and/or lateral femoral cutaneous nerve), pulmonary embolism, deep venous thrombosis, severe lower back pain, and trochanteric bursitis *(3,32,86,87)*. Previously, a high rate of position related complication was reported in 20% to 50% of cases *(76,88)*. However, recently the reported percentage of this complication is less than 3% due to shortening of the surgical time less than 5 h and meticulous protocols of patient protection during this type of surgery *(31,62,67)*. Anema et al. in a review of 185 patients who had extended lithotomy position with a mean position time of 287 min (4.7 h) found that length of stricture, duration of surgery, and lithotomy position are all statistically significant risk factors *(76)*. However, Angermeier et al. *(89)* demonstrated the safety of exaggerated lithotomy position when carefully applied in less than 5 h of surgical time, as only 1.7%, 2.3%, and 15.8% of the

177 patients, has had severe back pain, deep venous thrombosis and transient numbness /parasthesia of the lower extremities respectively. Anema et al. *(76)* confirmed the same observation, as only 2% (4/185) of patients has had severe complications which needed prolonged hospitalization and/or additional outpatient treatment. With meticulous positioning, we have a rate of temporary positioning complications that is lower than 2%, and a rate of permanent positioning complications approaching 0%. We use a gel-padded bean bag, sequential compression devices, compression stockings, arm padding, and keep surgical time as short as possible *(1)*. Anema et al. *(76)* suggested that elements of the surgical procedure that can be done with the patient in supine position, such as buccal mucosa graft harvesting, should be completed in supine position then reposition patient in high lithotomy position.

Appendix

Preferred Instruments and Suture of RA Santucci

Specialty Instruments

8 inch Debakey needle driver
7 inch serrated curve fine Metzenbaum scissors (Sontec, Maxicut, Englewood, CO)
Andrews suction tip
Bougies a boule
7.75 inch fine tipped Debakey forceps × 2
3.5 inch Bishop Harmon forceps
6.75 inch serrated straight Mayo scissors (Sontec Maxicut, Englewood, CO)
40 mm eye calipers
Jordan retractor system (C&S Surgical, Slidell, LA) for Bookwalter retractor system (Codman, Raynam, MA)

General Instruments

19F Rigid cystoscope
22F Red Robinson catheter
Bipolar and monopolar cautery
0.5% bupivacaine (Marcaine/Sensorcaine)

Suture

5-0 and 6-0 PDS (glycolic acid) or Maxon (poly-dioxanone)
General sutures 2-0, 3-0, 4-0 Vicryl (polyglycolic acid and 2-0 chromic gut on a SH needle.

References

1. Al-Qudah HS, Santuci RA (2005) Extended complications of urethroplasty. Int Braz J Urol 31:315
2. Flynn BJ, Delvecchio FC, Webster GD (2002) Perineal repair of posterior urethral stricture and defect: Experience in 79 cases in the last 5-years. J Urol 167
3. Santucci RA, Mario LA, McAninch JW (2002) Anastomotic urethroplasty for bulbar urethral stricture: analysis of 168 patients. J Urol 167:1715
4. Elliott SP, Metro MJ, McAninch JW (2003) Long-term followup of the ventrally placed buccal mucosa onlay graft in bulbar urethral reconstruction. J Urol 169:1754
5. Pansadoro V, Emiliozzi P, Gaffi M, et al. (2003) Buccal mucosa urethroplasty in the treatment of bulbar urethral strictures. Urology 61:1008
6. Andrich DE, Leach CJ, Mundy AR (2001) The Barbagli procedure gives the best results for patch urethroplasty of the bulbar urethra. BJU Int 88:385
7. Heyns CF, Steenkamp JW, De Kock ML et al. (1998) Treatment of male urethral strictures: is repeated dilation or internal urethrotomy useful? J Urol 160:356
8. Pansadoro V, Emiliozzi P (1996) Internal urethrotomy in the management of anterior urethral strictures: long-term followup. J Urol 156:73
9. Greenwell TJ, Castle C, Andrich DE et al. (2004) Repeat urethrotomy and dilation for the treatment of urethral stricture are neither clinically effective nor cost-effective. J Urol 172:275
10. Heyns CF, S. J., De Kock ML,Whitaker P (1998) Treatment of male urethral strictures: is repeated dilation or internal urethrotomy useful? J Urol 160:356
11. Jakse G, Marberger, H (1986) Excisional repair of urethral stricture. Follow-up of 90 patients. Urology 27:233
12. Jezior JR, Schlossberg SM (2002) Excision and primary anastomosis for anterior urethral stricture. Urol Clin North Am 29:373–380
13. Martinez-Pineiro JA, Carcamo P, Garcia Matres MJ, et al. (1997) Excision and anastomotic repair for urethral stricture disease: experience with 150 cases. Eur Urol 32:433
14. Azoury BS, Freiha FS (1976) Excision of urethral stricture and end to end anastomosis. Urology 8:138
15. Schlossberg SM (2000) Anastomotic urethral reconstruction. Presented at the American Urologic Association postgraduate course, Atlanta, Georgia
16. Barbagli G, G. G., Palminteri E, Lazzeri M. (2006) Anastomotic fibrous ring as cause of stricture recurrence after bulbar onlay graft urethroplasty. J Urol 176:614

17. Wessells H, McAninch JW (1996) Use of free grafts in urethral stricture reconstruction. J Urol 155

18. Andrich DE, Mundy AR (2001) Substitution urethroplasty with buccal mucosal-free grafts. J Urol 165

19. Barbagli G, Selli C, Tosto A et al. (1996) Dorsal free graft urethroplasty. J Urol 155:123

20. Palminteri E, Lazzeri M, Guazzoni G, Turini D, Barbagli G (2002) New 2-stage buccal mucosal graft urethroplasty. J Urol 167:130

21. Dubey D, Kumar A., Mandhani A, Srivastava A, Kapoor R, Bhandari M (2005) Buccal mucosal urethroplasty: a versatile technique for all urethral segments. BJU Int. 95:625–629

22. Gupta NP, A. M., Dogra PN, Tandon S (2004) Dorsal buccal mucosal graft urethroplasty by a ventral sagittal urethrotomy and minimal-access perineal approach for anterior urethral stricture. BJU Int 93:1287

23. Fichtner J, Filipas D, Fisch M, et al. (2004) Long-term outcome of ventral buccal mucosa onlay graft urethroplasty for urethral stricture repair. Urology 64:648

24. Zinman L (2003) The use of buccal mucosal graft onlay in urethral reconstruction. Am J Urol Rev 1:45

25. el-Kasaby AW, Fath-Alla M, Noweir AM, el-Halaby MR, Zakaria W, el-Beialy MH (1993) The use of buccal mucosa patch graft in the management of anterior urethral strictures. J Urol 149:276–278

26. Barbagli G, Palminteri E, Guazzoni G, et al. (2005) Bulbar urethroplasty using buccal mucosa grafts placed on the ventral, dorsal or lateral surface of the urethra: are results affected by the surgical technique? J Urol 174:955

27. Dubey D, S. A., Srivastava A, Mandhani A, Kapoor R, Kumar A (2005) Buccal mucosal urethroplasty for balanitis xerotica obliterans related urethral strictures: the outcome of 1 and 2-stage techniques. J Urol 173:463

28. Heinke T, Gerharz EW, Bonfig R, et al. (2003) Ventral onlay urethroplasty using buccal mucosa for complex stricture repair. Urology 61:1004

29. Elliott SP, Metro MJ, McAninch JW (2002) Long-term follow-up of the ventrally placed buccal mucosa onlay graft in bulbar urethral reconstruction. J Urol 167

30. Andrich DE, Dunglison N, Greenwell TJ, et al. (2003) The long-term results of urethroplasty. J Urol 170:90

31. Kane CJ, Tarman GJ, Summerton DJ, et al. (2002) Multi-institutional experience with buccal mucosa onlay urethroplasty for bulbar urethral reconstruction. J Urol 167:1314

32. Kellner DS, Fracchia JA, Armenakas NA (2004) Ventral onlay buccal mucosal grafts for anterior urethral strictures: long-term followup. J Urol 171:726

33. Barbagli G, P. E., Guazzoni G, Montorsi F, Turini D, Lazzeri M. (2005) Bulbar urethroplasty using buccal mucosa grafts placed on the ventral, dorsal or lateral surface of the urethra: are results affected by the surgical technique? J Urol 174:955

34. Bhargava S, C. C. (2004) Buccal mucosal urethroplasty: is it the new gold standard? BJU Int 93:1191

35. Venn SN, Mundy AR (1998) Early experience with the use of buccal mucosa for substitution urethroplasty. Br J Urol 81:738

36. Al-Qudah HS, C. A., Santucci RA. (2005) Early catheter removal after anterior anastomotic (3 days) and ventral buccal mucosal onlay (7 days) urethroplasty. Int Brazil J Urol 31:459

37. Coursey JW, Morey AF, McAninch JW et al.(2001) Erectile function after anterior urethroplasty. J Urol 166:2273

38. Barbagli G, Selli C, di Cello V, et al. (1996) A one-stage dorsal free-graft urethroplasty for bulbar urethral strictures. Br J Urol 78:929

39. Yucel S, B. L (2003) Neuroanatomy of the male urethra and perineum. BJU Int 92:624

40. Andrich DE, Mundy AR (2000) Urethral strictures and their surgical treatment. BJU Int 86:571

41. Dubey D, Kumar A, Bansal P, Srivastava A, Kapoor R, Mandhani A, Bhandari M. (2003) Substitution urethroplasty for anterior urethral strictures: a critical appraisal of various techniques. BJU Int 91:215–218

42. Dublin N, Stewart LH (2004) Oral complications after buccal mucosal graft harvest for urethroplasty. BJU Int 94:867–869

43. Raber M, Naspro R, Scapaticci E, Salonia A, Scattoni V, Mazzoccoli B, Guazzoni G, Rigatti P, Montorsi F (2005) Dorsal onlay graft urethroplasty using penile skin or buccal mucosa for repair of bulbar urethral stricture: results of a prospective single center study. Eur Urol 48:1013–1017

44. Wood DN, Allen SE, Andrich DE, Greenwell TJ, Mundy AR. (2004) The morbidity of buccal mucosal graft harvest for urethroplasty and the effect of nonclosure of the graft harvest site on postoperative pain. J Urol 172:580–583

45. Morey AF, McAninch JW (1996) Technique of harvesting buccal mucosa for urethral reconstruction. J Urol 155:1696

46. Eppley BL, Keating M, Rink R. (1997) A buccal mucosal harvesting technique for urethral reconstruction. J Urol 157:1268–1270

47. Kamp S, Knoll T, Osman M, Hacker A, Michel MS, Alken P. (2005) Donor-site morbidity in buccal mucosa urethroplasty: lower lip or inner cheek? BJU Int 96:619–623

48. Tolstunov L, Pogrel MA, McAninch JW (1997) Intraoral morbidity following free buccal mucosal graft harvesting for urethroplasty. Oral Surg Oral Med Oral Pathol Oral Radiol Endod 84:480–482

49. Barbagli G (2004) When and how to use buccal mucosa grafts in penile and bulbar urethroplasty. Minerva Urol Nefrol 56:189

50. Meneghini A, Cacciola A, Cavarretta L, et al. (2001) Bulbar urethral stricture repair with buccal mucosa graft urethroplasty. Eur Urol 39:264

51. Pressman D, G. D. (1953) Reconstruction of the. perineal urethra with a free full thickness skin graft from the prepuce. J Urol 69:677

52. Jordan GH, Schlossberg SM (2002) Surgery of the penis and urethra, in Walsh P Retik AB, Vaughan ED, et al. (eds) Campbell's urology (ed 8). Philadelphia, Saunders, pp 3886–3954

53. Mundy AR (1995) The long-term results of skin inlay urethroplasty. Br J Urol 75:59

54. Koraitim M (2003) Failed posterior urethroplasty: lessons learned. Urology 62:719

55. Greenwell TJ, Venn SN, Mundy AR (1999) Changing practice in anterior urethroplasty. BJU Int 83:631

56. McAninch JW, Morey AF (1998) Penile circular fasciocutaneous skin flap in 1-stage reconstruction of complex anterior urethral strictures. J Urol 159:1209

57. Bhandari M, Dubey D, Verma BS (2001) Dorsal or ventral placement of the preputial/penile skin onlay flap for anterior urethral strictures: does it make a difference? BJU Int 88:39

58. Morey AF, Tran LK, Zinman LM (2000) Q-flap reconstruction of panurethral strictures. BJU Int 86:1039

59. Mundy AR (1993) Results and complications of urethroplasty and its future. Br J Urol 71:322

60. Baskin LS, Erol A, Li YW, Cunha GR (1998) Anatomical studies of hypospadias. J Urol 160: 1108–1115

61. Kessler TM, Fisch M, Heitz M, Olianas R, Schreiter F.(2002) Patient satisfaction with the outcome of surgery for urethral stricture. J Urol 167:2507–2511

62. Micheli E, Ranieri A, Peracchia G, Lembo A. (2002) End-to-end urethroplasty: long-term results. BJU Int 90:68–71

63. Roehrborn CG, McConnell JD (1994) Analysis of factors contributing to success or failure of 1-stage urethroplasty for urethral stricture disease. J Urol 151:869

64. Park S, McAninch JW (2004) Straddle injuries to the bulbar urethra: management and outcomes in 78 patients. J Urol 171:722

65. Barbagli G, Palminteri E, Bartoletti R, et al. (1997) Long-term results of anterior and posterior urethroplasty with actuarial evaluation of the success rates. J Urol 158:1380

66. Morey AF, Kizer W (2006) Proximal bulbar urethroplasty via extended anastomotic approach—what are the limits? J Urol 175:2145–2149

67. Jordan GH, Virasoro R, Eltahawy EA (2006) Reconstruction and management of posterior urethral and straddle injuries of the urethra. Urol Clin North Am 33:97–109

68. Chapple C, Barbagli G, Jordan G, Mundy AR, Rodrigues-Netto N, Pansadoro V, McAninch JW (2004) Consensus statement on urethral trauma. BJU Int 93:1195

69. Mouraviev VB, Santucci R (2005) Cadaveric anatomy of pelvic fracture urethral distraction injury: most injuries are distal to the external urinary sphincter. J Urol 173:869–872

70. Morey AF, McAninch JW (1997) Reconstruction of posterior urethral disruption injuries: outcome analysis in 82 patients. J Urol 157:506

71. Brandes S (2006) Initial management of anterior and posterior urethral injuries. Urol Clin North Am 33:87

72. Koraitim MM (2005) On the art of anastomotic posterior urethroplasty: a 27-year experience. J Urol 173:135

73. Mouraviev VB, Coburn M, Santucci RA.(2005) The treatment of posterior urethral disruption associated with pelvic fractures: comparative experience of early realignment versus delayed urethroplasty. J Urol 173:873–876

74. Mundy AR (1996) Urethroplasty for posterior urethral strictures. Br J Urol 78:243

75. Pratap A, A. C., Tiwari A, Bhattarai BK, Pandit RK, Anchal N (2006) Complex posterior urethral disruptions: management by combined abdominal transpubic perineal urethroplasty. J Urol 175:1751

76. Anema JG, Morey AF, McAninch JW, et al.(2000) Complications related to the high lithotomy position during urethral reconstruction. J Urol 164:360

77. Koraitim MM (1996) Pelvic fracture urethral injuries: evaluation of various methods of management. J Urol 156:1288

78. Berger AP, D. M., Bartsch G, Steiner H, Varkarakis J, Gozzi C (2005) A comparison of one-stage procedures for post-traumatic urethral stricture repair. BJU Int 95,1299

79. Netto Junior NR, Lemos GC, Claro JF (1989) Internal urethrotomy as a complementary method after urethroplasties for posterior urethral stenosis. J Urol 141:50

80. Dhabuwala CB, Hamid S, Katsikas DM, et al.(1990) Impotence following delayed repair of prostatomembranous urethral disruption. J Urol 144:677

81. Flynn BJ, Delvecchio FC, Webster GD (2003) Perineal repair of pelvic fracture urethral distraction defects: experience in 120 patients during the last 10 years. J Urol 170:1877

82. Armenakas NA, McAninch JW, Lue TF, et al. (1993) Posttraumatic impotence: magnetic resonance imaging and duplex ultrasound in diagnosis and management. J Urol 149:1272

83. Shenfeld OZ, Verstandig AG, Kiselgorf D, et al. (2002) Erectile dysfuction after pelvic fractures: Is it neurogenic or arteriogenic? J Urol 167

84. Aboseif SR, Lue TF (1996) Impotence after urethral injury, in Traumatic and reconstructive urology. Philadelphia, W.B. Saunders Company, pp 455–462

85. Andrich DE, Mundy AR (2001) The nature of urethral injury in cases of pelvic fracture urethral trauma. J Urol 165:1492

86. MacDonald MF, Santucci RA (2005) Review and treatment algorithm of open surgical techniques for management of urethral strictures. Urology 65:9

87. Wessells H, Morey AF, McAninch JW (1997) Single stage reconstruction of complex anterior urethral strictures: combined tissue transfer techniques. J Urol 157:1271–1274

88. Price DT, Vieweg J, Roland F, Coetzee L, Spalding T, Iselin C, Paulson DF (1998) Transient lower extremity neurapraxia associated with radical perineal prostatectomy: a complication of the exaggerated lithotomy position. J Urol 160:1376

89. Angermeier KW, Jordan GH (1994) Complications of the exaggerated lithotomy position: a review of 177 cases. J Urol 151:866

90. el-Kasaby AW, Alla MF, Noweir A, et al. (1996) One-stage anterior urethroplasty. J Urol 156:975

91. Lindell O, Borkowski J, Noll F, et al. (1993) Urethral stricture repair: results in 179 patients. Scand J Urol Nephrol 27:241

20
Postprostatectomy Strictures

James K. Kuan and Hunter Wessells

Contents

1. Background and Epidemiology.. 229
2. Mechanisms and Risk Factors 230
3. Evaluation and Preoperative Management... 230
   3.1. Management of Strictures 231
4. Surgical Management: Endourological.. 232
   4.1. After TURP.. 232
   4.2. After RRP.. 233
5. Surgical Management: Open... 234
   5.1. After TURP.. 234
   5.2. After RRP.. 235
Editorial Comment... 236
References... 238

Summary   Complications of open and transurethral prostate surgery are the most common cause of iatrogenic posterior urethral strictures. Although the number of transurethral resections of the prostate (TURPs) performed in the United States has decreased dramatically, surgery for prostate cancer has proportionately increased in frequency such that Urologists will continue to treat many strictures of the bladder neck, prostatic fossa, and vesicourethral anastomosis. Individualized therapy is required based on etiology, local tissue factors, and incontinence risk. This chapter reviews the epidemiology, mechanisms, and optimal treatment of acquired postprostatectomy strictures of the posterior urethra and bladder neck.

Keywords   Stricture, post prostatectomy, bladder neck, TURP, refractory.

1. Background and Epidemiology

First-line management of benign prostatic hyperplasia (BPH) currently consists of pharmacotherapeutic agents, and this shift has been associated with a reduction in the number of men undergoing surgery for lower urinary tract symptoms (LUTS) secondary to BPH. However, many men will still require surgical intervention for failure of medical management or development of complications. Today, endourological intervention is the preferred modality, and the urologist can choose among a variety of procedures to relieve obstruction from BPH. Among them is transurethral resection of the prostate, which continues to represent the gold standard *(1)*.

Several large retrospective series provide data regarding the incidence of urethral stricture and bladder neck contracture after TURP. Anterior urethral

From: *Current Clinical Urology: Urethral Reconstructive Surgery*
Edited by: S.B. Brandes © Humana Press, Totowa, NJ

stricture, after transurethral intervention for BPH, has been reported to occur in 1.5–3.8% of patients *(2–4)*. However, posterior urethral strictures predominate. In general, a bladder neck contracture (BNC) incidence of 2–2.4% is reported *(5–7)*, although meta-analysis of randomized controlled trials of surgical therapy for BPH report the rate to be as high as 7% *(8)*. When followed long-term, patients may develop BNC as a late complication *(5)*, but usually these occur early, within 2–6 mo *(9,10)*. The rate of BNC and prostatic fossa stricture after laser ablation of the prostate is in the range of 1–2% *(11)*, but further study in larger numbers of patients is required. Neither standard TURP nor laser ablation/enucleation technologies appear to provide an advantage with regards to urethra stricture *(12)*.

The likelihood of bladder neck contracture after radical prostatectomy ranges from 1.3% to 27% of patients. Most contemporary series report BNC rates of 5–10% *(13,14)*. In one large multi-institutional series, 28% of patients self-reported bladder neck strictures after RRP, but only 2.8% were persistent *(15)*. The robotic laparoscopic prostatectomy has been heralded as a technique associated with earlier continence and lower complication rates; publications to date *(16)* suggest that BNC rates of 1–3% are common; however, longer follow-up is needed to confirm these results.

In 2000, 87,400 TURPs were performed in nonfederal hospitals *(1)*. In the following year, more than 80,000 radical retropubic prostatectomies (RRPs) were being performed in the United States; it is likely that this number will continue to increase. Using conservative estimates from the literature, it is calculated that more than 5000 men will require treatment each year for post prostatectomy strictures of the posterior urethra and bladder neck. Thus, although this chapter focuses on surgical treatment, further investigations are needed to understand the pathogenesis of post prostatectomy stricture so that preventive measures can be introduced.

2. Mechanisms and Risk Factors

The occurrence of a BNC after TURP may be related to extensive resection, undermining or fulguration of the bladder neck, and over-resection of a small prostate. Some authors have used weight of the prostate chips as a surrogate marker of initial gland size and suggest that for anticipated resections <10 g, transurethral incision of the prostate may yield fewer bladder neck contractures *(17,18)*. Alternatively, large resection loops may generate excessive heat producing a hypertrophic scar in a small intraurethral adenoma. Urethra-resectoscope disproportion and stray current *(10)* caused by the use of faulty loops, faulty insulation, or non-conductive lubricating gels with non-insulating lubricant *(19)*, are suggested as other mechanisms of urethral injury. Duration of catheterization *(20)* and extravasation of urine *(21)* are proposed as additional risk factors; colonization or infection of urine remains an unsubstantiated causative factor. Clearly, multiple etiologies exist and likely co-exist in individual patients.

After radical prostatectomy, vesicourethral anastomotic strictures are usually the result of scar tissue encircling and narrowing the reconfigured bladder neck *(13,22)*. Proposed mechanisms include anastomotic tension, inflammation from urinary extravasation, poor tissue handling, and ischemia. Risk factors identified in previous studies include excessive blood loss, type of bladder neck dissection, postoperative urinary leakage, adjuvant radiotherapy, and prior TURP *(13,22,23)*. It is likely that multiple factors contribute to the development of BNC post-RRP.

3. Evaluation and Preoperative Management

Development of a bladder neck contracture is usually associated with de novo, recurrent or persistent LUTS. The main complaint may relate to an obstructed voiding pattern, such as a reduced force of stream, although other obstructive and or irritative symptoms may predominate. After TURP, deterioration of symptoms may become manifest after initial improvement after outlet reducing surgery. Bladder neck contracture can occur weeks to years after the primary treatment and may not be associated with severe symptomatology. It is our practice to observe patients for 8–12 wk after TURP, awaiting resolution of the LUTS. After RRP, obstructive symptoms are rare and should immediately suggest bladder neck contracture.

Careful evaluation before the initiation of secondary treatment should be undertaken. It is well established that many men after TURP will have persistent storage and emptying issues. It is important thus to distinguish between functional bladder problems and those related to obstruction. When they persist despite conservative measures, investigation for stricture is indicated. In general evaluation of suspected posterior urethral stricture post prostatectomy include the following:

1. Urinalysis: the presence of hematuria may indicate bladder tumor or complications of bladder outlet obstruction, such as a bladder calculus.
2. Urine culture: this test is essential before instrumentation; infection may represent or contribute to the underlying cause of the voiding symptoms
3. Uroflowmetry and postvoid residual measurement
4. Combined retrograde urethrography (RUG) and voiding cystourethrography (VCUG): In general, imaging is reserved for cases in which complete cystourethroscopy cannot be performed because of various reasons (multiple strictures encountered, complete urethral obliteration, patient unwilling to undergo procedure in ambulatory setting). Performed separately, each provides useful information in evaluating the level of the stricture, but it is our preference to obtain both simultaneously, allowing evaluation of the whole urinary tract proximal and distal to the level of stricture (**Fig. 20.1**).

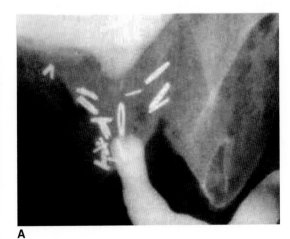

A

FIG. 20.1. Combined RUG and VCUG of a post-RRP stricture

5. Cystoscopy: allows the surgeon to evaluate the lower urinary tract to assess for prostatic regrowth after TURP, anterior urethral pathology, and sphincteric and bladder neck integrity. This examination should be performed on all patients with suspected iatrogenic stricture post-TURP or RRP.
6. Urodynamic evaluation is reserved for specific cases. After TURP, the presence of concomitant risk factors for neurological dysfunction or where a patient fails to become catheter free after TURP should indicate urodynamics. Despite limited use of urodynamic evaluation, the goal is to document obstruction in the setting of a functioning bladder prior further operative intervention. After RRP, urodynamics should be considered before proceeding to aggressive electrosurgical incision of refractory strictures of the vesicourethral anastomosis, as these patients will likely require subsequent anti-incontinence surgery (see discussion to follow).

Thorough evaluation allows accurate delineation of the stricture, and our diagnostic algorithm is presented in **Fig. 20.2**. Disease classifications should document incremental anatomic severity and should ultimately predict treatment and outcome, such that higher-grade lesions are associated with greater morbidity, warrant more aggressive treatment, and have poorer prognoses. Pansadoro et al. *(24)* have proposed a classification of posterior urethral strictures. However on the basis of their experience, it is suggested that all injuries are best managed in the same fashion, using bladder neck incision, thus this anatomic classification addresses only two of these requirements of a valid grading system. It is provided here:

Type I: Fibrous tissue involves the bladder neck only, termed "bladder neck contracture."

Type II: Stricture is localized to the median part of the prostatic fossa, with open bladder neck and spared verumontanum.

Type III: Complete prostatic urethral obliteration.

3.1. Management of Strictures

The definitive management of strictures in the posterior urethra generally requires endourological or open surgical interventions. Conservative tactics are used as temporizing measures until definitive

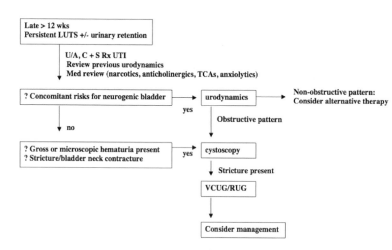

FIG. 20.2. Algorithm for clinical evaluation of suspected iatrogenic posterior urethral strictures

management of the stricture can be achieved. Urinary drainage per urethra or a suprapubic tract may be necessary in cases of retention secondary to obstruction.

Local urethral dilatation using male urethral sounds or other forms of dilators may facilitate placement of a urethral drainage catheter or allow initiation of an intermittent self-catheterization protocol. Simple dilation may prove successful for vesicourethral anastomotic strictures after RRP, but rarely is successful after TURP (25).

A critical consideration in the treatment of BNC is the risk of urinary incontinence. After TURP, bladder neck contracture treated by transurethral incision, even using electrocautery, does not significantly increase the risk of urinary incontinence. In contrast, formal electrosurgical incision of BNC after RRP is very likely to cause urinary incontinence.

4. Surgical Management: Endourological

Interruption of the scarred bladder neck fibers is the central premise of endourological procedures for bladder neck contracture. This can be accomplished by resection or incision of the bladder neck. For resection, electrocautery with a loop resectoscope is described. The success of this type of procedure is reported to be 54%, with recurrence of the stricture defining failure (25). Thus, use of this technique is discouraged and incision is the preferred method. A multitude of techniques have been described and include the use of various

energy sources or a cold-knife incision. The risk of incontinence must be discussed frankly with any patient who has undergone prior prostatectomy and now faces incision of the bladder neck.

4.1. After TURP

The most commonly used energy is monopolar electrocautery or laser incision with Ho:YAG or Nd:YAG lasers. Our practice is to use bilateral incisions at the 5- and 7-o'clock position s originating at the bladder neck, extending to the level of the verumontanum. A full-thickness incision is made through the scar to the level of the circular bladder neck fibers, leaving an intervening segment of "normal" urothelium. This achieves release and opening of the bladder neck and promotes secondary epithelialization from the spared median strip of epithelium (**Fig. 20.3**). A catheter is placed for 24–72 h.

The principles of bladder neck incision are well described by Pansadoro and Emiliozzi's report (24) on 122 patients with iatrogenic posterior urethral strictures, with 47% occurring after TURP. Using a technique similar to ours, they report an overall success of 92% (range, 76% for type III and 98% for type II strictures). The non-TURP patients had undergone open suprapubic prostatectomy and similar success is reported, although none of the type III strictures occurred after open adenectomy. In this series, 17% of patients experienced complications, including urinary tract infection (11%), incontinence (4%), stress incontinence (4%), and severe bleeding (1%). Retrograde ejaculation is clearly a concern after TURP and is to be expected

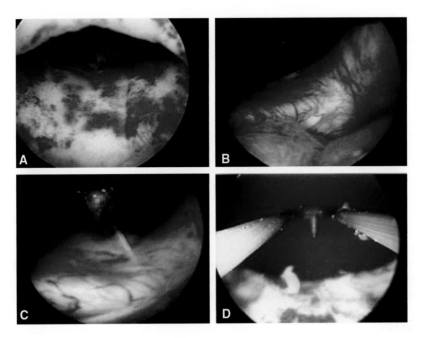

FIG. 20.3. (A) Cystoscopic appearance of bladder neck contracture prior to intervention, status-post TURP 16 weeks previously. (B) Positioning of the endoscope prior to incision of the bladder neck at 5 o'clock. (C) Initiation of bladder neck incision using a Collins' knife and monopolar electrocautery. (D) Appearance of bladder neck and prostatic fossa after bilateral incisions, noting preserved median strip of urothelium

after bladder neck incision for iatrogenic posterior urethral strictures.

Cold knife incision has a success rate of approximately 90% (25) and may be as high as 100% (26,27). When urethrotomy is coupled with self-dilatation postoperatively, improved success has been reported in small series. Most series of laser bladder neck incision are reports of postradical prostatectomy vesicourethral anastomotic stricture. In one report of laser urethrotomy in 450 patients undergoing 900 urethrotomies, 62.8% of whom had posterior urethral strictures, a recurrence rate of 70% is reported. Nearly 50% of strictures recurred within one year post incision. Because of the inferior results of this series, no clear advantage is seen over electro-incision of the bladder neck.

Urethral stenting has been proposed, although currently it is used sparingly because of challenges with tissue regrowth or intrusion and migration into the bladder. Removal of the prosthesis is challenging and, when regrowth is encountered, transurethral resection of the intruding adenoma to the level of the stent is indicated and performed usually without difficulty. Although not currently approved by the U.S. Food and Drug Administration, thermoexpandable nickel titanium coiled stents, which are placed temporarily and can be removed with minimal accessory trauma using an endoscope, may provide an adjunct to bladder neck incision. However, more investigation is required to fully appreciate the potential benefits of this device.

4.2. After RRP

After radical prostatectomy, electrosurgical incision of a bladder neck contracture is reserved for patients who have failed dilation, cold-knife incision, and require ongoing manipulation. In contrast to anterior urethral strictures, in which the concept of the reconstructive ladder has been supplanted, we advocate a stepwise approach with the goal of preserving urinary continence.

Most anastomotic strictures after RRP occur within 6 mo. We and others differentiate between early "immature" strictures that occur days to weeks after catheter removal from "mature" scarring (23). For early postoperative BNC, urethral dilation with sounds or filliforms and followers is indicated. In both cases, cystoscopic placement of a guide wire or long filiform reduces the risk of false passage or disruption of a recent anastomosis. Dilation allows spontaneous voiding while the scarred region stabilizes. The success of dilation in these circumstances is low *(23)*, although some series report long-term favorable outcomes with this approach *(13)*.

For strictures that fail initial dilation or occur more than 6 wk after radical prostatectomy, we recommend cold-knife direct vision internal urethrotomy (DVIU) of the vesicourethral anastomotic stricture. Our technique is based on that described by Dalkin and associates *(28)*. In brief, deep incisions at the 4- and 8-o'clock positions are made from the proximal area of the contracture to the distal extent of the stricture. Care is taken to avoid injury to the normal striated sphincter muscle fibers. The incisions are carried down to bleeding tissue; a monopolar cautery electrode can be used if hemostasis is required. Catheter drainage is necessary for 24 h. Voiding, urinary bother, continence, and quality of life were no different in men after DVIU for vesicourethral anastomotic stricture when compared with a control group of asymptomatic men after RRP *(29)*.

Transurethral incision using electrocautery is recommended only when all more conservative interventions have failed, including dilation, DVIU, and a course of intermittent self catheterization. In such circumstances, the much greater risk of incontinence must be weighed against the likelihood of long-term urethral patency. In most cases, these patients are highly symptomatic and willing to accept the risks of incontinence and the high likelihood of needing either artificial urinary sphincter (AUS) or male sling surgery. However, a small subset is discovered incidentally during workup of post-prostatectomy incontinence. Regardless of the scenario, aggressive incision is carried out using a technique identical to that described previously for post-TURP bladder neck contractures. After incision, we reevaluate the bladder neck 6 wk postoperatively, and proceed with AUS placement.

5. Surgical Management: Open

In cases of refractory post-TURP strictures and the most severe post-RRP anastomotic strictures, an aggressive reconstructive approach is warranted.

A temporary diverting suprapubic catheter should be placed while plans are made for the optimal type of reconstruction or diversion. For certain selected patients, suprapubic drainage may be the best long-term management strategy when faced with severe medical comorbidities, a complex stricture requiring urinary diversion, or recurrent advanced prostate carcinoma.

In an appropriately selected patient, the options are twofold: 1) open resection with reanastomosis or 2) urinary diversion. Selection of the appropriate procedure requires consideration of surgical exposure, the amount of scar to be excised, and sources of healthy vascularized tissue for transfer into the diseased bladder neck region. Patient age, prior surgery or radiotherapy, cancer stage, and life expectancy must be assessed before intervention for this formidable complication.

Adequate exposure of the bladder neck region is vital for successful reconstruction of stricture after prostatectomy. A standard perineal incision may not afford sufficient visualization of the stricture, and we advocate combined above and below approach to the stricture *(29)*. This goes against current concepts in delayed repair of posterior urethral disruption injuries, in which initial perineal mobilization of the bulbar urethra usually allows reapproximation without pubectomy. Radical prostatectomy changes the local anatomy, making the bladder less mobile and creating a potential for tension on the anastomosis. The length of stricture to be excised and replaced may warrant pubectomy early in the operation.

5.1. After TURP

Open reconstruction for post-TURP posterior urethral stricture is a complex undertaking. If urinary diversion is used, the principles remain standard in terms of selection of diversion type and timing. For open reconstruction, the primary objective is complete resection of the scar, which frequently involves the entire length of the prostatic urethra. As such, an abdominal approach usually is required to adequately access the diseased tissue and gain mobilization of the bladder to facilitate a tension-free anastomosis to the membranous urethra. For strictures that involve the length of the membranous urethra a combined abdominal-perineal approach may be required, with perineal mobilization of the bulbar urethra to gain length to bridge the anastomotic gap. As with post-RRP bladder neck reconstruction, de novo urinary incontinence may occur post-operatively. Simultaneous AUS placement has been described *(30)*, but our preference is to delay placement of an AUS until a complete assessment of the urinary incontinence can be performed after reconstruction. Few patients will require such aggressive surgical undertaking. Inherent in this procedure are significant risks, including rectal injury, incontinence, need for artificial urinary sphincter, urinary retention requiring self-catheterization, erectile dysfunction, vesicourethral anastomotic stricture, and only well selected, motivated patients should be considered for this type of reconstruction. In performing this type of operation, adherence to reconstructive principles is paramount: complete resection of the scar, watertight anastomosis, and complete urinary drainage.

5.2. After RRP

The majority of men with vesicourethral anastomotic strictures after RRP can undergo successful excision of the stricture and reanastomosis. Two main schools of thought predominate. One favors a perineal approach, such as used for radical perineal prostatectomy, excising vesicourethral scar and performing reanastomosis *(10,31)*. Minimal mobilization of the distal urethra is performed in this method, thus preserving remnant urethral sphincteric function as is possible. Although this approach is feasible in case with relatively short strictures, long defects may require more extensive mobilization of the distal urethra.

Our approach has been more aggressive, recognizing the multiple prior interventions to which these patients have been subjected, and assumes that the striated sphincter is destroyed. The primary goal is patency, with most men requiring AUS at a later date. Men in this situation must be willing to accept the need for multiple surgeries to be free from obstruction. We use a combined abdominal and perineal approach, mobilize the bulbar urethra distally to the suspensory ligament, and excise the scarred stricture, which usually encases and obliterates any remnant sphincter

and membranous urethra. Reanastomosis then can be performed either from above or below. We favor end-to-end anastomosis when possible (**Fig. 20.4**) but have used grafts and flaps (**Fig. 20.5**) as indicated to achieve a patent urethral lumen. Catheterization for 3 weeks followed by voiding cystourethrography ensures complete urethral healing prior to catheter removal. Using this approach in a series of four patients all of the patients maintained urethral patency, although artificial sphincter placement was usually required to achieve continence *(29)*.

We reserve diversion for patients with radiation necrosis, severe neurogenic bladder dysfunction, complex fistulae, or other factors that make reconstruction of the urethra impractical or impossible *(32)*. We achieve cephalad mobilization of the bladder base after resection of the vesicourethral anastomosis (or prostate if present after TURP or radiation), incorporate an intestinal segment into the bladder neck, and create a cutaneous stoma (**Fig. 20.6**). No attempt is made to close the distal urethra. Intestinal tissue is anastomosed to the bladder neck without any tension using a single layer closure with 2-O polyglycolic acid suture. The appendix or tapered ileum is used according to the Mitrofanoff principle for continent catheterizable diversion (**Fig. 20.6**). A continence

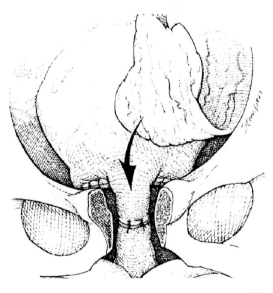

Fɪɢ. 20.4. Post-RRP stricture reconstruction using a bladder tube

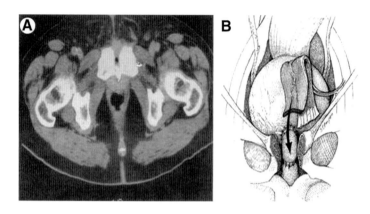

FIG. 20.5. Post-RRP stricture reconstruction using a free graft and rectus flap

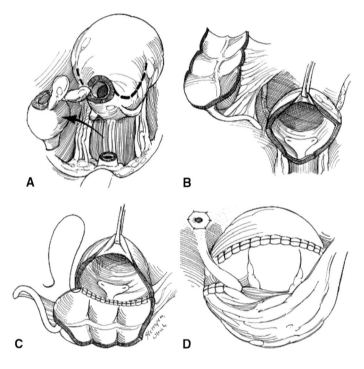

FIG. 20.6. Diversion procedure. (A) The bladder neck is incorporated into a transversely oriented clamshell cystotomy leaving the ureterovesical junctions undisturbed (B). The appropriate segment of bowel was then mobilized and incorporated directly into the bladder neck, either as (C) an augmentation or as (D) a continent catheterizable stoma, depending on patient wishes and manual dexterity

mechanism based on the ileocecal valve can also be used. The bladder is drained with a catheter through the stoma as well as a suprapubic catheter in the augmented bladder. Closed suction drains are maintained in the region of the bladder neck until output is less than 30 ml per day. Contrast cystography confirmed the absence of extravasation prior to removal of catheters.

Editorial Comment

Elliot et al. (J Urol 178:529–534, 2007), in an analysis of the CaPSURE database, recently reported that the incidence of urethral strictures after primary management of localized prostate cancer was 344 of 6597 cases (5.2%, range 1.1–8.4%). Median follow-up was 2.7 years. Most strictures were short and thus managed by dilation (63%). Previous reports of bladder neck contracture after radical prostatectomy range from 2.7% to 25.7%. Historically, risk factors include low surgeon volume, increased blood loss, and current smoking. Good mucosa-to-mucosa apposition is believed to be essential for preventing bladder neck contracture, although there are conflicting data about whether urinary extravasation is a risk factor. Detailed in **Table 20.1** are the rates of urethral stricture development by the type of prostate cancer therapy. The highest rates occur after radical prostatectomy and brachytherapy plus external-beam radiation therapy. As you can see from the actuarial life table analysis of **Table 20.2**, radical prostatectomy strictures typically occur in the first 6 mo postoperatively, with the rates tapering off by 1 yr and totally flatten out after 2 yr. In contrast, postradiation therapy strictures incidence was initially very low but over time increased at a

gradual and steady rate, from an initial zero up to 5% to 16% at 4 years. Body mass index and age were significant predictors of needing a subsequent urethral stricture surgery. That obese patient had more urethral strictures may be due to technical difficulties of achieving a good anastomosis or the higher Gleason rate and positive margins noted in the obese. Urethral strictures refractory to dilation or urethroplasty were not included in their search, so such strictures were thus underreported.

Our technique for managing recurrent bladder neck contractures after prostatectomy is similar to the technique detailed above by Kuan and Wessells, with some notable differences. Urethral strictures that occur within the 3-mo postoperative period we dilate over a wire. We avoid urethrotomy in the early postsurgical period because it risks bothersome and permanent urinary incontinence. After a period of at least 6 mo afer surgery, we feel more comfortable that the anastomosis is mature and take the patient for a transurethral incision of the bladder neck (TUIBN) with a resectoscope. Initially, we cystoscope the patient and place a guide wire across the stricture into the bladder. If we are not confident that the wire is in the bladder we will retrograde fill the bladder and then place a suprapubic percutaneous peel away sheath. Through the sheath, we cystoscope the bladder and either place the wire antegrade and out the urethra or place the wire retrograde and use graspers to pull the wire through the SP tact. Through–through access gives excellent control of the urethra. We prefer a super stiff guide wire to prevent a false passage during dilation. We typically dilate the urethra to 24 or 26 French with either Heyman or Amplatz dilators. Once dilated, a 24-French

TABLE 20.1. Urethral stricture incidence after therapy for prostate cancer (From, Elliott et al. (2007) J Urol, 159–534).

Treatment	No. Pts/No. Stricture (%)
RP	3,310/277 (8,4)
RP+EBRT	73/2 (2.7)
Cryosurgery	199/5 (2.5)
BT	799/14 (1.8)
BT+EBRT	231/12 (5.2)
EBRT	645/11 (1.7)
ADT	961/19 (2.0)
WW	378/4 (1.1)
Total	6,597/344 (5.2)

Followup not considered.

TABLE 20.2. Actuarial table of stricture free rates after prostate cancer therapy. (From, Elliott et al. (2007) J Urol, 159–534).

Primary Treatment	% Stricture Treatment Free (95% CI)			
	6 Mos	1 Yr	2 Yrs	4 Yrs
RP	93 (92–94)	91 (90–93)	91 (89–92)	89 (86–91)
RP+EBRT	97 (88–99)	95 (85–98)	95 (85–98)	86 (46–97)
Cryotherapy	96 (92–98)	96 (92–98)	95 (89–98)	87 (66–95)
BT	96 (94–97)	94 (92–96)	93 (90–95)	89 (80–94)
BT+EBRT	96 (92–98)	92 (87–95)	88 (91–93)	84 (71–92)
EBRT	99 (97–99)	98 (96–99)	96 (93–97)	95 (90–98)
Hormones	96 (94–97)	94 (92–96)	93 (90–95)	92 (87–95)
WW	99 (97–100)	99 (97–100)	98 (95–99)	98 (68–99)

Log rank test p < 0.01.

noncontinuous flow resectoscope is placed and a Orandi blade hot knife at 160 watts of pure cut is used to incise the epithelium from just lateral of the ureteral orifices through the bladder neck, till the distal edge of the white scarred urethra, at both 4 and 8 o'clock. Intravenous indigo carmine and a diuretic are given before BN incision to help identify the ureteral orifices, which are typically distorted and/or displaced after prostatectomy. We confirm adequate incision when the resectoscope can freely be moved in all directions. If the scope feels stiff or held in position, the bladder neck has not been sufficiently incised. We then use a Williams' needle and inject 10 ml of 40 mg/ml of triamcinolone into the urethrotomy sites. A 20- or 22-French Foley catheter is typically placed and maintained for 5 to 7 d.

If such a TUIBN and biological modifier injection fails, we repeat the TUIBN. If this fails, we have little success nor experience with formal bladder neck reconstruction. Instead, we will consider the patient for an off label placement of a wire endourethral prothesis (Urolume) stent. The only problem with placing a UroLume in a radiated field is that it may not get completely covered and endothelialized. Exposed wires may predispose to stone and stricture formation. Furthermore, it is often tricky to properly position the stent without the edge extending into the bladder. A Holmium laser with side-firing arm is useful to incise off these intravesical edges of tines. Also, hypertrophic scar regrowth of urethral stricture into the lumen may occur after placement. Once this happens, the UroLume is difficult to manage. At first we dilate the hypertrophic scar over a wire. With a resectoscope on 75 W pure cut, we scrape the scar tissue, until the wire mesh is exposed. For patients who fail the salvage stent scraping, we advocate a supravesical urinary diversion of some sort—either a suprapubic tube, neobladder with catherizable stoma, augmentation cystoplasty and catherizable Monti or Mitrofanoff, ileal vesicostomy or ileal conduit (after Bricker) urinary diversion.—S.B. Brandes

References

1. Wei JT, Calhoun E, Jacobsen SJ (2005) Urologic diseases in America project: benign prostatic hyperplasia. J Urol 173:1256–1261

2. Uchida T, Ohori M, Soh S, et al. (1999) Factors influencing morbidity in patients undergoing transurethral resection of the prostate. Urology 53:98–105

3. Madersbacher S, Marberger M (1999) Is TURP still justified? Br J Urol 83:227–237

4. Mcconnell J, Barry M, Bruskewitz R: Benign prostatic hyperplasia: diagnosis and treatment. Clinical practice guidelines, No 8. AHCPR Publication No 94—582. Rockville, MD, Agency of Health Care Policy and Research, Public Health Service, US Department of Health and Human Services.

5. Varkarakis J, Bartsch G, Horninger W (2004) Long-term morbidity and mortality of transurethral prostatectomy: a 10-year follow-up. The Prostate 58:248–251

6. Ala Opas MY, Aitola PT, Metsola EJ (1993) Evaluation of immediate and late results of transurethral resection of the prostate. Scand J Urol Nephrol 27:235–239

7. Zwergel U, Wullich B, Lindenmeir U, et al. (1998) Long term results following transurethral resection of the prostate. Fur Urol 33:476–480

8. Roehrborn, CG, McConnell JD, Barry MJ (2003) Chapter 3. Results of the Treatment Outcomes Analyses" in Guideline on the Management of Benign Prostatic Hyperplasia (BPH). American Urological Association Education and Research, Inc.

9. Greene LF, Leary FJ (1967) Contracture of the vesical neck following transurethral prostatic resection. Surg Gynecol Obstet 124:1277–1282

10. Nielsen KK, Nordling J (1990) Urethral stricture following transurethral prostatectomy. Urology 35:18–24

11. Elzayat EA, Elhilali MM (2006) Holmium laser enucleation of the prostate (HoLEP): the endourologic alternative to open prostatectomy. Eur Urol 49:87

12. Tan AHH, Gilling PJ, Kennett KM, et al. (2003) A randomized trial comparing holmium laser enucleation of the prostate with transurethral resection of the prostate for the treatment of bladder outlet obstrction secondary to benign prostatic hyperplasia in large glands (40 to 200 grams). J Urol 170:1270–1274

13. Besarani D, Amoroso P, Kirby R (2004) Bladder neck contracture after radical retropubic prostatectomy. BJU Int 94:1245–1247

14. Borboroglu PG, Sands JP, Roberts JL, et al. (2000) Risk factors for vesicourethral anastomotic stricture after readical prostatectomy. Urology 56:96

15. Kao TC, Cruess DF, Garner D, et al. (2000) Multicenter patient self-reporting questionnaire on impotence, incontinence and stricture after radical prostatectomy. J Urol 163:858

16. Gonzalgo ML, Pavlovich CP, Trock BJ, et al. (2005) Classification and trends of perioperative morbidities following laparoscopic radical prostatectomy. J Urol 174:135

17. Hellstrom P, Lukkarinen O, Kontturi M, et al. (1986) Bladder neck incision or transurethral electroresection for the treatment of urinary obstruction caused by a small benign prostate? Scand J Urol Nephrol 20:187–192

18. Edwards L, Bucknall T, Pittam M, et al. (1985) Transurethral resection of the prostate and bladder neck incision: a review of 700 cases. Br J Urol 57:168–171

19. Sofer M, Vilos GA, Borg P, et al. (2001) Stray radiofrequency current as a cause of urethral strictures after transurethral resection of the prostate. J Endourol 15:221–225

20. Robertson GS, Everitt N, Burton P, et al. (1991) Effect of catheter material on the incidence of urethral strictures. Br J Urol 68:612–617

21. Lentz HC Jr, Mebust WK, Foret JD, et al. (1977) Urethral strictures following transurethral prostatectomy: review of 2223 resections. J Urol 117:194–197

22. Surya BV, Provet J, Johanson KE, et al. (1990) Anastomotic strictures following radical prostatectomy: risk factors and management. J Urol 143:755

23. Dalkin BL (1996) Endoscopic evaluation and treatment of anastomotic strictures after radical retropubic prostatectomy. J Urol 155:206

24. Pansadoro V, Emiliozzi P (1999) Iatrogenic prostatic urethral strictures: classification and endoscopic treatment. Urology 53:784–789

25. Sikafi Z, Bulter MR, Lane V et al. (1985) Bladder neck contracture following prostatectomy. Br J Urol 57:308–310

26. Varkarakis J, Bartsch G, Horninger W (2004) Long-term morbidity and mortality of transurethral prostatectomy: a 10-year follow-up. The Prostate 58:248–251

27. Wettlaufer JN, Kronmiller P (1976) The management of post-prostatectomy vesical neck contracture. J Urol 116:482–483

28. Yurkanin JP, Dalkin BL, Cui H (2001) Evaluation of cold knife urthrotomy for the treatment of anastomotic stricture after radical retropubic prostatectomy. J Urol 165:1545

29. Wessells H, Morey A, McAninch JW (1998) Obliterative vesicourethral strictures following radical prostatectomy for the treatment of prostate cancer: reconstructive armamentarium. J Urol 160:1373

30. Theodorou C, Katsifotis C, Stournaras P, et al. (2000) Abdomino-perineal repair of recurrent and complex bladder neck-prostatic urethra contractures. Eur Urol 38:734–741

31. Schlossberg S, Jordan G, Schellhammer P (1995) Repair of obliterative vesicourethral stricture after radical prostatectomy: a technique for preservation of continence. Urology 45:510

32. Ullrich NF, Wessells H (2002) A technique of bladder neck closure combining prostatectomy and intestinal interposition for unsalvageable urethral disease. J Urol 167:634

21
Urethral Stricture and Urethroplasty in the Pelvic Irradiated Patient

Kennon Miller, Michael Poch, and Steven B. Brandes

Contents

1. Radiobiology 241
2. Grading of Radiation Morbidity 242
3. Incidence, Risk Factors, and Presentation 242
4. Histology 244
5. Evaluation 245
6. Management of Radiation-Induced Urethral Strictures 245
7. Illustrative Cases 247
    7.1. Case Study 1 247
    7.2. Case Study 2 247
    7.3. Case Study 3 247
    7.4. Case Study 4 248
References 249

Summary The overall incidence of bulbo-membranous urethral stricture or bladder neck contracture after radiation therapy is roughly 3–16%. Time to stricture presentation is usually delayed (24 months) and insidious. Radiation urethral strictures typically have an unhealthy or pale appearance on cystoscopy, with varying degrees of local tissue induration or dense fibrotic scarring. Radiation induced urethral strictures are often refractory to urethrotomy or dilation, and more likely complex management dilemmas. Management methods include urethrotomy and intermittent self-catheterization, off-label use of an endourethral prosthesis, excision and primary urethral anastomosis urethroplasty, salvage prostatectomy with anastomotic urethrovesical urethroplasty, combined abdominal-perineal urethroplasty, onlay flap urethroplasty, and supravesical urinary diversion surgery. Grafts should generally be avoided in the radiated field unless buttressed by a muscle flap.

Keywords bladder neck contracture, ischemia, fibrosis, onlay flap urethroplasty, anastomotic urethroplasty, supravesical urinary diversion, endourethral prosthesis

1. Radiobiology

Radiation causes cell death in multiple ways, and active investigation is still under way to fully understand this process. Radiation damage can be directly ionizing or indirect when free radicals are formed as radiation interacts with intracellular water. The ultimate effect is free radical damage to

From: *Current Clinical Urology: Urethral Reconstructive Surgery*
Edited by: S.B. Brandes © Humana Press, Totowa, NJ

deoxyribonucleic acid, causing impaired replication and protein synthesis. The effect of ionizing radiation on normal tissues is dependent on radiation total dose, dose fraction size, total volume treated, and elapsed time.

Radiation causes both acute and chronic effects on tissue. Acute effects usually occur within 2–3 wk of therapy, whereas chronic effects can manifest months and, indeed, years later. Tissues with a rapid cell turnover such as skin and mucous membranes are most susceptible to the acute effects of radiation. Chronic tissue damage is characterized by cell ischemia and fibrosis. Multiple theories have been postulated to explain chronic effects, including microvascular damage and stem cell injury. The result is vascular damage characterized by endothelial proliferation and an obliterative endarteritis leading to ischemia and fibrosis of the effected and surrounding tissue.

Onset of subacute and chronic complications after radiotherapy is typically from 6 to 24 mo (1). However, some chronic complications, such as bleeding, fibrosis, and scarring, can occur even after decades. In general, some of the comorbid conditions that predispose to radiation complications and vascular damage are diabetes mellitus, hypertension, cardiovascular disease, prior surgery, and concomitant radiation sensitizing chemotherapy.

There have been tremendous advances in tumor localization with radiation therapy during the last 20 yr. Originally, radiation oncologists used skeletal anatomy to guide the radiation beams. Prostate cancer was treated by aiming the beams at the area between the pubic symphysis and femoral heads. Computed tomography (CT) scanning, more widely used in the 1990s, allowed three-dimensional visualization of the target organ. This lead to more advanced techniques, termed conformal radiation, which use sophisticated software to allow the radiation to "conform" to the shape of the target organ. The end result of these advances is to maximize cancer control while greatly limiting the amount of radiation delivered to surrounding organs.

Prostate brachytherapy (BT) achieves a high radiation dose to the prostate with a rapid fall off in the juxtaposed and interposed adjacent normal tissue (2). Seed are typically placed in a distribution to generally "spare" the prostatic urethra. The number and percent of men treated with BT has increased dramatically since the 1990s. Preimplant prostate volume and severe lower urinary tract symptoms (as evidenced by a high American Urological Association Symptom Score [AUA SS]) are associated with greater post-BT urinary toxicity. Published rates of urethral morbidity are from the most experienced providers and centers and thus the true incidence of complications are probably higher and underreported—in particular the most severe complications.

Intensity-modulated radiotherapy is the most current and advanced form of conformal radiation that uses a combination of CT scanning and computer software to deliver an unprecedented level of radiation to the target tissue while minimizing exposure to surrounding organs.

2. Grading of Radiation Morbidity

The Radiation Therapy Oncology Group established a grading system for radiation complications. The system is based largely on the patients' performance status and what level of intervention is required. Although general, it has been modified to describe morbidity to the urinary tract (Table 21.1). In essence, grades 1–2 describe minor treatment-related morbidities that require only outpatient care. Grades 3–4 can result in more serious sequelae and require either hospitalization or surgical intervention (Fig. 21.1).

3. Incidence, Risk Factors, and Presentation

The overall incidence of bulbomembranous urethral stricture or bladder neck contracture (BNC) after radiation therapy is roughly 3–16% (1).

TABLE 21.1. Modified RTOG urinary toxicity scale.

Grade	Description
1	Symptomatic nocturia and/or frequency requiring no therapy
2	Early obstructive symptoms requiring α-blockade and phenazopyridine
3	Requiring indwelling catheters or intermittent catheterization
4	Requiring postimplantation TURP, TUIP, urethral dilation, or suprapubic catheter placement

* TUIP = transurethral incision of the prostate; TURP = transurethral resection of the prostate
(From Mayo Clin Proc. (2004);79:314–317).

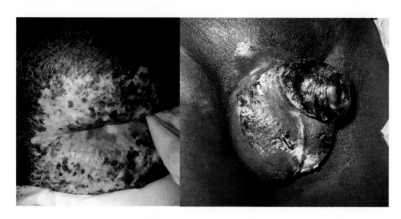

FIG. 21.1. Pendulous urethral stricture, urinary retention and penile dry gangrene after pelvic RT for clinically localized prostate cancer, in a diabetic with severe peripheral vascular disease. A. RT skin changes of buttock B. Penile dry gangrene

Time to presentation is typically 12–36 mo (mean, roughly 24 mo), and the typical presentation occurs with obstructive and irritative voiding symptoms. However, at longer follow-up and the inclusion of a significantly greater number of patients, stricture disease has been documented up to 6 yr after BT. Elliot et al. *(1)* in their analysis of the CaPSURE database (mostly community practices) noted that postradiation therapy strictures incidence was initially very low but, over time, increased at a steady rate, from an initial near zero, up to 5–16% by 4 yr. In other words, as in other areas of radiotherapy (RT) damage, the RT effects on the urethra and bladder neck are typically delayed and insidious. This study, however, grossly underestimated the incidence of urethral stricture because they surveyed only strictures that were amenable to dilation or urethroplasty, and not obliterative strictures. Although refractory radiation induced strictures and their management were not included, it is precisely this population that is a management dilemma and often require major reconstruction or urinary diversion.

The overlap with radiation cystitis symptoms can lead to misdiagnosis or delayed diagnosis of the stricture. Multiple risk factors for the development of strictures have been examined. History of TURP before radiation therapy has been implicated as a cause of stricture and BNC *(3)*. Greskovich et al. *(4)* reported a higher rate of stricture in patients who underwent prior transurethral resection of the prostate (TURP) and Seymore et al. *(1)* noted that 72% of the patients who developed bladder neck contractures after RT to 68 Gy had prior TURP (mean

33 d before). The likely mechanism of stricture formation is ischemia and microfibrosis after cautery use (especially at the bladder neck, resulting in relative inability of the area to repair endothelial damage caused by radiation). To reduce the risk of such strictures, they recommended an interval between surgery and prostate RT of at least 6 wk. There are numerous other studies that also note that previous TURP increases the incidence of radiation induced strictures.

Merrick et al. *(2)* examined a series of 1186 patients who underwent BT and noted that the overall radiation dose to the bulbomembranous urethra and the use of concurrent external beam therapy correlated with urethral stricture formation (see Fig. 2 in Merrick et al. *[2]*) The greater the average urethral dose of radiation, the greater the rate of stricture (**Fig. 21.2**). All strictures involved the bulbo-membranous urethra and <1 cm from the apex of the prostate. This stresses the need for very careful preplanning for BT and the use of supplemental external beam RT (EBRT) in a judicious manner. Careful seed placement and prostatic apical urethral sparing are essential. Merrick et al. *(2)* reported 3.6%, 9-yr actuarial risk of urethral stricture disease, with a mean time to presentation of 2.6 ± 1.3 yr. These patients presented with gross or microscopic hematuria, increase in IPSS score, late-onset dysuria, or an increase in post void residual. Strictures were diagnosed by cystoscopy alone. Furthermore, of those who developed strictures, roughly one-third had recurrent strictures after initial management. Wallner et al. *(5)* also reported

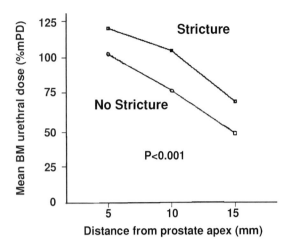

an association of the late urethral toxicity and maximum urethral dose from I^{125} BT. For patients with Grade 2 and 3 toxicities, average maximal urethral dose was 592 cGy, compared with only 447 cGy for zero-to-minimal late toxicities.

In a recent study by Astrom et al. *(6)* of 214 patients receiving high-dose BT for localized prostate cancer, 13 (7%) developed urethral strictures, 1 of whom, an obliterative stricture requiring urinary diversion. The median latency time was approximately 3 yr *(5)*. Zelefsky et al. *(7)* noted that 248 patients who underwent I^{125} BT had a 10% 5-yr actuarial stricture rate. All their strictures occurred within the first 24 mo (mean time till stricture 18 mo). Galalae et al. *(7)* describe a 2.7% incidence of urethral stricture after BT (4 of 148 pts), with a median 5-yr follow-up. All four of those patients had TURP before radiation therapy. Demanes et al. *(8)* reported a 6.7 % stricture rate after high-dose BT. However, 8% had pre-existing strictures. Martinez et al. *(9)* reported a 5-yr actuarial risk of 7%. Of interest, Albert et al *(10)* reported a urethral protective effect of magnetic resonance imaging-guided BT such that the seeds are directed away from the prostatic urethral mucosa. In their multicenter trial, there were no urethral strictures found over a median 2.8-yr follow-up period *(10)*.

Therefore, overly aggressive implantation of BT seeds in the peri-apical region increase the risk for urethral stricture. With careful attention to planning and implant technique, including extensive use of the sagittal plane for intraoperative deposition of the seeds, it is possible to implant the apex within a 5-mm margin without excessive doses to the urethra. Clearly, surgeon skill and dose planning are key to avoiding urethral morbidity.

4. Histology

There is little in the literature that describes the histopathology of the urethral strictures *(11)*. Early changes in the formation of anterior urethral stricture are initial ulceration with subsequent proliferation of a stratified squamous epithelium with infiltration of elongated myofibroblasts and clumps of multinucleated giant cells. The proliferation of myofibroblasts have been proposed as causative factors for stricture formation and giant cells are thought to promote collagen synthesis in the strictured area. Chronic radiation changes are characterized by obliterative endarteritis, tissue ischemia and fibrosis. Extravasation of urine through a leaky urethral epithelium is another potential cause for fibrosis and narrowing of the urethral lumen. Inflammatory strictures may form as a result of microabscess formation in periurethral glands extending deep into the corpus spongiosum.

More recently, reports by Baskin et al. *(11)* describe an increase in the ratio of type I and type III collagen deposition within urethral strictures compared to the normal urethra. Cavalcanti and Yucel *(12)* also describe the functional role of nitric oxide in wound healing and collagen deposition within the bulbar urethra. They postulated a causal relationship between the loss of smooth muscle and increase in collagen deposition and lack of responsiveness to nitric oxide. Those patients were thought to have injury to the neuronal innervation of the bulbar urethra leading to a decreasing responsiveness to nitric oxide. In addition, surrounding corpora spongiosum was less vascular.

It is uncertain whether the aforementioned histologic changes can be applied categorically to RT strictures. The available models of stricture are either traumatic or idiopathic in these studies. Radiation therapy is known to cause fibrotic changes which, in the setting of stricture, mimics or even intensifies the process that worsens its clinical course. Therefore, the radiation itself may not initiate the stricture, but it certainly exacerbates even the slightest insult (ischemic, traumatic, or inflammatory) to result in a more clinically relevant stricture process.

5. Evaluation

Typically, evaluation begins with thorough history and physical examination. Often patients treated with RT can have a component of radiation cystitis that may present with irritative symptoms. However, even at that time one should have a high suspicion for the presence of stricture. Urinalysis and urine culture should be tested routinely because these patients may present with urinary tract infections or hematuria.

Endoscopic and sonourethrography are helpful tools to determine length of stricture and degrees of stenosis. Endoscopy should be performed with extreme care and avoid dilation of strictured areas. Pediatric or flexible ureteroscopes should be employed if an adult flexible cystourethroscope cannot be passed.

Retrograde urethrography is the gold standard for evaluation and can help not only with diagnosis but management decisions as well. It should always be performed under the direct supervision of the urologic surgeon who will be managing the stricture to obtain a full understanding of the length, thickness, and caliber of the stricture. In general, the visual appearance of the epithelium (pink or grey) and the elasticity of the tissue will help determine the degree of spongiofibrosis and possible radiation injury.

Newer studies that use magnetic resonance imaging are currently being investigated for stricture and appear to provide additional information regarding the relationships of soft tissues, including prostate and bladder neck. Although they have shown to influence choice of procedure and appear to be promising results, they have not been evaluated in those patients with a history of radiation therapy. It is unclear whether the presence of radiation seed implants will affect the study.

6. Management of Radiation-Induced Urethral Strictures

In general, radiation impairs the healing potential of tissues, particularly as a result of end arteritis hypo vascularity, decreased intrinsic cellular vitality and interstitial fibrosis. Radiation urethral stricture typically has a unhealthy or "wash leather" appearance on cystoscopy and have varying degrees of local tissue induration or dense fibrotic scarring.

Merrick et al. (2) noted that 29 of 1186 patients developed a membranous or proximal bulbar urethral stricture after prostate BT. All 29 strictures were initially managed by dilation or urethrotomy. Roughly one-third (9/29) had recurrent strictures requiring repeat urethrotomy and intermittent self-catheterization to prevent restenosis. Of these nine, three became obliterative and refractory strictures, and thus were eventually managed with suprapubic urinary diversion. (**Fig. 21.3, A** and **B**) Thus, it appears that roughly one-third of BT-related urethral strictures are recurrent

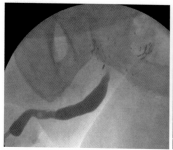 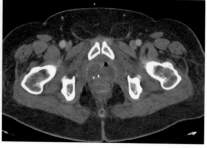

A   **B**

Fig. 21.3. A, B. Prostate liquefaction and obliterative prostatic and membranous urethral strictures after prostate brachytherapy. Note poor distribution of seeds due to tissue liquefaction

and, of these, one-third are devastating, requiring a urinary diversion. Of all the BT-treated patients, the need for supravesical diversion translates to a 0.25% incidence. Others have also noted that most post-BT urethral stricture are minor and can be managed by an endoscopic means. Ragde et al. *(13)* noted 12% bulbomembranous strictures at a median follow-up of 69 mo. Of all their urethral strictures, most were short and managed by urethral dilation with and without self catheterization.

In contrast, Moreira et al. *(14)* reported their experience with severe BN contractures after I^{125} BT in seven patients. All seven had recurrent contractures, each of whom had failed at least three or more intraoperative transurethral incisions. Final management consisted of self catheterization in one, indwelling Foley catheter in one, and open reconstruction and supravesical urinary diversions in the remaining four of seven. Of these diversions, three underwent enterocystoplasty and continent catherizable stomas, and one a salvage cystoprostatectomy and Florida pouch catherizable urinary diversion. All the diversion patients reported successful urinary control and improved quality of life after reconstruction

In our experience, radiation induced urethral strictures have been refractory to urethrotomy or dilation, and thus more mimic the South Florida experience noted previously in this chapter *(14)*. The large proportion of radiation urethral strictures we have treated are typically complex and management dilemmas; yet, this may have more to do with our referral practice, rather then to conclude that minor strictures do not occur after RT. The methods that we have used over the years with our refractory radiation induced strictures have been urethrotomy and intermittent self-catheterization (**Fig. 21.4**), off-label use of the Urolume endourethral prosthesis, excision and primary urethral anastomosis urethroplasty, salvage prostatectomy with anastomotic urethrovesical urethroplasty, combined abdominal-perineal urethroplasty, onlay flap urethroplasty, and supravesical urinary diversion surgery.

In general, urethroplasty for RT strictures should use excision and primary anastomosis (for short bulbar strictures) or an onlay flap. Grafts should be avoided in the radiated field because grafts rely on the host bed for vascularity (imbibition and inosculation), which is typically compromised in the pelvic irradiated patient. Instead, a pedicle island skin

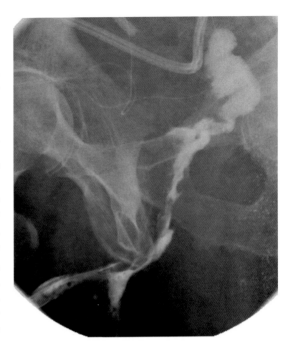

FIG. 21.4. Radiation induced bulbar urethral stricture after EBRT for prostate cancer, managed successfully by urethrotomy and BID intermittent self catheterization x 2 years. RUG demonstrates traumatic self catheterization resulting in proximal bulbo-rectal fistula. Rocky septic course eventually managed by end colostomy, abdominal wash out and SP tube diversion

flap is a good method for reconstructing the radiated stricture, because it has its own blood supply and can be sewn into place as an readily available onlay flap. Another option for urethral reconstruction is the use of extragenital skin that has been grafted onto a gracilis muscle flap and then used as an onlay flap. See chapter 16 in this text by Dr. Zinman for details of this technique.

Hyperbaric oxygen (HBO) therapy had been shown to help stimulate angiogenesis, which can help to physiologically repair the baseline obliterative endarteritis induced ischemia. Treatment typically requires breathing 100% oxygen at two atmospheres of pressure for 2 to 3 h per day for a total of 40 to 60 sessions. HBO has been used with varying results with bladder complications and fair results with grade 2 and 3 rectal complications. Theoretically, HBO could be used as an adjunctive method to promote angiogenesis of the urethra and thus improve the success of a subsequent urethroplasty or a staged reconstruction. However,

Theodorescu et al. *(15)* recently reported on the uniform failure of HBO for Grade 4 RTOG urinary complications. The practical value of HBO for urethral stricture surgery, thus appears to be small.

7. Illustrative Cases

To illustrate some of the surgical methods for dealing with radiation induced urethral strictures, we present a few select cases.

7.1. Case Study 1

J.H. was a 55-yr-old gentleman with a history of hypertension who was diagnosed with Stage T2A Gleason 7(3+4) prostate cancer. He was initially treated with I^{125} brachytherapy in March 2001, followed by a boost of 4500 cGy of EBRT in 25 fractions. He also underwent hormone ablation therapy for a total of 3 yr. His prostate-specific antigen decreased to <0.1. Initial postoperative complications were relatively minor. By December 2003, he developed both obstructive and irritative voiding, with an AUA SS of 27/35 and a Qmax flow rate of 6 mL/s (voided volume 288 mL). Endoscopy noted a membranous stricture to roughly 8 Fr. The patient refused formal urethroplasty, so during the next 2 yrs he was managed with urethral dilation twice and internal urethrotomy once. Subsequent recurrence managed by urethral dilation and Urolume stent. Hyperplastic tissue in growth quickly obstructed the stent after 6 mo. Stricture managed by transurethral resection on a low cutting current (**Fig. 21.5**). *See* Chapter 24 by Brandes in this volume for more details as to managing Urolume stent problems. Currently the stricture has not recurred, yet his AUA SS is moderate at 11 and complains of bothersome postvoid dribbling.

7.2. Case Study 2

M.C. is a 76-yr-old man with peripheral vascular disease, hypertension, and gout with T_{1C} Gleason 8 prostate cancer managed with I^{125} brachytherapy, a boost of EBRT in 2000, followed by hormone ablation therapy. Severe obstructive lower urinary tract symptoms after the radiation until urinary retention in 2002. Membranous and prostatic urethral stricture managed during the next 2 yr by urethral dila-

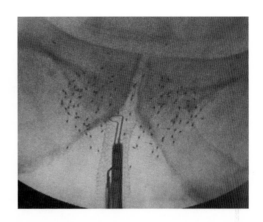

FIG. 21.5. Transurethral resection of hyperplastic ingrowth obstructing Urolume stent placed for prostate brachytherapy induced membranous urethral stricture 6 months before

tion × 2, optical urethrotomy × 2, and TURP × 2, and a failed "cut-to the-light" procedure. Retention developed despite intermittent self-catheterization. In 2005, urethrography noted a 4-cm obliterative membranous and prostatic urethral stricture; confirmed by cystoscopy from above and below (**Fig. 21.6, A** and **B**). Suprapubic tube is placed. Bladder is very friable and he develops hemorrhagic cystitis, eventually responding to 20 treatments of hyperbaric oxygen (discontinued prematurely due to barotrauma). He was unable to keep the SP tube plugged due to small bladder capacity and suffers from bothersome bladder spasms. Because of bladder bother and radiation cystitis, M.C. underwent palliative supratrigonal cystectomy and transverse colo-conduit urinary diversion.

7.3. Case Study 3

N.K. is a 68-yr-old healthy man with only glaucoma who had a history of a bulbar urethral stricture managed by a two stage Johanson urethroplasty in 1980 and 1981. He was voiding well with minimal complaints until being treated for T_{1C} Gleason 6 prostate cancer with three-dimensional conformal EBRT to a total dosage of 78 stage Gy, completed in May 2002. Subsequently, he developed a mid-bulbar urethral stricture and severe obstructive voiding, which was managed initially with optical urethrotomy in January of 2004 and again in 2005. Obstructive voiding reoccured and urethrography was performed, at which we noted a 6-cm midbulbar urethral stricture

FIG. 21.6. A, B. Obliterative prostatic
and membranous urethral strictures
after prostate brachytherapy. Managed
by supravesical diversion; initially by
SP tube, and later by ileal-vesicostomy

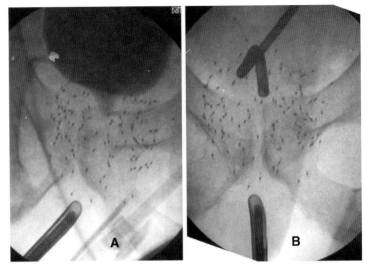

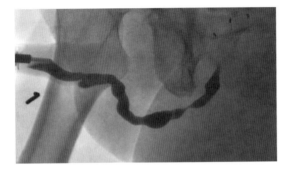

FIG. 21.7. Radiation induced mid bulbar urethral stricture
(6cm) after radiotherapy for Gleason 6 prostate cancer

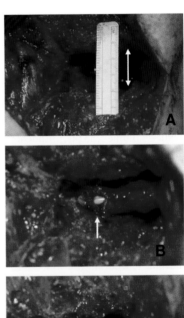

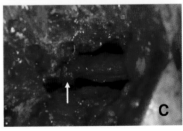

(**Fig. 21.7**). Because of the patient's pelvic irradiation, a fasciocutaneous island flap of penile skin was
selected and sewn in as an onlay flap, through a
scrotal window. His current peak urinary flow rate is
17 mL/s and AUA sympton score is minor at 7.

7.4. Case Study 4

W.L. is a 68-yr-old man with hypertension and GE
reflux who underwent I^{125} brachytherapy in for T_{IC}
Gleason 7 (3+4) prostate cancer. He developed a
dense proximal bulbar-membranous urethral stricture
initially managed by internal urethrotomy on two
occasions. After the second urethrotomy, he developed
an obliterative stricture that was managed by a SP
tube. Urethrography noted a proximal 3-cm postradiation stricture. At the time of his planned perineal
approach urethroplasty, the stricture was too dense
and long to feel through transmission of the antegrade
placed sound. An abdomino-perineal approach was

FIG. 21.8. A–C Abdominoperineal urethroplasty approach
with pubectomy (2.5cm excision) and primary anastomosis, for an obliterative membranous urethral stricture after
pelvic RT

thus performed, which required a total pubectomy to
adequately expose the apex on the prostate (**Fig. 21.8,
A–C**). The urethra was routed through the pubic bone.
The anastomosis subsequently remained open yet he

developed bothersome stress incontinence, requiring two to three large pads per day. Ten months later, a distal bulbar urethral artificial urinary sphincter was placed, which eroded 7 mo later. The plan is for a transcorporal artificial urinary sphincter in the near future.

References

1. Elliot SP, Meng MV, Elkin EP, McAninch JW, Duchane J, Carroll PR (2007) Incidence of urethral stricture after primary treatment for prostate cancer: data From CaPSURE. J Urol 178:529–534
2. Merrick GS, Butler WM (2006) Risk factors for the development of prostate brachytherapy related urethral strictures. J Urol 175:1376–1380
3. Sandhu AS, Zelefsky MJ (2000) Long-term urinary toxicity after 3-dimensional conformal radiotherapy for prostate cancer in patients with prior history of transurethral resection. Int J Radiat Oncol Biol Phys 48:643–647
4. Greskovich, FJ (1991) Complications following external beam radiation therapy for prostate cancer: an analysis of patients treated with and without staging pelvic lymphadenectomy. J Urol 146:798–802
5. Wallner K, Roy J, Harrison L (1995) Dosimetry guidelines to minimize urethral and rectal morbidity following transperineal I-125 prostate brachytherapy. Int J Radiat Oncol Biol Phys 32:465–471
6. Astrom L, Pedersen D (2005) Long-term outcome of high dose rate brachytherapy in radiotherapy of localised prostate cancer. Radiother Oncol 74:157–161
7. Zelefsky MJ, Yamada Y, Cohen G, Venkatraman ES, Fung AY, Furhang E, Silvern D, Zaider M (2000) Postimplantation dosimetric analysis of permanent transperineal prostate implantation: improved dose distributions with an intraoperative computer-optimized conformal planning technique. Int J Radiat Oncol Biol Phys 48:601–608
8. Demanes DJ, Rodriguez RR (2005) High-dose-rate intensity-modulated brachytherapy with external beam radiotherapy for prostate cancer: California endocurietherapy's 10-year results. Int J Radiat Oncol Biol Phys 61:1306–1316
9. Martinez AA, Pataki I (2001) Phase II prospective study of the use of conformal high-dose-rate brachytherapy as monotherapy for the treatment of favorable stage prostate cancer: a feasibility report. Int J Radiat Oncol Biol Phys 49:61–69
10. Albert M, Tempany CM, Schultz D, Chen MH, Cormack RA, Kumar S, Hurwitz MD, Beard C, Tuncali K, O'Leary M, Topulos GP, Valentine K, Lopes L, Kanan A, Kacher D, Rosato J, Kooy H, Jolesz F, Carr-Locke DL, Richie JP, D'Amico AV (2003) Late genitourinary and gastrointestinal toxicity after magnetic resonance image-guided prostate brachytherapy with or without neoadjuvant external beam radiation therapy. Cancer 98:949–954
11. Baskin LS, Constantinescu SC (1993) Biochemical characterization and quantitation of the collagenous components of urethral stricture tissue. J Urol 150:642–647
12. Cavalcanti AG, Yucel S (2004) The distribution of neuronal and inducible nitric oxide synthase in urethral stricture formation. J Urol 171:1943–1947
13. Ragde H (1997) Brachytherapy (seed implantation) for clinically localized prostate cancer. J Surg Oncol 64:79–81
14. Moreira SG Jr, Seigne JD, Ordorica RC, Marcet J, Pow-Sang JM, Lockhart JL (2004) Devastating complications after brachytherapy in the treatment of prostate adenocarcinoma. BJU Int 93:31–35
15. Theodorescu D, Gillenwater JY, Koutrouvelis PG (2000) Prostatourethral-rectal fistula after prostate brachytherapy. Cancer 89:2085–2091

22
Complex Rectourinary and Vesicoperineal Fistulas

Steven B. Brandes

Contents

1. Introduction.. 252
2. Fistula Etiology.. 252
3. Rectourinary Fistulas 252
    3.1. Signs and Symptoms.. 252
    3.2. Diagnosis.. 253
    3.3. Preoperative Assessment and Decision-Making... 254
    3.4. Urinary and Fecal Diversion 254
    3.5. Specific Reconstruction Methods.. 255
4. Large and Complex Fistulas 258
    4.1. Trans-Perineal Approaches 258
    4.2. Gracilis Muscle Flap *(2, 7)* 260
    4.3. Transabdominal Approaches.. 264
5. Rectovesical and Urinary-Perineal Fistulas 265
6. Complex Urinary Fistulas in Patients with Poor Performance Status or Limited Life Expectancy 266
    6.1. Embolization Technique 266
    6.2. Embolization Costs and Outcomes 268
References.. 268

Summary The management and reconstruction of complex rectourinary and vesicoperineal fistulas are some of the most difficult problems to deal with in Urology. To decide on the proper management of such fistulas, a detailed knowledge of the fistula etiology, integrity of the anal and external urethral sphincters, functional status of the bladder, extent of rectal radiation damage, size and location of the urinary fistula, and the overall performance and nutritional status of the patient is needed. Few surgeons have had a large experience with such fistulas, and this is why there is no clear standard surgical repair approach. Treatment needs to be tailored to the specifics of the fistula, the etiology, and the patient.

Fistulas that result from radiation therapy are more complex and more difficult to reconstruct than those developing after other forms of treatment, with the frequent concomitant problems of urinary and fecal incontinence, and/or urethral strictures. Small, non-radiated fistulas often are successfully managed by the transanal or York-Mason approach. Complex fistulas that are large, or of radiation or cryotherapy etiology, are often best managed either by primary repair, buttressed with a gracilis interposition flap, or by proctectomy and colo-anal pull through, or supravescial urinary diversion. Here-in we have detailed the varying surgical methods for fistula repair, as well as for salvage.

From: *Current Clinical Urology: Urethral Reconstructive Surgery*
Edited by: S.B. Brandes © Humana Press, Totowa, NJ

Keywords rectourinary, vesicoperineal, fistulas, York Mason, transsphincteric approaches, Gracilis muscle flap, colo-anal pull through

1. Introduction

To decide on the proper management of a rectourethral fistula (RUF), a detailed knowledge of the fistula etiology, integrity of the anal and external urethral sphincters, functional status of the bladder, extent of rectal radiation damage, size and location of the urinary fistula, and the overall performance and nutritional status of the patient is needed. Small, nonradiated fistulas often are successfully managed by the transanal or York-Mason approach. Complex fistulas that are large or of radiation or cryotherapy etiology are often best managed either by primary repair, buttressed with a gracilis interposition flap, proctectomy and colo-anal pull through, or if the bladder and sphincter function is poor, then by supravesical urinary diversion.

2. Fistula Etiology

By definition, a fistula is an extra-anatomic, epithelialized channel between two hollow organs or a hallow organ and the body surface. Acquired RUFs are uncommon and are usually the result of trauma, pelvic radiation therapy, iatrogenic injury during pelvic surgery (such as laparoscopic and open radical prostatectomy, prostate cryotherapy, or abdominal perineal resection), or an infectious or malignant tumor cause. Concomitant urethral and rectal injuries from blunt abdominal trauma and pelvic fracture or penetrating missile injury has been reported as a cause (yet, admittedly rare cause) for RUFs. Potential infectious causes of RUF include Crohn's disease, fistula in ano, perirectal infections, or tuberculosis. With the increased usage of brachytherapy and its combination with external beam radiotherapy boost, particularly devastating fistulas can occur. Most of the reported cases in the literature are from radical retropubic (laparoscopic or open) or perineal prostatectomy, with an incidence of 1–3.6% for the former and up to 11%, for the later. Rectourethral fistulas after brachytherapy are reported in up to 0.4–0.8% of cases, and for brachytherapy plus external beam radiation therapy (EBRT), up to 2.9% *(1)*. Such radiation fistulas are more common

when being used as salvage therapy or if the anterior rectal wall has been biopsied after RT. Transanal rectal wall or rectal ulcer biopsies (via sigmoidoscope) in the pelvic RT patient are unwise and have a high chance of eliciting a RUF. Reported average time from last RT session until RUF diagnosis is roughly 2 yr. Mean time from a rectal procedure till RUF is 4 mo. Few surgeons have had a large experience with RUF and, thus, there is no clear standard surgical repair approach. Treatment needs to be tailored to the specifics of the fistula, the etiology, and the patient. Fistulas that result from radiation therapy are more complex and more difficult to reconstruct than those developing after other forms of treatment, with the frequent concomitant problems of urinary and fecal incontinence, and/or urethral strictures.

3. Rectourinary Fistulas

3.1. Signs and Symptoms

The presence of a RUF fistula is typically readily apparent. The most common symptoms are watery stools (in roughly 90%), urinary incontinence, irritative voiding complaints, and pneumaturia and fecaluria (in roughly 60%). To a lesser degree, patients present with dysuria, fever, discolored or feculent urine, recurrent urinary tract infections (usually poly-organism), or with an associated metabolic acidosis from systemic absorption (via the colon) of the urine. One of the initial signs of a developing RUF after RT or cryotherapy typically is severe rectal pain, which resolves when the necrotic/ischemic tissue eventually breaks down and the fistula occurs. Although uncommon, pelvic an abdominal sepsis can also be the presenting event (in roughly 10% of cases)

3.2. Diagnosis

Methods used to diagnose a RUF includes endoscopic and radiographic means. (**Fig. 22.1**) Cystoscopy is used to determine the degree of radiation damage to the bladder as to capacity and compliance and the location of the fistula in relation to the ureteral orifices and the bladder neck. Proctoscopy is used to determine the level of rectal entry, to identify the fistula, fistula proximity to the anal sphincter, and to rule out other rectal-colon pathology

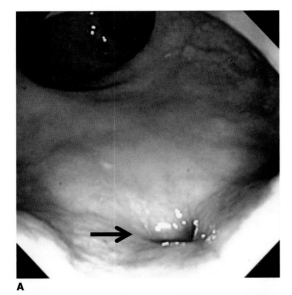

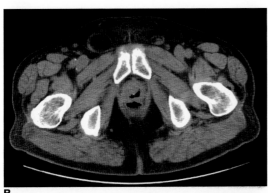

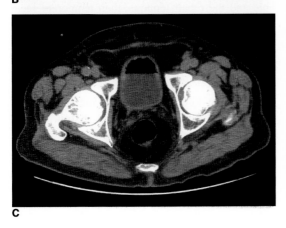

(radiation proctitis, concomitant colon cancer). Other important evaluation methods are examination under anesthesia, digital rectal exam, and retrograde urethrography (RUG) and voiding cystourethrography (VCUG; **Fig. 22.2**). Computed tomography (CT) of the pelvis is typically fairly sensitive and specific qualitatively for diagnosing a fistula, with the note of air in the bladder (without any prior instrumentation), but not readily for location and size of the fistula. Rectovesical fistulas on CT imaging will typically show a thickened trigone and posterior bladder wall and nonspecific bladder air (without being instrumented). For cases of high index of suspicion but negative studies, an oral charcoal slurry test followed by urinalysis for charcoal can be performed. The Bourne test is also helpful in making a diagnosis. Here, oral contrast is consumed by the patient, or a hypaque enema performed, and the urine collected, centrifuged, and X-rayed. Radio-opaque material in the radiograph confirms the presence of a fistula. When the fistula is small, flow through the fistula is typically in "one way," from the high-pressure to low-pressure system. The low trans-sphincteric RUF of Crohn's disease or an anterior rectal space

Fig. 22.1. Prostato-rectal fistula after cryotherapy for low stage prostate cancer. (A) Colonoscope view of fistula (arrow marks fistula). (B) Pelvic CT of the fistula. Note air in prostate and rectum (noninstrumented system). (C) CT demonstrating air in bladder (noninstrumented system)

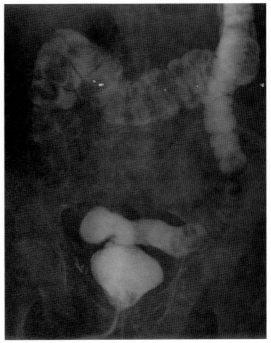

Fig. 22.2. Cystogram demonstrating vesico-rectal fistula

infection is difficult to diagnose and often demand magnetic resonance imaging of the pelvis, combined with meticulous transanal examination.

3.3. Preoperative Assessment and Decision-Making

To decide how to manage and repair RUF, it is essential to preoperatively determine the function of the anal and external urethral sphincters, the presence of a concomitant urethral stricture or bladder neck contracture, the visible and palpable health of the tissue adjacent and near the fistula, and the size and location of the fistula (particularly in its proximity to the ureteral orifices). Another important factor to determine preoperatively is patient nutritional status, performance status, and overall condition. Cigarette smoking will greatly impair the chances for a successful fistula repair and reconstruction. We routinely send such patients to a smoking-cessation program.

The function and capacity of the bladder is also important to determine. Unfortunately, urodynamics is usually difficult, if not impossible, to perform in patients with a large RUF. Although others claim that a Fogarty balloon can be passed to occlude the fistula and then perform a urodynamics study, we have not had success with this technique.

Instead, we typically rely on the visual appearance of the bladder urothelium as a surrogate measure of bladder radiation damage and postfistula repair poor bladder capacity. Urothelium that appears white/blanched, or hemorrhagic (friable with multiple telangiectasias) often demonstrates bladder dysfunction and radiation damage. Such visual changes do not portend well for good postsurgical bladder capacity.

3.4. Urinary and Fecal Diversion

3.4.1. Indications for Diversion

Patients who present with RUF but without evidence of surrounding inflammation or sepsis, fecal, and urinary diversion are not essential prior to fistula repair and can be delayed till the time of fistula surgery. However, if the patient is particularly symptomatic and suffers from recurrent sepsis, despite suppressive antibiotics, severe rectal pain, or overwhelming urinary and/or fecal incontinence,

then fecal and urinary proximal diversion should be performed and the patients nutritionally supplemented. Conversely, if a patient with a radiation RUF has not been diverted before presentation, such patients typically undergo fecal and urinary diversion to prevent sepsis and to reduce inflammation around the fistula track.

In rare and fairly select cases, some small surgical fistulas (up to 25%) will close spontaneously with just urinary (suprapubic or Foley catheter) and/or rectal diversion and suppressive antibiotics. Such conservative therapies are usually reserved for poor surgical candidates *(2)*.

Moreover, if the rectal sphincter is irreversibly injured or incompetent, an end colostomy is usually the better option for fecal diversion. If a reconstructive procedure is a potential option, a temporary loop ileostomy (up stream segment of bowel), which can easily be performed laparoscopically is also performed. Laparoscopic loop ileostomy is a quick, less invasive, and readily reversible form of diversion without the need for a staged laparotomy for reversal. For cases of tenuous repair, previous failed attempts at fistula repair, complex (radiation or cryotherapy induced), or large fistulas that cannot be closed primarily and require adjunctive procedures such as a patch graft and/or muscle interposition flap, fecal diversion is generally mandatory for a successful outcome. A general rule of thumb is that if the tissues are friable and the repair tenuous, then temporary fecal diversion should be part of the reconstruction.

3.4.2. Anatomy of the Anal Sphincter and Rectum

An intimate knowledge of the rectal and anal anatomy allows for successful fistula repair, with limited morbidity. The levator ani muscles are divided in a lateral and medial division: the medial division is the puborectalis sling, which forms a muscular sling that arises from the pubic bone and encircles the anorectal flexure. This sling is crucial to maintaining fecal continence. The most caudal part of the sling forms the longitudinally oriented external anal sphincter (**Fig. 22.3**). The blood supply to the levator ani and the external and internal anal sphincters is the pudendal artery, while the nervous innervation comes from the pelvic plexus, from the

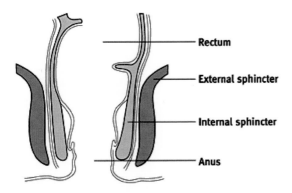

FIG. 22.3. Muscles of the anal sphincter

— Rectum

— External sphincter

— Internal sphincter

— Anus

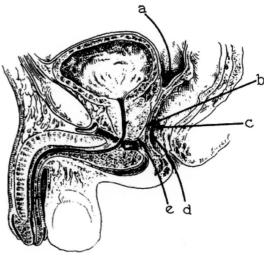

FIG. 22.4. Approaches for repair of rectourethral fistulas. (A) Transabdominal. (B) Kraske laterosacral. (C) Posterior transsphincteric (York Mason). (D) Transanal. (E) Perineal. From Wood TW (1990) Middleton: single-stage transrectal transsphincteric (modified York Mason) repair of rectourinary fistulas. Urology 35:27–30

S2–S4 nerve roots. The nerves and vasculature to the rectum are enclosed within a fascial capsule, known as Waldeyer's fascia. The ventral aspect of Waldeyer's fascia is more commonly known as Denonvier's fascia.

3.5. Specific Reconstruction Methods

As to evidence that there is no one correct method and that there is uncertainty as to what the best approach for repair is, is that there are numerous surgical procedures detailed for fistula repair. The surgical technique selected is largely dictated by the surgeon's preference, as well as the size, location, and etiology of the fistula (**Fig. 22.4**).

3.5.1. Transanal Rectal Advancement Flap

A sliding rectal advancement flap performed transanally is an effective method for small nonradiated, low-lying prostate-rectal fistulas (3). The procedure is very well tolerated and relatively minimally invasive. Reported success rates range from 75% to 100%. The patient is placed jackknife prone, the anus dilated, and a speculum and/or Lonestar retractor used to expose the fistula in the anterior wall of the rectum. The tissue surrounding the fistula (lateral and distal) is de-epithelized. A "U"-shaped incision is made in the rectal wall, to create a full-thickness rectal wall flap that is advanced distally to cover the fistula and sutured to the edges of the caudal denuded rectal mucosa. (**Fig. 22.5**). The fistula is closed primarily with interrupted absorbable polyglactin (vicryl) sutures. No suture lines are overlapping. We have had particularly good success with

this technique for surgical fistulas after open or laparoscopic radical prostatectomy. As a relatively minimally invasive procedure, proximal fecal diversion is typically not performed. For failures, the advancement flap can be repeated, along with a diverting loop ileostomy and urinary diversion. The other option for failures, which prefer, is the anterior trans-perineal approach, buttressed with gracilis muscle flap.

3.5.2. Posterior-Sagittal Approach

For fistulas that are too low to approach from the abdominal incision and too high to access from below, the posterior-sagittal approach was described in the late 1800s. Kraske popularized this technique, where a posterior midline incision is made extending to the left paramedian aspect of the coccyx and sacrum, that often required coccygectomy and sacrectomy. Here, the rectum is swept laterally to avoid dividing the anal sphincter.

3.5.3. York Mason Repair

The York Mason technique is a posterior, mid-sagittal, trans-anosphincteric approach to RUF repair (4). It is the most reported and widely used

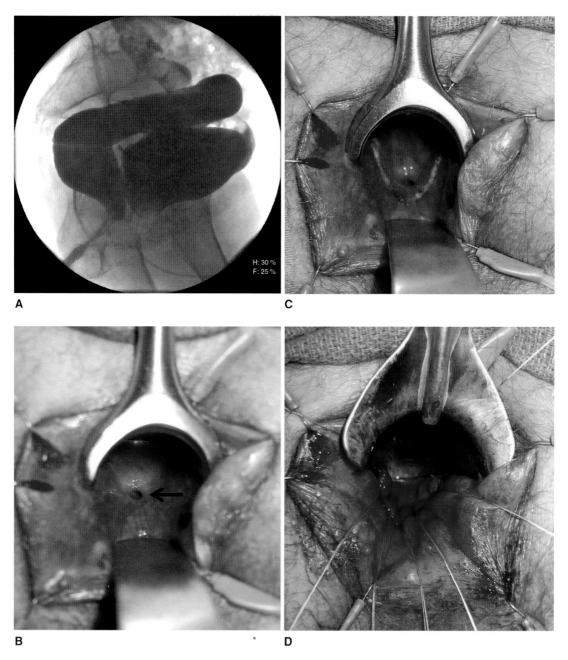

FIG. 22.5. Bladder neck-rectal fistula after salvage radical prostatectomy for post HIFU local recurrence. (A) Hypaque enema demonstrating bladder filling. (B) Transanal view of fistula (arrow). (C) Sliding flap marked out. (D) Sliding rectal flap advanced distally and sewn into place with interrupted sutures

repair method. It is often not necessary to perform concomitant fecal and urinary diversion at the time of the fistula repair. In general, York Mason repairs are useful and successful in small postsurgical fistulas (especially those that follow radical prostatectomy) that are too proximal and thus hard to reach with a sliding rectal flap. York Mason is not a suitable for large, complex (radiation, cryotherapy etc.) fistulas that may require an interposition muscle flap, concurrent urethral reconstruction, or patch grafting. Other relative contraindications for the York-Mason are prior anorectal dysfunction or impaired wound healing (e.g., after RT, or in patients with HIV). In the properly selected patient, York Mason had good success without severe bowel dysfunction or fecal incontinence, except for a higher incidence of impaired flatulence control.

The key to preventing fecal incontinence is a midline trans-sphincteric incision, careful tagging of the sphincteric muscle, followed by an anatomical restoration of the rectal wall. The patient initially is cystoscoped and a wire and subsequent catheter placed across the fistula. The patient is then placed prone, jackknife, the buttocks taped laterally and an incision made from the tip of the coccyx to the anal verge (**Fig 22.6**, inset). The posterior anal sphincter is divided and each layer is carefully tagged for subsequent reconstruction. The anterior rectum and fistula are well exposed once the posterior rectal mucosa is divided (**Fig. 22.6**). The main advantage to the York Mason approach it that it allows rapid

access through unscarred tissue and provides a wide working space to operate in. The posterolateral rectal innervations, urinary continence, and potency are consistently preserved by staying in the midline and avoiding the lateral pelvic and pararectal space. The fistula is sharply excised, and the rectum and urinary tracts are separated and undermined. After closure of the fistula in the urethra, a full-thickness rectal wall flap is developed and sutured down in a "vest over pant" method. In so doing, the suture lines do not overlap. Alternatively, a fish-mouth-shaped excision of the fistula, followed by primary closure can be made. The rectum is closed in two layers with absorbable interrupted sutures. Each of the paired anal sphincter sutures is then tied, and the rectal wall and the sphincteric muscle components carefully restored. A pre-sacral drain is left in place for 2 d. Urethral catheterization is maintained for 3 wk or until cystourethrography demonstrates no leak. This approach, in the properly selected patient, has a low recurrence rate, and demonstrates that anal sphincter can be divided, and not result in fecal incontinence.

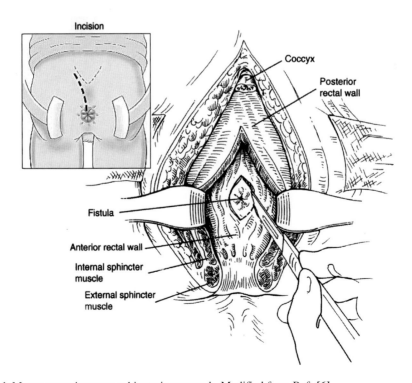

FIG. 22.6. York Mason posterior trans-sphincteric approach. Modified from Ref. *[6]*

4. Large and Complex Fistulas

For large prostato-rectal or perineal urinary fistulas in radiated field, salvage prostatectomy sounds
at first like a good idea. However, in our hands,
we have found that salvage prostatectomy typically
results in vesicourethral anastomotic stricture and/
or severe urinary incontinence. Therefore, we
prefer either to repair such urinary fistulas by the
methods detailed in this section, or to perform an
exenterative pelvic surgery with concomitant ileal
or colo-conduit, or at times, a continent catherizable stoma/neobladder *(5)*.

4.1. Trans-Perineal Approaches

For repair of RUF, we prefer to use an anterior perineal approach augmented with a gracilis muscle flap
for bulk and vascular tissue interposition. Obviously,
fistula size, etiology, location, failed prior attempts
of repair, and concomitant urethral or bladder neck
stricture, determine the specific procedure.

4.1.1. Trans-Sphincteric Anterior Approaches

We have found the trans-sphincteric method of
Gecetler et al. *(6)* to be successful for small fistulas of postsurgical (after open or laparoscopic
prostatectomy) or trauma (pelvic fracture) etiology
and/or when a simultaneous urethral stricture and
reconstruction is planned. A normal anal sphincter
and lack of any anorectal pathology is essential. The
patient is placed in the lithotomy position with stirrups. The patient is cystoscoped and the fistula cannulated with a wire, which is subsequently pulled
out the rectum and used as a guide for Fogarty or
Foley placement through the fistula, via the rectum.
An incision is made in the midline perineum from
the scrotal base to the anal verge. The transverse
perinei, the perineal body, and the anal sphincter
(through both the external and internal anal sphincter and rectal wall) are divided in the posterior
midline, in the same manner as a York Mason.
Each of the components of the internal and external
anal sphincter are carefully tagged with sutures in
pairs for subsequent anatomic reconstruction of the
sphincters (**Fig. 22.7**). A bulbar or membranous
urethral stricture can be repaired at this time either
by excision with primary urethral anastomosis (for a
short stricture) or by a substitution method of graft

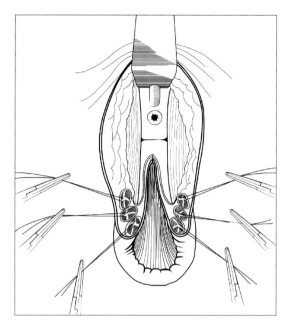

FIG. 22.7. Transsphincteric anterior approach to a RUF
(after Gectler). Note tags on divided anal sphincter

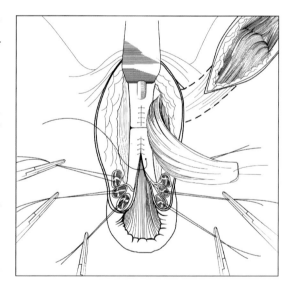

FIG. 22.8. Gracilis interposition flap to repair fistula

or flap (for longer, more complex, strictures). The
fistula is repaired primarily of with a free graft,
followed by a buttress of a gracilis muscle flap,
transferred from the posterior medial thigh (**Fig. 22.8**).
The sphincters are reconstructed and the rectum
closed in two layers with with absorbable polyglactin suture. Catheters are maintained for minimum

of 3 wk, or until the cystogram shows no leak. Anal sphincteric control of solid stool takes roughly 3 wk, whereas control of liquid and gas typically takes 6 or more weeks. If a fecal diversion has been performed, we usually delay reversal for at least 3 mo after fistula repair, when cystoscopy and or urethrography demonstrates a healed rectal and urethral lumen and the anal sphincter is intact and functional.

4.1.2. Anterior Perineal Approach

In general, the anterior perineal approach buttressed with gracilis muscle is our preferred method for repairing RUF (**Fig. 22.9**) *(7)*. The patient is placed in the lithotomy position, and a classic inverted "U" incision (perineal prostatectomy like incision) is made in the perineum (**Fig. 22.9A**). A transverse incision is made 3 cm anterior to the anal verge, and then carried medial to the ischial tuberosities, and posteriorly to lie lateral to the sphincter at 3 and 9 o'clock. The ischio-rectal fossa are then dissected out bilaterally bluntly and with electrocautery. The central tendon is isolated bluntly and then divided (**Fig. 22.9B**). Dissection is then performed between the longitudinal rectal fibers on the ventral aspect of the rectal wall and the external anal sphincter. A finger in the rectum helps control the depth of dissection. The longitudinal fibers of the rectum are followed to the rectourethralis muscle, which attaches to the rectum to the posterior GU diaphragm. The rectourethralis is then divided. A plane is dissected between the rectum and the prostate and bladder to the level of the peritoneal reflection. The dissection starts superior to the anal sphincter and is then carried down onto the rectum. By avoiding any

lateral or posterior dissection, the innervation of the anal sphincter is preserved. A Lowsley prostatectomy sound (retractor) can be placed in the urethra and into the bladder to help localize and palpate the prostate and the fistula. A blue colored Foley catheter (modified into a Council with a distal hole) placed into the bladder over a guide wire, greatly facilitates dissection. Often times, the Lowsley can be difficult to place because the pelvis/prostate are often fixed. Otherwise, under cystoscopic guidance, a wire and subsequent small council tipped catheter or Fogarty is placed across the fistula. If the fistula is small, it can be dilated with sounds until a size that a small catheter can be placed across. The rectum, urethra and prostate are widely separated (**Fig. 22.10**). The rectum is widely mobilized and preferentially closed transversely in two-layered closure to prevent anal stenosis. The fistula margins are typically debrided till a supple margin. The hole on the urinary side is closed primarily with interrupted suture, if the fistula is small. When the defect is too large to be easily closed primarily, a tailored buccal graft is placed on the urethra or prostate fistula defect. When there is only a fistula, even if large, some do not sew a graft into the fistula, but instead feel that the interposition muscle flap is sufficient for tissue in-growth from the sides. We have no experience with this technique modification.

When there is a concomitant stricture of the membranous urethra, the urethrotomy can be extended ventrally from the level of the fistula and through the stricture. Into the defect (stricturotomy) a muscle flap augmented buccal graft or only flap are typically placed. The proximal graft is covered with a well vascularized gracilis muscle

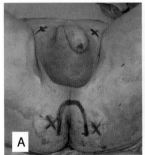 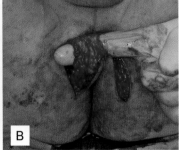 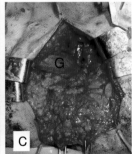

FIG. 22.9. Rectourethral fistula. (A) Exposure in lithotomy position by inverted "U" incision. "x" marks ischial tuberosities. (B) Transection of central tendon as is done with perineal prostatectomy. (C) Gracilis flap from right thigh shown mobilized and placed as an interposition flap and fistula coverage

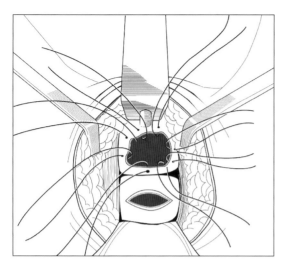

FIG. 22.10. Perineal approach and exposure of prostate-rectal fistula. Note wide separation of the prostate and rectum and stay sutures placed in the prostate to "parachute" a buccal graft

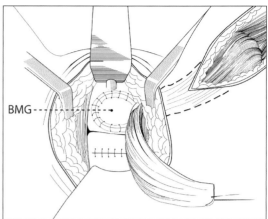

FIG. 22.11. Completed buccal graft to prostatic fistula. On the right is a gracilis muscle flap mobilized as an interposition flap and to provide buccal graft vascularity

flap while the proximal bulbar areas can be covered by the corpus spongiosum (as in a spongioplasty; **Fig. 22.11**). The grafts are fenestrated and quilted/sutured to the gracilis muscle. In so doing, the muscle acts as the vascular bed for the graft. The muscle flap is the main reason that the fistula repair is successful, by separating the rectal and urethral suture lines, filling the dead space, and interposing well vascularized nonradiated tissue that can act as a host bed. The transperineal approach with muscle flap interposition has a reported success of roughly 87%. The transperineal approach is best suited when the rectum and perirectal tissues are not overly damaged and will allow adequate healing and primary closure of the rectum.

Potential complications of this method include minor fecal soiling (up to 8%), anal stenosis (4%, managed by periodic dilation), and urinary incontinence (29–50%) (*2*). For stress urinary incontinence, these have been successfully managed by artificial urinary sphincters. However, urge incontinence, because of a small contacted radiated bladder, is very refractory to conservative treatments, such as anticholinergics. Such patients will require adjunctive procedures such as augmentation cystoplasty or exenterative procedures and urinary diversion. In our recent review of our last 17 patients with RUF, we concluded that patients that are pelvic radiation

naïve, RUF can successfully be managed by rectal sliding advancement flaps (*8*). However, complex RUF in patients treated with pelvic radiation, at times may be better served by exenterative surgeries, due to severe underlying bladder and sphincter dysfunction. Therefore, proper patient selection is the key. Although it is often difficult to determine preoperative bladder capacity or sphincter function, this is essential to determine the optimal surgery so that social urinary continence can be achieved.

4.2. Gracilis Muscle Flap (*2,7*)

The gracilis muscle is long and thin, tapering from its widest point superiorly to a tendinous insertion on the medial knee inferiorly. It acts as a thigh adductor and a flexor of the knee joint, but when mobilized causes no significant donor functional loss. It is an expendable muscle since the adductor longus and magnus totally replace the function of adduction of the thigh. The medial thigh scar is slightly posterior to the midline and relatively inconspicuous. The consistent vascular anatomy and relative ease of dissection make this muscle an excellent choice for perineal and urethral reconstruction. See **Table 22.1** for a summary of gracilis muscle flap characteristics.

4.2.1. Anatomy

The origin of the gracilis muscle starts with a tendinous aponeurosis to the ischiopubic ramus and

TABLE 22.1. Gracilis muscle flap characteristics.

Function	Adducts the thigh and flex the knee
Origin	Ischium and inferior ramus of pubis
Insertion	Medial tibia
Nerve supply	A branch of the obturator nerve (L2, 3, 4)
Size	4–8 cm wide; length = Patient's inner thigh length
Blood supply	Single artery off profunda femoral artery
Artery	Small; <1–2 mm
Vein(s)	2 venae, 1 often larger than the artery
Pedicle length	Usually no more than 4 cm

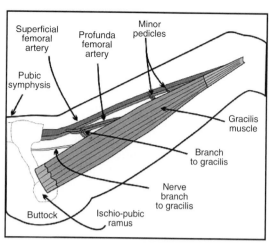

FIG. 22.13. Gracilis muscle blood supply. Note main pedicle from profunda femoral artery and secondary minor pedicles distally. (From Buntic R. Gracilis Muscle Flap. www.microsurgeon.com)

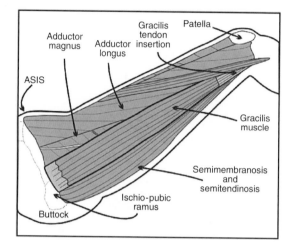

FIG. 22.12. Gracilis origin on ischiopubic ramus and insertion distally on medial tibia at adductor tubercle. Muscle lies on adductor magnus. (From Buntic R. Gracilis Muscle Flap. www.microsurgeon.com)

distally, inserts into the adductor tubercle (medial condyle) of the tibia. Depending on patient leg length, the gracilis muscle is approximately 24 to 30 cm in length and roughly 6 cm wide, proximally and 4 cm, distally. The width of the muscle can be extended by splitting the investing epimysium, which will increase the width an additional 30 to 50%. The muscle lies on the adductor magnus along most of its course, with the adductor longus superiorly and the sartorius inferiorly (**Fig. 22.12**). At the gracilis muscle's distal aspect, the saphenous vein lies just superficial and anterior to it. The muscle is innervated by the anterior branch of the obturator nerve. The nerve enters the muscle slightly more cephalad and superior to the upper aspects of the vascular pedicle. A long leash of nerve can usually be dissected free (up to 6–7 cm). Under loupe magnification, the nerve can even be

dissected intraneurally, so that the muscle can be split into smaller anterior and posterior segments, if so needed.

4.2.2. Vascular Anatomy

The gracilis has a single dominant and secondary minor vascular pedicle. The primary pedicle is very consistently located about 8–12 cm (mean, 10 cm) distal to the bony origin. The main arterial supply is the medial circumflex femoral, which is a proximal branch of the profunda femoral vessels in most cases, running between the adductor longus and magnus muscles and then enters the undersurface of the gracilis. The artery is surprisingly small in comparison to most muscle flaps, with an external diameter of less than 1 millimeter in pediatric patients, and ranging from 1 to 2 mm in the adult. It has two veins, often smaller than the artery, although occasionally one is larger. On rare occasions, the gracilis is supplied by two arteries and with an origin from the adductor pedicle. The medial circumflex femoral pedicle measures 7 to 10 cm in length and emerges between the adductor brevis and the adductor longus, with small branches to both muscles. The artery enters the gracilis and branches into four or five branches, which pass proximally and distally along the muscle. The muscle also has two distal, relatively insignificant arterial branches, which can be routinely sacrificed (**Fig. 22.13**).

4.2.3 Surgical Dissection

The patient is typically placed in the lithotomy position, and the entire lower extremity is prepped and draped and positioned with the leg abducted and the knee flexed (**Fig. 22.14**). It is wise to prep out both legs since one gracilis muscle may have insufficient bulk to cover the fistula repair. The gracilis can also be harvested in the prone position (**Fig. 22.15**). The muscle location is marked by first drawing a line from the pubic tubercle to the medial tibial condoyle of the knee. We then measure from the inguinal crease distally and place a mark on the skin at 8 to 10 cm. This marks the likely insertion site of the vascular pedicle.

The incision is then made two to three finger breaths posterior and parallel to this line and distal to the pedicle insertion. The incision site often appears to be overly posterior to the untrained eye. The muscle is easily identified at the base of the wound after the subcutaneous fat and muscular fascia are divided. On the anterior border of the muscle the vascular pedicle and nerve can be identified 8 to 10 cm distal to the ischiopubic ramus entering the deep surface of the gracilis (**Fig. 22.16**). Early identification of the pedicle enables the dissection to proceed more rapidly. Since the vessels to the gracilis are so small, we refer to use a hand-held Doppler to help confirm

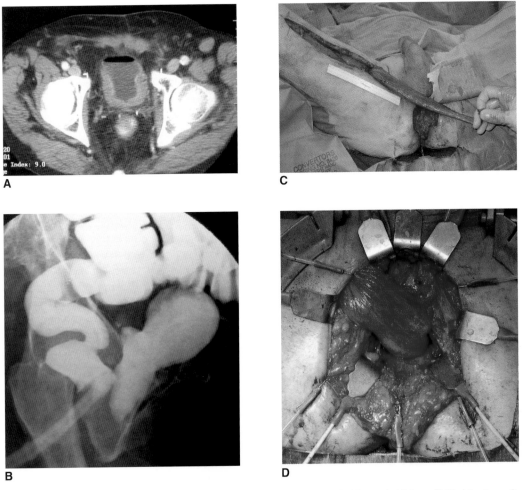

A

C

B

D

Fig. 22.14. Prostatorectal fistula. (A) CT of pelvis. Note typical air in bladder and thick wall bladder base from chronic infections. (B) Hypaque enema noting bladder filling. (C) Gracilis mobilized from right inner thigh. Note muscle length and mobility. (D) Completed gracilis flap to fistula site

FIG. 22.15. Gracilis muscle mobilized in the prone position. Note main incision and small distal counter incision

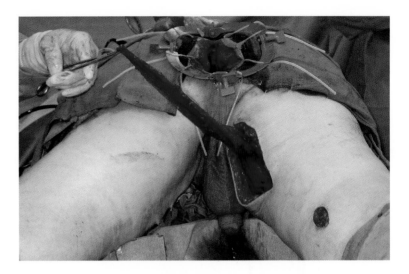

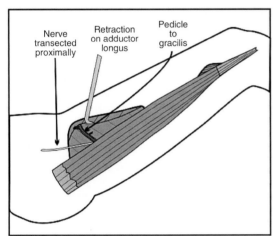

FIG. 22.16. Adductor longus freed and retracted away from underlying magnus to expose pedicle. Note vascular pedicle and nerve. (From Buntic R. Gracilis Muscle Flap. www.microsurgeon.com)

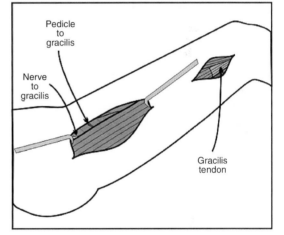

FIG. 22.17. Distal counter incision to identify and dissect free the gracilis tendinous insertion. (From Buntic R. Gracilis Muscle Flap. www.microsurgeon.com)

their location. The proximal dominant pedicle is preserved, but not skeletonized, so as to avoid vascular spasm and injury. A Penrose drain is placed around the muscle and used as a handle to facilitate dissection. A small counter-incision is then performed over the distal leg to identify and dissect free the tendinous insertion (**Fig. 22.17**).

Alternatively, both incisions can be joined to form a single large exposure. The distal accessory pedicles are difficult to discern and vascular control is easily achieved with electrocautery. Counter-traction on the muscle helps to ensure the tendon dissected out is in continuity with the

gracilis muscle. The gracilis tendon can be easily distinguished by being distinctively long and its insertion on the medial tibial tubercle (**Fig. 22.18**). The semitendinosis and semimembranosis tendons are thicker, more posterior, and shorter then the gracilis tendon.

With the distal tendon transected, the muscle is freed up by blunt finger dissection and electrocautery. The fascial attachments of the adductor longus to the adductor magnus are freed superior and inferior to the pedicle, and the adductor longus is retracted away from the magnus. The gracilis muscle is mobilized enough in order to

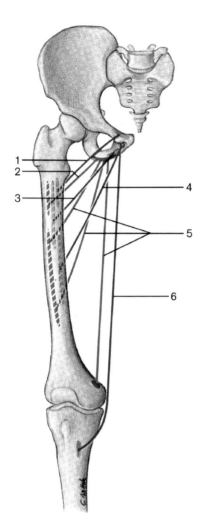

FIG. 22.18. Course of adductor muscles demonstrating origin and insertions. 1 = pectineus 2 = adductor minimus; 3 = adductor brevis; 4 = adductor longus; 5 = adductor magnus; 6 = gracilis, note long and distal tendon insertion onto tibial condyle. (From Rohen JW, Yokochi C, Igaku-Shoin (ed) Color Atlas of Anatomy. New York, 1983.)

reach into the perineum. The thigh incisions are closed in 3 layers, with the skin by a running subcuticular stitch. A single suction drain and a light compressive dressing are placed to help prevent seroma formation. Post surgery, the drain is removed when serous output is minimal and anticoagulants are stopped. Patient ambulation can begin as soon as it is indicated with regard to the reconstruction.

4.3. Transabdominal Approaches

The trans-abdominal approach uses an omental or rectus muscle flap for repair or a colo-anal sleeve pull through procedure (after Park's or Turnball-Cutait). *See* Chapter 26 in by Brandes in this volume on ometum, which details the anatomy and methods for mobilizing and lengthening the omentum. The other advantage of the trans-abdominal approach is that a simultaneous fecal diversion can be performed. Limitations of trans-abdominal are that the pelvis can be deep and narrow and make exposure poor, particularly because most rectourethral fistulas are below the level of the levator ani. Furthermore, abdominal surgery is more morbid and more of a cardiovascular stressor then perineal surgery. Fistulas that are rectovesical or vesico-perineal can be more easily exposed abdominally the rectourethral fistulas.

4.3.1. Abdomino-Perineal Approach (Turnball-Cutait Colo-Anal Pull Through)

When the rectum is extensively damaged by radiation that will not allow primary rectal closure due to severe radiation proctitis or extensive tissue loss, these fistulas are often better managed by proctectomy and pull through of healthy rectum. The patient is initially placed in the prone jack-knife position and a proctectomy and buccal graft closure of the urinary fistula performed. The patient is then positioned supine and a midline abdominal incision made. The rectosigmoid colon is divided intra-abdominally as is the distal rectum at the dentate line (preserving the anal sphincter). The proximal sigmoid colon is then pulled through to cover the patched or repaired fistula and in so doing provides an excellent vascular bed to insure healing and take of the graft, and suture lines are not overlapping. The sigmoid is left emanating from the anus is moist gauze. In a delayed fashion, the segment of exteriorized colon is transected and the colon is sutured to the dentate line, with the mesentery facing the urethral side. By doing such a delayed pull through operation, there are no overlapping suture lines. After a few days, the distal colon has adhered in place, and then the anastomosis is performed.

5. Rectovesical and Urinary-Perineal Fistulas

We place such patients jack-knife prone (**Fig. 22.19**). Open the perineum and the intragluteal fold. Such fistulas typically occur after abdomino-perineal rectal resection (APR). Such patients have often received neoadjuvant pelvic radiation and chemotherapy. Often, a coccygectomy will need to be performed for exposure. Under cystoscopy, the fistula is cannulated and a Fogarty of small Foley is placed across ans secured. Oftentimes, the fistulas are cephalad and

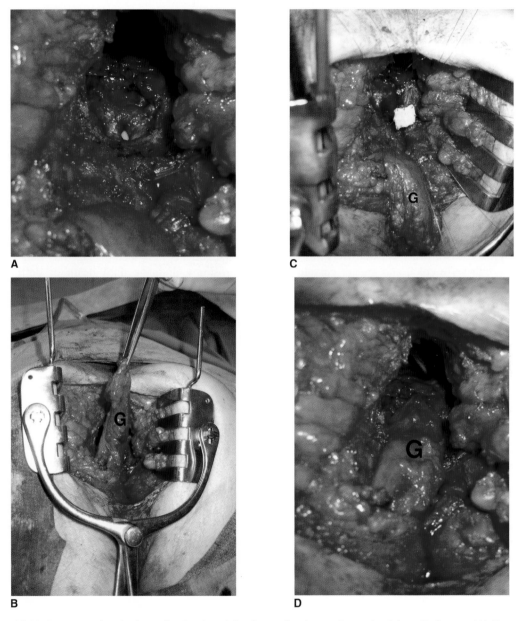

FIG. 22.19. Prostatoperineal urinary fistula after abdomino-perineal resection and pelvic radiotherapy. (A) Prostatic fistula exposed via paracoccyxygeal incision in prone position. (B) Gracilis muscle mobilized into perineal wound. Note "Bear claw" retractor for excellent exposure. (C) "Parachuting" in the buccal graft to the prostatic fistula. "G" denotes gracilis muscle flap. (D) Gracilis flap in place over buccal graft

that under the sacrum. Here a sacrectomy may be needed for exposure. To fill the dead space once an abdominal incision is made, a paddle of de-epithelialized skin and subcutaneous fat based on a pedicle of the gracilis muscle can be used. The inferior gluteus maximus can be mobilized to fill the space, once detached from ileal sacral ridge. Our institution's plastics surgeons, however, feel that the gluteus muscle does not have sufficient mobility; so, we have little experience with this technique. *See* Chapter 16 by Zinman in this volume for more details on the gluteal muscle flap. The recto-vesical fistula typically drains into a radionecrotic cavity, which then fistulizes to the perineum. Once the radionecrotic cavity is exposed, it should be curetted of its poorly vascularized tissue. Rectovesical fistulas are typically cephalad and difficult to reach perineally. Furthermore, the gracilis flap often-times will not be long enough to reach, or is tethered by a high or distal vascular pedicle.

When the dead space to fill is large, tissue transfer methods to fill the gap are: a rectus abdominal muscle flap, bilateral gracilis (gracilis with a de-epithelized myocutaneous paddle) or by omentum (when it is robust), which is extensively mobilized off the transverse colon and greater curvature of the stomach to lengthen it. Another management option is a proctectomy and closure of the defect or supravesical urinary diversion.

6. Complex Urinary Fistulas in Patients with Poor Performance Status or Limited Life Expectancy

Patients with complex urinary fistulas and urinary incontinence need to have a decent performance status to undergo a major surgical reconstruction and repair of the fistula. Patients who have multiple comorbidities and, thus, poor surgical candidates with limited life expectancy, have limited options for managing their urinary fistulas. Typically a suprapubic tube is initially placed to divert the urine away from the urethral-rectal or urethral perineal fistula, as long as the internal urinary sphincter is intact. However, if the bladder neck is open or the urinary fistula is in the bladder, then the only noninvasive method to proximally divert the urine is bilateral percutaneous nephrostomy tube

placement. Although in most cases the nephrostomies can divert the urine, in some instances the majority of the urine still travels down the ureters. An effective and durable method for managing such urinary fistulas and incontinence, is bilateral percutaneous nephrostomy tube placement, followed by trans-ureteric embolization of the distal ureters with a combination of Giantuco coils (steel coils) and Gelfoam (gelatin sponge; **Fig. 22.20**).

During the last 12 yr, we have managed 29 patients (23 women and 6 men; mean age 59 years, SD 16) with complex urinary fistulas from the bladder or urethra, that were refractory to nephrostomy drainage alone *(9)*. One patient had a history of severe perineal trauma, and the remaining 28 had a history of cancer. None of the patients were surgical candidates because of severe co-morbidities or had a limited life expectancy. Seventeen fistulas occurred in the setting of previous surgery. Twenty patients had received adjunctive pelvic irradiation, and 11 had had chemotherapy. In all, refractory urinary incontinence was managed by embolization of 52 ureters. Patients were then managed by long-term nephrostomy drainage until death or definitive reconstructive surgery.

6.1. Embolization Technique

In brief, the procedure is done with the patient under local anesthesia and conscious sedation. A nephrostomy tube is placed into both kidneys before embolization. Each nephrostomy tube is replaced at the time of embolization with an access sheath of comparable outer diameter (**Fig. 22.20A**). A nephrostogram is performed and a 4- or 5-French end-hole catheter advanced co-axially into the distal ureter A nest of 0.9 mm stainless-steel coils (Gianturco Coils, Cook, Bloomington, IN) is created with various sizes of 5 to 12 mm in diameter (**Fig. 22.20B**). Between 4 and 12 coils are typically needed to occlude the ureter. In some cases, gelatin sponge pledgets (Gelfoam) were also sandwiched among the coil nests, to hasten lumen occlusion. An antegrade nephrostogram is then taken to confirm occlusion of flow at the level of the coils (**Fig. 22.20C**). The access sheath is then replaced with a 10- or 12-French (depending on surgeon preference)

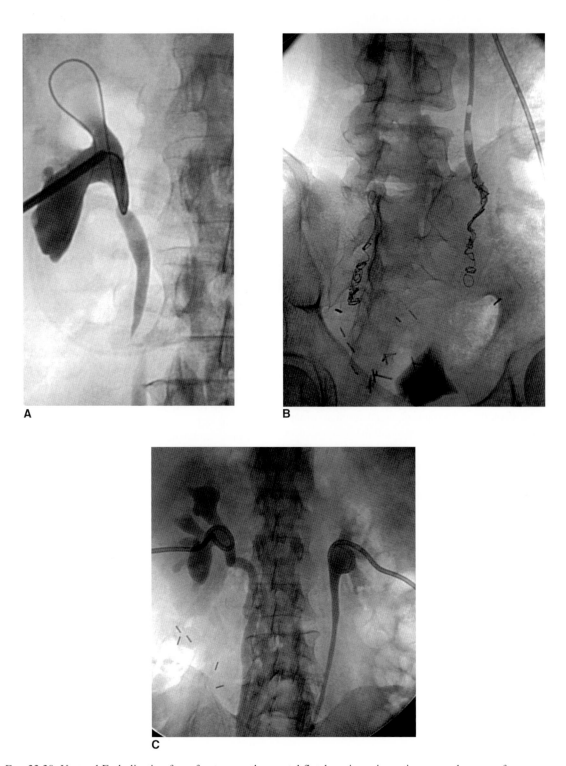

FIG. 22.20. Ureteral Embolization for refractory urethro-rectal fistula, urinary incontinence, and poor performance status. (A) Access sheath placed percutaneously into renal pelvis. (B) Deployed Gianturco coils into distal ureters. Left nephrostogram notes obstruction. (C) Nephrostomy tube placement after ureter embolization

nephrostomy tube and placed to gravity drainage. Subsequently, nephrostomy catheters are exchanged, typically every 8 wk. The advantages of this procedure are the ease of using an existing nephrostomy tract and the ready availability and familiarity with the necessary equipment.

6.2. Embolization Costs and Outcomes

The results with stainless-steel coils are superior to those obtained with cyanoacrylate glues or detachable ureteric balloons. The procedure is also relatively inexpensive. At our institution, steel coils cost roughly $25 (U.S.) each and nephrostomy tubes cost roughly $50 (U.S.). The total material cost is thus $150–350 (U.S.) per embolized renal unit. The other equipment used for the procedure is commonly available in most interventional radiology suites. With a mean follow-up of 43.8 (38) mo, occlusion was successful in all cases, with complete or near-complete (<1 pad/d) dryness within 3 days. No repeat embolizations were required and there were no significant complications. Twenty-three patients died from cancer at a mean of 8.1 ± 11.5 months after embolization. Four patients were alive, three having had staged surgical urinary diversions (colonic or ileal conduit) at a mean of 6 mo after ureteric embolization. Ureteric embolization is a viable option for managing complex lower urinary tract fistula in patients with a poor performance status. Moreover, it can be used as definitive management in patients with a limited life-expectancy (<1 yr).

References

1. Lane BR, Stein DE, Remzi FH, Strong SA, Fazio VW, Angermeier KW (2006) Management of radiotherapy induced rectourethral fistula. J Urol 175:1382–1387
2. Zinman L (2004) The management of the complex recto-urethral fistula. BJU Int 94:1212–1213
3. Jones IT, Fazio VW, Jaqelman DG (1987) The use of transanal rectal advancement flaps in the management of fistulas involving the anorectum. Dis Colon Rectum 30:919–923
4. Renschler TP, Middleton RG (2003) 30 Years of experience with York-Mason repair of recto-urinary fistulas. J Urol 170:1222–1225
5. Moreira SG, Seigne JD, Ordorica RC, et al (2004) Devastating complications after brachytherapy in the treatment of prostate adenocarcinoma. Br J Urol Int 93:31–35
6. Gecelter L (1973). Transanorectal approach to the posterior urethra and bladder neck. J Urol 109:1011–1016
7. Zmora O, Potenti FM, Wexner SD, et al (2003) Gracilis muscle transposition for iatrogenic rectourethral fistula. Ann Surg 237:483–487
8. Ferguson GG, Brandes SB (2007) Surgical management of rectovesical fistulas: An evaluation of treatments at washington university J Urol 177: 28A
9. Shindel AW, Zhu H, Hovsepian DM, Brandes SB (2007) Ureteric embolization with stainless-steel coils for managing refractory lower urinary tract fistula: a 12-year experience. BJU Int 99:364–368

23
Reconstruction of Failed Urethroplasty

Steve W. Waxman and Allen F. Morey

Contents

1. Introduction..269
2. Causes of Failure..270
3. Evaluation 270
4. Preparation and General Considerations.................................271
5. Urethral Meatus 272
6. Pendulous Urethra..272
7. Bulbar Urethra 273
8. Posterior Urethra..274
References...275

Summary   While initial open urethroplasty has a success rate of approximately 90%, salvage repairs do not fare as well, having a success rate of roughly 80% on average. Failed anastomotic repairs are usually the result of an inadequate excision of fibrotic tissue and/or inadequate distal urethral mobilization, resulting in an anastomosis performed under tension. The mainstay of treatment for recurrent penile urethral strictures remains a flap procedure with penile shaft skin. It is crucial to resect redundant sacculations, residual scar, or hair-bearing tissue remaining from prior procedures at the time of reconstruction. If distal stenosis should occur after a flap procedure, extended meatotomy is highly effective. Strictures most amenable to excision with re-anastomosis are those in the proximal bulb–these allow for maximal use of the elastic properties of the distal bulbar urethra to bridge the gap created once the scarred segment is excised. For strictures greater than 3 cm. in length located in the distal bulb, patch graft (penile skin or buccal mucosa) is the most effective and efficient approach. The primary reason for failure of a primary open urethroplasty of the posterior urethra is inadequate exposure of the prostatic apex, resulting in incomplete excision of scar tissue. Urethral stenosis may recur after any of the above types of open urethral reconstruction—fortunately the recurrent stricture is often short and web-like, and usually responds well to a single urethral balloon dilation or direct visual internal urethrotomy, because it is associated with less underlying spongiofibrosis.

Keywords   recurrent stricture, salvage urethroplasty, onlay flap, patch grafting, extended meatotomy, penile skin

1. Introduction

During the past two decades, open urethroplasty increasingly has been used for the treatment of urethral stricture disease. Effective new techniques have resulted in success rates for initial repair ranging from 80% to 90% in most contemporary

From: *Current Clinical Urology: Urethral Reconstructive Surgery*
Edited by: S.B. Brandes © Humana Press, Totowa, NJ

series *(1,2)*. Substitution urethroplasty procedures have fared worse than anastomotic procedures, with long-term success rates approximating 50% *(2)*. Still, although recurrent stenosis may develop after open urethroplasty with the best of surgeons, many failures can be salvaged with a second reconstructive procedure. This chapter will focus on the reasons for primary urethroplasty failure, along with the workup and subsequent treatment of these challenging patients in need of salvage surgery.

2. Causes of Failure

Most open urethroplasties follow one or more urethral dilations or urethrotomies. As the number of previous dilations or open repairs increases, so does the amount of spongiofibrosis. Repeated endoscopic procedures and dilations have no role in the treatment of most strictures nowadays and may actually compromise salvage urethroplasty success rates. Diabetes, hypertension, malnutrition, spinal cord injuries, tobacco abuse, and other co-morbidities may also adversely affect tissue healing and contribute to failure.

Previous open repair has been shown to be an independent risk factor for subsequent salvage urethroplasty failure *(3)*. Failed anastomotic repairs usually are the result of an inadequate excision of fibrotic tissue and/or inadequate distal urethral mobilization, resulting in an anastomosis performed under tension. Inappropriate choice of repair may also contribute to urethroplasty failure. An excisional repair, flap, or graft may be appropriate for one stricture and not another depending on its location, length and character.

Anterior repairs can fail due to inadequate extension of the urethrotomies into normal healthy urethra on both ends of the stricture prior to patching with graft or flap. A common area for failure of buccal mucosa graft urethroplasties is at the distal aspect of the repair. Usually, the recurrent stricture in these cases is thin and web-like and may respond to a simple dilation or visual urethrotomy. Consideration of a urethral biopsy is warranted to rule out malignancy in refractory and advanced stricture cases.

Failure of posterior urethroplasty is nearly always the result of inadequate resection of scar tissue at the site of complete urethral distraction defects *(4)*. We believe that inadequate fibrosis resection

results from difficulties achieving adequate exposure of the proximal urethral segment, such as in cases where pubic bone fragments have lead to distortion or displacement of the prostate within the retropubic space.

3. Evaluation

Long-term postoperative follow-up from urethroplasty is important because of the occasional occurrence of late failure. Typically, patients with stricture recurrence experience decrease in the force of stream or new onset of split stream. The American Urological Association Symptom Score Index has proven effective as screening tool, along with urinary flow rate testing, for men with a history of urethral reconstruction surgery *(5)*. Urinary tract infection with prostatitis or epididymitis symptoms may also occur, although we have observed that most men with recurrent stricture do not have elevated post void residual. Urethral palpation may demonstrate significant induration associated with spongiofibrosis.

The use of retrograde urethrogram (RUG) is the gold standard for determining the recurrence of stricture. RUG should be performed at 3–6 mos after urethroplasty and then again at 12–18 mo to assess for late failure. Imaging will show the location and length of the stricture, along with associated findings such as proximal urethral dilation or reflux into Cowper's ducts.

Recent imaging before salvage repair is essential because the length and location of the stricture may have changed significantly from previous regenerative or open procedures. A simultaneous RUG and cystogram per suprapubic catheter should be performed in patients with obliterative strictures of the urethra that have necessitated the placement of a suprapubic tube *(4)*. Oblique views are crucial in the determination of the length of the stricture or defect. Radiographic irregularities may be commonplace after urethroplasty, even in asymptomatic patients.

When recurrent stricture is suggested on the basis of clinical findings and urethrography, we advocate the use of flexible cystoscopy as the gold standard. If a 15-French scope passes into the bladder without difficulty, the patient may be safely observed without surgery. For posterior urethral or

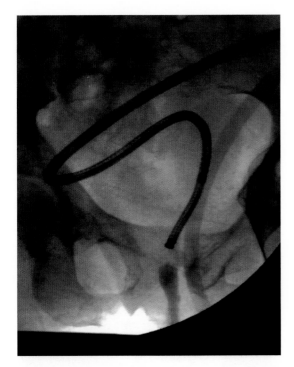

FIG. 23.1. A flexible cystoscope passed suprapubically delineates the fibrotic segment in conjunction with a retrograde urethrogram in this patient who has failed a previous posterior urethroplasty

proximal bulbar strictures, imaging of the prostatic urethral segment may be difficult when the bladder neck does not open during cystography; the flexible scope may be used in combination with radiographic imaging to provide an "up-and-down-o-gram" to demonstrate the length of the fibrotic segment (**Fig. 23.1**).

Sonourethrography has revealed that approximately one-third of strictures initially appearing amenable to end-to-end urethroplasty will be found to be too long on ultrasound, thus warranting a substitution repair (*6*). Biopsy of the scarred urethra to rule out malignancy is prudent in advanced or unusual cases.

4. Preparation and General Considerations

Patient counseling is crucial such that expectations are realistic. Although initial open urethroplasty has a success rate of approximately 90% depending

on the study quoted, salvage repairs do not fare as well, having a success rate of roughly 80% on average (*7*). Although it is true that the options for salvage repair are nearly identical to primary repair, scarring and lack of available genital tissue may limit the potential procedures which are available. We will focus on the differences and modifications of salvage repair as compared to primary urethroplasties in this chapter.

Many men are reluctant to undergo urethral surgery of any kind because of concerns about potential pain or sexual dysfunction. Nonoperative candidates or those who refuse surgery may wish to perform clean intermittent catheterization to calibrate and/or dilate the strictured area. In our experience, most young men will not remain compliant with long-term self-catheterization for stricture and/or will soon find the catheter nonpassable. For these reasons, self-catheterization is rarely a viable strategy for long-term stricture management.

If the stricture is short and web-like after previous repair, it usually responds well to a single urethral balloon dilation or direct visual internal urethrotomy because it is associated with less underlying spongiofibrosis. Long and/or dense recurrent strictures have a poor response rate to dilation or urethrotomy compared to sort, web-like, or previously unmanipulated strictures. Once surgery is selected as the course of action, the reconstructive surgeon must tailor repair to the length, location, and character of the current stricture.

Procedure selection is of paramount importance, and patient positioning, exposure, instrumentation, tissue handling, and choice of repair can all affect the success or failure of a salvage repair. A watertight closure tension-free anastomosis is crucial to increasing the chance for surgical success. Tissue at the anastomotic site must be well-vascularized, hairless, and supple to ensure a successful outcome.

Optical magnification with loupes is strongly advised to ensure that a careful mucosal anastomosis is ensured. Sharp dissection is preferred with limited use of electrocautery. For perineal cases, the Lone Star self-retaining retractor has provided ample perineal exposure in several hundred cases in our experience. A headlamp promotes maximal visualization during deep dissection. A plastic surgical instrument tray including fine instruments such as calipers, Gerald forceps, and tenotomy scissors. We typically use 5-O and 6-O polydioxanone for our anastomotic sutures. A drain is not typically needed and patients are generally discharged to home on the morning of the first post-operative day. A 16-French silastic catheter is placed for 2 to 3 wk postoperatively with a voiding cystourethrogram or pericatheter urethrogram being done at the time of catheter removal. Suprapubic urinary drainage has not proven necessary.

5. Urethral Meatus

Recurrent urethral meatal stenosis can occur with or without urethral stricture. One of the most common reasons for failed primary treatment of meatal stenosis is the missed fossa navicularis stricture. We have found that penile skin flap repairs work extremely well for discreet fossa navicularis strictures 2.5 cm or less in length. A penile fasciocutaneous skin flap tunneled under the ventral aspect of the glans works very well and provides excellent cosmesis *(8)*.

Lichen sclerosus (LS) has a pathognomonic whitish peri-meatal thickening and is an adverse prognosticator which may influence treatment strategies. When LS is suspected, it is reasonable to document its presence by sending a specimen for histopathologic biopsy confirmation. We have found that an extended meatotomy (first-stage Johanson procedure) provides a simple, reasonable approach for perimeatal stenosis that extends beyond the fossa navicularis (**Fig. 23.2**). Such patients must be warned about the potential for sprayed or split stream. Many reoperative patients of middle age will gladly accept a hypospadiac cosmetic appearance in conjunction with alleviation of their voiding difficulties, and we believe this scenario is far preferable to perineal urethrostomy. Many experts now advocate a staged approach to all balanitis xerotica obliterans-related strictures of the fossa navicularis and pendulous urethra.

6. Pendulous Urethra

The mainstay of treatment for recurrent penile urethral strictures remains a flap procedure with penile shaft skin. Various configurations may be used as described by Orandi, Quartey, and McAninch *(9–11)*. Excision with end to end anastomosis

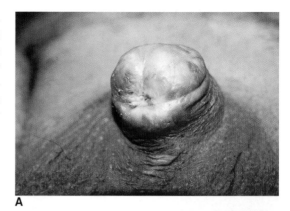

A

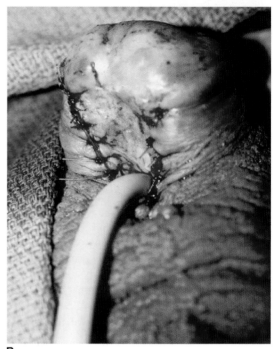

B

FIG. 23.2. Extensive perimeatal LS is noted in conjunction with an extensive stricture of the pendulous urethra and fossa navicularis

should be avoided on the penile shaft to avoid the risk of penile shortening and distortion.

One key to salvage repair is extension of the urethrotomy well into normal caliber urethra proximal and distal to the stricture—we usually open the stricture until a 24-French bougie passes without resistance. Even with previous open urethroplasy in the pendulous urethra or circumcision, there is usually enough extra penile skin distally or circumferentially to allow one of the above stated flaps.

We prefer the circular penile fasciocutaneous flap as described by McAninch because it is extremely versatile and effective. It is crucial to resect redundant sacculations, residual scar, or hair-bearing tissue remaining from prior procedures at the time of reconstruction (**Fig. 23.3** *[1]*).

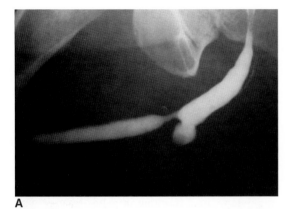

A

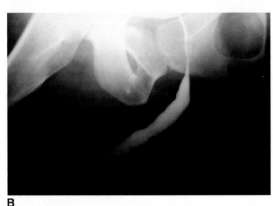

B

FIG. 23.3. (A) Sacculation of previous scrotal skin flap near recurrent stricture. (B) Postoperative appearance after excision of redundant hair-bearing tissue in conjunction with a 4-cm circular penile skin flap onlay during revision urethroplasty

When genital skin is lacking, buccal mucosa provides the optimal graft tissue because of its robust nature, reliability, availability, and ease of harvest *(12–16)*. Lingual grafts have also recently been successfully used for urethroplasty and may be an appropriate choice in advanced cases in lieu of repeat cheek harvesting, which may be difficult *(17)*. Grafts may be placed ventrally or dorsally depending on surgeon preference with equally good results, although our preference remains ventral onlay *(18,19)*. Although grafts have traditionally been discouraged in the pendulous urethra because of the limited vascularity of the distal corpus spongiosum, we have found buccal mucosa grafts to perform very well for pendulous reconstruction in a salvage setting and now utilize tunica vaginalis flaps (obtained via a scrotal counter-incision) to support these distal grafts.

Care must be taken to ensure an adequate urethral plate width during any onlay repair for advanced stricture disease. When found to be inadequate (<1 cm in width), urethral plate "salvage" via a dorsal buccal mucosa graft may be accomplished in conjunction with ventral skin flap onlay as an alternative to flap tubularization (which should be avoided whenever possible, **Fig. 23.4** *[20]*). Hairless scrotal flaps and/or staged procedures as described by Schreiter may be considered for severe, refractory strictures, although these options are almost never used in our experience *(21)*.

7. Bulbar Urethra

Excision of fibrotic urethra with end to end anastomosis is the mainstay of bulbar urethroplasty, even for salvage repairs if the excised

FIG. 23.4. (A) Focally severe (5 Fr) distal stricture (oval) located at distal end of pendulous stricture. (B) Dorsal buccal mucosa graft (arrow) used for urethral plate salvage at terminal end of ventral penile skin flap onlay repair. The subcoronal meatus location is prudent to avoid subsequent meatal stenosis in reoperative cases

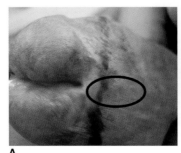

A

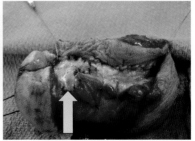

B

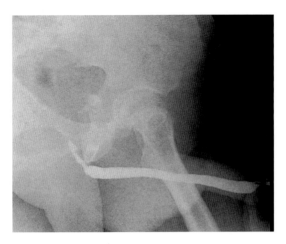

FIG. 23.5. Proximal bulbar stricture 3.5 cm in length after prior penile skin graft urethroplasty successfully reconstructed via complete excision with primary anastomosis

segment is not so long as to preclude a tension free anastomosis (22,23). Strictures most amenable to primary excision with reanastomosis are those which are located in the proximal bulb (**Fig. 23.5**). This allows for maximal use of the elastic properties of the distal bulbar urethra to bridge the gap created once the scarred segment is excised. Conditions favorable for an extended anastomotic urethroplasty include stricture location in the proximal half of the perineum and normal stretched penile length (13 cm or greater [24]). Excision with end-to-end anastomosis has the highest success rate both short and long term.

If the stricture is too long or not proximal enough, tension on the anastomosis can result, leading to failure. For strictures greater than 3 cm. in length located in the mid-bulb, patch graft (penile skin or buccal mucosa) is the most effective and efficient approach (1). The presence of multiple prior endoscopic urethrotomies is commonly associated with longer strictures not amenable to complete excision whereas we have found that uninstrumented "virgin" strictures are often more amenable to anastomotic repair.

Although flaps have the advantage of carrying their own blood supply, the extensive genital dissection required to transfer a distal penile skin flap to the perineum makes this a formidable undertaking. Further, sexually active young men are prone to complaints of penile shortening or ventral

tethering when penile flaps are used for bulbar reconstruction (25).

Grafts may be performed in the bulb for both primary and salvage urethroplasty because the thick ventral spongiosum is an ideal recipient site and these procedures are extremely well tolerated. Although we prefer ventral graft placement because it is more straightforward, a dorsally placed graft may be preferred if the spongiosum is deficient (18). Grafts may also be used to augment a partial anastomosis in the bulbar urethra if the stricture is focally stenotic but too long for end-to-end anastomosis (26).

8. Posterior Urethra

Posterior urethral injuries are usually the result of pelvic trauma, resulting in pelvic fracture with urethral distraction at the membranous portion. If treated acutely via early primary realignment over a catheter, most men will eventually develop a short stricture amenable to a simplified anastomotic repair. Longer strictures and those associated with fistula, abscess, or other complicating factors may require extensive dissection with not only perineal but also simultaneous suprapubic and/or transpubic dissection (27).

The primary reason for failure of a primary open urethroplasty of the posterior urethra is inadequate exposure of the prostatic apex, resulting in incomplete excision of scar tissue. When performing salvage posterior urethroplasty, the amount of fibrosis and length of defect will ultimately determine the dissection necessary to achieve a tension free anastomosis. If the recurrent stricture is relatively short, a perineal anastomotic repair with excision of fibrotic tissue and end-to-end anastomosis is performed. Complete excision of the "plug" of fibrotic tissue separating the prostatic apex and healthy bulbar urethra is essential before performing the anastomosis. In all but the most severe injuries, the bulbar urethra remains well vascularized via retrograde blood flow, allowing repair of defects up to 5 cm in length.

Intraoperative cystoscopy is essential during revision posterior urethroplasty to 1) detect eggshell calculi which may form on longstanding suprapubic catheter balloons (**Fig. 23.6**) and

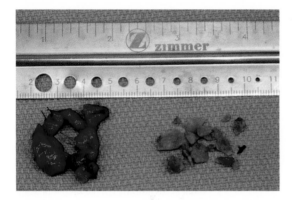

FIG. 23.6. Numerous eggshell calculi removed cystoscopically in conjunction with repeat posterior urethroplasty

2) visualize the prostatic apex to ensure the correct proximal anastomotic site (**Fig. 23.7**). The progressive repair popularized by Webster involves separation of the corporal bodies, inferior pubectomy, and/or supracrural re-routing of the urethra. We have found the maneuver of sharp scalpel dissection between the proximal corporal bodies, through fibrotic tissue, directly to the inferior pubis, essential in reoperative cases.

We have found a perineo-abdominal approach with or without pubic bone resection to be helpful in reoperative and/or pediatric posterior urethroplasty *(28,29)*. Several factors arguing for this combined approach include: a long urethral defect (>3 cm), a chronic periurethral cavity, recto-cutaneous and periurethral bladder fistula, or an associated anterior urethral stricture *(30–32)*. Good mobilization of the bulbar urethra to the level of the suspensory ligament of the penis promotes tension-free urethral distraction defect repair. Omentum may be brought down to protect the anastomosis and fill dead space *(33)*. Finally, the timing of a salvage repair is important as one should optimally wait at least 3 to 6 mo from any urethral instrumentation to allow for maximal healing and thus increase the pliability of the tissues.

References

1. Morey AF, Duckett CP, McAninch JW (1997) Failed anterior urethroplasty: guidelines for reconstruction. J Urol 158:1383–1387
2. Andrich DE, Dunglison N, Greenwell TJ, Mundy AR (2003) The long-term results of urethroplasty. J Urol 170:90–92

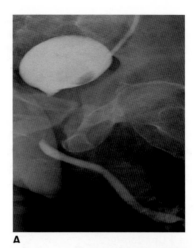

A

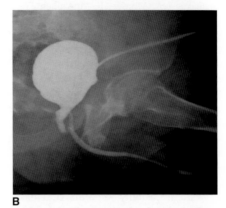

B

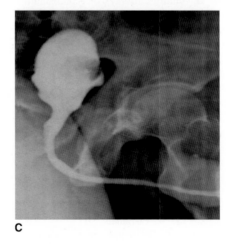

C

FIG. 23.7 (A) Preoperative combined cystogram/retrograde urethrogram shows long posterior urethral defect after pelvic fracture. (B) Appearance after initial repair (complicated by brisk periurethral hemorrhage, during which intraoperative cystoscopy was not performed) shows bulbar urethra anastomosed to anterior prostate. (C) Repeat perineal urethroplasty in same patient demonstrates bulbar urethra anastomosed correctly to prostatic apex

3. Roehrborn CG, McConnell JD (1994) Analysis of factors contributing to success or failure of 1-stage urethroplasty for urethral stricture disease. J Urol 151:869

4. Koraitim MM (2005) On the art of an astomotic posterior urethroplasty: a 27-year experience. J Urol 173:135–139

5. Morey AF, McAninch JW, Duckett CP, Rodgers R (1998) AUA symptom index in assessment of urethroplasty outcomes. J Urol 159:1192–1194

6. Morey AF, McAninch JW (1997) Role of preoperative sonourethrography in bulbar urethral reconstruction. J Urol 158:1376–1379

7. Barbagli G, Selli C, Tosto A (1996) Reoperative surgery for recurrent strictures of the penile and bulbous urethra. J Urol 156:76

8. Armenakas NA, Morey AF, McAninch JW (1998) Reconstruction of resistant strictures of the fossa navicularis and meatus. J Urol 160:359–363

9. McAninch JW, Morey AF (1998) Penile circular fasciocutaneous skin flap in 1-stage reconstruction of complex anterior urethral strictures. J Urol 160:2164–2167

10. Orandi A (1968) One-stage urethroplasty. Br J Urol 40:717

11. Quartey JKM (1983) One-stage penile/preputial cutaneous island flap urethroplasty for urethral stricture: a preliminary report. J Urol 129:284

12. Kane CJ, Tarman GJ, Summerton DJ, Buchmann CE, Ward JF, O'reilly KJ, Ruiz H, Thrasher JB, Zorn B, Smith C, Morey AF (2002) multi-institutional experience with buccal mucosa onlay urethroplasty for bulbar urethral reconstruction J Urol 167:1314–1317

13. Andrich DE, Mundy AR (2001) Substitution urethroplasty with buccal mucosal free grafts. J Urol 165,1131

14. Heinke T, Gerharz EW, Bonfig R, Riedmiller H (2003)Ventral onlay urethroplasty using buccal mucosa for complex stricture repair. Urology 61:1004

15. Pansadoro V, Emiliozzi P, Gaffi M, Scarpone P, DePaula F, Pizzo M (2003) Buccal mucosa urethroplasty in the treatment of bulbar urethral strictures. Urology 61:1008

16. El-Kasaby AW, Fath-Alla M, Noweir AM, El-Halaby MR, Zakaria W, El-Benaly MH (1993) The use of buccal mucosa patch graft in the management of anterior urethral strictures. J Urol 149:276

17. Simonato A, Gregori A, Lissiani A, Galli S, Ottaviani F, Rossi R, Zappone A, Carmignani G (2006) The tongue as an alternative donor site for graft urethroplasty: a pilot study. J Urol 175:589

18. Barbagli G, Selli C, Tosto A, Palminteri E (1996) Dorsal free graft urethroplasty. J Urol 155:123

19. Wessells H (2002) Ventral onlay graft techniques for urethroplasty. Urol Clin North Am 29:381

20. Morey AF (2001) Urethral plate "salvage" with dorsal graft promotes successful penile flap onlay reconstruction of severe pendulous strictures. J Urol 166:1376–1378

21. Schreiter F, Noll F (1989) Mesh graft urethroplasty using split thickness skin graft or foreskin. J Urol 142,1223

22. Mundy AR (1993) Results and complications of urethroplasty and its future. Br J Urol 71:322

23. Joseph JV, Andrich DE, Leach CJ, Mundy AR (2002) Urethroplasty for refractory anterior urethral stricture. J Urol 167:127–129

24. Morey AF and Kizer WS (2006) Proximal bulbar urethroplasty via extended anastomotic approach: What are the limits? J Urol 175:2145–2149

25. Coursey JC, Morey AF, McAninch JW, Summerton DJ, Secrest C, White P, Miller K, Pieczonka C, Armenakas NA, Hochberg D (2001) Erectile function after anterior urethroplasty J Urol 166:2273–2276

26. Guralnick ML, Webster GD (XXXX) The augmented anastomotic urethroplasty: indications and outcome in 29 patients J Urol 165:1496–1501

27. Morey AF, McAninch JW (1997) Reconstruction of posterior urethral disruption injuries: outcome analysis in 82 patients. J Urol 157:506–510

28. Pratap A, Agrawal CS, Tiwari A, Bhattarai BK, Pandit RK, Anchal N (2006) Complex posterior urethral disruptions: management by combined abdominal transpubic perineal urethroplasty. J Urol 175:1751–1754

30. Waterhouse, K Abrams, JI, Grover, et al (1973) The transpubic approach to the lower urinary tract. J Urol 109:486

31. Webster GD, Ramon J, Kreder KJ (1990) Salvage posterior urethroplasty after failed initial repair of pelvic fracture membranous urethral defects. J Urol 144:1370

32. Turner-Warwick R (1977) Complex traumatic posterior urethral strictures. J Urol 118:564

33. Turner-Warwick R (1976) The use of the omental pedicle graft in urinary reconstruction. J Urol 116:341

24
Urethral Stent Complications and Methods for Explantation

Steven B. Brandes

Contents

1. Introduction... 277
2. Complications Specifics... 278
   2.1. Overlapping Stent Separation 278
   2.2. Recurrent Stricture 278
   2.3. Hyperplasia 279
   2.4. Chronic Pain and/or Chordee.. 279
   2.5. Postvoid Dribbling 279
   2.6. Stent Encrustation 279
3. Urolume Explantation.. 279
   3.1. Endoscopic Methods.. 279
   3.2. Open Surgical Methods.. 281
References.. 283

Summary The UroLume endourethral prosthesis (American Medical Systems) is a braided wire mesh cylinder that self expands upon endoscopic placement. Indications for the urethral stent are very limited and narrowed to recurrent and short bulbar strictures that are distal to the external sphincter, in patients who are older or have co-morbidities that severely increase anesthetic risk. Contraindications to urethral stent placement include pendulous urethral strictures, traumatic membranous strictures, meatal strictures, strictures that cannot be cut or dilated sufficiently, active urinary tract infection, urethral fistula or cancer, and perineal urethrostomy. Relative contraindications that predispose to failure and severe complications are prior urethroplasty, prior pelvic irradiation, and long stricture length. Re-stenoses usually occur within the first year of implantation. Typical complications include recurrent stricture, chronic pain, chordee, post void dribbling, and stent encrustation. It is the off-label use of the UroLume that leads to the most severe complications. Detailed here-in are surgical methods for managing the complex problem of failed UroLume stent, in particular explantation and subsequent urethral reconstruction.

Keywords endourethral prosthesis, recurrent stricture, chronic pain, encrustation, post void dribbling, explantation

1. Introduction

The Urolume endourethral prosthesis (American Medical Systems, Minnetonka, Minnesota) is a braided wire mesh super-alloy cylinder that is placed endoscopically. It self expands after deployment and epithelializes in 6 wk to 12 mo. Epitheliazation is essential to prevent stent encrustation, stone formation, urethritis. and dysuria. As noted in Chapter 8 by Yachia and Markovic in this

From: *Current Clinical Urology: Urethral Reconstructive Surgery*
Edited by: S.B. Brandes © Humana Press, Totowa, NJ

volume, the indications for the Urolume stent are limited and narrowed to recurrent and short bulbar strictures <3 cm length and >7 mm distal to the external sphincter, in patients who are older than 55 years of age or have co-morbidities that increase their surgical risk for anesthesia. Such strictures are in the location and length of strictures that are typically amenable to open anastomotic urethroplasty, which has well documented and durable (decades of) success. Older patients often do better with the Urolume, however, not only because time till stricture recurrence may be longer the their life expectancy, but that they are not as bothered by postvoid dribbling, are less physically active, and oftentimes are not sexually active. Contraindications (and thus an off-label uses) to urethral stent placement include pendulous urethral strictures, traumatic membranous strictures, meatal strictures, strictures that cannot be cut or dilated to 26 French, active urinary tract infection, urethral fistula or cancer, and perineal urethrostomy. Relative contraindications that are predispositions to failure and severe complications are prior urethroplasty, prior pelvic irradiation, and strictures >3 cm length.

When the Urolume is used for its limited indications, there is a well-reported and recognized complication and failure rate. Urolume failures often are surgical reconstructive challenges. The North American Multicenter Urolume Trial (NAUT) is the largest and longest follow-up study of the Urolume and bulbar urethral strictures. Shah et al. *(1)* reported on 179 patients in a prospective, open-label study. Follow-up was poor at 11 yr, with only 24 patients (13%). A total of 87% (n = 155) dropped out after the 5-yr approval study. Of the limited number available for long-term follow-up, 33.3% (8/24) failed, required transurethral resection (TUR) or restenting. The majority (78%) of the recurrences occurred within 1 yr of stenting. Moreover, Shah et al. *(2)* reported in 2003 on the NAUT experience with Urolume explantation, noting that of 465 patients, 69 (14.9%) required removal after 7 yr, with stents removed according to etiology: 5% for bulbar stricture, 22% for DSD, and 23% for benign prostatic hyperplasia. All stricture restenoses occurred within the first year of implantation. Restenosis was primarily hyperplastic ingrowth and focal inflammation. Risks for stent explanation for bulbar stricture were highest for prior urethroplasty and prior pelvic irradiation.

In 1996, Milroy et al. *(3)* presented their long-term results with 50 patients treated with stent placement for bulbomembranous strictures. Restenosis requiring retreatment developed in 8 patients (16%), insignificant intraluminal narrowing developed in 1 patient (2%), and extraluminal stricture developed in 9 patients (18%) who also required additional treatment. Most restenoses occurred in strictures with a traumatic etiology or history of prior urethroplasty. A recent long-term study from London, reported that only 45% of the patients were free of recurrence and complications, and 45% suffered multiple complications after Urolume placement.

2. Complications Specifics

2.1. Overlapping Stent Separation

If overlapping stents do not sufficiently cover each other, a gap will develop between them, as the implanted stents shorten as they expand *(4)*. One of the stents can also become displaced. Regardless, hypertrophic scar typically forms between the separated stents, leading to lumen obstruction. To mange such scar, the scar can be resected by transurethral loop resection at 75 W pure cut, followed by another stent to span the separation, long enough to overlap 1 cm on each end. The additional stent should epithelize at the expected rate and extent as the other Urolume stent, as long as it is not in a radiated field.

2.2. Recurrent Stricture

The location and length of the recurrent stricture after stent placement dictates the treatment (2). Short strictures proximal to the stented area can be managed by an additional overlapping stent, as long as the stent is in the bulbar urethra and >0.5 cm distal to the external sphincter. Short strictures distal to the stent can also be managed by an overlapping stent, as long as the distal end is before the penoscrotal junction. In both areas, the stent should overlap the prior stent by at least 1 cm and be long enough to extend beyond the stricture by 1 cm (**Fig. 24.1**). Thus, a 3-cm Urolume is typically needed.

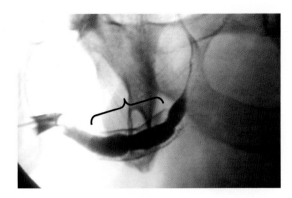

FIG. 24.1. Retrograde urography of second overlapping stent placed for recurrent stricture at the edge of prior Urolume. Bracket outlines stent limits

2.3. Hyperplasia

After Urolume placement, a narrowed lumen in follow-up can either be from hyperplastic tissue growing through the stent mesh or recurrence of the stricture due to fibrotic ingrowth. Most restenoses occur within the first year of implantation and within the stent is from hyperplastic ingrowth and inflammation (4). Some have reported that judicious TUR of the hyperplasia can be effective. Supposedly, with each TUR, the hyperplastic reaction and the need for repeat TUR gets better with time. We have not had the opposite experience. Although we have had short-lived success with TUR of hyperplastic ingrowth, and in our anecdotal experience with a half dozen patients, we have noted that with each recurrence of hyperplastic growth, the time period till recurrence often gets shorter, not longer.

2.4. Chronic Pain and/or Chordee

After implantation, there are reports of chronic perineal pain, despite proper placement in the bulbar urethra. Upon sitting (particularly when on a hard surface), most patients report a discomfort or "poking" feeling in the perineum. Off-label placement of the Urolume in the pendulous urethra will result in painful erections, and either tethering of the penis and urethra and painful erections. Distally placed stent are furthermore palpable and create an abnormal cosmetic and dysfunctional result.

2.5. Postvoid Dribbling

Most patients notice some postvoid dribbling incontinence for the first 6 to 8 wk after Urolume stent placement. The dribbling resolves spontaneously in most, but persists in roughly 20%. Persistent dribbling typically is not severe enough to require the use of an incontinence pad, yet appears to be worst in those stented with multiple Urolumes (e.g., >3 cm overall stricture). It is likely that the problem relates to a combination of serous exudate from the hyperplastic epithelium covering the stent, together with the pooling of urine in the bulb, due to the rigid and inelastic tissue (preventing tissue coaptation), and to the mid bulb's dependent nature. Resolution of the hyperplasia may explain the spontaneous resolution of this postoperative symptom in some patients.

2.6. Stent Encrustation

When the Urolume stent is placed in a patient with prior pelvic radiation, the stet is much less likely to endothelialize. Without epithelial coverage, the wires can act as a nidus/wick for stone formation. Such stones are typically soft, phosphate stones. Such stones can be successfully cleared with the use of EHL lithotripsy.

3. Urolume Explantation

It is the off-label use of the Urolume that leads to the most severe complications and are the most difficult challenges to reconstruction (**Fig. 24.2**). From our national practice patterns study of U.S. board-certified urologists, the Urolume stent is a commonly used method (23.4% per year) for recurrent bulbar strictures. Furthermore, from our survey, it appears that the off-label use of the Urolume is common. Herein we detail the endoscopic and open surgical methods for managing severe complications—most of them after an off-label use.

3.1. Endoscopic Methods

In the initial postoperative period, before stent epitheliazation, stent explantation can be fairly easily performed cystoscopically, by dislodging and elongating the stent. Once the stent is epithelialized and

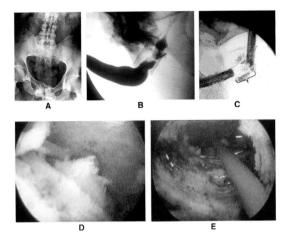

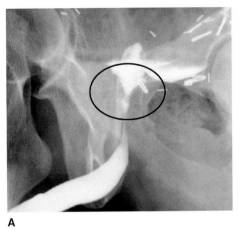

A

FIG. 24.2. 52 year-old with posterior urethral injury after pelvic fracture from a motorcycle accident. (A) AP films of pelvic fracture (after reduction). (B) Failed multiple urethrotomies and now Urolume. (C) Antegrade and retrograde endoscopy confirming stricture and length. (D) Hyperplastic obstructing ingrowth. (E) TUR down to the wires. Eventually undergoes definitive EPA and open stent removal

fixed in position, Urolume stent removal is not easy and entails TUR of the epithelium or hyperplastic tissue until the wires of the stent are completely exposed. To do so, we first place a "Superstiff" guidewire across the stenotic urethra cystoscopically into the bladder and dilate the stenosis to 24 or 26 French with Heyman or Amplatz dilators. A noncontinuous flow resectoscope is then placed and using a low current setting (e.g., 75 W pure cut) the resectoscope loop is used to remove ("resect") the scar and overlying epithelium (**Fig. 24.3**). The hot loop is used to resect the tissue within the Urolume until the metal tines of the stent can be seen circumferentially. The cutting current is reduced to in order to prevent the tines from melting. Once the tines melt and separate, the whole stent will start to unravel and poke out into the lumen of the urethra. We have had a similar negative experience with the Holmium (HO) laser. Although at first using the laser to resect the hypertrophic scar seems to make good sense—the laser too easily will cut the wire tines of the stent and cause it to unravel. The only instances in which we have used the HO laser is when a Urolume has been placed at the bladder neck for a recalcitrant contracture, and the stent is too long, jutting into the

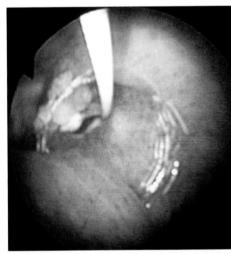

B

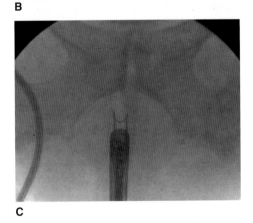

C

FIG. 24.3. (A) Recurrent BN contracture and hyperplastic ingrowth into Urolume stent after off label use for recurrent BN contracture after RRP. Note circle. (B) Wire placed across stricture. Note non-endothelialized Urolume. (C) TUR of hyperlastic tissue ingrowth

bladder lumen. These exposed tines are a nidus for stone formation and infection and be cut off with the HO laser.

Once the wires are all exposed, with the use of an alligator forceps and a cystoscope, the distal three to five diamonds of the stent mesh are grasped. As it is pulled, the stent should elongate and narrow, yet still keep its orientation due to the preplaced guidewire. We prefer to do such procedures under combined fluoroscopy and cystoscopy to ensure that the remaining urethra is not injured. At one point, American Medical Systems had developed an endoscopic device to grasp and facilitate Urolume removal; however, it never became commercially available.

An alternative method is initially the same with guidewire placement and TUR down to the wires. Then, with a grasper, instead the distal end of the stent is pulled cephalad to dislodge the stent in to the bladder. The distal end of the guidewire is then grasped with an alligator forceps and pulled into the lumen. With both ends of the guide wire coming out the end of the scope, both wire ends can be pulled, forcing the Urolume to be deformed and pulled into and out the scope lumen. An alternative method to remove the Urolume is to again resect the epithelium and scar first and then use the HO laser to make radial incisions into the stent wires. The stent will unravel and loose its structural integrity. With alligator forceps, the wires can be removed piecemeal. This is a very tedious and cumbersome process, and requires both visual and fluoroscopic guidance.

3.2. Open Surgical Methods

Zinman has described a method to explant a Urolume by open surgery, by cutting first exposing the spongiosum and then the wires with a ventral urethrotomy at 12 o'clock and then pulling the wires of the unraveled stent out individually (**Fig. 24.4**). This method is tedious but leaves a potential urethral plate that can then be augmented by a ventral graft (if there is sufficient vascular spongiosum to cover the graft) or by a skin island flap (also placed ventral). An alternative method is to place a buccal or skin graft onto the opened spongiosum as a first stage and allow it to heal and mature until subsequent reconstruction in a second stage 6–12 mo later. An alternative method would be to perform a two-stage Schreiter-type urethroplasty. Mundy described such a two-stage method of stent excision, with the epithelium and some of the spongiosum. Here, most of the spongiosum is retained along with the tunica of the spongiosum. To the remaining vascular bed, a skin graft or buccal graft in sutured and quilted to the tunical edges in a one-stage Schreiter type first stage, followed by tubularization after graft maturation in 6 to 12 mo.

Another alternative method, which we initially described in 2004 (5), entails complete en-bloc excision of the Urolume and the overlying urethra and spongiosum. This leaves a large gap of missing urethra (typically at least 3 cm). If the stricture and stent are at the proximal bulbar urethra then urethral mobilization and a progressive approach can bridge the gap with a primary anastomosis (**Fig. 24.5**). For a more distal or tandem stent excision, the urethra can be reconstructed by the combination of a dorsal buccal graft and ventral skin island flap (**Fig. 24.6**). We have recently performed such surgeries on six patients. All patients had hyperplastic tissue ingrowth and stent encrustation, causing recurrent stenosis. Average

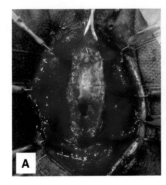 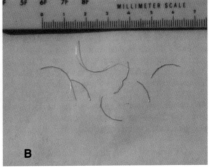

FIG. 24.4. (A) Ventral urethrotomy made through Urolume.
(B) Urolume wires pulled out individually, leaving scarred urethral plate. Eventual reconstruction was with a onlay flap

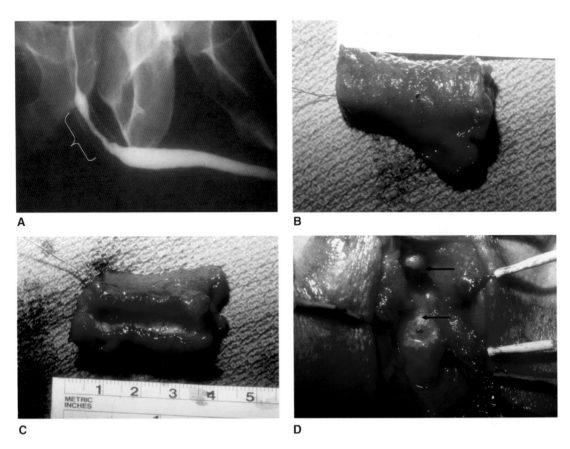

FIG. 24.5. (A) Intrastent bulbar stricture through Urolume. Bracket outlines stent limits. (B) Urolume and spongiosum excised. (C) Excised Urolume and spongiosum opened. Note wires. (D) Transected edges of urethra. Arrows at distal and proximal ends. Repair by BMG augmented anastomosis

age was 49 yr (range, 36–53 yr) with a mean of 1.8 Urolumes (range, 1–3). Urolume locations were two membranous, three bulbar, and one pendulous and bulbar urethra. Stricture etiology for the initial stricture were off-label uses, with four traumatic (two straddle injuries, two pelvic fracture and bulbomembranous disruptions) and two iatrogenic. The patient with the Urolumes in the pendulous urethra suffered from ventral chordee and painful erections. Stricture length ranged from 2 to 9 cm. Five of the six were initially managed by urethral dilation followed by transurethral resection of the scar down till exposure of the woven mesh of the stent, followed by periurethral injection of triamcinolone (a biological modifier).

After TUR, all strictures recurred within 6 mo. All six then underwent open surgical excision and explantation of the stent and surrounding spongiosum and urethra. The urethral defect was bridged by natural elasticity and mobilization of the proximal urethra, for an anastomotic urethroplasty for the two membranous strictures. In the remaining four, the defect was too long to bring the edges together, so a combination of a buccal graft (quilted dorsally) and a circular fasciocutaneous island skin flap (ventrally in the technique of Morey (6). At a mean follow-up of 23 mo, there have been no recurrences (as determined by flexible cystoscopy). Although the American Urological Association Symptom Score nicely decreased to 6/35 and flow rates increased to a mean of 21 mL/s, one-half (3/6) had bothersome postvoid dribbling, requiring a small incontinence pad and/or perineal urethral milking. Penile pain and chordee resolved in all

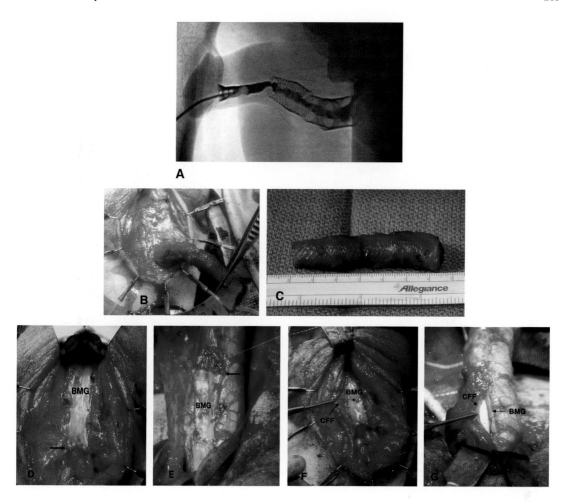

FIG. 24.6. Graft and flap urethral reconstruction for failed, sequential Urolumes x 3, for a bulbar and proximal pendulous stricture. (A) Long intra-stent stricture on urethrography (B) Urethra and Urolume mobilized. Note forceps on Urolume. (C) Urolumes excised. (D) Buccal graft to perineum (arrow at proximal anastomosis). (E) Second buccal graft to penile shaft (arrow at distal anastomosis). (F) Onlay flap to buccal plate in perineum. (G) Onlay flap to buccal graft on penis

patients and were able to resume normal sexual function after stent explantation. Gelman et al. *(7)* recently reported a similar successful experience with one stage reconstruction of the urethra after explantation. In their experience with 10 patients and 51 months' follow-up, the urethra was reconstructed with three dorsal buccal grafts and one skin island flap to a residual plate, one combined dorsal and ventral buccal graft, and five primary anastomoses (for three membranous and two proximal bulbar strictures). Therefore, Urolume stent excision and open explantation followed by a one-stage reconstruction is technically feasible and with durable results.

References

1. Shah DK, Paul EM, Badlani GH, North American Study Group (2003) 11-year outcome analysis of endourethral prostheses for the treatment of recurrent bulbar urethral stricture. J Urol 170:1255

2. Shah DK, Kapoor R, Badlani GH (2003) Experience with urethral stent explantation. J Urol 169: 1398–1400.

3. Milroy E, Allen A (1996) Long-term results of urolume urethral stent for recurrent urethral strictures. J Urol 155:904–908.

4. Wilson TS, Lemack GE, Dmochowski RR (2002) UroLume stents: lessons learned. J Urol 167: 2477–2480

5. Brandes SB (2004) Managing the complications of the urolume endourethral prosthesis: use of one stage urethroplasty. J Urol 171:71A

6. Morey AF (2001) Urethral plate salvage with dorsal graft promotes successful penile flap onlay recon-

struction of severe pendulous strictures. J Urol 166:1376–1378

7. Gelman J, Rodriguez E Jr (2007) Stricture recurrence after urethral stent placement. J Urol 177:188–191

25
Reoperative Hypospadias Surgery and Management of Complications

Douglas E. Coplen

Contents

1. Introduction.. 285
2. Surgical Complications... 286
    2.1. Urethrocutaneous Fistula 286
    2.2. Urethral Diverticulum 286
    2.3. Persistent Chordee... 286
3. Complex Reoperative Hypospadias Techniques 287
    3.1. Urethral Plate Retubularization... 287
    3.2. Adjacent Genital Tissues... 288
    3.3. Extragenital Tissues 288
    3.4. Squamous Epithelium 290
    3.5. Bladder Mucosal Graft.. 290
    3.6. Buccal Mucosal Graft.. 291
4. Postpubertal and Adult Complications 291
    4.1. Urethral Hair 292
References.. 294

Summary Re-operative hypospadias surgery is often complicated by the general lack of healthy tissue for urethroplasty and skin coverage. The penile skin that is present is typically scarred and has a variable and poorly defined blood supply. Each case is different and demands individualized evaluation and care. Re-operation is delayed at least 6 months after the last repair, in order to maximize tissue healing and vascularity. Earlier attempts at definitive repair are often fraught with more complications. Common post hypospadias repair complications are urethrocutaneous fistula, urethral diverticulum, persistent chordee, and urethral stricture. Successful reconstruction of such refractory, post-surgical strictures, requires the whole surgical armamentarium, namely vascularized onlay flaps, buccal mucosal grafts, and planned staged procedures.

Key words urethrocutaneous fistula, chordee, buccal mucosal graft, onlay flap, complications, staged urethroplasty, urethral stricture

1. Introduction

Current hypospadias techniques set a high standard for functional and cosmetic outcomes. In all but the most severe cases, a slit-like meatus in an orthotopic position on a conical glans can be achieved with a single operation with the expectation of a low incidence of minor or major complications. The most important factor that impacts reoperative hypospadias is the presence of healthy tissue that is needed for urethroplasty and skin coverage. There is usually a paucity of penile skin that is scarred and has a variable and poorly defined blood supply.

From: *Current Clinical Urology: Urethral Reconstructive Surgery*
Edited by: S.B. Brandes © Humana Press, Totowa, NJ

Natural tissue planes often are disrupted, and dissection may damage the blood supply to the penile skin. Each case requires individual evaluation and management based upon sound plastic surgical principles.

In general, reoperative surgery should be delayed at least 6 mo after the last repair to eliminate any residual inflammation and allow complete healing. Time allows in growth of new blood supply to relocated penile skin. Earlier attempts at definitive repair may actually create a more significant complication. The glansplasty is the key to a normal postoperative appearance so urethrocutaneous fistulae, diverticula, or urethral strictures in the presence of a normal glandular urethra may be technically easier and more successfully repaired than cases where post-operative disruption of the glansplasty has occurred.

2. Surgical Complications

2.1. Urethrocutaneous Fistula

When a fistula is identified, the urethra and meatus are examined under anesthesia prior to making any incisions. The urethra is calibrated with bougie-a-boule to exclude meatal stenosis and any urethral irregularity. Depending upon the age of the patient and the previous surgical technique used, urethroscopy may be indicated to exclude urethral hair or encrustations that would complicate the fistula closure. The urethra is pressurized with saline or water through a catheter to confirm the location and number of fistulae.

We pass a small lacrimal duct probe through the fistula tract and out the urethral meatus. This step helps to define the tract and identifies the exact point of communication with the urethra. Lidocaine with epinephrine is infiltrated around the fistula site. Electrocautery is rarely if ever required during these cases and should be discouraged.

The principles of fistula closure include dissection of the tract flush with the urethra, excision of unhealthy tissues, an inverting watertight closure, and placement of one or more barrier layers between the urethra and the skin (1). A Dartos-based subcutaneous pedicle flap can usually be advanced to cover the fistula closure, although tunica vaginalis may be used in more complex cases (2,3).

Small fistulae on the penile shaft can be circumscribed and excised flush with the urethra. However, subcoronal or glandular fistulae may require a more extensive dissection because of a paucity of healthy adjacent tissues. In these cases, a takedown of the glansplasty may be required to facilitate fistula excision. A distal urethroplasty can then be performed, followed by interposition of a Dartos pedicle and reapproximation of the glans wings. Simple fistula closures without meatal reconstruction rarely require a postoperative catheter, but when distal edema may increase urethral voiding pressure a catheter or urethral stent are preferable.

2.2. Urethral Diverticulum

Diverticular formation after hypospadias surgery may be indicative of urethral meatal stenosis but, in most cases, calibration reveals no evidence of narrowing. Repair is most accurately performed after degloving the phallus. A feeding tube is passed transurethrally and the diverticulum is distended with saline (**Fig. 25.1**). This tube facilitates dissection by defining the appropriate plane between the diverticulum and skin while sparing the blood supply to the urethra. The diverticulum is opened in the ventral midline along its entire length (**Fig. 25.2**). Calipers are used to mark the appropriate urethral width (10–12 mm in a prepubertal male and 20–24 French postpubertal) on the dorsal urethral wall. Redundant epithelium is sharply excised while sparing the subcutaneous blood supply. The urethra is closed with a running and interrupted inverting suture line. The redundant subcutaneous tissue is an excellent covering layer and can be approximated over the urethroplasty in a pant over vest fashion. Because of the length of the closure catheter drainage is advisable.

Repair of a urethral diverticulum using plication has been reported (4). This approach, however, does not remove the redundant mucosa and since absorbable sutures are used the diverticulum might recur. Definitive excision and urethroplasty are recommended to eliminate potential long-term concerns.

2.3. Persistent Chordee

Persistent penile curvature may be a result of ventral skin tethering, corporal disproportion and urethral foreshortening (5–7). Historically, the urethral plate

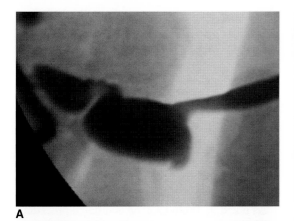

A

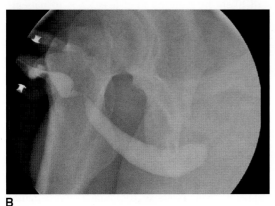

B

Fig. 25.1. Retrograde urethrograms reveal post hypospadias surgery urethral diverticula (A) and strictures (B). (Courtesy of S.B. Brandes.)

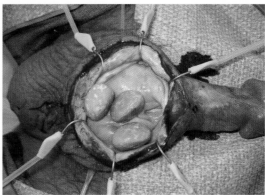

Fig. 25.2. Three large calculi are found in a large urethral diverticulum after marsupialization in the ventral midline. The redundant epithelium can be sharply excised with preservation of the underlying vascular tissue that provides an excellent barrier layer to prevent subsequent fistula formation. (Courtesy of S.B. Brandes.)

was divided to correct penile curvature. However, in the 1990s, Duckett and others popularized the concept of corporal disproportion as the primary etiology of penile curvature *(8)*. Histological evaluation of the urethral plate usually reveals healthy spongy tissue that clinically is very elastic.

Curvature may recur years after the initial hypospadias repair even when corporoplasty (plication and/or ventral grafting) was used to successfully correct chordee at the first surgery. There are no good data showing whether or not free graft urethroplasties are at greater risk for recurrence of curvature when compared with vascularized flaps or primary plate tubularizations. However, a urethral graft with some fibrosis is less likely to grow in concert with the rest of the phallus at puberty. Even if the urethral plate was not previously divided because of a normal appearance, it is possible that

the primary surgeon did not appreciate its contribution to curvature.

At reoperation, an artificial erection is induced intraoperatively. The urethra is inspected to determine whether it is supple or a "bowstring" (indicative of fibrosis). When urethral tethering is suspected then the urethra should be transected and fibrous tissue resected. A repeat erection after transection may show persistent curvature in up to 50% of cases, indicating coexisting corporal disproportion. Either ventral dermal grafting or dorsal plications can be used to correct the curvature in these cases. In cases where the urethra is normal, then a primarily dorsal approach to correction is indicated. In some cases, prior dorsal plications may have disrupted but it is also possible that the intrinsically disproportionate corporal growth pattern persisted at puberty.

3. Complex Reoperative Hypospadias Techniques

3.1. Urethral Plate Retubularization

Tubularized incised plate (TIP) hypospadias repair was introduced in 1994 and is the operation of choice for distal hypospadias repair in many centers.

There is good evidence that the preserved urethral plate can be used in reoperative hypospadias (9–14). Extensive experience with the primary procedure is helpful when assessing the quality of the urethral plate. If the plate appears supple without scarring or evidence of a prior incision, then tubularization is reasonable. The complication rate with tubularization of the plate in secondary operations is similar to the rate when used in primary repairs (**Table 25.1**).

Previous surgery that involved incision of the urethral plate might alter the blood supply and decrease the success of a second tubularization. In addition, a failed TIP may be indicative of an intrinsic abnormality with the plate and spongiosum that precludes a second attempt at urethroplasty using the same technique. Because of these factors, there has been reluctance to perform a repeat TIP, although literature reports show that a repeat TIP does not appear to be associated with a higher complication rate in experienced hands (**Table 25.1**).

The plate can always be incised at the time of reoperation. If it is apparent after the incision that fibrosis is present that precludes a healthy tension free urethral closure, adjacent genital tissues or a free graft can be utilized. Incision of the plate does not burn a bridge and exclude other operative approaches (15).

The most common complication with retubularization is fistula formation so the use of a barrier flap is very important in these reoperative cases. If a circumcision was not performed at the time of the prior hypospadias repair a dartos subcutaneous is available for neourethral coverage. Otherwise, adjacent ventral dartos or tunica vaginalis flaps are useful barriers.

3.2. Adjacent Genital Tissues

If the urethral plate is not suitable for retubularization, then the use of vascularized adjacent genital tissues may be possible (**Fig. 25.3** *[6,16–22]*). Local flaps may be preferable to grafts because the former does not rely upon the reestablishment of vascularity. Care must be taken when harvesting the flap in the presence of scarring from multiple prior procedures. Both meatal-based and Dartos pedicle flaps can be used for the urethroplasty, but ventral blood supply is often more highly compromised than tissues that are laterally or dorsally positioned. Scrotal skin is often well vascularized, but it is usually hair bearing and is associated with a high incidence of future urethral complications.

As noted in **Table 25.2**, an additional procedure will likely be required in at least 25% of patients when a vascularized flap is used for the urethroplasty. This complication rate is clearly higher than the outcomes when flaps are used in a primary repair. The penile skin adjacent to the meatus is often not well vascularized at the hinge of the flip-flap. If this technique is utilized, the dartos pedicle from the prior Byar's flap is preserved as the blood supply for the ventral flap.

Although skin is usually available, there is a significant incidence of postoperative fistulas, stricture's and glansplasty breakdown when adjacent skin is used for repeat hypospadias repairs. Some authors express concern that the glansplasty and meatal appearance are abnormal after flap urethroplasty but with appropriate glans wing dissection an orthotopic vertical meatal opening can be achieved. The limiting factor for a normal appearing glans is the degree of glans scarring and contraction after the prior repairs.

3.3. Extragenital Tissues

Frequently, a paucity of genital tissue is available in reoperative hypospadias. A skin graft

TABLE 25.1. Outcomes after TIP repair in reoperative hypospadias.

	No plate incision		Prior plate incision	
	Number	Complication	Number	Complication
Borer et al. (9)	24	25%	1	0
Shanberg et al. (10)	12	17%	1	0
Yang et al. (11)	18	17%	7	57%
El-Sherbiny et al. (12)	30	17%	4	25%
Nguyen et al. (13)	13	23%	18	22%
Cakan et al. (14)	28	25%	9	11%

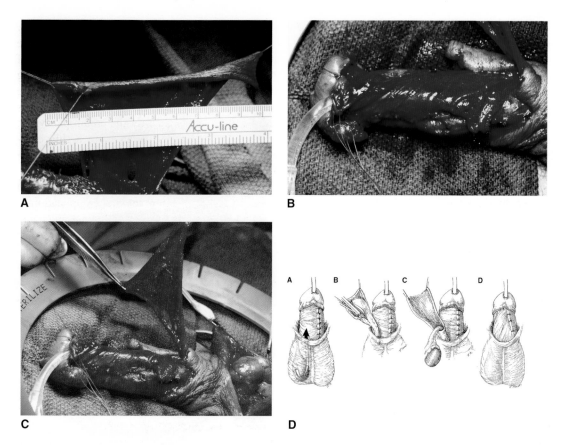

FIG. 25.3. (A and B) A 10-cm vascularized flap urethroplasty is performed. (C) A tunica vaginalis flap is harvested from the left hemiscrotal compartment and transposed with its vascular supply to cover the urethroplasty. (D) Illustration of tunica vaginalis flap dissection. (Courtesy of S.B. Brandes.)

TABLE 25.2. Surgical outcomes after the use of adjacent genital tissue in reoperative hypospadias.

	Technique	No. patients	Success rate (%)
Jayanthi et al. *(16)*	Flip-flap	28	71
	Vascularized flap	16	43
Teague et al. *(17)*	Flip-flap	9	89
Emir et al. *(18,19)*	Flip-flap	55	75
	Vascularized flap	33	58
Secrest et al. *(20)*	Flip-flap	34	53
	Vascularized flap	35	71
Simmons et al. *(21)*	Flip-flap	17	76
	Vascularized flap	36	86
Soutis et al. *(22)*	Vascularized flap	21	76
Zargooshi *(23)*	Vascularized flap	20	85

urethroplasty using either squamous *(6,23–26)*, transitional (bladder mucosa *[27–29]*), or pseudostratified (buccal mucosa *[26,30–34]*) is then required. Most hypospadias surgeons are somewhat uncomfortable with this approach because they are now trained in primary repairs that consist of either primary plate tubularization or vascularized flaps.

Grafts can be approached with a one- or two-stage operation. A graft must establish vascularity to survive. In reoperations, this neovascularity comes from the scarred recipient bed. Graft take is theoretically more reliable in a staged approach because the corporal bodies are likely healthier than the shaft skin that would be important in supplying blood to the ventral aspect of an onlay or tube graft. If a tube graft is used, a tunneled placement may cause less disruption to the ventral blood supply.

Bracka uses a staged grafting technique for most primary hypospadias and this same technique is very useful in reoperative repairs (23). During the first operation, the scarred urethral plate and unhealthy ventral tissue are excised. The graft is secured to the corporal bodies from the proximal urethral opening to the tip of the glans. The graft can be quilted onto the corporal bodies and a gentle compression dressing that immobilizes the graft. This prevents hematoma formation and the shear forces that inhibit the development of blood supply. Graft take can be assessed before a second tubularization at least 6 mo later.

A staged approach may give a better cosmetic result to the patient (23,33). When a hypospadias repair fails, the glans wings often contract and there is not sufficient width or mobility to achieve an orthotopic meatus after the second procedure. Glanular scarring can be excised and the graft can be interposed between the corporal bodies to give a deep groove for subsequent glansplasty and distal urethroplasty.

A barrier layer is required and this can be challenging when there is a paucity of local skin. A tunica vaginalis or subcutaneous scrotal flap has an excellent blood supply and can usually be mobilized to give a barrier layer (**Fig. 25.4**) The use of small intestinal submucosa has been described but in some series did not inhibit fistula formation and there was the subjective assessment of increased fibrosis ventrally.

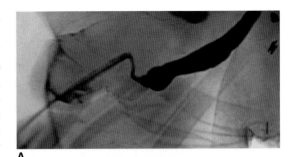

A

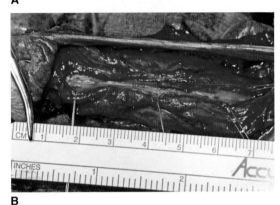

B

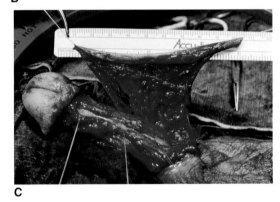

C

FIG. 25.4. A distal urethral stricture is visualized on a retrograde urethrogram (A). The narrowed urethra is opened in the ventral midline (B) and a dartos pedicle (circular skin flap) is isolated and an onlay urethroplasty is performed (C). (Courtesy of S.B. Brandes.)

3.4. Squamous Epithelium

Nonhair-bearing squamous epithelium has historically been the graft material of choice. Bracka uses the inner preputial skin for staged repairs but the prepuce is frequently unavailable in reoperative cases (23). Single-stage skin graft urethroplasty in these cases has a 30–50% failure rate with complete graft loss in up to 25% of cases. A split thickness technique has been described but the grafted area is usually very small so meshing may not be required to achieve coverage (24,25).

3.5. Bladder Mucosal Graft

Bladder mucosal urethral replacement was poplarized in the middle of the 1980s. Penile dissection and correction of chordee is completed before harvesting of the bladder mucosa. A Pfannestiel incision is used to harvest the bladder. Distending the bladder and sharply excising the muscle giving the typical "blue-domed cyst" appearance of the bulging mucosa best performs this. The bladder mucosa is very thin and difficult to handle.

Urethral meatal prolapse is a unique complication with bladder mucosa urethroplasty. The exposed transitional epithelium becomes sticky and hypertrophic *(28)*. Construction of a 20-French urethral meatus, prolonged catheter drainage, anchoring of graft to the corporal bodies, and a distal skin graft may reduce this complication. A greater than 75–85% success rate has been described with bladder mucosal urethral replacement. Certainly transitional epithelium is a natural choice for urethral replacement since it is normally exposed to urine. The need for the lower abdominal incision has led to the use of other graft materials.

3.6. Buccal Mucosal Graft

Buccal mucosa is a thick epithelium with good tensile strength and a very vascular submucosal plexus that favors graft take *(30)*. The thickness aids in dissection and subsequent manipulation of the graft material. The buccal mucosa can be harvested from either the inner cheek or lip. The harvest minimizes fat and avoids dissection into muscle. The inner cheek donor site is usually left open while the inner lip is allowed to heal by secondary intention. In the early 1990s, there were several reports of short-term success with single-stage buccal mucosal grafts in complex urethroplasty. Surprisingly, tube grafts seemed to do better than onlays, but the overall complication rate was as much as 60% with long-term follow-up *(33)*.

Buccal graft urethroplasty using the staged technique described by Bracka has improved outcomes when compared with single-stage buccal repairs *(34)*. In this technique, the initial graft take is probably better because it is dependent only upon the corporal bodies and not upon the previously operated ventral skin. The ability to inspect the graft prior to retubularization allows regrafting when clinically indicated. This likely decreases the development of urethral strictures.

Critics of staged procedures correctly note that some patients did not require two additional surgeries. Dorsal grafting of an attenuated yet supple plate has been described as part of a single stage repair. The decision to proceed with this approach require as appropriate assessment of the recipient bed.

4. Postpubertal and Adult Complications

A summary of our treatment algorithm for recurrent stricture after prior hypospadias repair is detailed in **Table 25.3**. Adult hypospadias surgery is associated with a much greater complication rate even in de novo cases *(35)*. Even though the techniques are similar, there are clear differences in wound healing, infections, and overall success rate. A number of steps may be taken to reduce the risk of complications in adults. All adults presenting for hypospadias repair should have a urine culture with directed treatment for positive cultures. Chronically infected or hair-bearing tissue should be removed at the time of surgery.

A postoperative suprapubic diversion may be beneficial from both a comfort and healing standpoint. A urethral catheter has a tendency to pull on the phallus and this can be very uncomfortable in the post-operative period. This distal tension may also disrupt the glansplasty.

The adult "cripple" has an abnormal meatus, a scarred glans, curvature that is either intrinsic or related to ventral urethral contraction, an absent foreskin and very thin or scarred ventral shaft skin that is usually adherent to the underlying urethra. Any future surgery is complicated because well-vascularized skin is not available for flaps and the lack of a good vascular bed hinders the success of free grafts (**Fig. 25.5**).

Strictures often develop long after an apparently successful hypospadias repair. This may be secondary to failed growth at puberty but Bracka suggests that balanitis xerotica obliterans is causative in at least 30% of late hypospadias failures and strictures *(37)*. In these cases, a skin graft is doomed to failure and buccal mucosa should be used as the graft material.

Surgical experience is a key to success and ideally the extent of the problem can be determined

TABLE 25.3. Treatment algorithm for reoperative hypospadias surgery.

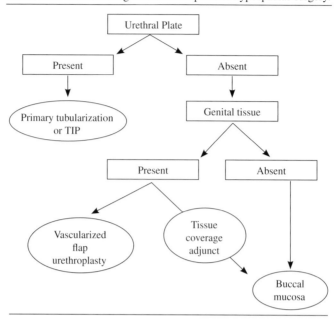

preoperatively. Abnormalities of only the distal shaft and glans are more readily corrected than cases where the entire urethra needs to be replaced. In theory, even in re-operative cases, the glans (spongiosum) has excellent blood supply. If there is minimal glans injury a deep cut into the ventrum gives an excellent vascular bed for a free graft.

If the urethral abnormality extends proximal to the glans then the region between the glans and the more proximal normal spongiosum is at risk for recurrent fistula, stricture, or complete breakdown. A planned-staged procedure is preferable in these cases. The advantages of a staged repair are more reliable and secure graft revascularization. In addition, one can observe graft take or contraction prior to completing the secondary tubularization.

The phallus should be degloved and all ventral fibrotic tissues should be sharply excised. If curvature persists then dorsal plications are usually performed. If the phallus if foreshortened and ventral grafting is performed, then a third operation will be required because a graft will not survive when placed on another graft. Snodgrass has described multiple transverse "feathered cuts" in the ventral corporal bodies at the time of a first stage buccal mucosal graft. This is successful only if the graft is aggressively quilted to eliminate hematomas under the graft and improve the take.

After the curvature is corrected, the entirety of the denuded tunica albuginea is grafted. The results of this procedure are assessed 6 mo later for adequacy of graft take, depth of the glans cleft and suppleness of the surrounding tissues. Tubularization of the urethra is completed only if these are satisfactory. A tunica vaginalis flap is usually available to cover this urethroplasty.

4.1. Urethral Hair

Urethral hair is an annoying complication that occurs when hair bearing skin is inadvertently incorporated into a urethroplasty. Infections, calculi, and trichobezoar (hair ball) may result (**Fig. 25.6**). Obviously, the use of nonhair-bearing skin flaps or free grafts is preferable. Preemptive epilation of hair bearing skin has been described but electrocoagulation of the dermal papillae is usually ineffective because of poor depth of penetration. The Nd:YAG laser has 4- to 5-mm penetration and destroys hair follicles more effectively.

However, if hair-bearing skin has been previously used, eradication and prevention of recurrence is very important. When isolated

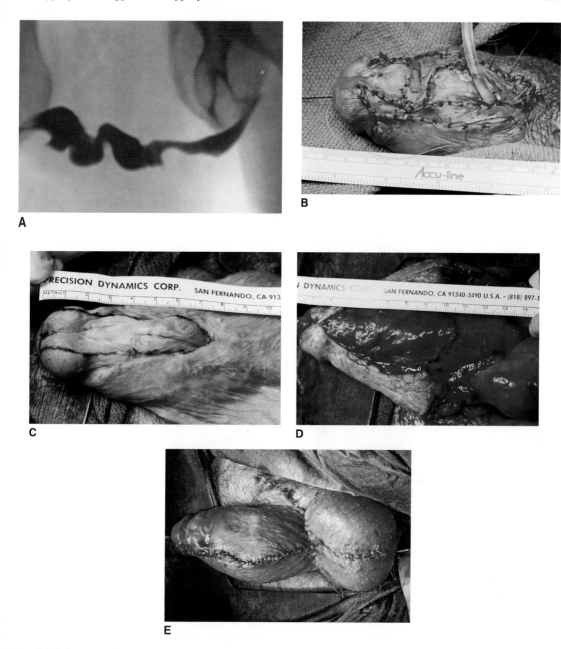

FIG. 25.5. A retrograde reveals distal tortuosity, stricture and mild diverticular formation after prior hypospadias surgery (A). The phallus is degloved and the ventral urethra is opened. The tissue is rearranged distally, advanced into a deep glans cleft and allowed to heal in preparation for a second stage (B). Six months later, there is a nice supple template available for tubularization and glansplasty (C, D, and E). Although this was the result of inlay of vascular tissue this is also the appearance after a free graft when adjacent genital skin is not available. (Courtesy of S.B. Brandes.)

hair is identified, endoscopic removal with laser coagulation of the base may be effective. When hair growth is more abundant, a urethrotomy should be performed. One has to decide whether the urethral segment needs to be replaced with a nonhair-bearing graft (in a staged fashion) or if the hair can be removed and the segment effectively depilated. If the segment then it should be closely followed for regrowth and chemical depilation can be attempted using reducing agents that break the cross-linkage disulfide bonds in keratin (38).

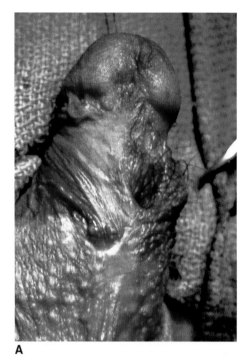

A

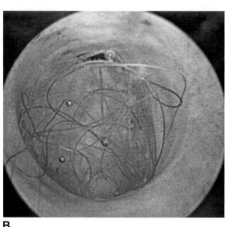

B

FIG. 25.6. (A) Hair extrudes from a distal shaft meatus. (B) The endoscopic appearance of urethral hair and urethrocutaneous fistula is shown. (Courtesy of S.B. Brandes.)

References

1. Waterman BJ, Renschelt T, Cartwright PC, et al (2002) Variables in successful repair of urethrocutaneous fistula after hypospadias surgery. J Urol 168:726–730
2. Churchill BM, Van Savage JG, Khoury AE, McLorie GA (1996) The dartos flap as an adjunct in preventing urethrocutaneous fistulas in repeat hypospadias surgery. J Urol 156:2047–2049
3. Landau EH, Gofrit ON, Meretyk S, et al. (2003) Outcome analysis of tunica vaginalis flap for the correction of recurrent urethrocutaneous fistula in children. J Urol 170:1596–1599
4. Heaton BW, Snow BW, Cartwright PC (1994) Repair of urethral diverticulum by placation. Urology 44:749–752
5. Vandersteen DR, Husmann DA (1998) Late onset recurrent penile chordee after successful correction at hypospadias repair. J Urol 160:1131–1133
6. Secrest CL, Jordan GH, Winslow BH, et al (1993) Repair of complications of hypospadias surgery. J Urol 150:1415–1418
7. Soylet Y, Gundogdu G, Yesildag E, Emir H (2004) Hypospadias reoperations. Eur J Ped Surg 14:188–192
8. Baskin LS, Duckett JW, Ueoka K, et al (1994) Changing concepts of hypospadias curvature lead to more onlay island flap procedures. J Urol 151:191–196
9. Borer JG, Bauer SB, Peters CA, et al. (2001) Tubularized incised plate urethroplasty: expanded use in primary and repeat surgery for hypospadias. J Urol 165:581–585
10. Shanberg AM, Sanderson K, Duel B (2001) Re-operative hypospadias repair using the Snodgrass incised plate urethroplasty. BJU Int 87:544–547
11. Yang SSD, Chen SC, Hsieh CH, Chen YT (2001) Re-operative snodgrass procedure. J Urol 166:2342–2345
12. El-Sherbiny MT, Hafez AT, Dawaba MS, et al (2004) Comprehensive analysis of tubularized incised-plate urethroplasty in primary and re-operative hypospadias. BJU Intl 93:1057–1061
13. Nguyen MT, Snodgrass WT (2004) Tubularized incised plate hypospadias reoperation. J Urol 171:2404–2406
14. Cakan M, Yalcinkaya F, Demirel F, et al (2005) The midterm success rates of tubularized incised plate urethroplasty in reoperative patients with distal or midpenile hypospadias. Pediatr Surg Int 21:973–976
15. Hayes MD, Malone PS (1999) The use of dorsal buccal mucosal graft with urethral plate incision (Snodgrass) for hypospadias salvage. BJU Int 84:508–509
16. Jayanthi VR, McLorie GA, Khoury AE, Churchill BM (1994) Can previously relocated penile skin be successfully used for salvage hypospadias repair? J Urol 152:740–743
17. Teague JL, Roth DR, Gonzales ET (1994) Repair of hypospadias complications using the meatal based flap urethroplasty. J Urol 151:470–472
18. Emir L, Erol D (2003) Mathieu urethroplasty as a salvage procedure: 20-Year experience. J Urol 169:2325–2327
19. Emir L, Bermiyanoglu C, Erol D (2003) Onlay island flap urethroplasty: a comparative analysis of primary versus reoperative cases. Urology 61:216–9

20. Simmons Br, Cain MP, Casale A, et al (1999) Repair of hypospadias complications using the previously utilized urethral plate. Urology 54: 724–726

21. Soutis M, Papandreou E, Mavridis G, Keramidas D (2003) Multiple failed urethroplasties: Definitive repair with the Duckett island-flap technique. J Pediatr Surg 38:1633–1636

22. Zargooshi J (2004) Tube-onlay-tube tunica vaginalis flap for proximal primary and reoperative adult hypospadias. J Urol 171:224–228

23. Bracka A (1995) A versatile two-stage hypospadias repair. Br J Plastic Surg 48:345–342

24. Ehrlich RM, Alter G (1996) Split-thickness skin graft urethroplasty and tunica vaginalis flaps for failed hypospadias repairs. J Urol 155:131–134

25. Schreiter F, Noll F (1989) Mesh graft urethroplasty using split thickness graft or foreskin. J Urol 142:1223–1226

26. Amukele SA, Stock JA, Hanna MK (2005) Management and outcome of complex hypospadias repairs. J Urol 174:1540–1543

27. Koyle MA, Ehrlich RM (1987) The bladder mucosal graft for urethral reconstruction. J Urol 138:1093–1095

28. Ransley PG, Duffy PG, Oesch IL, et al (1987) The use of bladder mucosa and combined bladder mucosa/preputial skin grafts for urethral reconstruction. J Urol 138:1096–1098

29. Decter RM, Roth DR, and Gonzales ET (1988) Hypospadias repair by bladder mucosal graft: an initial report. J Urol 40:1256–1258

30. Duckett JW, Coplen D, Ewalt D, Baskin LS (1995) Buccal mucosal urethral replacement. J Urol 153:1660–1663

31. Li L-C, Zhang X, Zhou S-W, et al. (1995) Experience with repair of hypospadias using bladder mucosa in adolescents and adults. J Urol 153:1117–1119

32. Ahmed S, Gough DCS (1997) Buccal mucosal graft for secondary hypospadias repair and urethral replacement. Br J Urol 80:328–330

33. Metro MJ, Wu H-Y, Snyder HM. Et al (2001) Buccal mucosal grafts: lessons learned from an 8-year experience. J Urol 166:1459–1461

34. Snodgrass W, Elmore J. (2004) Initial experience with staged buccal graft (Bracka) hypospadias reoperations. J Urol 172:1720–1724

35. Hensle TW, Tennenbaum SY, Reiley EA, Pollard J (2001) Hypospadias repairs in adults: adventures and misadventures. J Urol 165:77–77

36. Barbagli G, De Angelis M, Palminteri E, aLazzeri M (2006) Failed hypospadias repair presenting in adults. Eur Uroly 49:887–895

37. Depasqualie I , Park AJ, Bracka A (2000) The treatment of balanitis xerotica obliterans BJU Int 86:459–65

38. Singh Iqbal, Hemal AK (2001) Recurrent urethral hairball and stone in a hypospadiac: management and prevention J Endourol 15:645–7

26
Use of Omentum in Urethral Reconstruction

Steven B. Brandes

Contents

1. Introduction... 297
2. Anatomy of Omentum 299
3. Surgical Mobilization of Omentum 300
References.. 302

Summary The omentum is a well-vascularized organ that can be utilized to maximize surgical success and promote wound healing in urethral reconstruction and fistula repair. Omentum can act as a bulking flap to fill the dead space, as a physical barrier between reactive tissues, as well as a vascular blood supply and lymphatic drain to support tenuous tissues and to help resolve infections and tissue inflammation. In one-third of cases the omentum is long enough to reach the pelvis, without any mobilization. In the other two-thirds of cases, methods in omental lengthening include dissecting the omentum off the transverse colon, dissecting the omentum off the stomach, and basing the blood supply on the right gastroepiploic artery.

Keywords gastroepiploic artery, vascular arcade, physiologic drain, lymphatics, omental artery

1. Introduction

In reconstructive urology, the use of a well-vascularized interposition flap helps to insure surgical success and promote wound healing. Aside from muscle flaps like the gracilis or rectus, the omentum is a wonderful organ with multiple uses when it comes to urethral reconstruction (after posterior urethroplasty) and fistula (mainly vesical) closure

surgery. Furthermore, unlike the omentum, striated muscle tissue has a low resistance to infection. The omentum can serve many purposes: as bulk to fill the dead space, as a physical barrier between reactive tissues (such as in retroperitoneal fibrosis), and as a vascular blood supply support for tissue of tenuous vascularity (such as infected, radiated, or prior surgical fields). Omentum is unique in that it can help resolve infections and tissue inflammation by its characteristics of abundant blood supply, efficient lymphatic drainage, and because of its mobility and suppleness. The omentum is the main area of active lymphatic drainage in the abdomen (acting as a physiologic drain). The only instance that the omentum is naturally absent is in developmental anomalies of the fore-gut.

To properly use omentum flaps, an intimate knowledge of its anatomy and vasculature are required. In roughly one-third of cases, the omental apron is long enough to reach the perineum without any mobilization of either vacular pedicle. To use the omentum in lower urinary tract reconstruction, the omentum typically has to be lengthened to reach the pelvis. The first way to gain omental length is to dissect the omentum off the transverse colon from left to right along the avascular plane. By lifting the omentum cephalad, the dissection usually begins on the left to the right in a bloodless

From: *Current Clinical Urology: Urethral Reconstructive Surgery*
Edited by: S.B. Brandes © Humana Press, Totowa, NJ

Cross-sectional View

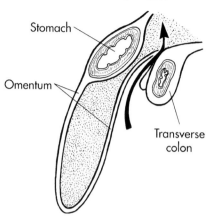

Stomach

Omentum

Transverse
colon

FIG. 26.1. Cross-sectional view of the dissection planes
between the omentum and transverse colon. (From Yu
GW and Miller HC: Critical operative maneuvers in
urologic surgery. Mosby Publ., St. Louis.)

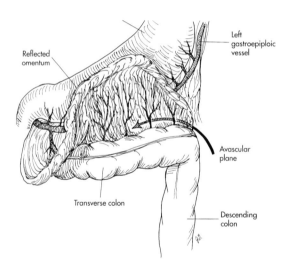

Reflected
omentum

Left
gastroepiploic
vessel

Avascular
plane

Transverse colon

Descending
colon

FIG. 26.2. Lifting the entire omentum cephalad helps to
delineate the avascular plane between the left omentum and
transverse colon (left to right) (From Critical Maneuvers in
Urologic Surgery (1996), Mosby, St. Louis.)

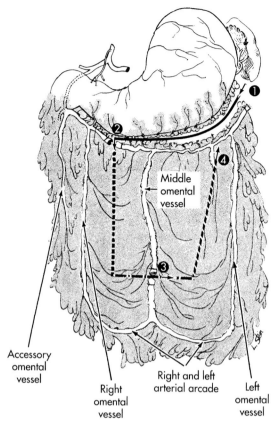

Middle
omental
vessel

Accessory
omental
vessel

Right
omental
vessel

Right and left
arterial arcade

Left
omental
vessel

FIG. 26.3. The typical blood supply to the omentum consists of the right and left gastroepiploic vessels, which
form the gastroepiploic arcade, which further divides
into a middle, left, right, and accessory omental artery
(From Ref. [2])

plane between the omentum and transverse colon
(**Figs. 26.1 and 26.2**). We typically perform this
step with electrocautery on a low setting (as opposed
to the short gastrics, which must be ligated). This
maneuver of freeing the omentum from the colon
will typically lengthen the omental length, considerably; typically till the pelvic inlet or beyond.

When the omentum is short or insufficient,
despite mobilization of the transverse colon (which

occurs in roughly 40%), length can be gained only
by dissecting the omentum off the stomach. To
do so, the short gastrics are taken down and the
vascular pedicle to the omentum is based on the
right or left gastroepiploic artery (which forms a
vacular arcade that is the main blood supply for the
omentum; **Fig. 26.3**) In most, the right gastroepiploic
artery is much larger then on the left, and its vertical branches supply more then two-thirds of the
omental apron. Omental lengthening dissection
is usually based on the right pedicle, because in
10% of patients the gastroepiploic arteries do not
anastomose to form an arcade (*1*). In such patients,
if mobilization is based on the left gastroepiploic
arteries, the pedicle will become ischemic. (**Fig.
26.4, A** and **B**) We strongly discourage dividing
the omentum transversely, across the apron, below
the gastroepiploic arch because that will potentially

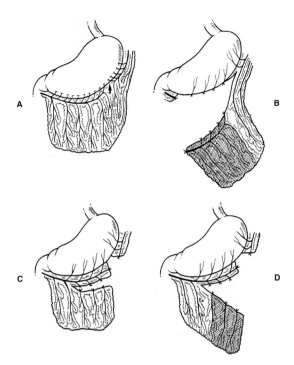

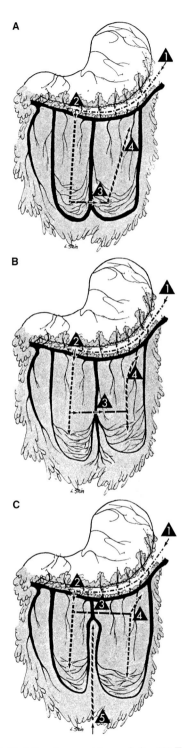

FIG. 26.4. (A, B) Omental mobilization based on the left gastroepiploic artery can result in distal omental ischemia. In 10% of patients, the right and left gastroepiploic arteries do not anastomose (note arrow). (C, D) Transverse division across the omental arcade often leads to distal ischemia. (From Turner Warwick R, Kirby RS (1993) Principles of sphincteroplaty, in Webster G, Kirby R, King L, Goldwasser B (eds) Reconstructive urology. Boston, Blackwell Scientific Publications)

compromise an already tenuous arcade, and lead to distal ischemia (**Fig. 26.4, C** and **D**).

2. Anatomy of Omentum

In general, there are four arterial branches off the gastroepiploics (the left, middle, right, and accessory omental vessels), of which later anastomose (in varying degrees) at the distal aspect of the omentum (**Fig. 26.5A**). Five major variations in the arcade have been noted and are based on the absence or presence of the middle omental artery and the level of its bifurcation. The right gastroepiploic artery is a branch of the gastroduodenal artery, and occasionally from the superior mesenteric. The left gastroepiploic artery is a branch from the splenic artery. Alday and Goldsmith (2), in their classic paper, detailed the

FIG. 26.5. Variations in omental vascularity. (A) Type 1: the middle omental artery bifurcates near the lower end of the omental apron. (B) Type 2: the middle omental artery bifurcates midway between the gastroepiplic arch and the lower end of the omental apron. (C) Type 3: the middle omental artery bifurcates 2 to 3cm from gastroepiploic arch (From Ref [2])

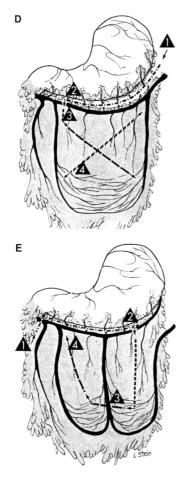

D

E

L Stein

Fig. 26.5. (continued) (D) Type 4: no middle omental artery. (E) Type 5: the left omental artery is a direct branch off the splenic artery. The right gastroepiploic artery supplies the middle omental artery (From Ref *[2]*)

loic arch (3%). In type 4, there is no middle omental artery. The right and left omental arteries form the arcade (1%). Finally, in type 5, an uncommon pattern (0.7%), the terminal branch of the splenic artery is not part of the gastroepiploic arch but instead connects directly into the left omental artery. The right gastroepiploic artery diminishes in caliber as it traverses the lower portion of the greater curvature of the stomach and never develops communication with the short gastric vessels. The middle omental artery arises from the right gastroepiploic artery.

3. Surgical Mobilization of Omentum

By holding the omentum up and trans-illuminating it, the arcade pattern can be determined. After dividing one of the gastroepiploic arteries (usually the left), serially ligate the short gastrics, favoring the stomach side to preserve the vascular arcade of the omentum. (**Fig. 26.6**) There are roughly 20–40 short gastric branches of the right gastroepiploic vessels to the stomach and each of these needs to be ligated to carefully and fully mobilize the omentum. The short gastrics on the greater curvature of the stomach are arranged in two distinct rows, anterior and posterior. Meticulous hemostasis is mandatory in order to avoid an omental hematoma. We typically ligate the omental pedicle vessels with 2-O absorbable (polyglactin) sutures. We discourage the use of

omental vasculature patterns in 136 cadavers. They determined that the omental blood supply arcades could be divided into five main types (**Fig. 26.5, A–E**). Furthermore, they described surgical methods for how to develop omental length for each of the 5 types of arcades. The 5 types are divided by the level of the bifurcation or the presence or absence of the middle omental artery (**Fig. 26.5, A–E**). Type 1 is by far the most common (85%) pattern and is where the middle omental artery bifurcates near the caudal end of the apron. In type 2, the middle omental artery bifurcates or trifucates midway between the gastroepiploic arch and the lower end of the apron (10%). In type 3, the middle omental artery bifurcates or trifurcates roughly 2 to 3 cm below the gastroepip-

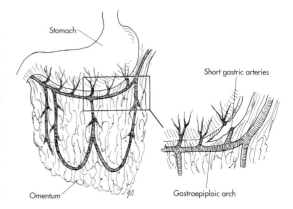

Fig. 26.6. To free the omentum from the stomach, the short gastric arteries are divided close to the stomach (From Yu GW and Miller HC: Critical Operative Maneuvers in Urologic Surgery (1996), St. Louis, Mosby)

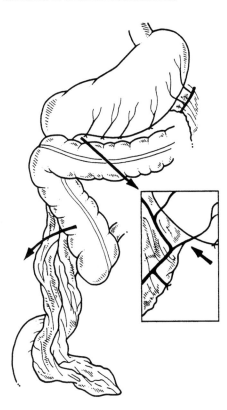

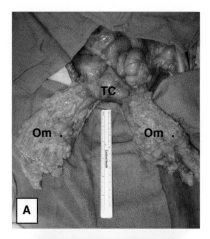

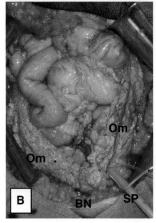

FIG. 26.7. Omental mobilization into the colic gutter. Mobilizing the right gastroepiploic vessel to its gastroduodenal origin avoids rupture of the lateral undivided branches (arrow). (From Webster G et al. (1993). Reconstructive urology. London, Blackwell)

liga-clips on the short gastrics because they often get caught in the tissues and become avulsed. Electrocautery for omental hemostasis (during mobilization), is typically not effective because the vessels walls are too thin and short, and they do not electro-obliterate easily. Furthermore, as the omentum is mobilized off the stomach, mobilization of the right gastroepiploic artery should be extended all the way to the left, at the level of the gastroduodenal origin. In so doing, when the omentum is pulled caudally into the pelvis, excessive tension on the pedicle and the potential for rupturing off the last few lateral, undivided branches to the pyloric area are prevented (**Fig. 26.7**). An excellent use of such an omental flap is after pubectomy and primary anastomosis during a posterior urethroplasty. Here, omentum facilitates the anastomotic blood supply, and thus success, as well as fills the dead space (**Fig. 26.8**).

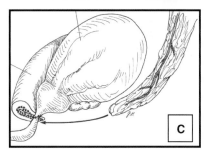

FIG. 26.8. Pubectomy and transabdominal urethroplasty patient. (A) Long omentum is split in midline. (B) Via the colic gutters, omentum is brought to pelvis, for bulking and vasculature. (C) Omental interposition at pubectomy site

Once the omental pedicle is mobilized, we usually run it along the colic gutter to reach into the pelvis (**Fig. 26.9**). The ascending colon is typically mobilized medially and the omentum placed behind it. This will help prevent potential bowel entrapment

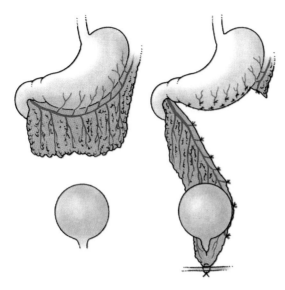

FIG. 26.9. Full-length mobilization of the vascular pedicle of the omentum. (From Turner-Warwick R, Chapple C (2002) Functional reconstruction of the urinary tract and gynaeco-urology. Oxford, Blackwell Science, pp 164)

and subsequent bowel obstruction. Because full mobilization of the right gastroepiploic pedicle often results in a period of ileus and abdominal and gastric distention, temporary nasogastric drainage and bowel rest for at least 24 to 48 h is warranted. Although usually excessive and unnecessary, as an alternative to nasogastric drainage tube placement, a temporary gastrostomy tube (G tube) can be done at the time of the omental surgery. A G tube, however, is often unnecessary, and some consider it excessive, since bowel rest is typically short-lived. Moreover, early gastric distention can potentially avulse ties on the ligated short gastrics. If a G tube is selected, make the Witzel tunnel start off on the left and exit on the right. Otherwise, the G tube can be pushed through the pylorus and into the duodenum. The long gastric tunnel over the catheter helps prevent leakage after the tube is removed. Surgical failure after omental flap interposition is usually due to one of the four possibilities: 1) failure to mobilize a sufficient bulk of omentum; 2) inappropriate omental mobilization resulting in impairment of the blood supply; 3) failure to properly anchor the omentum down and/or placing it effectively as an interposition flap; and 4) not avoiding overlapping suture lines.

References

1. Turner–Warwick R (1976) The use of the omental pedicle graft in urinary tract reconstruction. J Urol 116:341–347
2. Alday ES, Goldsmith HS (1972) Surgical techniques for omental lengthening based on arterial anatomy. Surg Gynecol Obstet 135:103.

27
Female Urethral Reconstruction

Jason Anast, Steven B. Brandes, and Carl Klutke

Contents

1. Introduction... 303
2. Anatomy and Function.. 304
    2.1. Anatomy of the Urethra 304
    2.2. Function of the Urethra... 304
3. Pathology of Female Urethra Injury 304
    3.1. Iatrogenic 304
    3.2. Trauma 305
4. Preoperative Evaluation 305
5. Treatment for Urethral Injuries and Incontinence.. 306
    5.1. Surgery for Urethral Loss... 306
    5.2. Female Urethral Stricture Reconstruction.. 309
6. Overall Outcomes 311
7. Transvaginal Closure of the Bladder Neck 311
References... 313

Summary Female urethral injury is an uncommon issue, though frequently requiring complex surgical reconstruction. Appropriate diagnosis and treatment of female urethral injuries requires an adequate understanding of female urethra anatomy and function, causes of female urethra injury, diagnostic evaluation of the female urethra, and proper surgical treatments of female urethral injuries. Most injuries are due to iatrogenic causes, childbirth, or pelvic fracture. Injuries that result in urethral loss can be corrected with urethroplasty utilizing vaginal tissue advancement or advancement of a flap of bladder tissue. Placement of a sling for coexisting incontinence can be performed simultaneously with autologous fascia; sling placement in patients without stress incontinence, though frequently practiced, is controversial. Depending on the location, urethral strictures can be treated with meatotomy, endoscopic incision, or graft urethroplasty. For the most severe cases, urine can be diverted suprapubically, with the bladder closed transvaginally with a tight obstructing autologous sling or via surgical closure of the bladder neck. Surgical repair of female urethral injuries is usually a successful procedure with durable outcomes.

Keywords urethra, vagina, injury, stricture, repair

1. Introduction

Female urethra injury is a rare problem, frequently requiring complex reconstruction. Appropriate diagnosis and treatment of female urethral injuries requires competency of female urethra anatomy

From: *Current Clinical Urology: Urethral Reconstructive Surgery*
Edited by: S.B. Brandes © Humana Press, Totowa, NJ

and function, causes of female urethra injury, diagnostic evaluation of the female urethra, and proper surgical treatments of female urethral injuries. Each of these topics is reviewed in detail below.

2. Anatomy and Function

2.1. Anatomy of the Urethra

The urethra is a thin fibromuscular tube, 2 to 5 cm in length, responsible for both drainage of urine from the bladder and continence. The female urethra comprises several tissue layers. The proximal two-thirds of the female urethra is lined by transitional cells that are a continuation from the urothelial lining of the bladder. In the distal urethra, the urothelial lining transitions into stratified squamous epithelial cells. The mucosa is redundant with multiple folds, which contribute to continence by acting as a seal. Deep to the urothelial lining lies the lamina propria, a soft tissue layer of longitudinally organized collagen and elastin fibers, as well as a venous plexus, which has been postulated to contribute to continence by increasing the resting pressure of the urethra. The musculature of the female urethra is comprised of an inner smooth layer and a striated external layer. The inner smooth layer runs longitudinally along the entire urethra. The proximal third of the external sphincter completely encircles the urethra. The middle of the external urethral sphincter covers the ventral surface of the urethra in a horseshoe shape, increasing in size distally to envelop the distal vagina and has been called the urethrovaginal sphincter. The relative lack of musculature in the distal third of the female urethra allows it to act as a nozzle to direct the flow of urine.

2.2. Function of the Urethra

The urethra plays a major role in continence and storage of urine. In addition to the intrinsic anatomical features mentioned previously, the structure of the female pelvis contributes to continence. The proximal and mid urethra provides the majority of baseline continence due to tonic contraction of the circumferential external sphincter. Additionally, the urethra rests upon a supportive layer of endopelvic fascia and anterior vaginal wall, gaining additional structural stability through lateral attachments to the arcus tendineus and

levator ani muscle. Pressure from above compresses the mid-urethra against this hammock-like supportive layer, constricting its lumen closed and preventing urine leakage during cough *(1)*. Micturition is initiated by relaxation of the external urethra followed by parasympathetic mediated contraction of the detrusor. Contraction of urethral smooth muscle contributes to micturition by shortening the urethra and opening the bladder neck.

3. Pathology of Female Urethra Injury

Female urethral impairment requiring reconstruction can generally be attributed to two major sources: traumatic injury and postsurgical iatrogenic injury. In developing countries, trauma is most commonly caused by obstetrical complications of prolonged childbirth, whereas in industrial countries is usually related to injury from pelvic fracture. Urethral injury in developed countries is more likely to be due to iatrogenic injury from urogynecological surgery, such as diverticulectomy or synthetic sling placement. Less common causes of urethral injury are urethral destruction or erosion from chronic urethral catheterization, pelvic radiation, or locally advanced carcinoma.

3.1. Iatrogenic

In developed countries, anterior vaginal or urethral surgery is the most common cause of urethral fistula or erosion. In a review of 98 cases with urethral damage, previous vaginal or urethral surgery was the primary insult in 86 (88%) of the cases, with transvaginal bladder neck suspension, urethral diverticulectomy, and anterior colporraphy the most common. Synthetic urethral sling placement has become greatly used during the past decade and, although rare, urethral erosion is potential complication after synthetic sling placement. The most common presenting symptoms include hematuria, irritative voiding complaints, recurrent stress incontinence, and periurethral discomfort *(2)*. Patients may also present with urinary retention, with urethral erosion thought to be secondary to trauma caused by recurrent urethral catheterization and/or dilation, or urethral necrosis due to excessive sling tensioning or poor tissue regenerative properties (i.e. radiated tissue, estrogen deficiency, or immunosuppressive state). Symptoms of erosion may not present for several months, with some erosions not presenting until up to 15 years after sling placement. Interestingly, most cases to date have involved urethra erosion without evidence of fistula formation *(3)*. If suspicion of urethral erosion arises after sling placement, urethroscopy can be performed to visualize intraluminal sling material. The bladder should be inspected at the same time to rule out intravesical sling violation. Treatment of urethral sling erosion is detailed later in this chapter.

3.2. Trauma

3.2.1. Obstetrical

Obstetrical trauma of the urethra is the result of maternal-fetal head disproportion leading to prolonged fetal head compression of the bladder and urethra against the pelvic bones, causing extensive ischemic necrosis and subsequent fistula formation. Modern obstetrical techniques have virtually eliminated this type of injury in developed countries; however, it may be seen in up to 4 women per 1000 vaginal deliveries in some non-industrialized areas. While most fistulas occur between the bladder and vagina, injury to the proximal urethra involves as much as 17% of all obstetric fistulas. Because of the involvement of the proximal urethra, virtually all patients present with total urinary incontinence as their major complaint. Most urethral fistulas due to obstetric complications are 1.5 cm in diameter or greater, and therefore are usually easily seen on vaginal examination. Proximal urethra injuries can be categorized as either partial or complete absence of the proximal urethra: partial absence is identified by the ability to pass a catheter into the bladder with the inferior aspect of the catheter entering the bladder able to be seen in the vagina, whereas complete absence of the proximal urethra is identified by a blind ending distal urethra and a communication between the bladder and anterior vagina. Rarely, ischemic injury can lead to complete urethra sloughing *(4)*.

3.2.2. Pelvic Fracture

Injury to the female urethra due to pelvic fracture is less common than that for similar injuries in males (0–6% in modern series vs 10% in males), likely

as the result of greater mobility, relatively protected, and shorter length of the urethra in females. Urethral injury may be more common in pediatric than adult females with similar injuries. Inability to void, urinary incontinence through the vagina, hematuria, or blood at the introitus in the setting of pelvic trauma should raise concern that there is an associated urethral injury.

Perry noted that most female urethral injuries were longitudinal lacerations, in patients with less severe mechanisms of injury *(5)*. Such lacerations are more easily overlooked since such patients can usually be catheterized. In contrast, Venn *(6)*, and later Podesta *(7)* both noted that most of their female urethral injuries were avulsion, distraction injuries, and associated with major trauma and other severe injuries. Such avulsion injuries are less likely to be overlooked, because of inability to catheterize and higher chance for concomitant vaginal (up to 87%) or rectal laceration and blood per vault. Recommended options for management of urethral avulsions were: 1) primary urethral realignment (endoscopic); 2) unstable patient, i.e., suprapubic tube and delayed reconstruction; 3) prepubertal girls (combined abdominal-vaginal approach with partial pubectomy); and 4) pubertal and post puberty, i.e., abdominal approach.

4. Preoperative Evaluation

Patients suspected of having a urethral injury or defect, initial evaluation always consists of thorough physical examination. The patient should be examined in the lithotomy position. Although a pelvic examination with a vaginal speculum should always be performed, many urethral defects are visible upon inspection of the anterior vagina. Flexible cystoscopy in the office should be performed to evaluate for a mucosal defect or foreign body, particularly if a sling procedure has been performed. Difficulty with cystoscope insertion may be indications of a urethral stricture. With a flexible cystoscope the location of the stricture (mid, distal, proximal, bladder neck) can be determined. A voiding cystourethrography will help determine the length of the stricture (**Fig. 27.1**). Signs and symptoms that will suggest a urethral stricture include a history of pelvic fracture, previous urethral surgery (such as urethral dilation or diverticulectomy), and obstructive voiding, as

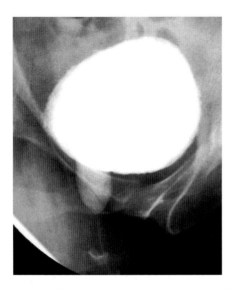

FIG. 27.1. Voiding cystourethrogram reveals a distal urethral stricture

evidenced by a poor peak flow on uroflometry and obstructive voiding complaints on American Urological Association symptom score. Patients with previous pelvic malignancy or concern of concurrent malignancy should undergo biopsy of the fistula tract prior to any surgical reconstruction. A novel test to determine the location of urinary-vaginal fistula is the double dye test: after insertion of a tampon into the vagina, phenazopyridine is taken orally and methylene blue is injected into the bladder via a catheter. Blue discoloration of the distal tampon suggests a urethral–vaginal fistula, whereas a blue discoloration of the middle of the tampon and orange discoloration of the proximal tampon suggests a vesicovaginal or uretral–vaginal fistula, respectively. Imaging can be helpful in determining the extent of injury, particularly when office examination is equivocal. Voiding cystourethrography and pelvic ultrasound have traditionally been the imaging study of choice to document female urethral fistula or stricture. Endovaginal magnetic resonance imaging is slowly becoming the modality of choice for imaging the female pelvis, being more sensitive and specific than urethrography, urethroscopy, or ultrasound for a variety of urethral abnormalities (in particular, urethral diverticulum). Urine culture should be obtained before any scheduled surgical procedure. If concern exists for pelvic malignancy, obtaining a urine cytology should also be considered.

5. Treatment for Urethral Injuries and Incontinence

The goals of urethral reconstruction are to create a continent neourethra that will allow urine to flow freely and is of sufficient length so that the patient does not void into the vagina. Most patients who present with an iatrogenic urethral injury have undergone one or more prior vaginal surgeries and have troublesome urinary incontinence. The vagina is usually severely scarred. Prior to surgery it is important to assess the full extent of tissue loss and the ability of local tissue to be utilized for reconstruction. In general, the urethra can be reconstructed with an anterior vaginal wall flap. If the vaginal tissue is very scarred or insufficient, a perineal or labial pedicel flap is often used. Furthermore, a well vascularized labial fat pedicle flap (Martius flap) is also mobilized to buttress the reconstructed urethra. Rarely, a gracilis or rectus muscle flap is need.

5.1. Surgery for Urethral Loss

5.1.1. Urethral Sling Injury

The patient is placed in dorsal lithotomy position, sterilely prepped and draped, and a a weighted speculum placed into the vagina. An inverted U-shaped incision is then made on the anterior vagina. A 16-French Foley catheter is placed. Necrotic and ischemic tissue is débrided. All eroding sling material should be carefully identified and dissected out. We typically only excise the offending segment of sling and a small amount on either side, leaving the majority of the sling intact. Next, the urethral defect is primarily closed with interrupted absorbable sutures. An incision is then made over one of the labia majora and a labial fat pad (Martius flap) is mobilized. The fat pad is brought over the urethral repair and sutured into place, taking care not to place any significant tension on the flap (**Fig. 27.2**). The vaginal mucosa is advanced over the defect and closed in several watertight nonoverlapping layers. Post-operatively, the patient is continued on antibiotics for 1 to 2 weeks, and the catheter is left in place for at least 2 weeks.

Although this procedure will work for most cases of urethral injury, obviously the repair should be individualized to each patient's specific problem and anatomy. A variety of novel surgical

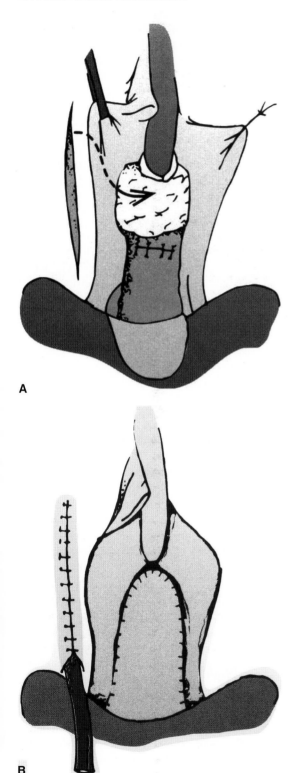

A

B

FIG. 27.2. Martius Fat Pad. A. A labial fat pad is mobilized and advanced to cover the urethra. B. The vaginal and labial incisions are closed and a drain placed within the labia dissection

approaches to repair the damaged female urethra have been reported. Friedman et al. *(8)* described crossing the bulbocavernosal muscles under the urethra to cover the defect. Instead of just using a labial flap, Davis et al. *(9)* described rotating an intact flap of labial mucosa and fat over the defect, which may be provide less tension on the tissue than the Martius procedure but is likely less cosmetically appealing. The variety of techniques used to replace the repair the female urethra highlights the need to individualize the procedure to each patient. Bruce et al. *(10)* described the use of a rectus muscular flap for use in complicated or recurrent urethrovaginal fistulas, with no recurrences in six patients and five of six patients continent. Mundy *(11)* reported on a tubularized pedicle flap of labial fat or omentum.

5.1.2 Open Urethroplasty

5.1.2.1. Vaginal Flap Urethroplasty

When the periurethral vaginal tissue is not adequate, a vaginal flap (akin to the Mathieu "flip-flap" repair for hypospadias) can be rotated to reconstruct a functional urethra. A ventral and midline urethrotomy is made until the urethra open up to a normal caliber and the epithelium is supple and pink. Bougies a boule are useful here to calibrate the urethra and determine if the urethrotomy needs to be extended. A "U"-shaped incision is then made in the adjacent and cephalad vaginal wall that is felt to be supple enough to be raised and rotated. Once the "U" flap of epithelium is mobilized, it is flipped distally and sutured as a dorsal onlay flap to create a tubular neourethra over a Foley catheter. (**Fig. 27.3**). The anterior vaginal wall harvest site is then closed primarily. When there is insufficient vaginal wall for coverage a labial or local thigh flap can be raised and mobilized into the field. If any extravasation is noted on imaging, a Foley catheter is replaced for another 2 weeks.

5.1.2.2. Vaginal Wall Urethroplasty

When there is adequate peri-urethral vaginal tissue, two parallel incisions are made in the lateral vaginal wall, on either side of the urethral catheter; with the addition of an inverted "U" shaped vaginal wall flap (**Fig. 27.4**). The flaps of vaginal tissue are mobilized from lateral to medial and rolled into a tube over a urethral catheter and sutured together

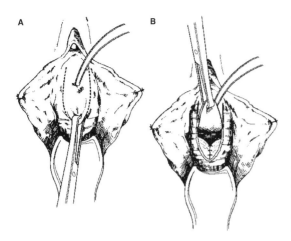

FIG. 27.3. Vaginal Flap Urethroplasty. A. "U"-shaped incision into healthy anterior vaginal tissue and advanced distally around the urethra. B. Vaginal wall flap is "flipped" anteriorly and sutured around the catheter to lengthen the urethra. (From Rosenblum N, Nitti VW: Female urethral reconstruction. Atlas Urol Clin NA 12:213–223, 2004)

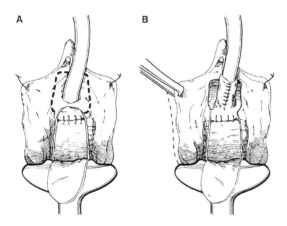

FIG. 27.4. Vaginal wall urethroplasty. A. Anterior vaginal "U" shaped wall flap and periurethral parallel vaginal wall incisions are made B. Vaginal wall tubularized around the catheter to create a neourethra. "U" flap then advanced to cover the neourethra. (From Rosenblum N, Nitti VW: Female urethral reconstruction. Atlas Urol Clin NA 12:213–223, 2004)

in the midline with absorbable suture. When there is extensive scarring, a flap of labia minora can be raised and tubularized to create a neourethra. A Martius fat pad flap is then mobilized from the labia majora and tunneled underneath the vaginal epithelium and sewn into place to cover the suture

line of the neourethra. If a single labial fat flap does not provide adequate urethral coverage, a second flap should be dissected from the contralateral labia. If the contralateral labia is still deficient, an alternative is a gracilis muscle flap from the inner thigh. To provide additional suburethral support, a pubovaginal sling of autologous fascia can be harvested from the anterior abdomen and placed at this time. An alternative and readily available source for autologous fascia is the tensor fascia lata from the lateral thigh. Blavis (12) has reported good success with concomitant sling placement. We prefer, however, to delay the sling or incontinence procedure to a later day when we can better assess the nature of any incontinence and so as not to potentially compromise our urethroplasty surgery. The initial and inverted "U" shaped vaginal incision is then advanced to cover the entire reconstructed urethra. Again, a vaginal pack is placed for 24 to 48 hours and a voiding cystourethrogram performed after 2 to 3 weeks to insure urethral healing.

5.1.3. Pubovaginal Sling for Associated Stress Incontinence

In patients with concomitant stress urinary incontinence, a simultaneous pubovaginal sling can be performed with neourethral reconstruction. The sling material of choice here is autologous fascia. Synthetic grafts should be avoided. Although allografts and xenografts (such as small intestine submucosa) can be used, there is little support in the literature for this practice. The autologous fascia, 2 cm wide, is harvested from the anterior rectus sheath via a Pfannenstiel incision, (**Fig. 27.5**) and then placed over the reconstructed urethra and Martius flap. The sling is secured without tension to the rectus fascia on either side.

5.1.4. Bladder Flap

The female urethra can also be reconstructed with a bladder flap for more proximal urethral injuries or complete urethral loss. Hemal et al. (13) detailed this technique of urethral reconstruction for injuries after pelvic fracture. Starting at the bladder neck, oblique or vertical bladder incisions are made. Vertical bladder flaps provide more length then oblique flaps, which are limited by the location of

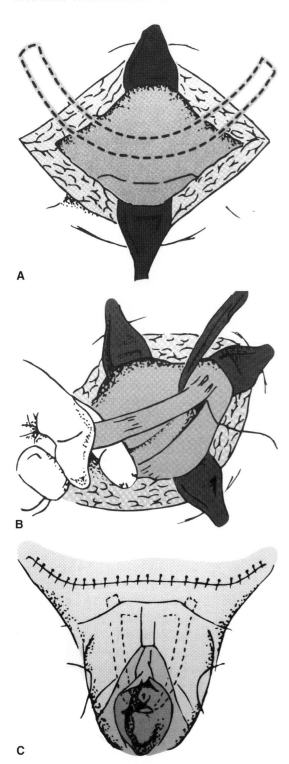

the ureteral orifices. The flap is then tubularized over a catheter. Space between the anterior vaginal wall and the pubic bone is created by sharp dissection to allow routing of the urethra into the vestibule. This can be surgically challenging, however, because the tissue planes may be obliterated and the bladder adherent to the pubic bone after prior pelvic fracture. Tanahgo *(14)* also described a similar tubularized anterior bladder flap for urethral reconstruction. Concomitant pubovaginal sling can be performed to improve urine control from stress incontinence. However, we typically defer sling placement till after a prolonged recovery from the major surgery.

5.2. Female Urethral Stricture Reconstruction

At first, it is important to rule out a primary or direct extension malignancy etiology for the stricture. Urethral cancers are rare, and present as a palpable urethral mass or induration and/or for smelling urethral discharge in women older than 50. In contrast to male urethral strictures, where a treatment plan and outcomes are more readily available, the female urethral stricture algorithm is not well defined. Nonmalignant causes of female stricture disease most commonly are observed after pelvic radiation for GYN malignancy (e.g., cervical) and iatrogenic (e.g., diverticulectomy or instrumentation). In general, stricture repairs can be either open or endoscopic. Because the female urethra is relatively short (roughly 4 cm), stricture excision and primary anastomosis is typically not feasible.

5.2.1. Distal Urethral Stricture

Women with stenoses or stricture of the distal urethra typically present with obstructive voiding. Such distal strictures typically occur after traumatic instrumentation of the urethra, endoscopic procedures, after radiotherapy to the pelvis of vulva, and more commonly in postmenopausal women with vulvar dystrophy or significant vaginal atrophy. Female urethral strictures are very uncommon and typically managed by recurrent urethrotomy and urethral dilation.

Meatotomy can be performed to treat distal strictures by simple incision of the meatus. In general,

Fig. 27.5. Pubovaginal Sling. A, B. The anterior rectus sheath fascia is harvested through a Pfannenstiel incision. C. The fascia is placed over the urethra and secured to the rectus fascia without tension

circumferential and distal urethrectomy and advancement meatoplasty works well for distal urethral strictures (a distal stricture being within 5 to 10 mm of the meatus). Interrupted absorbable sutures are first placed at four quadrants, into the more proximal, healthy urethral mucosa (proximal to the strictured segment), so that the mucosa does not retract (**Fig. 27.6**). A circumferential excision of the distal urethra and meatus is performed sharply and the cut edges sutured to the vaginal epithelium. A Foley catheter is typically left indwelling for 1–3 days. As an adjunct to promote healing, daily intravaginal estrogens cream placement is often helpful.

5.2.2. Mid-Urethral Strictures

5.2.2.1. Endoscopic Repair

Midurethral strictures can be managed by visual internal urethrotomy. Incisions in the scar tissue are usually made at the 3- and 9-o'clock position, with an occasional additional 12-o'clock incision. After urethrotomy, a urethral catheter is typically maintained for several days to a week. Some advocate clean intermittent catheterization after urethrotomy to help prolong or "prevent" that risk of stricture recurrence. However, in general, the concept that self catheterization will help stabilize a stricture is often untrue; time until stricture recurrence is only delayed as long as the catheterization is still regularly preformed. We thus do not commonly recommend self-catheterization.

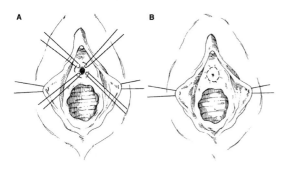

FIG. 27.6. Distal Urethral Stricture Repair. A. Four quadrant traction stitches are placed in the urethra proximal to the stricture to prevent retraction. B. Stricture is circumferentially excised and the healthy proximal urethra sutured to the vaginal epithelium. (From Rosenblum N, Nitti VW: Female urethral reconstruction. Atlas Urol Clin NA 12:213–223, 2004)

Obliterative mid-urethral strictures that are not amenable to a simple urethrotomy have been managed in a few cases with a "cut to the light" procedure. This procedure often is performed (from above and below) with simultaneous above and below cystoscopy, under direct visualization and fluoroscopic guidance. Two surgeons are typically needed, and finding the "true" lumen is often difficult or unclear. Such procedures require prolonged Foley catheter drainage to ensure urethral epitheliazation. Furthermore, post procedure, indefinite intermittent catheterization will usually be needed, otherwise the stricture will recur.

5.2.2.2. Graft Urethroplasty

Buccal mucosa grafts for male urethral reconstruction have been successful and durable and thus intuitively should work well for female strictures.

5.2.2.2.1. Dorsal Placement The patient is placed lithotomy and a guidewire is placed across the stricture. The dorsal aspect of the distal urethra is then dissected from the surrounding tissue through a suprameatal incision and the urethral wall incised dorsally at the 12-o'clock position until normal urethral tissue and lumen size are reached. Mean incision urethral length is 2–3 cm from the meatus *(15)*. The proximal urethra is then calibrated with a large (30-Fr) bougie. We prefer to harvest our free graft from the inner cheek. As for male urethroplasty the buccal graft needs to be defatted and thinned to facilitate 'take" in a vascular host bed.

5.2.2.2.2. Ventral Placement The urethra can also be reconstructed with a ventral buccal graft. However, the main disadvantage of placing the graft ventrally is the greater risk for urethrovaginal fistula formation *(16)*. Further argument favoring dorsal graft placement is that if an anti-incontinence procedure is ultimately needed, it will be easier and more effective if the ventral aspect of the urethra is intact and the anterior vaginal wall is free from prior dissection (**Fig. 27.7**).

Park and Hendren *(17)* reported on their experience with a tubularized full thickness buccal graft (for cases where the local tissue was fibrotic and unsuitable for creating a supple new urethra). However, as a concept, tubularized grafts usually

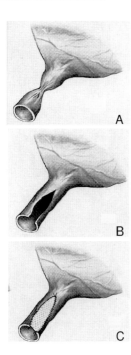

Fig. 27.7. Buccal Graft Urethroplasty A. Schematic of a mid-urethral stricture. B. Dorsal urethral stricturotomy. C. Buccal graft sutured into the incised defect. (From Ref. *[5]*)

do poorly because there is often insufficient well vascularized tissue to circumferentially cover the graft. As an alternative to the ventral buccal graft, McKinney used a ventrally placed, full thickness vaginal wall graft for urethral reconstruction *(18)*.

6. Overall Outcomes

In general, reconstruction of the female urethra is a successful procedure, with 47–100 % reporting cure with most greater than 75%, and 48–100% of patients reporting urinary continence (**Table 27.2**). In the majority of reported cases, surgeons used primary closure, with most also using a vaginal fat pad interposition (Martius flap). Reports from several studies have suggested that the use of a Martius flap improves outcomes. Webster et al. *(19)* treated four patients with urethral fistula with a primary repair only with only one patient cured, compared with four patients treated with primary repair and a Martius flap with all four patients without recurrence. Similarly, Ragnekar reported that only one of four patients with primary repair only was cured compared with seven of eight cured who underwent Martius flap interposition in addition to primary repair.

Table 27.1. Technical principles of female urethral reconstruction.

Débridement of ischemic and/or necrotic tissue
Excision of foreign bodies when applicable
Meticulous and careful dissection of the involved structures
Use of vascularized tissue flaps
Watertight, nonoverlapping, multilayer closure of urethra and
  vagina
Adequate postoperative bladder drainage
Infection prophylaxis

Table 27.2. Outcomes of female urethral reconstruction.

	Patients	Percent cured	Percent continent
Friedman, 1969 *(8)*	4	100	75
Keetel, 1978 *(22)*	24	88	n/a
Davis, 1980 *(9)*	3	100	100
Webster, 1984 *(9)*	8	63	n/a
Lee, 1988 *(23)*	53	47	n/a
Tancer, 1993 *(24)*	26	96	92
Blavias, 1996 *(12)*	49	87	87
Rangnekar, 2000 *(20)*	12	75	92
Flisser, 2003 *(25)*	74	93	87
Pushkar, 2006 *(21)*	71	90	48

The placement of a urethral sling at the time of urethra repair is controversial. Blavias reported that he routinely places a fascial sling at the time of urethra repair since his early failures without a sling (approximately 50% continence rate) were all cured with a subsequent fascial sling *(12)*. Pushkar et al. *(21)* reported on the use of a synthetic transobturator sling in three patients reporting stress incontinence after surgery, with no subsequent complications related to the synthetic sling. Patients who present with incontinence after the primary procedure may benefit from fascial sling.

7. Transvaginal Closure of the Bladder Neck

When the female urethra is extensively injured and fixed open, and not amenable to surgical repair, surgical closure of the bladder neck is often warranted. In general, we initially prefer to close the bladder neck by a tight pubovaginal sling tensioned over the rectus muscles, since the urethra can still be catheterized, as a safety "pop-off valve." When the sling approach fails, we will typically close the bladder neck using a transvaginal approach, thereby avoiding the more invasive transabdominal incision and closure. Transvaginal bladder neck closure is also a reasonable choice for ileal-vesicostomy, augmentation cystoplasty or suprapubic catheter patients with persistent post reconstruction incontinence *(26)*.

To close the bladder neck transvaginally, the patient is placed in the lithotomy position and a suprapubic tube typically placed, unless another form of bladder drainage had been previously performed (such as a continent catherizable stoma (e.g., Mitrofanoff *[27]*) or an incontinent ileal-vesicostomy). An inverted U-shaped incision is made in the anterior vaginal wall, circumscribing the damaged urethra and extending onto the anterior vaginal wall, to create a vaginal wall flap (**Fig. 27.8**).Dissection of the bladder neck is extended laterallyto the endopelvic fascia and pubic rami. The endopelvic fascia is perforated sharply to facilitate bladder neck and bladder base mobilization. During closure of the bladder neck, to prevent ureteral ligation, intravenous indigo carmine is given to facilitate ureteral orifice visualization. The remaining urethra is excised and the bladder neck closed in two layers. The second suture line extends from the bladder neck to the anterior bladder wall (behind the pubic symphysis). In so doing, the closed bladder neck is placed in the retropubic space. By avoiding overlapping suture lines, the chance for subsequent urinary fistula is minimized. As a third layer, an anterior vaginal wall advancement flap is developed. Patients with preoperative chronic infections or pelvic radiation, a Martius labial fat pad flap should be interposed over the bladder neck closure, in order to buttress the repair. A vaginal pack covered in estrogen cream is typically placed for 24–48 hours.

FIG. 27.8. Transvaginal Bladder Neck Closure A. The urethra is circumscribed and an anterior vaginal wall, inverted "U" - shaped flap constructed. B. The urethra is dissected back to the bladder neck and excised. C. The bladder neck is sutured closed vertically. D. A second layer of horizontal absorbable suture provides a more water tight closure. E. Anterior vaginal wall flap advanced and sutured into place (From Rosenblum N, Nitti VW: Female urethral reconstruction. Atlas Urol Clin NA 12:213–223, 2004)

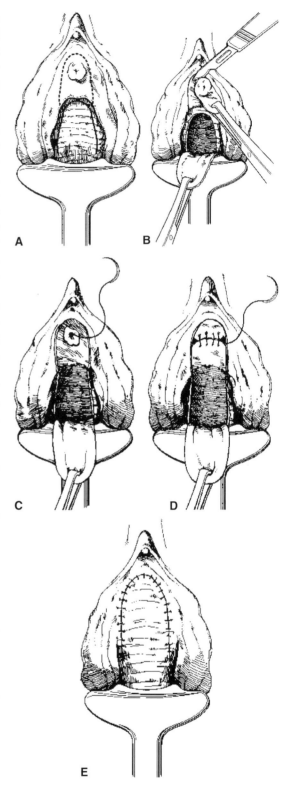

References

1. DeLancey JO. Structural support of the urethra as it relates to stress urinary incontinence: the hammock hypothesis. Am J Obstet Gynecol 1994, 170:1713–1720; discussion 1720–1723.

2. Wai CY, Atnip SD, Williams KN, Schaffer JI. Urethral erosion of tension-free vaginal tape presenting as recurrent stress urinary incontinence. Int Urogynecol J Pelvic Floor Dysfunct. 2004, 15:353–355.

3. Amundsen CL, Flynn BJ, Webster GD. Urethral erosion after synthetic and nonsynthetic pubovaginal slings: differences in management and continence outcome. J Urol 2003, 170:134–137.

4. Roenneburg ML, Wheeless CR Jr. Traumatic absence of the proximal urethra. Am J Obstet Gynecol 2005, 193:2169–2172.

5. Perry MO, Husmann DA. Urethral injuries in female subjects following pelvic fractures. Urethral injuries in female subjects following pelvic fractures. J Urol. 1992, 147:139–143.

6. Venn SN, Greenwell TJ, Mundy AR. Pelvic fracture injuries of the female urethra. BJU Int. 1999, 83:626–630.

7. Podestá ML, Jordan GH. Pelvic fracture urethral injuries in girls. J Urol. 2001, 165:1660–1665.

8. Friedman EA, Leventhal ML. Urethral reconstruction. Am J Obstet Gynecol. 1969, 104:108–113.

9. Davis RS, Linke CA, Kraemer GK. Use of labial tissue in repair of urethrovaginal fistula and injury. Arch Surg. 1980, 115:628–630.

10. Bruce RG, El-Galley RE, Galloway NT. Use of rectus abdominis muscle flap for the treatment of complex and refractory urethrovaginal fistulas. J Urol. 2000, 163:1212–1215.

11. Mundy AR. Urethral substitution in women. Br J Urol. 1989, 63:80–83.

12. Blaivas JG, Heritz DM. Reconstruction of the damaged urethra. In: Raz S, ed. Female Urology. Philadelphia: WB Saunders, 1996:584–597.

13. Hemal AK, Dorairajan LN, Gupta NP. Posttraumatic complete and partial loss of urethra with pelvic fracture in girls: an appraisal of management. J Urol 2000, 163:282–287.

14. Tanagho EA. Bladder neck reconstruction for total urinary incontinence: 10 years experience. J Urol. 1981, 125:321–326.

15. Migliari R, Leone P, Berdondini E, De Angelis M, Barbagli G, Palminteri E. Dorsal graft urethroplasty for female urethral stricture. J Urol 2006, 176:611–613.

16. Palou J, Caparros J, Vicente J. Use of proximal based vaginal flap in stricture of the female urethra. Urology 1996, 47:747–749.

17. Park JM, Hendren WH. Construction of female urethra using buccal mucosa graft. J Urol. 2001, 166:640–643.

18. McKinney DE. Use of full thickness patch graft in urethrovaginal fistula. J Urol 1979, 122: 416.

19. Webster GD, Sihelnik SA, Stone AR. Urethrovaginal fistula: a review of the surgical management. J Urol 1984, 132:460–462.

20. Ragnekar NP, Imdad-Ali N, Kaul SA, Pathak HR. Role of the Martius procedure in the management of urinary-vaginal fistulas. J Am Coll Surg 2000, 191:259–263.

21. Pushkar DY, Dyakov VV, Kosko JW, Kasyan GR. Management of urethrovaginal fistulas. Eur Urol. 2006, 50:1000–1005.

22. Keettel WC, Sehring FG, deProsse CA, Scott JR. Surgical management of urethrovaginal and vesicovaginal fistulas. Am J Obstet Gynecol. 1978, 425–431.

23. Lee RA, Symmonds RE, Williams TJ. Current status of genitourinary fistula. Obstet Gynecol. 1988, 72:313–319.

24. Tancer ML. A report of thirty-four instances of urethrovaginal and bladder neck fistulas. Surg Gynecol Obstet. 1993, 177:77–80.

25. Flisser AJ, Blaivas JG. Outcome of urethral reconstructive surgery in a series of 74 women. J Urol 2003, 169:2246–2249.

26. Zimmern PE, Hadley HR, Leach GE, Raz S. Transvaginal closure of the bladder neck and placement of a suprapubic catheter for destroyed urethra after long-term indwelling catheterization. J Urol 1985, 134:554–556.

27. Khoury AE, Agarwal SK, Bagli D, Mergurian P, McLorie GA. Concomitant modified bladder neck closure and Mitrofanoff urinary diversion. J Urol 1999, 162:1746–1748.

28
Follow-up Strategies After Urethral Stricture Treatment

Chris F. Heyns

Contents

1. Follow-Up Strategies 316
2. Noninvasive Evaluations... 316
    2.1. Urinary Flow Rate.. 316
    2.2. Patient-Reported Symptoms 317
    2.3. AUA Symptom Score and Urinary Flow Rate 318
3. Invasive Evaluations... 318
    3.1. Urethral Calibration and Bouginage 318
    3.2. Cystoscopy 319
    3.3. Urethrography.. 319
4. Follow-up Frequency 319
    4.1. Length of Follow-Up.. 319
Editor's Comment 319
References.. 320

Summary

Follow-up strategies after urethral stricture treatment include noninvasive (symptom assessment, urinary flow study) and invasive methods (retrograde urethrography, urethral calibration/bouginage and urethrocystoscopy). Urinary flow rate measurement is often used as an objective test. The presence of a urethral stricture is suggested by a peak urinary flow rate (Qmax) <10 mL/s and a uroflow tracing which is flat and box-shaped, whereas the absence of a stricture is indicated by a Qmax >15 mL/s.

Using a combination of the American Urological Association Symptom Severity Index (AUA-SSI) and Qmax may avoid invasive testing. There is a significant inverse correlation between the AUA-SSI and urethral diameter as well as Qmax, and a positive correlation between urethral diameter and Qmax. Using cut-off values of an AUA-SSI >10 and Qmax <15 mL/s second provides about 93% sensitivity and 68% specificity for predicting the presence of a stricture, and avoids further invasive testing in 34% of patients.

Urethral calibration is considered more accurate than urethrography, since the urethra may look narrow radiologically, but still easily admit a 16-18F catheter. Some define a significant urethral stricture as one that will not easily accept a 16-18F flexible cystoscope. Others feel that endoscopy could underestimate stricture recurrence and that urethrography should be the gold standard.

From: *Current Clinical Urology: Urethral Reconstructive Surgery*
Edited by: S.B. Brandes © Humana Press, Totowa, NJ

There is no consensus about the optimal intervals and duration of follow-up. Since most stricture recurrence occurs in the first 12 months after treatment, 3-4 monthly follow-up for 24 months and then yearly seems reasonable. After anastomotic urethroplasty patients should be followed for at least 5 years and after substitution urethroplasty for 15 years.

Keywords   Urethra, Stricture, Treatment, Follow-up, Urinary flow rate, Symptom score

1. Follow-Up Strategies

The evaluation of urethral stricture disease post-treatment typically includes urethrocystoscopy retrograde urethrography, voiding cystourethrography, urinary flow studies, and urethral calibration/bouginage. Although these techniques can define the objective criteria for stricture diagnosis, they are often found to be invasive and costly to the patient. In general, many patients who undergo urethral surgery are reluctant to undergo follow-up invasive diagnostic procedures, as long as they are voiding at acceptable levels.

2. Noninvasive Evaluations

Measurement of the urinary flow rate combined with determination of the post-void residual volume by ultrasound are often the most useful tests in the study of any voiding disorder.

2.1. Urinary Flow Rate

The urinary flow rate is typically recorded on an electronic flow meter which plots the flow pattern in a graphic representation of flow rate (mL/s) vs voiding time. The peak flow rate is an objective measure of functional bladder outlet obstruction and it is directly dependent on the volume voided (**Fig. 28.1**). Peak flow rates with voided volumes <150 mL are typically inaccurate. The shape of the urinary flow tracing when the urethra and bladder outlet are unobstructed is a characteristic smooth, hyperbolic, bell-shaped curve (**Fig. 28.2**). When the shape of the uroflow tracing is flat and box shaped, this is characteristic of a urethral stricture (**Fig. 28.3**).

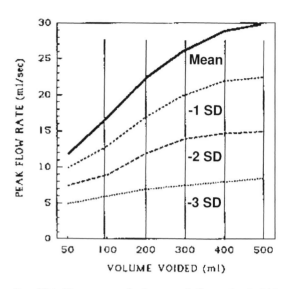

FIG. 28.1. Nomogram of urinary peak flow rates (mL/s) by voided volumes (from Siroky MB, Olsson CA, Krane RJ (1980) The flow rate nomogram: II. Clinical correlation. J Urol 123(2): 208–10)

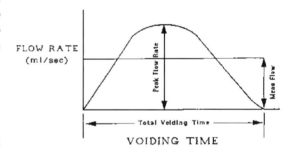

FIG. 28.2. Typical hyperbolic, bell-shaped urinary flow rate curve of a normal, unobstructed urethra

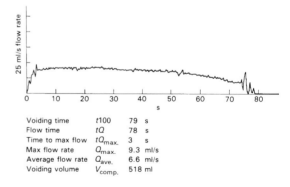

Voiding time	$t100$	79	s
Flow time	tQ	78	s
Time to max flow	$tQ_{max.}$	3	s
Max flow rate	$Q_{max.}$	9.3	ml/s
Average flow rate	$Q_{ave.}$	6.6	ml/s
Voiding volume	$V_{comp.}$	518	ml

FIG. 28.3. Typical flat, box-shaped flow rate tracing in the presence of a urethral stricture (from Blandy JP, Fowler C. Urethra and Penis Inflammation. In Urology. Blackwell Science, Oxford (1996) p. 479)

Examples of stricture definition in different studies are the following: patient symptomatic and peak urine flow rate (Q_{max}) <6 mL/s (1); Q_{max} <15 mL/s and urethra not permitting the passage of a 21-French (F) cystoscope (2); Q_{max} <10 mL/s (with a micturition volume greater than 100 mL) and a characteristic flow curve (3); inability to pass an 18F catheter into the bladder (4–6); obstructive symptoms, Qmax <10 mL/s (with a voided volume >150 mL), obstructive urine flow pattern, and/or impossible dilation (7).

Based on the assumption that the mean caliber of the normal adult male bulbar urethra is 33 F to 36 F, Stormont and associates considered "large-caliber" bulbar strictures to be greater than 20 F, with narrow caliber strictures less than or equal to 20 F. In 65% of their patients the bulbar urethral stricture diameter was more than 20 F, which would certainly not qualify as a stricture by the definition of some reports in the literature (4,8).

Examples of definitions of successful stricture treatment are the following: Q_{max} ≥15 mL/s with a normal urethrogram (9); Q_{max} ≥15 mL/s, voiding urethrogram normal and urine sterile (10); patient satisfied and Q_{max} >10 mL/s (2); no clinical symptoms and Q_{max} ≥15 mL/s (11); satisfactory voiding, normal retrograde urethrogram and VCUG, and Q_{max} ≥15 mL/s (12).

Controversy exists as to whether strictures with a caliber larger than 18 F are symptomatic (13–15). Especially in elderly men with benign prostatic hyperplasia it is impossible to determine whether symptoms are due to urethral stricture or benign prostatic hyperplasia, unless the symptoms completely disappear after successful stricture treatment.

There is evidence that, in relatively young men (mean age <50 years), a Q_{max} <10 mL/s has a positive predictive value of about 95% for the presence of a urethral stricture (6,14). Heyns and Marais showed that a urethral diameter of 18 F or larger correlates well with a Q_{max} >15 mL/s and an American Urological Association Symptom Severity Index (AUA SSI) <10, confirming the view that a Q_{max} >15 mL/s indicates the absence of a significant stricture (6,14).

2.2. Patient-Reported Symptoms

There is no consensus about the best protocol for follow-up after urethrotomy or urethroplasty to detect stricture recurrence. Some authors contend that the most practical and meaningful criteria of therapeutic efficacy are recurrent symptoms (8). A recent study used only mailed International Prostate Symptom Score and quality of life questionnaires (16). However, it is known that clinical assessment alone will detect fewer recurrences than when uroflowmetry is used (3). Uroflowmetry often-times appears to be a better objective measure of success than urethrography (17). In the pediatric population, follow-up by means of patient or parent reported symptoms may be preferable to invasive tests such as cystoscopy, urethrography, postvoid residual volume measurement, and uroflowmetry (18).

Most authors advocate using periodic objective tests such as urinary flow rate measurement and assessment of the flow pattern (a flat, plateau-like flow curve, instead of the normal hyperbolic curve), retrograde urethrography, urethral calibration, urethro-cystoscopy and urinalysis (1,8,9,19). Some authors have suggested doing urethrocystography only with a Q_{max} <15 mL/s (14).

Lipsky and Hubmer (9) commented on the close correlation between symptomatology and urine flow rates. In a quantitative study of 49 urethral stricture patients with an average age of 48 yr, Heyns and Marais (6) found a significant negative linear correlation of urethral diameter with the AUA-SSI (**Fig. 28.4**). There was a significant positive linear correlation of maximum urine flow (Q_{max}) with urethral diameter (**Fig. 28.5**) and a significant negative correlation of the AUA-SSI with Q_{max} (**Fig. 28.6**).

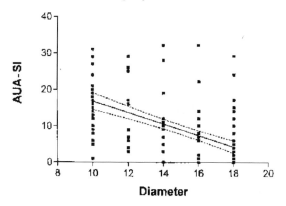

FIG. 28.4. Correlation between urethral diameter and AUA-SI; dotted lines indicate 90% CI (from reference [6])

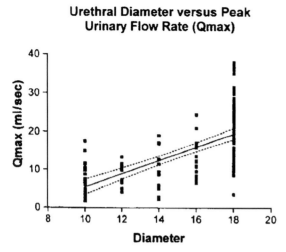

Urethral Diameter versus Peak Urinary Flow Rate (Qmax)

FIG. 28.5. Correlation between urethral diameter and peak urinary flow rate; dotted lines indicate 90% CI (from reference *[6]*)

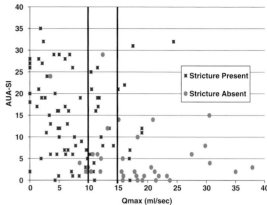

FIG. 28.7. AUA Symptom score and peak urinary flow rate in men with and without a urethral stricture (from reference *[6]*)

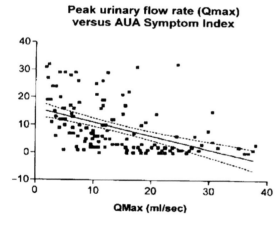

Peak urinary flow rate (Qmax) versus AUA Symptom Index

FIG. 28.6. Correlation between AUA symptom index and peak urinary flow rate; dotted lines indicate 90% CI (from reference *[6]*)

only 72% specificity (**Fig. 28.7**). However, it would avoid further invasive testing in 37% of patients, while missing only 6% of strictures with a diameter of 14 F or less. At the other extreme, an AUA-SSI greater than 10 and a Q_{max} less than 10 mL/s (i.e., when both of these were present) had a specificity of 98% for the presence of a stricture but only 37% sensitivity. It would avoid further invasive testing in 79% of patients, but would miss 27% of strictures with a diameter 14 F or smaller *(6)*. The best combination to maximize both sensitivity and specificity appeared to be an AUA-SSI of greater than 10 plus Q_{max} of less than 15 mL/s. This provided 93% sensitivity and 68% specificity, avoided further invasive studies in 34% of patients and missed only 4.3% of recurrent strictures.

Figure 28.7 clearly shows that using an AUA-SSI >15 or a Q_{max} <15 mL/s would capture the most men with a stricture present and would exclude a significant proportion of those without a stricture.

2.3. AUA Symptom Score and Urinary Flow Rate

Heyns and Marais *(6)* suggested using a combination of the AUA-SSI and urinary Q_{max} to predict the presence or absence of a stricture. The criteria of an AUA-SSI greater than 15 or a Q_{max} less than 15 mL/s (i.e., if either one of these was present) had a sensitivity of 91% for the presence of a stricture, but

3. Invasive Evaluations

3.1. Urethral Calibration and Bouginage

Urethral calibration is more accurate than urethrography in determining if stenoses are significant, since the urethra may look narrow radiologically, but still easily admit a 16 to 18 F catheter or bougie without difficulty *(8)*.

3.2. Cystoscopy

There is some controversy about the definition of a urethral stricture and about the definition of success after treatment. Some define a significant urethral stricture as urethral lumen that will not easily accept a flexible cystoscope, or in other words, a lumen less then or equal to 16 F. Others feel endoscopy could underestimate the presence of stricture recurrence and feel that any narrowing on urethrography denotes recurrence.

3.3. Urethrography

See Chapter 4 by Peterson et al. in this volume on urethral imaging.

4. Follow-up Frequency

There is no consensus about the optimal intervals and duration of objective testing, which have varied from three to four monthly for 12–24 mo in different reports, although it is well recognized that late stricture recurrence may sometimes occur more than 5 yr after direct vision internal urethrotomy or dilation *(4,20,21)*.

4.1. Length of Follow-Up

There is a clear correlation between the duration of follow-up and the risk of recurrence, with most recurrences occurring within 6 to 12 mo after DVIU *(9,11)*. In pediatric patients the length of follow-up was the most important risk factor for recurrence: 19% at 6 mo and 65% after 4 yr *(22)*.

Editor's Comment

Clearly, most experts would consider urethrography to be the gold standard when evaluating the urethra for stenosis; however, it is often difficult to gauge the functional significance of narrowing on an x-ray in an asymptomatic patient. As noted already, the literature appears to support the use of AUA SSI and urinary flow rate as surrogates for urethral caliber and thus for significant stricture recurrence after urethrotomy. How about after urethroplasty?

Are the noninvasive studies of flow rate and AUA SSI equally accurate?

Morey et al. *(23)* also reviewed their experience with the AUA SSI in 50 patients who underwent urethroplasty surgery. In general, the AUA SSI is a validated instrument with internal consistency (Cronbach's alpha = 0.85) and test–retest correlation (reliability) of 0.93., that provides a quantitative estimate of subjective voiding symptoms. Successful urethroplasty outcomes were noted in follow-up when the AUA SSI was minimal (<7). Such correlation with urethroplasty success and symptom score decrease was shown for all types of surgical reconstruction: namely excision with primary urethral anastomosis, buccal graft, fasciocutaneous onlay flap, and posterior urethroplasty (Table 28.1). Stricture recurrence, as confirmed by radiographic means, correlated well when the symptom score was in the severe range (>20). Symptom score had a strong inverse correlation with maximum urinary flow rate (*see* **Fig. 28.8**). The AUA SSI can thus be reliably used as an inexpensive and quick screening tool to assess the need for more invasive testing. When post-urethroplasty AUA-SSI does not go into the minor range and no stricture is noted on invasive testing, then the etiology is either benign prostatic hyperplasia-lower urinary tract symptoms or neurogenic bladder. Bullock and Brandes *(24)* recently published a nationwide survey of U.S. urologists as to their routine follow-up after urethral stricture surgery (**Table 28.2**). Practicing urologists mostly use flow rate (63%) to determine if the stricture has recurred. Urologists less often use cystoscopy (33.2%), urethral calibration (27.6%), and the AUA SSI (27.6%) to identify stricture recurrence.

TABLE 28.1. Successful Urethroplasty, regardless of type, demonstrates a significant reduction in AUA symptom score (from reference *[23]*)

Comparison of mean AUA symptom index scores by type of urethroplasty

Type	No. Pts.	Mean Score	
		Preop.	Postop.
End to end	19	25.7	5.4
Graft	8	27.1	3.0
Fasciocutaneous flap	11	25.3	3.8
Prostatomembranous	12	*	4.1

* Patients with prostatomembranous urethral disruption injuries required suprapubic urinary diversion preoperatively.

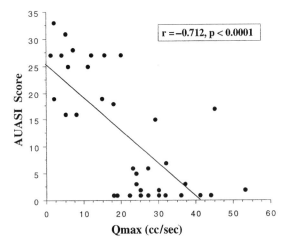

FIG. 28.8. Correlation between AUA symptom score and peak urinary flow rate (Qmax) demonstrates significant inverse correlation before and after successful urethroplasty (from reference *[23]*)

TABLE 28.2. Methods used by U.S. urologists to evaluate urethral strictures after urethral surgery (from reference *[24]*)

Method	Frequency	Percentage
Urinary flow rate	271	62.9
Cystoscopy	143	33.2
Urethral calibration	119	27.6
AUA SSI/IPSS	119	27.6
RUG/VCUG X-ray	57	13.2
Ultrasonography	11	2.6
Other	21	4.9

IPSS, International Prostate Symptom Score; RUG, retrograde urethrogram; VCUG, voiding cystourethrogram.

After urethroplasty, for how many years should they be followed? It is evident from the literature that anastomotic urethroplasty is highly successful and has sustained durable results. Here, stricture recurrence slightly rises from 1 to 5 yr of follow-up and is then relatively stable at 10 and 15 yr. It seems reasonable then, that anastomotic urethroplasty patients should be followed for 5 yr (after 5 yr is debatable). In contrast, substitution urethroplasty has progressive and ever increasing rates of failure with time (even up to 15 yr after surgery). Thus, follow-up for the substitution urethroplasty patient should be essentially for life. In our own practice, post-urethroplasty, we perform a baseline urinary flow rate, postvoid residual urine by ultrasound, AUA SSI and flexible cystoscopy at 3 mo follow-up. If all the parameters are normal at that time, the patients are then followed on a yearly basis.

We have not been eliminating the yearly flexible cystoscopy. However, many authors only utilize noninvasive studies in follow-up, and only when they are abnormal are invasive studies, such as flexible cystoscopy or retrograde urethrography performed.—S.B. Brandes

References

1. Holm-Nielsen A, Schultz A, Moller-Pedersen V (1984) Direct vision internal urethrotomy. A critical review of 365 operations Br J Urol 56:308–312
2. Schultz A, Bay-Nielsen H, Bilde T, Christiansen L, Mikkelsen AM, Steven K (1989) Prevention of urethral stricture formation after transurethral resection of the prostate: a controlled randomized study of Otis urethrotomy versus urethral dilation and the use of the polytetrafluoroethylene coated versus the uninsulated metal sheath J Urol 141:73–75
3. Bodker A, Ostri P, Rye-Andersen J, Edvardsen L, Struckmann J (1992) Treatment of recurrent urethral stricture by internal urethrotomy and intermittent self-catheterization: a controlled study of a new therapy J Urol 148:308–310
4. Steenkamp JW, Heyns CF, De Kock ML (1997) Internal urethrotomy versus dilation as treatment for male urethral strictures: a prospective, randomized comparison J Urol 157:98–101
5. Heyns CF, Steenkamp JW, De Kock ML, Whitaker P (1998) Treatment of male urethral strictures: is repeated dilation or internal urethrotomy useful? J Urol 160:356–358
6. Heyns CF, Marais DC (2002) Prospective evaluation of the American Urological Association symptom index and peak urinary flow rate for the followup of men with known urethral stricture disease J Urol 168:2051–2054
7. Tunc M, Tefekli A, Kadioglu A, Esen T, Uluocak N, Aras N (2002) A prospective, randomized protocol to examine the efficacy of postinternal urethrotomy dilations for recurrent bulbomembranous urethral strictures. Urology 60:239–244
8. Stormont TJ, Suman VJ, Oesterling JE (1993) Newly diagnosed bulbar urethral strictures: etiology and outcome of various treatments. J Urol 150:1725–1728
9. Lipsky H, Hubmer G (1977) Direct vision urethrotomy in the management of urethral strictures Br J Urol 49:725–728
10. Boccon-Gibod L, Le Portz B (1982) Endoscopic urethrotomy: does it live up to its promises? J Urol 127:433–435
11. Albers P, Fichtner J, Brühl P, Müller SC (1996) Long-term results of internal urethrotomy J Urol 156:1611–1614

12. Giannakopoulos X, Grammeniatis E, Gartzios A, Tsoumanis P, Kammenos A (1997) Sachse urethrotomy versus endoscopic urethrotomy plus transurethral resection of the fibrous callus (Guillemin's technique) in the treatment of urethral stricture. Urology 49:243–247

13. Kinder PW, Rous SN (1979) The treatment of urethral stricture disease by internal urethrotomy: a clinical review. J Urol 121:45–46

14. Pansadoro V, Emiliozzi P (1996) Internal urethrotomy in the management of anterior urethral strictures: Long-term followup. J Urol 156:73–75

15. Walton JK, Wright WL, Robinson RG, Nacey JN (1984) The meatal problem with TUR prostate: the value of post-operative self-dilation. Br J Urol 56:202–207.

16. Kamp S, Knoll T, Osman MM, Kohrmann KU, Michel MS, Alken P (2006) Low-power holmium: YAG laser urethrotomy for treatment of urethral strictures: functional outcome and quality of life. J Endourol 20:38–41

17. Hjortrup A, Sorensen C, Sanders S, Moesgaard F, Kirkegaard P (1983) Strictures of the male urethra treated by the Otis method. J Urol 130:903–904

18. Hsiao KC, Baez-Trinidad L, Lendvay T, Smith EA, Broecker B, Scherz H, Kirsch AJ (2003) Direct vision internal urethrotomy for the treatment of pediatric urethral strictures: analysis of 50 patients. J Urol 170:952–955

19. El-Abd SA (1995) Endoscopic treatment of posttraumatic urethral obliteration: experience in 396 patients. J Urol 153:67–71

20. Hossain AZ, Khan SA, Hossain S, Salam MA (2004) Holmium laser urethrotomy for urethral stricture. Bangladesh Med Res Counc Bull 30:78–80

21. Mandhani A, Chaudhury H, Kapoor R, Srivastava A, Dubey D, Kumar A (2005) Can outcome of internal urethrotomy for short segment bulbar urethral stricture be predicted? J Urol 173:1595–1597

22. Hafez AT, El Assmy A, Dawaba MS, Sarhan O Bazeed M. (2005) Long-term outcome of visual internal urethrotomy for the management of pediatric urethral strictures. J Urol 173:595–597

23. Morey AF, McAninch, Duckett CP, Rogers RS. (1998) American Urological Association Symptom Index in the assessment of urethroplasty outcomes. J Urol 159:1192–1194

24. Bullock TL, Brandes SB (2007) Adult anterior urethral strictures: a national practice patterns survey of board certified urologists in the United States. J Urol 177:685–690

29

General Technical Considerations and Decision Making in Urethroplasty Surgery

Steven B. Brandes

Contents

1. Introduction 323
2. Preoperative Assessment 324
    2.1. Stricture Versus Stricture Disease 324
    2.2. Imaging 324
    2.3. Timing of Surgery 325
3. Positioning 325
    3.1. Patient Positioning 325
    3.2. Scrub Tech Positioning 325
4. Anterior Urethroplasty 326
    4.1. General Concepts 326
5. Specific Methods 328
    5.1. Anastomotic Urethroplasty 328
    5.2. Substitution Urethroplasty and "Stricture Disease" 329
    5.3. Posterior Urethroplasty 332
Appendix 334
Suggested Readings 335

Summary General technical skills for urethroplasty surgery can often be learned fairly quickly by the trainee. The difficult skill to acquire, which often times requires years of experience, is the ability to make proper and sound, pre and intraoperative decision making. Here-in we have detailed how to properly and accurately evaluate urethral strictures by imaging, cystourethroscopy and physical examination. Operative tricks and tips, as to patient selection, timing of surgery, patient positioning and surgical technique specifics are elaborated. Key aspects of anterior and posterior urethroplasty surgical methods are detailed, in particular, the methods of excision and primary anastomosis, buccal mucosal grafting, and penile skin flaps.

Keywords surgical tricks, positioning, timing, patient selection, grafts, flaps, anastomotic urethroplasty

1. Introduction

The open surgical repair of urethral strictures has dramatically changed during the last 50 or so years. Today, nearly all urethral strictures, regardless of length, can be reconstructed in a one-stage operation. In patients with a normal penis, the penile skin, urethral plate, corpus spongiosum, and Dartos fascia are available for urethral reconstruction. Only a small proportion of patients, who have severely scarred or insufficient local tissues, associated skin infections

From: *Current Clinical Urology: Urethral Reconstructive Surgery*
Edited by: S.B. Brandes © Humana Press, Totowa, NJ

(or disease), or complex strictures and/or fistula, require a staged approach.

The length and location of the urethral stricture, the etiology of the stricture, and the history of previous urethral surgery or instrumentation helps one to decide which urethroplasty method to use. Before undertaking urethroplasty surgery, the urologist must be familiar with the use of numerous surgical reconstructive techniques to address any condition of the urethra that might surface at the time of surgery. Oftentimes, the preoperative surgical plan needs to be modified intraoperatively, when faced with unexpected findings. Open urethroplasty is the gold standard treatment of urethral strictures. Urethroplasty should not be withheld on the basis of age. Older men tolerate urethroplasty well and with comparable complication rates.

Management of urethral strictures should not be considered a reconstructive ladder. The practice of repeat dilations and urethrotomies before considering urethroplasty is backwards thinking and should be abandoned. The goal of stricture management should be for cure and not just temporary management. Open surgical urethroplasty has a high degree of long-term success and should be considered the gold standard that all other methods should be judged.

2. Preoperative Assessment

The first important step to performing urethroplasty surgery is adequate and accurate preoperative information as to the anatomy of the urethral stricture. It is key to know the number of urethral strictures, the location and length of each stricture, and the lumen diameter of each stricture. It is also important to know the functional significance of the stricture and degree of resulting voiding dysfunction.

Urethral stricture evaluation starts with a flow rate measuring Q_{max} and voided volume. For accurate readings a voided volume of at least 150 mL is preferred. Examine the shape of the tracings. Uroflow tracings that look like a flat mesa are typical of a urethral stricture. A stricture cannot stretch with increasing flow and thus does not give the typical bell like shape of the normal unobstructed urethra. In the office, we also obtain a postvoid residual by bladder scan and an American Urological Association Symptom Score on each patient. A formal ultrasound of the bladder taken to examine bladder wall thickness will help determine

the chronicity of the outlet obstruction. In other words, long-standing stricture and outlet obstruction will result in bladder muscle hypertrophy.

Another important means to evaluate the urethral stricture is in office flexible cystoscopy. A flexible ureteroscope or a pediatric cystoscope is also useful when there is a tight distal stricture and the proximal urethra needs evaluating. We encourage a liberal use of endoscopy to better define confusing urethrography results and to evaluate the pallor of the epithelium and the elasticity or rigidity of the stricture. In general, the worse the spongiofibrosis, the worse the distensibility. Endoscopy is useful for confirming or clarifying urethrography findings and can visually assess urethral mucosa and associated scarring.

2.1. Stricture Versus Stricture Disease

A key concept when it comes to managing urethral stenoses is to categorizing the stenoses into either "urethral stricture" or "urethral stricture disease." The two processes of stenoses have different characteristics, extent, and etiology. "Strictures" are typically short, focal, and of an acute nature, such as from an external blow or iatrogenic instrumentation. Here, the injury to the urethra is limited and thus the vascularity and general condition of the remaining urethra and spongoisum are typically normal. "Stricture disease" stenoses are typically long, involve broad areas of varying spongiofibrosis, and typically the result of inflammation or infection, rather then trauma. "Urethral stricture," therefore, is typically managed by an anastomotic urethroplasty while "stricture disease" by substitution urethroplasty.

2.2. Imaging

Imaging with both a retrograde urethrogram and a voiding cystourethrogram is essential. Proper positioning of the patient is vital, so that if the patient is not placed oblique enough, the overall stricture length will be underestimated. When the patient is positioned in the oblique position, sufficiently on his side, the proper image shows only one obturator fossa. We encourage the reader to perform the urethral imaging of one's patients under fluoroscopy oneself to assure good quality images. We like to use a suction device with an injection port in its center that is placed on the glans penis to perform the retrograde under fluoroscopy. This typically works better then a small Foley catheter in the fossa or a Brodney clamp.

Once the patient's bladder is full, a voiding study is performed. If the stricture is too tight to fill the bladder, a small pediatric feeding can be placed to fill the bladder antegrade. If a feeding tube cannot be placed, intravenous contrast at roughly 2 mL per kilo is given, the patient forces fluids, and the bladder is allowed to fill over the next hour or so.

From a technical view point, a false stricture at the penoscrotal junction may appear to be the result of external compression from the urinal. This is usually observed in the patient with a short phallus or the obese patient. When measuring the length of a stricture, measure from normal urethral lumen diameter to normal lumen to predict the actual length of graft or flap needed. Most imaging today is digital. Hard copies are usually not produced and, when they are, they are small and not actual size. A useful trick to measuring strictures is to first measure the pubic ramus width, which is typically 2 cm. This distance can then be used as a ruler to estimate stricture length. The other trick is to place a 1-cm radiopaque marker next to the urethra during the actual imaging. It will show up on the final images and can be used as a scale to properly measure stricture length.

When the imaging remains confusing, intraoperative examination under anesthesia with a rigid cystoscope (retrograde) and/or flexible cystoscopy (antegrade) can be very helpful to making an accurate diagnosis and a surgical plan. Placement of a percutaneous peel away sheath into the bladder is further useful for antegrade cystoscopy.

2.3. Timing of Surgery

Before any urethroplasty is performed, the patient's scar (stricture) should be stable and no longer contracting. Thus, we prefer that the urethra not be instrumented for 3 mo before any planned surgery. If the stricture patient goes into urinary retention or requires frequent intermittent self catheterization, then we typically place a percutaneous suprapubic tube. Proximal urinary diversion will allow for resolution of acute urethral inflammation and allow narrowed areas to declare themselves.

After a previous failed urethroplasty, we generally wait at least 6 mos before attempting another open repair. The long time interval is needed for the tissues to soften and become pliable and for the tissue planes to reform. "Re-do" surgery at an earlier interval is often very difficult and prone to failure. For the long stricture, it is important that the genital skin is not infected with candidiasis or similar skin disease because it is penile skin that is often used as an onlay flap for long strictures. Here, contemplated urethral reconstruction needs to be postponed until the skin infection resolves.

3. Positioning

3.1. Patient Positioning

To prevent sacral nerve stretch, we use a folded blanket and egg crate mattress to rotate the pelvis in the cephalad direction while in the "social" lithotomy position. Commercially available special tables are also available for this purpose. The patient's legs should be liberally and carefully padded, especially the lateral thigh to prevent perineal nerve injury and palsy. At all costs, we try to minimize the time our patients are in the exaggerated lithotomy position. We also strongly try to limit surgery time to less than 5 h, because this seems to be the upper limit for developing severe positioning complications. In general, it takes us roughly 2 to 3 h for an anastomotic urethroplasty and 3 to 4 h for a substitution urethroplasty (particularly a skin island flap).

To hold the legs, we prefer the Yellowfin stirrups because of the superb leg support and overall padding, as well as its ability to move the legs up or down during the surgery with ease. Thus, if a buccal graft needs to be harvested unexpectedly, the legs can be taken down during graft harvest, without redraping or prepping.

3.2. Scrub Tech Positioning

The scrub nurse should be positioned in front of the surgeon with the Mayo stand over the chest of the patient. The instruments can be passed to the surgeon in this position with ease and so facilitates the overall speed of the operation. If the scrub nurse stands behind the surgeon, it is more difficult for the scrub nurse to pass instruments and she cannot assist you in the surgery.

4. Anterior Urethroplasty

4.1. General Concepts

4.1.1. Lighting

A head lamp is very useful to illuminate the deep hole that the perineum can be, particularly for proximal bulbar urethral strictures. Loupe magnification glasses are very useful. I have had a pair of 2.5 power glasses for years, and have found that they provide sufficient visualization. We strongly encourage anyone who performs urethroplasty surgery to purchase a pair of surgical loupes, even if one's eyesight is "perfect." It is a worthy investment that that you can use throughout one's career. I even use such loupes for my open abdominal reconstructive surgery cases.

4.1.2. Incision

A midline perineal incision and the Lonestar retractor (Cooper Surgical, Trumbel, CT) provide excellent exposure of the bulbar urethra. We have not found the Lamda incision or extravagant retractors to be necessary for excellent exposure. Many experts, however, like the Jordan retractor system (C&S Surgical, Slidell, LA) for the Bookwalter for posterior urethroplasty. As to length of perineal incision, I have been liberal with the length and typically make the incision from the inferior aspect of the scrotum to roughly 1 to 2 cm above the anus. In rare circumstances of poor proximal exposure hampered by the incision size, I have extended the incision posterior and around the anus.

4.1.3. Intraoperative Endoscopy

With the liberal use of a pediatric cystoscope or flexible ureteroscope, the degree of urethral lumen elasticity and inflammation can be assessed. In general, the worse the spongiofibrosis, the worse the distensibility. Endoscopy is useful for confirming or clarifying urethrography findings and can visually assess urethral mucosa and associated scarring. We perform flexible cystoscopy during every urethroplasty. After the bulbar urethra has been initially exposed, at times it is difficult to determine the location and/or full extent (proximal as well as distal) of the stricture. If confused or not definite about the stricture, we strongly encourage intraoperative cystoscopy. Oftentimes you can see

the urethra trans-illuminated by the cystoscope light at the extent of the stricture. If unclear about the proximal extent of the stricture, a useful trick is to fill the bladder retrograde and percutaneously place a peel away sheath into the bladder (We prefer the Chiou suprapubic tube kit, Cook Urological (USA)). Antegrade cystoscopy can then be performed. If the scope is too short to reach the proximal stricture, a guidewire can be placed retrograde into the bladder and then grasped with the cystoscope and brought out the SP tract. With thru-and-thru access, a Councill tip Foley can then be placed antegrade and retrograde. Palpating the ends of each of the catheters will give you the true length and extent of the stricture.

Furthermore, with every urethroplasty, after we have made our urethrotomy, we routinely cystoscope the proximal and distal ends of the urethra (**Fig. 29.1**). We do so to look for a secondary stricture, radiolucent bladder stone or tumor, and to assess the quality and color of the remaining urethra. If the urethral epithelium is white and blanched, we will typically extend the urethrotomy until healthy-appearing pink epithelium is reached. Another important trick, is that if we plan on doing a substitution urethroplasty, before performing the urethrotomy (ventral or dorsal, no matter), we routinely cystoscope the urethra and place a guidewire into the bladder. With the guidewire in place you

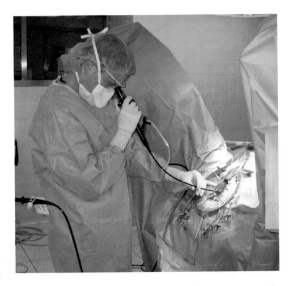

Fig. 29.1. Liberal use of intraoperative cystoscopy is essential to urethroplasty success

can guarantee that you can find the urethral plate (by palpation) and that it is being opened like a book, in the proper plane.

4.1.4. Urethral Mucosal Staining

Urethral injection of relatively pure methylene blue to stain the mucosa can be a very useful tool to facilitate proper suturing of mucosa to mucosa. Technically, we inject the blue dye with a catheter tip syringe into the penis and place a penile clamp to prevent leakage of the dye. Upon performing the urethrotomy, the mucosa will be stained blue. Since the spongiosum is white to pink, the same color as the urethral plate, the anatomical margins can be difficult to distinguish from each other. A blue mucosa gives us a roadmap or frame work to the proper placement of sutures.

4.1.5. Urethral Vascular Control

Oftentimes, when performing a urethral stricture excision and primary anastomosis, the cut ends of the nonscarred urethra bleed aggressively. A safe and effective way to control this bleeding is to place noncrushing straight "bulldog" vascular clamps on the proximal and distal aspects of the urethra. Only in a bloodless field can suturing be performed accurately and with leisure.

4.1.6. Bipolar Electocautery

Dissection of the urethral off the corporal cavernosal bodies can be tricky. There are many perforating vessels between the urethra and corporal body every centimeter or so. Liberal use of bipolar cautery will provide good hemostasis. We like to use the bayonet style with wide blades. Do not use unipolar cautery. We feel it unduly risks nerve or vessel injury that may effect penile sensation or sexual function.

4.1.7. Urethral Mobilization

The penile urethra is typically fairly adherent to the corpora. The urethra can be best separated from the corpora by a "split-and-roll" dissection method. This method is similar to the dissection technique one uses for caval mobilization for a retroperitoneal lymph node dissection for testis cancer. This is why we jokingly refer to the urethra as the "pena cava," To mobilize the proximal bulb effectively,

first the bulbospongiosus muscle fibers should be removed sharply and bluntly (with the use of a Kittner) off the tunica of the bulb, from medial to lateral. Once the spongiosis muscle is opened "like a book," the attachments to the perineal body needs to be divided. Typicality, we incise these attachments with our scissors directly posteriorly while holding anterior counter-traction on the bulb with forceps. This method will avoid accidentally injuring the tunica of the spongiosis and causing premature brisk bleeding. For a tension-free anastomosis, the urethra typically needs to be mobilized so that the cut edges overlap by 2 cm (one cm spatulation each, for the proximal and distal ends).

4.1.8. Urethral Elasticity

In his seminal work on fresh cadavers, Francisco Sampaio detailed the inherent elastic nature of the urethra and corpus spongiosum. With 25 fresh cadavers, penile extensibility was noted to be $51.1 \pm 7\%$, whereas mean urethral extensibility was $66.2 \pm 7.2\%$. Urethral extensibility was to the same degree for each urethral segment (namely penile, bulbar and membranous urethra). Maximal stretched urethral length without penile curvature with artificial erection was also calculated to a constant factor of 75.2%. They further calculated that to bridge each gap of 1 cm of excised urethra, the remaining normal urethra would have to be mobilized at least 4 cm (4:1 ratio). This ratio of mobilization to bridge a gap, changes with age, from a low of 1:3.2 for a 1-yr-old child, up to 1:6.6 for 70-yr-old man. In other words, penile and urethral extensibility reduces with advancing age (**Fig. 29.2**).

4.1.9. Straightening the Urethra (Shortening the Gap)

Anatomically the urethra is "S" shaped and makes a natural curve in the bulb around the pubic bone and corpora of the penis. The shortest path between two points is obviously a straight line. By mobilizing the urethra and making the urethra lie into a straight line, the excised gap in the urethra can be bridged (**Fig. 29.3**). This technique of straightening out the urethra is the key principle used with the progressive approach to posterior urethroplasty. Here, the urethra is straightened by the sequential methods of: splitting the corpora (developing the

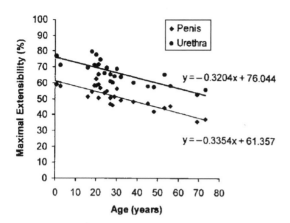

FIG. 29.2. Correlation of urethral and penile extensibility. Note that extensibility of the mobilized urethra is significantly longer then penile extensibility, as well as inter-variability by patient age. (From DaSilva EA, Sampaio FJB (2002) Urethral extensibility applied to reconstructive surgery, J Urol 167:2042–2045)

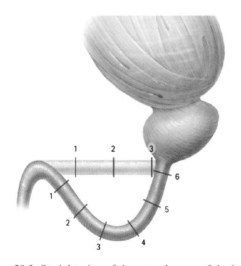

FIG. 29.3. Straightening of the natural curve of the bulbar urethra will help shorten the distance between the cut ends of the urethra by an additional 2 to 4 cm. (From Mundy AR (1996) Urethroplasty for posterior urethral strictures. Br J Urol 78:243–247)

inter-crural plane), performing an inferior pubectomy or, in extreme cases, re-routing the urethra around the superior pubic ramus. Each step helps to make the urethra progressively straighter, and thus progressively shorten the gap between the two ends of the urethra.

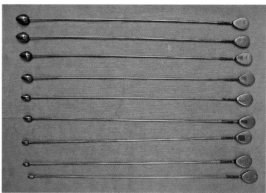

FIG. 29.4. Bouie a boules are essential to accurately calibrate and thus to adequately spatulate the urethra.

4.1.10. Urethral Calibration

Sound each of the cut ends of the urethra with bougie a boules to calibrate urethral size for proper and adequate spatulation, as well as to diagnose any secondary stricture up or downstream from the main stricture Bougie to 24 French for the penile urethra and to 36 French for the bulbar urethra (**Fig. 29.4**).

4.1.10. Urethral Orientation

Once the urethra is mobilized and excised, place stay sutures at the 3- and 9-o'clock positions in each of the cut ends of the urethra. This will greatly facilitate assist urethra orientation for proper spatulation and for subsequent suturing. For proximal bulbar or posterior urethra anastomotic urethroplasty, we use typically numbered mosquitoes (1 through 12, which correspond to the same location on the clock). This helps prevent the sutures from being tangled.

5. Specific Methods

5.1. Anastomotic Urethroplasty

Whenever possible, anastomotic urethroplasty is the preferred method of urethral reconstruction, because of its high success rate and durability. The successful bridging of the gap of excised tissue and performance of a tension-free anastomotic urethroplasty are dependent on urethral mobilization and inherent tissue elasticity to increase the urethra's overall length. The other means to bring the two cut edges together is to shorten the distance between then, by straightening out the urethra. Generally, we perform anastomotic urethroplasty only for bulbar strictures, proximal to the suspensory ligament, and less then 2.5 cm in length. Primary anastomosis for strictures of the penile urethra (distal to the suspensory ligament) typically risks bothersome chordee and should generally be avoided. Furthermore, extensive distal urethral dissection, beyond the suspensory ligament, risks penile tethering or urethral bow-stringing of the penis. Degrees of penile tethering range from a minor, straight erection that points down, to a more major, significant ventral chordee. To achieve a successful and durable urethroplasty result is a difficult undertaking, and thus we would never entertain taking down the anastomosis to correct chordee. Instead, such ventral chordee can be corrected by taking down the suspensory ligament in a secondary operation. By dividing the fulcrum where the penis is being held in position, helps to straighten it (**Fig. 29.5**).

When the stricture is very proximal, depending on patient anatomy, strictures longer then 2.5 cm stricture can often be bridged. Morey has suggested that the length of stenoses that can be bridged can be extended, based on whether the stricture is in the proximal or distal bulbar urethra and based on patient stretched penile length. Namely, patients with longer stretched penile urethral lengths (>15 cm) and stenoses in the proximal bulb, the longer the bulbar gap that can be bridged. Patients with short stretched

penile lengths (<15 cm) and distal bulbar stenoses are often better managed by a substitution urethroplasty. This makes intuitive sense if urethral dissection is carried distal to the suspensory ligament.

5.2. Substitution Urethroplasty and "Stricture Disease"

When the stricture is too long for stricture excision and primary anastomosis, a patch or flap of substitute material is interposed. The characteristics of the urethra of the patient who needs to undergo urethral substitution surgery are very different from the urethra of anastomotic urethroplasty. Here, the stenoses are just a manifestation of "urethral stricture disease" where the majority of the urethra is potentially "diseased" and the blood supply compromised in other areas of the urethra, proximal or distal to the obvious stricture. This distinction between "stricture" and "stricture disease" helps to explain the success and durability of anastomotic urethroplasty, whereas substitution urethroplasty, whatever material used, has consistent and progressive long-term recurrence.

As detailed in **Table 29.1**, it is evident that anastomotic urethroplasty is highly successful and durable. In contrast, substitution urethroplasty has progressive and ever increasing rates of failure with time (even up to 15 yr after surgery). The debate about the type, whether a flap or a graft should be used in the reconstruction, is thus often moot. Aside from having better and more durable success, anastomotic urethroplasty also has fewer complications then substitution urethroplasty. See the chapter in this text on Complications by Santucci, as well as **Table 29.2**, comparing the complication rates from a single institution in England.

Substitution urethroplasty entails three different surgical methods: 1) urethral stricture excision and missing segment replacement with an augmented anastomosis (a spatulated anastomosis on one side

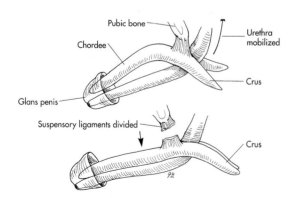

FIG. 29.5. Correction of iatrogenic chordee with suspensory ligament release. (From Yu GW, Miller HC (1996) Critical maneuvers in urologic surgery. St. Louis, Mosby)

TABLE 29.1. Stricture rates after anastomotic and substitution urethroplasty.

	1 yr	5 yr	10 yr	15 yr
Anastomotic	7%	12%	13%	14%
Substitution	12%	21%	30%	42%

Redrawn from Andrich DE, Dunglison N, Greenwell TJ, Mundy AR (2003) The long-term results of urethroplasty. J Urol 170:90–92.

TABLE 29.2. Complications reported after substitution and anastomotic urethroplasty.

	Substitution (%)	Anastomotic
Postvoid dribbling	28	-
Diverticulum/pouch	12	-
Urinary tract infection	5	-
Chordee	3	-
Urethro-utaneous fistula	3	-
Impotence	2	5%
Total	33	5%

Redrawn from Andrich DE, Dunglison N, Greenwell TJ, Mundy AR (2003) The long-term results of urethroplasty. J Urol 170:90–92.

and on the other, a graft or flap); 2) urethral stricture excision and missing segment replacement with a combination of a graft (dorsal) and a flap or graft (ventral); or 3) stricture incision (urethrotomy) either ventral or dorsal and patch the defect with an onlay graft or flap.

5.2.1. Flaps and Grafts

Penile skin flaps rely on the rich vascular collaterals within the tunica Dartos for its blood supply. The anterior lamella of Buck's fascia is elevated to ensure taking the entire Dartos. Elevation is basically along avascular planes and thus bloodless. Skin island flaps are versatile and can be mobilized to all areas of the anterior urethra. In general, make the flap at least 2 cm in width to insure that the final caliber of the reconstructed uretha is roughly 24 French, assuming the urethral plate is at least 0.5 cm to 1 cm in width, for a total circumference of 2.5 to 3 cm. When it comes to substitution urethroplasty, one-stage tube grafts or flaps should be avoided, due to their general lack of success and durability. Depending on the location and the length of the stricture, flaps can be ventral-longitudinal (for the pendulous urethra), ventral-transverse (for fossa strictures), or transverse-circumferential (for all aspects of the anterior urethra) and rotated to reach the defect. Proper mobilization will not put the flap on tension or cause penile torsion. From a practical viewpoint, when suturing the flap or graft to the open urethral plate it is essential to keep both the penis and the substitution material on stretch. Keeping the tissue stretched with traction and counter traction, avoids the complications of sacculations and diverticula,

which are prone to secondary infection and bothersome postvoid dribbling.

For substitution urethroplasty, there appears to be no advantage of using a flap over a graft when it comes to restricture rate. In fact, to date, there is no comparative, randomized prospective trial when it comes to comparing flaps or grafts. In general, grafts are quicker and easier to harvest and have less harvest donor site morbidity then flaps. For these reasons, buccal mucosa grafts are very popular and are the current substitution material of choice. In Wessells and McAninch's (1998) review and meta-analysis of 26 urethroplasty series, the restricture rates for grafts and flaps were not significantly different (15.7% and 14.5%, respectively). Urethral restricture rates seem to be highest for scrotal flaps and extragenital skin grafts and the lowest for posterior auricular grafts, buccal mucosa grafts, and penile skin flaps. Other distinct disadvantages of scrotal skin over penile skin are that it is more difficult to work with, tends to contact (more prone to sacculation), has a unilateral blood supply, and success rates are also worse.

In cases of bulbar strictures where there is inadequate penile skin or graft material, we therefore highly discourage the temptation to use a local scrotal skin flap; instead, we prefer a staged urethroplasty in such rare situations. Furthermore, each of the low re-stricture rate grafts and flaps appear to be equally effective and durable. Tissues that possess a thin dermis, dense subdermal vascular plexus, and thick epithelium make the ideal grafts –namely, penile skin, posterior auricular skin, or buccal mucosa. Such grafts are full-thickness grafts and are preferred to split-thickness grafts for urethroplasty. They contract less but have slightly less "take" than split-thickness grafts.

Buccal mucosa is currently the most popular substitution tissue in urethroplasty surgery. Buccal mucosa is the current preferred graft material because it can be quickly and easily harvested, is readily available, is tough and resilient to handling, can be harvested from either cheek or lip in large sized grafts, contracts little and has a high degree of "take" (epithelium is thick and elastin rich, whereas the lamina propria is thin and highly vascular), minimal donor site morbidity, concealed donor site scar, possesses anti-bacterial and anti-infective properties, thrives in a wet/moist environment, and is often resistant to skin diseases. It is clearly an ideal graft material and we employ it almost exclusively.

5.2.2. *Does Location of Buccal Graft Placement (Dorsal or Ventral) Really Make Any Difference?*

Theoretically, yes. In practice, not really. Admittedly, dorsal graft placement usually has less blood loss and avoids sacculations yet has the same relative long-term stricture-free rates and the same complication rates of post void dribbling (one in five) as ventral grafts. Ventral grafts, on the other hand, require less urethral dissection and mobilization, and are thus technically easier. Ventral versus dorsal is more a matter of surgeon preference. For proximal bulbar strictures, we prefer ventral buccal graft placement because dorsal grafts are typically more technically difficult to sew in a deep and proximal. However, in all other areas of the urethra, we prefer dorsal buccal graft placement. Regardless of where the graft is placed, many patients will have some minor post-coital semen pooling and post void dribbling; bothersome in up to one in five. Clearly, the keys are proper tailoring, proper defatting and preparation of the graft, placing the graft in a vascular bed, and keeping the graft fixed and in apposition to the host bed. As to the harvest site, we prefer the inner cheek and strongly discourage the use of the inner lip. With lower lip harvest there is a greater likelihood for troublesome neurosensory complications, such as persistent pain and/or perioral numbness. The lip mucosa is also more flimsy and less robust then cheek mucosa.

5.2.3. *Buccal Graft Harvest: Technique Specifics*

Before surgery, we always examine the mouth for mucosal lesions like ulcerations or lichen planus. Patients with poor dentition or who use tobacco chew are more likely to have mucosal disease. Our only cases where the harvested buccal graft had no structural integrity and fell apart are those who chew or with lichen planus. We would exclude such patients from buccal mucosal harvest. As to the harvest technique, we first have the anesthetist tape the endotracheal tube to one side. Nasotracheal intubation is unnecessary and we have had many

patients with nasal erosions and complaints of nasal pain after surgery, so we have stopped this practice. At first we wash the face and inner mouth with 1% hydrogen peroxide. This type of prep is more then adequate, for when our ENT colleagues harvest the buccal mucosa, many of then do no use a skin preparation at all. As to preoperative antibiotics, at one time we were giving intravenous penicillin, but are now giving just cephazolin, a first generation cephalosporin. First, we pack the tongue medially with a 4×4 gauze, mark Stensen's duct with a marking pen, and place stay sutures of 2-O Prolene, one cm lateral and posterior from the vermillion of the mouth. We then place a Steinhauser buccal mucosal stretcher (Walter Lorenz, Florida (USA)) on the cheek. We have modified the Steinhauser with a weight on the end (as in the manner of a weighted vaginal speculum) so it further can self hold the mouth open. We then place another mouth prop in the midline, and mark a graft roughly 2×5 cm, careful to make the cephalad margin away from Stensen's duct. The anterior margin of the graft is roughly one cm from the vermillion, so as to avoid the possibility of causing retraction and esthetic problems. With a 22-gauge spinal needle we inject 10 to 20 ml of 1:100,000 epinephrine solution as a submucosal wheel. Waiting a few minutes after injection before dissection, allows for excellent hemostasis. Pesky bleeding can be easily controlled with bipolar electrocautery. Since the facial nerves are in proximity, it is unwise to use monopolar energy here. We place two stay sutures of 3-O chromic on the corners of the graft and then use a no. 15 blade to harvest the graft superficial to the buccinator muscle. With the stay sutures giving traction, an index finger and a gauze soaked in epinephrine solution gives counter traction. Once the graft is harvested, we pack the mouth with epinephrine soaked gauze to facilitate hemostasis. On the back table, we de-fat the graft with the mid portion of the Metzenbaum scissors and cut while pressing the blades against an index finger. This removes the bulk of fat. The graft is then pinned to a vein board or silicone block (alternative: the needle counter foam pad) and scraped with the edge of a no. 15 blade. This emulsifies any residual fat. The graft is ready for placement when newsprint lettering can be visible through the graft. The graft is particularly resistant to infection and skin diseases. It seems counter intuitive to take the "dirty" buccal graft and sew it in to a sterile penile or perineal wound, but obviously they all seem to do fine. In fact, we have accidentally dropped a buccal graft or two onto the operating room floor over the years. Those cases were highly successful and did not develop a wound or urinary tract infection. As to the harvest site, many report today that they leave the mucosa open and allow it to heal by secondary intention. Many claim that the oral and perioral side effects are less. The main disadvantage of not closing the mucosa is that it precludes future buccal graft re-harvest. As an alternative to leaving the site open, some sew a graft of Alloderm, an acellular dermal matrix to promote epitheliazation. Instead, we have preferred to reapproximate the mucosa in a modified "Z" plasty fashion. A single skin hook is placed into the distal edge of the harvest site and the mucosa is stretched into a parallelogram shape. We then reapproximate the mucosa with a few interrupted 3-0 chromic sutures. Postoperatively we have the patients swish and spit with a mouth wash four times a day. Although we typically use the prescription Peridex (chlorhexidine gluconate 0.12% oral rinse typically used to treat gingivitis), we have also had good success with over the counter mouth washes.

5.3. Posterior Urethroplasty

Posterior urethral stenosis is not a true "stricture" but instead is scar tissue that fills the gap created by the distracted ends of the urethra. In contrast, anterior urethral stricture is epithelial scar tissue that contracts in length and width, with varying degrees of spongiofibrosis. Posterior urethroplasty is "urethral flap advancement surgery" that relies on bipedal corpus spongiosal blood supply. With the stricture being so proximal, the length of the urethral flap can be relatively long, up to the suspensory ligament, being 6cm or more. Detached from its proximal vascular supply the urethra is solely dependent on distal retrograde blood flow. It is not surprising then that patients with compromised retrograde flow, such as can occur with the impotent (symptom of potential penile vascular insufficiency) or hypospadiac patient, or with excessive distal urethral mobilization, have lower rates of anastomotic surgical success. Overall, the excellent efficacy and long-term durability rates reported for posterior urethral reconstruction is another example that stricture excision and primary anastomosis is always the preferred method, over a tissue "substitution" urethroplasty.

5.3.1. Technical and Surgical Specifics

First, we make a midline perineal incision from just anterior to the anus up to the scrotal margin. We can typically achieve excellent exposure of the urethra and don't consider a lambda incision necessary (**Fig. 29.6**). Although many authors like the Jordan Bookwalter for exposure for posterior urethroplasty, we have had good success with just the Lonestar retractor system. When using this system, mobilize the urethra from the perineal membrane till the penoscrotal junction. Do not mobilize the urethra distal to suspensory ligament; otherwise, you risk creating iatrogenic chordee. Mobilize the entire bulb and separate the bulb from the perineal body and rectum posteriorly. We typically use bipolar electrocautery liberally here to control pesky bleeding from small perforating vessel branches or from the bulbospongiosus muscle. We try to avoid using monopolar electrocautery out of concern of electrical scatter and potential injury to the nervous and vascular supply to the penis for tumescence. Then, place a hard 22-French Robnel catheter and palpate the proximal

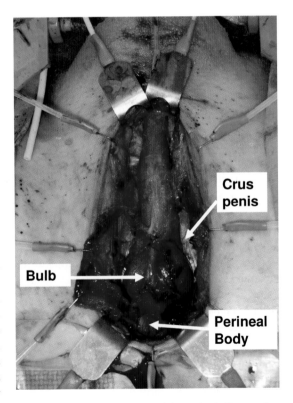

FIG. 29.6. Excellent exposure of the entire bulbar urethra via a midline incision and Lonestar rectractor

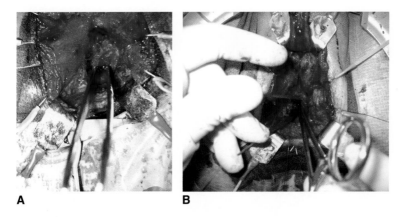

A   **B**

FIG. 29.7. A, B Debakey forceps placed "backwards" into the prostatic urethra to facilitate suturing

end of stricture. Transect the urethra just proximal to the palpable end of the Robnel with Mayo scissors. The urethra should not bleed too much if the cut is made through the scar. The bulbar arteries are usually obliterated already from the prior pelvic fracture. However, the bulbar urethra can bleed quite briskly, if the cut is not through the scar or if the bulbar arteries are intact. Once the urethra is transected, pack the fossa to temporarily to control bleeding and then over sew any bleeding bulbar arteries. Place a 24-French Van Buren sound via the SP tract and into the prostatic fossa and incise onto the palpable end of sound (use a scalpel). If the sound can't be felt confidently, we typically perform antegrade cystoscopy or open the bladder. When the sound cannot be felt it generally suggests that the stricture is long or the prostate is displaced off the midline. We typically inject methylene blue via the Robnel to stain the urethral mucosa prior to transection.

Scar tissue around the sound is then excised sharply until the tissue is supple and the antegrade placed sound can be easily rotated in all directions. Spatulate the prostatic/membranous urethra at 6 o'clock till the back handle of a Debakey forceps or nasal speculum can fit easily into the urethra (>32 French; **Fig. 29.7A**). The verumontanum can usually be easily seen at this time. To perform the anastomosis, we typically place eight sutures in the proximal urethra. Holding the end of the Debakey forceps open will facilitate suture placement (**Fig. 29.7B**). We first place sutures at 12, 6, 3, and 9 o'clock and then place another four sutures in between. We prefer 4-O PDS and will often bend the RB needle into a "ski" needle to facilitate

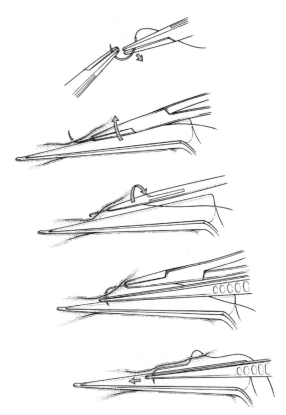

FIG. 29.8. The "ski" needle and Debakey forceps (alternative, gorgette) are useful to facilitate proximal sutures placement. (From Mundy AR (1997) Reconstruction of posterior urethral distraction defects: Atlas Uro Clin NA 5(1):139–174)

suture placement (**Fig. 29.8**). We serially place numbered labeled mosquitoes on all the sutures to enable proper orientation (**Fig. 29.9**). We then

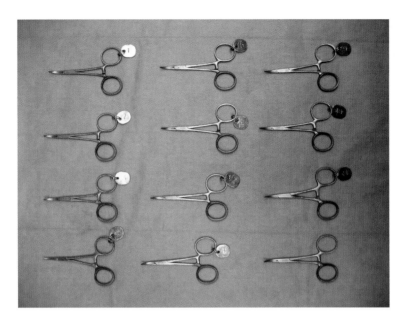

FIG. 29.9. Serially numbered mosquito clamps (1–12) to facilitate suture orientation

place a 16-French Silicone Foley catheter, followed by placing sutures into the distal urethra in numerical order in clockwise fashion (e.g., start at 12 o'clock proximal and sew to 6 o'clock distal). The sutures are then serially tied in numerical order in the same clockwise fashion. Turner-Warwick-isms we have not found useful are: complex acronyms, 12-French fenestrated catheter, lambda-shaped perineal incision, and so-called "specialty" instruments.

In 1983, Webster and colleagues popularized an elaborated perineal approach for reconstruction of pelvic fracture-related urethral distraction injuries wherein urethral mobilization is augmented as needed by progressing through the additional steps of corporal splitting, inferior pubectomy and urethral rerouting to bridge long urethral defects. We have found urethral rerouting to have a limited role and instead think that liberal urethral mobilization and corporal splitting alone are usually sufficient to bridge the gap. Moreover, most posterior urethral strictures are typically no more then 2–3 cm in length and, thus, the limits of the progressive approach are usually not required (1). As a salvage procedure for complex and long defects, we prefer and have had greater success with the abdominoperineal approach.

5.3.2. Informed Consent

An essential aspect of surgical planning is discussion with the patient about the risks and benefits of the procedure. When it comes to posterior urethroplasty, we tell each of our patients that the potential surgical side effects are stress urinary incontinence (minor degree, relatively common [up to 36%] whereas bothersome to more severe incontinence is rare [roughly 2%], urgency to void is common [up to 66%], temporary impotence is not uncommon [up to 26%], permanent impotence is possible but very rare [0–7% depending on the series], and positioning complications from being in lithotomy (such as perineal nerve palsy, sacral nerve stretch). We also quote to out patients that long term, durable success with posterior urethroplasty is roughly 85%.

Appendix

Preferred Instruments of SB Brandes

Instruments

1. Yellowfin stirrups
2. 3M-irrigation pouch, "Steri-drape" #1016. Suction tubing to bottom of pouch
3. Bipolar, "bayonet", wide tip cautery

4. Baby Yankauer-type suction, "Andrews" sucker
5. Bougie a boules from 10F to 32F
6. Lonestar retractor, #3308 (large ring) and corresponding hook: Blue ("dura") hooks, #3311 (5mm) × 6, and Four-arm yellow hooks , #3334 (14 × 20mm) × 4 (Cooper Surgical , Trumbel, CT)
7. 20F Robnel catheter
8. Stevens Tenotomy scissors, 6"
9. 0.5 Castro toothed forceps × 2
10. Jerold's forceps with teeth × 2
11. Van Buren sounds 20F-32F
12. Steinhauser mouth retractor/mucosal stretcher (Walter Lorenz Surgical Instruments, #01-0060)
13. Foam pad from needle counter or Vein board

Suture

1. 2-0 Prolene (polypropylene), SH needle, tapered × 1 (for glans penis traction or vermillion of mouth)
2. 4-0 chromic, RB-1, tapered
3. 4-0 PDS, tapered, single armed, RB-1
4. 16F Silastic Foley, 5cc balloon
5. 2-0 Vicryl (polyglactin), SH needle, tapered, 3-0 Vicryl (polyglactin) , SH needle, tapered, 3-0 chromic, SH needle, tapered

Suggested Readings

Andrich DE, Dunglison N, Greenwell TJ, Mundy AR (2003) The long-term results of urethroplasty. J Urol 170:90–92

DaSilva EA, Sampaio FJB (2002) Urethral extensibility applied to reconstructive surgery. J Urol 167:2042–2045

Johanson B (1953) Reconstruction of the male urethra in strictures: application of the buried intact epithelium tracking. Acta Clin Scand 176(suppl):1.

Kizer WS, Armenakas NA, Brandes SB, Cavalcanti AG, Santucci RA, Morey AF (2007) Simplified reconstruction of posterior urethral disruption defects: limited role of supracrural rerouting. J Urol 177:1378–1381

Mundy AR (1996) Urethroplasty for posterior urethral strictures. Br J Urol 78:243–247.

Quartey JKM (1983) One-stage penile/preputial cutaneous island flap urethroplasty for urethral stricture: a preliminary report. J Urol 129:284

Schreiter F, Noll F (1989) Mesh graft urethroplasty using a split-thickness skin graft of foreskin. J Urol 142:1223

Webster GD, Koerfoot RB, Sihelnik SA (1985) Urethroplasty management in 200 cases of urethral stricture: a rationale for procedure selection. J Urol 134:892

Waterhouse K, Abrahms JI, Gruber H, et al (1973) The transpubic approach to the lower urinary tract. J Urol 109:486.

30
Tissue Engineering of the Urethra

Anthony Atala

Contents

1. Introduction 337
2. Use of Cells for the Engineering of Urethral Tissues 338
3. Biomaterials for the Engineering of Urethral Tissues 338
    3.1. Selection 339
    3.2. Classes 339
    3.3. Acellular Tissue Matrices 339
    3.4. Synthetic Polymers 340
    3.5. Tissue–Regeneration Strategies 340
4. Engineering of Urethral Tissues with Acellular Matrices 340
5. Engineering of Urethral Tissues with Cell-Seeded Matrices 343
Editorial Comment 343
References 343

Summary Congenital abnormalities, trauma, infection, and cancer can all affect the urethra. In most of these cases, reconstructive procedures are eventually necessary. These procedures can be performed with native non-urologic tissues (skin, gastrointestinal segments, or mucosa), homologous tissues from a donor (cadaver or living donor kidney), heterologous tissues or substances (bovine collagen), or artificial materials (silicone, polyurethane, Teflon). However, these materials often lead to complications after urethral reconstruction. The implanted tissue is sometimes rejected, and often, the inherently different functional aspects of the different tissues or materials used in the reconstruction leads to improper or inadequate tissue development. The replacement of lost or deficient urethral tissues with functionally equivalent ones would improve the outcome of reconstructive surgery in the genitourinary system. This may soon be possible with the novel tissue engineering techniques described in this chapter

Keywords Acellular tissue matrix, biomaterials, synthetic polymers, tissue regeneration, all seeded matrices, urethra

1. Introduction

To address the problem of urethral reconstruction, tissue engineering has been proposed as a promising strategy. Tissue engineering may involve matrices alone, wherein the body's natural ability to regenerate is used to orient or direct new tissue growth, or the use of matrices with cells. Acellular collagen matrices derived from donor bladder submucosa have been used both experimentally and clinically for onlay urethral replacement with good success at our Institute. If a tubularized urethral repair is needed, the use of cells on the collagen matrix is essential for adequate tissue formation. Tissue engineering techniques as described in this chapter are useful for urethral reconstruction.

For both congenital and acquired etiologies, urethral reconstruction remains a challenge for most urologic surgeons. High success rates depend on having adequate tissues for reconstruction as well as appropriately trained surgeons. The difficulty in achieving adequate results is best represented by the myriad of articles published each year that attempt to explore new reconstructive techniques. There are more than 300 techniques described for the correction of hypospadias and urethral strictures, which illustrate the challenges and difficulties in the surgical correction of these anomalies. Considerable progress in the surgical correction of urethral defects has been made during the past 50 years as the result of the advances in microsurgical instrumentation, optical magnification, and development of fine, absorbable suture material *(1)*.

Some of the most challenging reconstructive problems for patients with hypospadias involve those with inadequate penile skin caused by unsuccessful surgical repairs or prior circumcision. In a review of 5882 newborn circumcisions, 35% of boys with hypospadias were circumcised *(2)*.

The most challenging reconstructive problems for patients with stricture disease involve long defects, which may be hard to manage with excision and primary anastomosis. Many tissues have been used for urethral reconstruction, including vascularized or free graft skin, bladder, buccal or rectal mucosa, dermal free grafts, and tunica vaginalis. All these tissues have been associated with numerous complications. Because of the problems associated with some of the tissues currently used, several investigators have sought alternate substances for urethral reconstruction.

Tissue engineering has been proposed as a strategy for urethral reconstruction *(3)*. Tissue engineering follows the principles of cell transplantation, materials science, and engineering toward the development of biological substitutes that restore and maintain normal function.

2. Use of Cells for the Engineering of Urethral Tissues

When cells are used for tissue engineering, donor tissue is dissociated into individual cells which are implanted directly into the host, or expanded in culture, attached to a support matrix, and re-implanted after expansion. The implanted tissue can be heterologous, allogeneic, or autologous. Ideally, this approach might allow lost tissue function to be restored or replaced *in toto* and with limited complications *(3)*. The use of autologous cells would avoid rejection, wherein a biopsy of tissue is obtained from the host, the cells dissociated and expanded in vitro, reattached to a matrix, and implanted into the same host *(3–17)*.

One of the initial limitations of applying cell-based tissue engineering techniques to urologic organs had been the previously encountered inherent difficulty of growing genitourinary associated cells in large quantities. In the past, it was believed that urothelial cells had a natural senescence which was hard to overcome. Normal urothelial cells could be grown in the laboratory setting, but with limited expansion. Several protocols were developed over the last two decades which improved urothelial growth and expansion *(9,18–20)*. A system of urothelial cell harvest was developed that does not use any enzymes or serum and has a large expansion potential. Using these methods of cell culture, it is possible to expand a urothelial strain from a single specimen which initially covers a surface area of $1 \, cm^2$ to one covering a surface area of $4202 \, m^2$ (the equivalent area of one football field) within 8 wk *(9)*. These studies indicated that it should be possible to collect autologous urothelial cells from human patients, expand them in culture, and return them to the human donor in sufficient quantities for reconstructive purposes. Normal human genitourinary epithelial and muscle cells can be efficiently harvested from surgical material, extensively expanded in culture, and their differentiation characteristics, growth requirements and other biological properties studied *(9,12,19–27)*.

3. Biomaterials for the Engineering of Urethral Tissues

Biomaterials in genitourinary tissue engineering function as an artificial extracellular matrix (ECM) and elicit biological and mechanical functions of native ECM found in tissues in the body. Native ECM brings cells together into tissue, controls the tissue structure, and regulates the cell phenotype *(28)*. Biomaterials facilitate the localization and delivery of cells and/or bioactive factors (e.g., cell adhesion peptides and growth factors) to desired sites in the body, define a three-dimensional space for the formation of new tissues with appropriate structure, and guide the development of new tissues with appropriate function (29). Direct injection of cell suspensions without biomaterial matrices have been used in some cases (30,31), but it is difficult to control the localization of transplanted cells. In addition, the majority of mammalian cell types is anchorage-dependent and will die if not provided with a cell-adhesion substrate. Biomaterials provide a cell-adhesion substrate and can be used to achieve cell delivery with high loading and efficiency to specific sites in the body. The configuration of the biomaterials can guide the structure of an engineered tissue. The biomaterials provide mechanical support against *in vivo* forces, thus maintaining a predefined structure during the process of tissue development. The biomaterials can be loaded with bioactive signals, such as cell-adhesion peptides and growth factors which can regulate cellular function.

3.1. Selection

The design and selection of the biomaterial is critical in the development of engineered urethral tissues. It must be capable of controlling the structure and function of the engineered urethral tissue in a predesigned manner by interacting with transplanted cells or host cells. Generally, the ideal biomaterial should be biocompatible, promote cellular interaction and tissue development, and possess proper mechanical and physical properties.

The selected biomaterial should be biodegradable and bioresorbable to support the reconstruction of normal urethral tissue without inflammation. Such behavior of the biomaterials would avoid the risk of inflammatory or foreign body responses which may be associated with the permanent presence of a foreign material in the body. The degradation products should not provoke inflammation or toxicity, and they must be removed from the body via metabolic pathways. The degradation rate and the concentration of degradation products in the tissues surrounding the implant must be at tolerable levels (32).

The biomaterials should possess appropriate mechanical properties to regenerate tissues with predefined sizes and shapes. The biomaterials

provide temporary mechanical support sufficient to withstand *in vivo* forces exerted by the surrounding tissue and maintain a potential space for tissue development. The mechanical support of the biomaterials should be maintained until the engineered tissue has sufficient mechanical integrity to support itself (3). This can be potentially achieved by an appropriate choice of mechanical and degradative properties of the biomaterials (29).

The biomaterials must be processed into specific configurations. A large surface area to volume ratio is often desirable to allow the delivery of a high density of cells. High porosity, interconnected pore structure, and specific pore sizes promote tissue ingrowth from the surrounding host tissue. Several techniques have been developed which readily control porosity, pore size, and pore structure.

3.2. Classes

Generally, two classes of biomaterials have been utilized for engineering urethral tissues: acellular tissue matrices (e.g., bladder submucosa and small intestinal submucosa), and synthetic polymers (e.g., polyglycolic acid [PGA], polylactic acid [PLA], and polylactic-co-glycolic acid [PLGA]). These classes of biomaterials have been tested for biocompatibility with primary human urothelial and bladder muscle cells (30). Naturally derived and acellular matrices have the potential advantage of biological recognition. Synthetic polymers are reproducible on a large scale with controlled properties of their strengh, degradation rate, and microstructure.

3.3. Acellular Tissue Matrices

Acellular tissue matrices are collagen-rich and prepared by removing cellular components from tissues. The matrices often are prepared by mechanical and chemical manipulation of a segment of bladder tissue (33,34). The matrices slowly degrade upon implantation and are replaced and remodeled by ECM proteins synthesized and secreted by transplanted or ingrowing cells. Acellular tissue matrices have proven to support cell ingrowth and regeneration of genitourinary tissues, including urethra and bladder, with no evidence of immunogenic rejection (18,35). Because the structure of the proteins (e.g., collagen and elastin) in acellular matrices is well conserved and normally arranged, the mechanical properties of the acellular matrices are not significantly different from those of native bladder submucosa (36).

3.4. Synthetic Polymers

Polyesters of naturally occurring α-hydroxy acids, including PGA, PLA, and PLGA, are widely used in tissue engineering. These polymers have gained approval from the Food and Drug Administration for human use in a variety of applications, including sutures (37). The ester bonds in these polymers are hydrolytically labile, and these polymers degrade by nonenzymatic hydrolysis. The degradation products of all three compounds are nontoxic, natural metabolites that are eventually eliminated from the body in the form of carbon dioxide and water (37). The degradation rate of these polymers can be tailored from several weeks to several years by altering crystallinity, initial molecular weight, and the copolymer ratio of lactic to glycolic acid. Because these polymers are thermoplastics, they can be formed easily into a three-dimensional scaffold with a desired microstructure, gross shape and dimension by various techniques, including molding, extrusion (2), solvent casting (23), phase separation techniques, and gas foaming techniques (24).

3.5. Tissue–Regeneration Strategies

Various strategies have been proposed over the years for the regeneration of urethral tissue. Woven meshes of PGA (Dexon) were used to reconstruct urethras in dogs. Three to four centimeters of the ventral half of the urethral circumference and its adjacent corpus spongiosum was excised, and the polymer mesh was sutured to the defective area. After 2 wk, the animals were able to void through the neourethra. At 2 mo, the urothelium was completely regenerated. The polymer meshes were completely absorbed after 3 mo. No complications occurred. However, the excised corpus spongiosum did not regenerate (38).

PGA has been also used as a cell transplantation vehicle to engineer tubular urothelium in vivo. Cultured urothelial cells were seeded onto tubular PGA scaffolds and implanted into athymic mice. At 20 and 30 d, polymer degradation was evident, and tubular urothelium formed in which cells were stained for a urothelium-associated cytokeratin (8).

PGA mesh tubes coated with polyhydroxybutyric acid (PHB) were used to reconstruct urethras in dogs. PHB is a biodegradable thermoplastic polymer produced microbially. PHB degrades by both hydrolysis and enzyme reaction. The hydrolized product, 3-hydroxybutyric acid, is a natural metabolite that is contained in human blood (39). Eight to twelve months after reconstruction, complete regeneration of urothelium and adjacent connective tissue occurred. All of the polymers disappeared after 1 yr, and there were no anastomotic strictures or inflammatory reactions (34).

4. Engineering of Urethral Tissues with Acellular Matrices

Small intestinal submucosa (SIS) was used as an onlay patch graft for urethroplasty in rabbits (19). SIS was compared with full-thickness preputial skin grafts and shams (simple urethrotomy and closure). Animals were sacrificed between 8 and 12 wk. Histologic evaluation demonstrated that SIS promoted urethral regeneration. Regenerated urethras contained three to four layers of stratified columnar urothelium that was indistinguishable from the normal rabbit urothelium. There was also evidence of circular smooth muscle regeneration underneath the urothelium. This regenerated muscle was contained within an abundant amount of collagen and fibrous connective tissue. Grossly, there was no evidence of diverticular formation. In contrast, all grafts in the preputial skin group had evidence of diverticulum formation.

A homologous free graft of acellular urethral matrix was used in a rabbit model (33). A 0.8- to 1.1-cm segment of the urethra was resected and replaced with an acellular matrix graft of 1.0 to 1.5 cm. Histological examination showed complete epithelialization and progressive vessel infiltration. At 3 mo, smooth muscle bundles were first observed infiltrating the matrix at the anastomosis; after 6 mo, the smooth muscle bundles had grown into one third of the matrix. By 8 mo, the host and implant could not be differentiated by urethrography.

All tissue components were seen in the grafted matrix after 3 mo, with further improvement over time; however, the smooth muscle in the matrix was less than that observed in normal rabbit urethra and was not well oriented.

A bladder-derived acellular collagen matrix has proven to be a suitable graft for repairing urethral defects both experimentally and clinically *(35)*. A ventral urethral defect measuring 1×0.7 cm (approximately half of the urethral circumference) was created in 10 male rabbits. The acellular collagen matrix was trimmed and used to replace the urethral defect in an onlay fashion. Serial urethrography was performed pre- and post-operatively at 0.5, 1, 2, 3, and 6 mo. Animals were sacrificed at 0.5, 1, 2, 3, and 6 mo after surgery. The retrieved implants were analyzed grossly, histologically, and with immunocytochemistry. All animals survived until sacrifice without any noticeable voiding dysfunction.

Serial urethrograms confirmed the maintenance of a wide urethral caliber without any signs of strictures. Gross examination at retrieval showed normally appearing tissue without any evidence of fibrosis. At retrieval, the distances between the marking sutures placed at the anastomotic margins remained stable, with no distance varying more than 10% in any axis, indicating the maintenance of the initial implant diameter. Histologically, the implanted matrices contained host cell infiltration and generous angiogenesis by 2 wk after surgery. Minimal infiltration of inflammatory cells was observed initially; however, complete disappearance of these cells was evident by the 3 mo postoperative time period. There was no evidence of fibrosis or scarring in the urethras at any of the retrieval time periods.

The presence of a complete transitional cell layer over the graft was confirmed 2 wk after the repair, and this was consistent throughout the study. The urothelial cell layers stained positively with the broadly reacting anti-pancytokeratins AE1/AE3 in all implants. There was no evidence of muscle fibers either at the 2-wk or 1-mo retrievals. Unorganized muscle fiber bundles were evident histologically 2 mo after implantation. The histologic patterns suggested that the ingrowth of muscle fibers occurred from all the adjacent native tissue areas, including the ends and sides of the grafts. These findings were confirmed using anti-α-actin antibodies. Increasing number of organized muscle

bundles were observed at 3 mo. Normal appearing organized muscle fiber bundles were evident 6 mo after implantation. These results demonstrated that the acellular collagen matrix could be a useful material for urethral repair in the rabbit *(35)*.

These results were confirmed clinically in a series of patients with a history of failed hypospadias reconstruction wherein the urethral defects were repaired with human bladder acellular collagen matrices *(17)*. The neourethras were created by anastomosing the matrix, which was trimmed to the appropriate size, in an onlay fashion to the urethral plate (**Fig. 30.1**). The size of the created neourethra ranged from 5 to 15 cm. After a 3-yr follow-up, three of the four patients had a successful outcome in regards to their cosmetic appearance and function. One patient, who had a 15 cm neourethra created, developed a subglanular fistula. Retrograde cystourethrograms, performed after 1 yr of repair were normal without any evidence of narrowing. Cystoscopic studies with urethral biopsies were also performed after 1 year of repair. Cystoscopic and cystographic studies showed adequate caliber conduits (**Fig. 30.2**). Histologic and immunocytochemical examination of

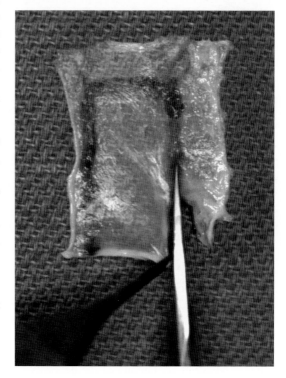

FIG. 30.1. Collagen matrix is rehydrated in a saline solution and trimmed to size at the time of surgical repair

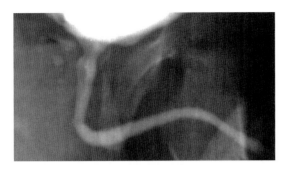

FIG. 30.2. Urethrogram of a patient 1 yr after hypospadias repair shows a normal caliber urethra

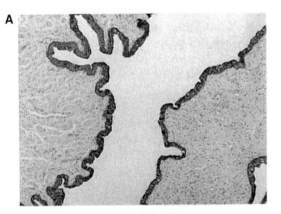

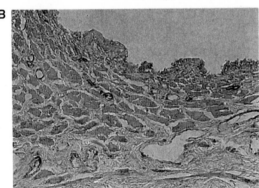

FIG. 30.3. Immunocytochemical analyses of neo-urethras show (A) normal urothelial layers staining positive for pancytokeratin antibodies AE1/AE3, and (B) normal-appearing muscle bundles which stain positively for α-actin antibodies

the biopsy specimens showed the typical urethral stratified epithelium (**Fig. 30.3**). The acellular collagen-based matrix eliminated the necessity of performing additional surgical procedures for graft harvesting. Operative time and the potential morbidity due to the harvest procedure are decreased.

Similar results were obtained in pediatric and adult patients with urethral stricture disease (7). Patients with a diagnosis of urethral stricture underwent reconstructive surgery using the collagen based inert matrix for urethral reconstruction. The matrix was trimmed to size as needed for each patient and the neourethras were created by anastomosing the matrix in an onlay fashion to the urethral plate with continuous 6-0 Vicryl sutures. The size of the created neourethra ranged from 1.5 to 16 cm (**Fig. 30.4**). Urethrograms were done routinely 4 mo postoperatively. Cystoscopic studies showed adequate caliber conduits and normal-appearing urethral tissues (**Fig. 30.5**). Histologic examination of the biopsy specimens showed the typical urethral stratified epithelium.

More than 60 pediatric and adult patients with urethral disease have been treated to date using the collagen based matrix. The results show that the use of a collagen-based acellular matrix appears to be beneficial for patients with hypospadias and stricture disease who may lack sufficient genital skin for reconstruction. The acellular collagen-based matrix

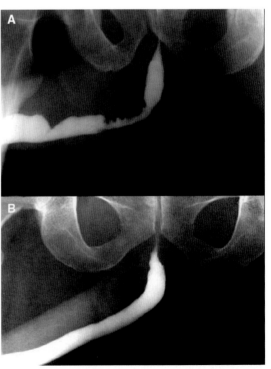

FIG. 30.4. Representative case of urethral stricture: (A) preoperative urethrogram and (B) urethrogram 6 mo after repair

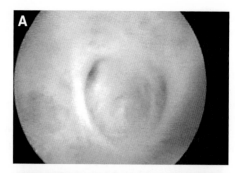

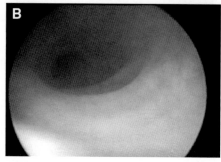

FIG. 30.5. Endoscopic view of the urethra, in a patient who presented with stricture disease, at the same location before urethral repair (A) and 1 yr after surgery (B).

eliminates the necessity of performing additional surgical procedures for graft harvesting. In addition, operative time and the potential morbidity due to the harvest procedure are decreased.

The acellular matrix was used only in an onlay fashion. The urethral segments reconstructed with the acellular matrices showed a normal cellular organization, indistinguishable from the native urethral tissue. Graft contracture or strictures did not occur.

5. Engineering of Urethral Tissues with Cell-Seeded Matrices

A series of experiments was performed to determine if the acellular matrix could be used for tubularized urethral repairs *(40)*. Autologous bladder smooth muscle cells from 10 rabbits were grown and seeded onto preconfigured tubular matrices. Approximately two thirds of the penile urethra was replaced in 20 male rabbits. Urethroplasties were performed with tubularized matrices seeded with cells in 10 animals and without cells in 10 animals.

Serial urethrography confirmed the maintenance of a wide urethral caliber without strictures in all animals implanted with cell seeded matrices. However, the urethral segments replaced with collagen scaffolds without cells demonstrated strictures at all time points. Gross examination of the urethral implants seeded with cells showed normal-appearing tissue without any evidence of fibrosis. Histologically, the implanted matrices contained normal urethral tissue by 1 month, consisting of a transitional cell layer surrounded by muscle cell fiber bundles with increasing cellular organization over time. Epithelial and smooth muscle phenotypes were confirmed with pAE1/AE3 and smooth muscle specific α-actin antibodies. Formation of a transitional cell layer was also confirmed in the matrices implanted without cells; however, only scant unorganized muscle fiber bundles were present at the anastomotic sites. Similar urothelial and smooth muscle differentiation were observed with the tissue engineered grafts compared to controls on Western Blot analyses. Organ bath studies demonstrated the capacity for contractility along with cholinergic and adrenergic specific receptors in the tissue-engineered scaffolds.

Although acellular collagen matrices can be used successfully for urethral repair in an onlay fashion, if tubularized they lead to poor tissue development and stricture formation. If a tubularized urethral repair is needed, the use of cells on the collagen matrix is essential for adequate tissue formation *(41)*.

Editorial Comment

Clearly, the future of urethral reconstructive surgery lies in tissue engineering and with an "off-the-shelf" graft repair. Although progress has been very slow, recent successful reports are encouraging, and will soon revolutionize not only urethral surgery, but all aspects of reconstructive surgery.—S.B. Brandes

References

1. Atala A, Retik AB (1996) Hypospadias, in Libertino JA, Zinman L (eds) Reconstructive urologic surgery. Baltimore, Williams and Wilkins, pp 467–481
2. Freed LE, Vunjak-Novakovic G, Biron RJ, et al. (1994) Biodegradable polymer scaffolds for tissue engineering. Bio/Technology 12:689–693
3. Atala A (1997) Tissue engineering in the genitourinary system, in Atala A, Mooney D (eds) Tissue engineering. Boston, Birkhauser Press, pp 149–149

4. Atala A, Schlussel RN, Retik AB (1995) Renal cell growth in vivo after attachment to biodegradable polymer scaffolds. J Urol 153:4

5. Atala A, Freeman MR, Vacanti JP, et al. (1993) Implantation in vivo and retrieval of artificial structures consisting of rabbit and human urothelium and human bladder muscle. J Urol 150:608–612

6. Atala A, Kim W, Paige KT, et al (1994) Endoscopic treatment of vesicoureteral reflux with chondrocyte-alginate suspension. J Urol 152:641

7. El-Kassaby AW, Retik AB, Yoo JJ, et al. (2003) Urethral stricture repair with an off-the-shelf collagen matrix. J Urol 169:170–173

8. Atala, A, Vacanti, JP, Peters, CA, et al. (1992) Formation of urothelial structures in vivo from dissociated cells attached to biodegradable polymer scaffolds in vitro. J Urol 148:658

9. Cilento, BG, Freeman, MR, Schneck, FX, et al. (1994) Phenotypic and cytogenetic characterization of human bladder urothelia expanded in vitro. J Urol 52:655

10. Solomon LZ, Jennings AM, Sharpe P, et al. (1998) Effects of short-chain fatty acids on primary urothelial cells in culture: implications for intravesical use in enterocystoplasties. J Lab Clin Med 132(4), 279–283

11. Fauza DO, Fishman S, Mehegan K, et al. (1998) Videofetoscopically assisted fetal tissue engineering: skin replacement. J Pediatr Surg 33:377

12. Fauza DO, Fishman S, Mehegan K, et al. (1998) Videofetoscopically assisted fetal tissue engineering: bladder augmentation. J Pediatr Surg 33:71

13. Amiel GE, Atala A (1999) Current and future modalities for functional renal replacement. Urol Clin N Am 26:235–246

14. Tobin MS, Freeman MR, Atala A (1994) Maturational response of normal human urothelial cells in culture is dependent on extracellular matrix and serum additives. Surg Forum 45:786

15. Oberpenning FO, Meng J, Yoo J, et al. (1999) De novo reconstitution of a functional urinary bladder by tissue engineering. Nat Biotech 17:2

16. Nguyen HT, Park JM, Peters CA, et al (1999) Cell-specific activation of the HB-EGF and ErbB1 genes by stretch in primary human bladder cells. In Vitro Cell Devel Biol 35:371–375

17. Atala A, Guzman L, Retik A (1999) A novel inert collagen matrix for hypospadias repair. J Urol 162:1148–1151

18. Probst M, Dahiya R, Carrier S, et al. (1997) Reproduction of functional smooth muscle tissue and partial bladder replacement. Br J Urol 79:505–515

19. Kropp, BP, Ludlow, JK, Spicer, D, et al. (1998) Rabbit urethral regeneration using small intestinal submucosa onlay grafts. Urology 52:138–142

20. Piechota HJ, Dahms SE, Nunes LS, et al. (1998) In vitro functional properties of the rat bladder regenerated by the bladder acellular matrix graft. J Urol 159:1717–1724

21. Liebert M, Wedemeyer G, Abruzzo LV, et al. (1991) Stimulated urothelial cells produce cytokines and express an activated cell surface antigenic phenotype. Semin Urol 9:124–130

22. Scriven S, Booth C, Thomas DF, et al. (1997) Reconstitution of human urothelium from monolayer cultures. J Urol 158:1147–1152

23. Mikos AG, Thorsen AJ, Czerwonka LA, et al (1994) Preparation and characterization of poly(L-lactic acid) foams. Polymer 5:1068–1077

24. Harris LD, Kim BS, Mooney DJ (1998) Open pore biodegradable matrices formed with gas foaming. J Biomed Mater Res 42:396–402

25. Puthenveettil JA, Burger MS, Reznikoff CA (1999) Replicative senescence in human uroepithelial cells Adv Exp Med Biol 462:83–91

26. Liebert M, Hubbel A, Chung M, et al. (1997) Expression of mal is associated with urothelial differentiation in vitro: identification by differential display reverse-transcriptase polymerase chain reaction Differentiation 61:177–185

27. Ponder KP, Gupta S, Leland F, et al. (1991) Mouse hepatocytes migrate to liver parenchyma and function indefinitely after intrasplenic transplantation. Proc Natl Acad Sci U S A 88:1217–1221

28. Alberts B, Bray D, Lewis J, et al. (1994) Molecular biology of the cell. New York, Garland Publishing, pp 971–995

29. Kershen RT, Atala A (1999) Advances in injectable therapies for the treatment of incontinence and vesicoureteral reflux. Urol Clin 26:81–94

30. Pariente JL, Kim BS, Atala A (2001) In vitro biocompatibility assessment of naturally derived and synthetic biomaterials using normal human urothelial cells. J Biomed Mater Res 55:33–39

31. Brittberg M, Lindahl A, Nilsson A, et al. (1994) Treatment of deep cartilage defects in the knee with autologous chondrocyte transplantation. N Engl J Med 331:889–895

32. Bergsma JE, Rozema FR, Bos RRM, et al. (1995) Biocompatibility and degradatin mechanism of pre-degraded and non-degraded poly(lactide) implants: an animal study. Mater Med 6:715–724

33. Sievert KD, Bakircioglu ME, Nunes L, et al. (2000) Homologous acellular matrix graft for urethral reconstruction in the rabbit: histological and functional evaluation. J Urol 163:1958–1965

34. Olsen L, Bowald S, Busch C, et al. (1992) Urethral reconstruction with a new synthetic absorbable device. Scand J Urol Nephrol 26:323–326

35. Chen F, Yoo JJ, Atala A (1999) Acellular collagen matrix as a possible "off the shelf" biomaterial for urethral repair. Urology 54:407–410
36. Dahms SE, Piechota HJ, Dahiya R, et al. (1998) Composition and biochemical properties of the bladder acellular matrix graft: comparative analysis in rat, pig and human. Br J Urol 82:411–419
37. Gilding DK(1981) Biodegradable polymers, in Williams DF (ed) Biocompatibility of clinical implant materials. Boca Raton, FL, CRC Press, pp 209–232
38. Bazeed MA, Thüroff JW, Schmidt RA, et al. (1983) New treatment for urethral strictures Urology 21:53–57
39. Holmes P (1985) Applications of PHB-α microbially produced thermoplastic Phys Technol 16:32–36
40. De Filippo RE, Yoo JJ, Atala A (2002) Urethral replacement using cell seeded tubularized collagen matrices J Urol 168:1789–1792
41. le Roux PJ (2005) Endoscopic urethroplasty with unseeded small intestinal submucosa collagen matrix grafts: a pilot study. J Urol 173:140–143

31

History of Urethral Stricture and Its Management From the 18th to 20th Century

Steven B. Brandes and Chris F. Heyns

Contents

1. Introduction 347
2. Stricture Etiology 347
3. Treatment Methods 348
4. Urethral Dilation 348
5. Caustics and Cauterization.. 350
6. External Urethrotomy 350
7. Stricture Diagnosis... 351
8. Alternative Methods for Treating Urethral Strictures 351
9. Internal Urethrotomy 352
10. Contemporary Urethrotomes 353
11. Urethroplasty.. 353
Appendix... 354
References... 354

Summary Urethral stricture management has evolved greatly over the last two centuries. We have come along way from the use of wax casts, caustics, cauterization, external urethrotomy, and stricture chairs. However, as much as we have advanced, we still actively utilize dilation and urethrotomy in current practice. Urethroplasty surgery stands on the shoulders of pioneering giants, such as Denis Browne, Hamilton Russel, Begnt Johanson, and Charlie Devine. For the second half of the 20th century, the urethral reconstruction pendulum has swung from mainly two-stage urethroplasty, then to grafts, then onto fasciocutaneous flaps, and currently, has swung back to grafts (buccal mucosa). Great promise lies with tissue engineering and regenerative medicine today. However, to know where we are going, it is often helpful to know where we have been.

Keywords dilation, urethrotomy, caustics, external urethrotomy, urethrotome, urethroplasty

1. Introduction

Until the Middle Ages, the treatment of urinary problems often was considered beneath the realm of physicians and was left to nonphysicians and itinerant practitioners who specialized in these conditions. At times, professors might lecture on diseases of the urinary trac, but rarely conceded to treat such maladies. Not until the 17th century were genitourinary diseases accepted as normal human aliments and thus regularly attended to by physicians and surgeons.

2. Stricture Etiology

It was originally thought that urethral strictures were the result of ulcers or carnosities. Ambrosie Pare, the great barber-surgeon, also believed this to be the cause. By the 18th century, such notions were discredited by the likes of John Hunter.

From: *Current Clinical Urology: Urethral Reconstructive Surgery*
Edited by: S.B. Brandes © Humana Press, Totowa, NJ

Several theories for the etiology of urethral strictures included a "plastic exudate" that reacted with
urine resulting in a "collar of swelling" by Tanchou
and Lallemand, a false membrane by Ducamp and
Laennec, or granular urethritis (1). In the 18th century, most articles with urethral stricture were only
concerned with urinary retention and complete
obstruction. Lesser degrees of stricture were not
emphasized.

The first classification system of urethral strictures was described by Charles Bell in 1810 into:
"simple, bridle, dilatable, spasmodic, callous, and
ulcerated" strictures (2). Bell felt that the etiology
of urethral strictures was inflammation and disa-
greed with John Hunter who believed the urethral
strictures were contractures of the "muscles" of the
urethra. In 1827, Ducamp logically deduced that as
"gonorrhea is the most frequent as well as the most
intense kind of inflammation to which the urethra
is subject, so it is the principal cause of stricture in
this canal." Furthermore, Amussat, the great French
physician of the early 1800s, classified strictures as
organic, spasmodic, or inflammatory (3). Other
common classifications used in the 1800s were
by Syme, "imaginary, slight, confirmed, irritable,
and contractile," and Thompson (1854), "organic,
inflammatory, and spasmodic."

3. Treatment Methods

Urethral stricture is one of the oldest known
urological diseases, and dilatation was the first
known form of treatment. In the earliest of
papyruses and clay tablets, urethral dilatation
is described. As the anatomy of the urethra and
the nature of urethral strictures became better
understood, instruments were designed to localize and treat them. However, dilatation was never
regarded as curative, and the high recurrence
rate probably gave rise to the somewhat cynical
remark: "Once a stricture, always a stricture."
In 1824, Lioult designed a sound with a tapered
bulb—essentially an early model of the modern
olive tipped bougie. By about 1830, bougies of
whalebone were made by Guillon, and in 1836,
Leroy E'tiolles invented the "bougie a boule."
These bougies were very similar to the urethral
bougies we use today, although they were not in
popular use at that time.

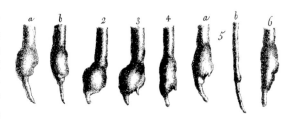

FIG. 31.1. Casts of strictures (Lallemand). (From Murphy
LJT (1972) The history of urology. Springfield, IL,
Charles C Thomas, pp 154)

In 1822, Ducamp introduced the "porte impreinte,"
an instrument to make casts of urethral strictures (4)
(Fig. 31.1). A bundle of silk threads impregnated in
wax was attached to the end of a sound or catheter
and inserted into the urethra and pressed against the
stricture. On removing the catheter, the wax would
be in the shape of the narrowed urethra and give a
rough idea of the anatomy (namely the stricture's
shape and any false passages). In the days before
roentgenology, this was a clever way to "visualize"
the anatomy of a stricture. Unfortunately, the wax
often became dislodged and acted as a plug that was
difficult to extract. Subsequently this method was
generally abandoned, yet was commonly practiced
by Lallemand and other prominent surgeons of the
time.

4. Urethral Dilation

There are three main methods in which dilatation
of the urethra has been performed over the ages is
namely gradual, continuous or forceable. The urethral dilation patient was never discharged. It was
a common doctrine that "once a stricture, always a
stricture." To improve the success of catheterization, attempts were made to medicate the bougies.
The word bougie came into English from the place
name of Bujiyah, Algeria. For it was this Algerian
port that came the best French wax candles, and
such candles with thin wax tapers were found to
make excellent urethral dilators. Soemmering was
the first to declare that the effects of medicated
bougies were only superficial, and thus helped to
discredit their use. To improve on serial dilation
methods, Ducamp introduced in 1822 a balloon
dilator, which consisted of a catheter with an inflatable cuff of calf intestine (1) (Fig. 31.2). He also

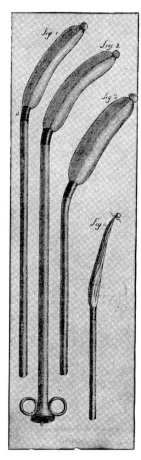

FIG. 31.2. Ducamp's dilating bougies, with inflatable bags of gold-beaters skin. (From Murphy LJT (1972) The history of urology. Springfield, IL, Charles C Thomas, pp. 156)

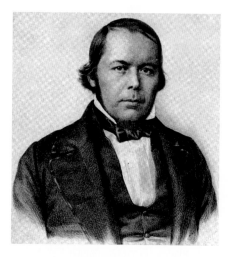

FIG. 31.3. Jacque-Gilles Maisonneuve (1809–1894). (From Murphy LJT (1972) The history of urology. Springfield, IL, Charles C Thomas, pp. 157)

used a fusiform, graduated dilator, called "bougie a ventr,e" with results that he reported as "good." Amussat furthered the principle of urethral dilation by using indwelling filliform bougies, adding another one each day until the bundle of sufficient size was inserted. Fine whalebone bougies were felt to be too rigid to be used safely. By 1834, Leroy d'Etiolles introduced the spiral tipped bougie.

The first filiform and followers to resemble modern versions were introduced by Maisonneuve in 1845 *(1)* (**Fig. 31.3**). He called them "instrumentation a la suite," or a system of filiform and detachable followers. The guiding filiform was soon used for multiple indications, including bougie placement, guiding dilators, as a caustic carrier, or to introduce a urethrotome. Filiforms were constructed from waxed linen or whalebone. Gouley's

bougies, guided by a whalebone filiform, was a particularly popular device in America.

In the early 19th century, in an attempt to find a method for urethral "cure" rather then "management," surgeons discarded gradual urethral dilation. Instead, they practiced and advocated forceable urethral dilation. Paget lamented that serial dilation was slow and that it often took a year before a patient could go for two weeks without treatment. In Paget's words, "[urethral] gradual dilation is tedious, liable to risk, and finally not curative." Unfortunately, many contemporary urologists still do not heed Paget's words of experience from nearly two centuries ago, and are known to still perform urethral dilation.

Although the technique of forceable dilation was generally successful in the hands of 19th-century experts like Desault and Boyer, there are multiple reports from that time of urethral rupture by Perreve. Mayor's (of Lausanne) words of condemning the use of force in urethral dilation still rings true today, when he stated that "I am always careful not to force a passage with a tapering or sharp sound. I am too frightened of causing false passages, lacerations and all kind of complications." Instead, Mayor used solid bougies and later switched to hollow bougies with two eyes. Interestingly, he felt that bloody drainage from the catheter was good, akin to the practice of using leeches to relieve "congestion." *(1)*

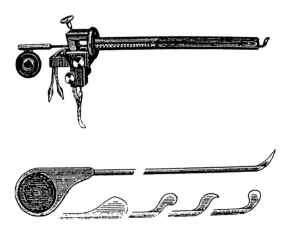

FIG. 31.4. Urethrotome of Oberlander, detailing the differing knife blades. (From Oberlander FM, Kollmann A (1910) Die chronische gonorrhoe der mannlichen harnrohre. Leipzig, Georg Thieme, pp. 73)

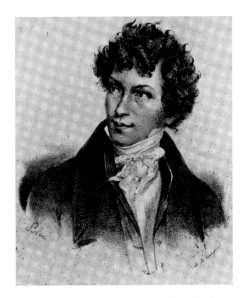

FIG. 31.5. Theodore Ducamp (1793–1823). (From Murphy LJT (1972) The history of urology. Springfield, IL, Charles C Thomas, pp. 159)

Other methods introduced at the later part of the 19th century were devices that caused rapid urethral stricture "rupture," "divulsion," and "distention." The rapid dilation method for opening up the recalcitrant stricture was introduced by Perreve, where a dilator with two parallel blades was forced apart to open up the stricture. Despite the dangers of forceable urethral dilation, the method was advocated for decades. Modeled on the work of Perreve, Bernard Holt introduced a "divulsor with graduated stilettes" where steel rods were pushed in a channel between two blades that forced them apart. Other dilating types of devices were the dilators of Oberlander and Kollmann, fitted with three and four dilating blades, respectively, and a screw mechanism that opened the blades (5) (**Fig. 31.4**). Thompson's two bladed instrument was designed to dilate rather then rupture the stricture.

5. Caustics and Cauterization

Cauterization of urethral strictures became the standard of practice during the early part of the 19th century. Hunter and Home's method of applying caustics injured healthy parts of the urethra. To prevent this, Whatley and, later, Arnott coated the caustic with a mucinous substance. The most popular of the cup-shaped caustic carriers was that of Theodore Ducamp (1793–1823; **Fig. 31.5**). Ducamp's method

included taking a mold of the stricture, passing a filiform bougie through an platinum open ended, hollow rod/catheter, and then dilating the stricture up enough to place the caustic carrier (4). Common caustics instilled in the urethra were silver nitrate (Advocated by Hunter, Home, Ducamp and Lallemand) and potash (advocated by Whatley). Caustics were typically complicated by severe urethritis, dysuria, bleeding, and rapid stricture recurrence. Use of caustics rapidly fell out of favor. With the advent of electrosurgery 50 years later, cauterization of urethral strictures saw a revival.

6. External Urethrotomy

External urethrotomy is one of the oldest surgical methods described for intractable, long urethral strictures. The first description of external urethrotomy was detailed by H. F. LeDran. During the last half of the 19th century, the treatment of recalcitrant urethral strictures by open surgery was strongly discouraged. Open surgery for urethral strictures was reserved only for desperate cases. It was often believed at the time that open urethral surgery was technically "formidable" and often failed, particularly if a guide could not be passed through the stricture. Such bias toward urethrotomy was particularly strong in America, and must less so in France and England, where open operations were performed more commonly for difficult urethral strictures. Gouley, a New York surgeon, was the first of numerous physicians who practiced such surgery and performed it with considerable success. Syme lauded external urethrotomy and felt that all strictures were penetrable and always operated with a sound. Furthermore, he felt that internal urethrotomy was "bloody, painful and dangerous procedures."

In Syme's operation, first described in 1853, a fine grooved staff was passed into the urethra and an incision was made onto the groove to marsupialize the urethra *(1)*. Occasionally, the bladder had to be opened and a sound passed down to the face of the stricture. A catheter was typically placed for 48 h (occasionally as long as 2 to 3 wk) and then the patient was dilated with bougies at regular intervals. Stricture recurrence is the typical course and thus dilation has to be kept up. Syme reported that he performed such surgery in 108 patients, with only 2 mortalities. The mortality rate for other surgeons, however, was reportedly much greater. In general, the technique entails performing a ventral urethrotomy proximally and distally into normal urethra. Periurethral scar is excised and the soft tissue reapproximated over a 26-French catheter. Recurrence rates are high, unless the urethra is self dilated.

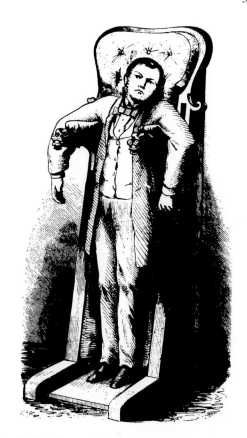

FIG. 31.6. Stricture chair. (From J. G. Beaney JG (1861) Contributions to practical surgery. Melbourne, Wilson & Mackinnon)

7. Stricture Diagnosis

The traditional method to diagnose a urethral stricture ahs been historically the passing of sounds and bougies, as well as Ducamp's porte-empreinte, and the early "urethrometers" *(1,4)*. By the late 1800s, there were multiple "urethrotomers" that were used to estimate urethral caliber (i.e., Otis' urethrometer). With the advent of the Nitze endoscope, stricture could be diagnosed and evaluated by direct vision. The use of retrograde urethrography was introduced by Cunningham in 1910 and Rubin Flocks in 1933. Around this time, many prominent surgeons of the day claimed to have never failed to place the instrument, even in the face of a dense urethral stricture. Syme and Thompson felt that no urethral stricture was impermeable. As to patient positioning for the procedures, some surgeons preferred the patient to stand. In fact, urethral stricture chairs were developed to support the position in the standing position (**Fig. 31.6**).

8. Alternative Methods for Treating Urethral Strictures

Of the various failed and curious treatment methods of the 19th century include suction, distension by gas, and electrolysis. Suction was a technique advocated by P. A. O'Connell in 1872, using suction applied to an open ended catheter and Politzer bulb catheter. Distension by gas involved the use of a solution of carbonate of soda and tartaric acid instilled into the urethra; the resulting gas was supposed to facilitate the passage of a sound to dilate the stricture. Electrolysis consisted as a linear filiform placed across the stricture and then a strong current applied. This method had little support when introduced in the 1860s but was revived in combination with a dilating instrument in the 1890s.

9. Internal Urethrotomy

Conceptually, the idea of cutting through (rather than just stretching) a fibrotic stricture appears to make more sense. The first urethrotome was described by the Philadelphia physician and surgeon, Philip Syng Physick. His technique consisted of a silver catheter placed into the urethra, through which a lancet was advanced and withdrawn to incise the stricture. By 1818, Dzondi, a German surgeon, used an olive-tipped sound with cutting edges that made longitudinal incisions in the stricture. Around the same time, from England, devices with retractable cutting blades for internal urethrotomy were introduced. Various other modifications to the urethrotome were introduced in the early 19th century, namely Amussat's and Reybard's (insertion guided with a small stylet; this was particularly dangerous and bleeding was often excessive). By 1823, Guillon introduced his "stricturotome." A urethrotome with a retractable blade at the bulbous end which cut from proximal to distal urethra. This device had many variations, going by such names as the Ricord coarctotome and the Petrequin, Mercier, Charriere, and Civiale urethrotomes. A whole array of competing instruments to perform urethrotomy arose for the next rough century.

Major improvements to urethrotomy involved combining a cutting blade with and expanding dilator and the addition of a calibrating device. In 1855 Jacques-Gilles Maisonneuve from Paris developed a urethrotome designed to cut the urethra *(5)*. In 1876, the American Fessenden N. Otis developed a dilating urethrotome with a calibrating device The Maisonneuve and Otis urethrotomes are still used today. These instruments can only be used if the caliber of the stricture is wide enough to admit them, they are passed blindly and the stricture is cut without vision. For this reason the Maisonneuve urethrotome incorporated a filiform bougie to avoid making a false passage. The potential complications arising from the Otis urethrotome are illustrated by the various devices he

recommended to controlling urethral hemorrhage; namely "Smith's Compressor", the perineal crutch, or the perineal tourniquet (**Fig. 31.7**).

In 1853, the French surgeon Antonin Jean Desormeaux succeeded in performing urethroscopy and, in 1865, he reported several cases in which he had incised urethral strictures using a thin knife that was introduced through a lateral opening of the endoscopic sheath. In 1881, the dermatologist Josef Grünfeld from Vienna reported 8 cases in which he had treated strictures by direct vision internal urethrotomy (DVIU). After the operation the patients were urged to perform daily intermittent catheterization to avoid scar retraction. Clearly, the concepts of DVIU and clean intermittent self-catheterization are not novel ideas. After 1900, internal urethrotomy became less popular, and most surgeons limited its use only to the bulbar urethra, resistant to dilation.

Felix Martin Oberländer designed the first direct vision urethrotome with an intracorporeal light source in 1892. This instrument was provided with a separate channel that allowed the introduction of different knives to cut urethral strictures under visual control. In 1896, Hurry Fenwick from London improved the operating urethroscope, while in America the Oberländer type of urethroscope with

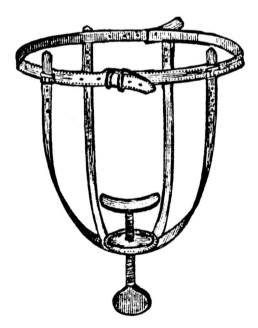

FIG. 31.7. Perineal tourniquet. (From Murphy LJT (1972) The history of urology. Springfield, IL, Charles C Thomas, pp. 469)

internal illumination was popularized by Ferdinand C Valentine from New York. Since 1903, George Luys from Paris used his modification of the urethroscope for incising strictures. In 1912, Erich Wossidlo from Berlin equipped the irrigation urethroscope with operating instruments allowing urethrotomy with a galvano-caustic hook.

10. Contemporary Urethrotomes

In the ensuing years, many combination cysto-urethroscopes were developed *(5)*. The most famous of them in America was the McCarthy panendoscope, and all of them were used for DVIU. In 1937, the German Karl Fischer designed an operating urethroscope which could be used to perform an exact incision of the urethral stricture. DVIU with electric diathermy was tried by Ravasini in 1957. Keitzer and associates (1961) first described the use of a blade fitted to a resectoscope loop for the incision of bladder neck contractures under direct vision.

Hans Sachse from Nürnberg, Germany, designed a new instrument with a sharp blade that could cut the stricture under direct vision. At the time, the electric knife was the method of choice, and Sachse noted that the necrosis ans subsequent re-scarring could be avoided by a simple sharp incision. In June 1971, he conducted the first operation with the prototype of his cold knife urethrotome built by the Karl Storz Company. Sachse reported a high success rate and initiated the resurgence of enthusiasm for endoscopic stricture treatment. In April 1977, the first endoscopic laser urethrotomy in humans was performed by Hartwig Bülow from Würzburg, Germany. To date, lasers have not been found to be superior to the cold knife urethrotomy of Sachse.

11. Urethroplasty

The first urethroplasty, where the urethral stricture was excised and the edges re-anastomosed by suture was carried out by Huesner in 1883 *(1)*. Similar excision and primary anastomosis (EPA) like urethral surgeries were carried out for short length stenoses by Mayo Robson in 1884 and later reported in 1892 by Guyon, Quenu, and Jouon at the French Congress of Surgery,

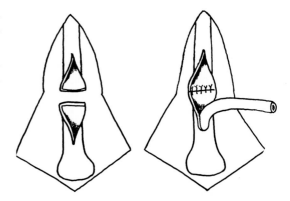

FIG. 31.8. Hamilton Russell's repair of the roof of the urethra after stricture excision. (From Murphy LJT (1972) The history of urology. Springfield, IL, Charles C Thomas, pp 471)

and by F Koenig in 1899. In 1906, Pasteau and Iselin reported on their experience with staged urethroplasty. Initially, the stricture was excised and the urethral ends marsupialized to the skin, followed by a second stage tubularization of the intervening skin, along with proximal urinary diversion by suprapubic tube.

Russell reported a variation of this staged, buried strip regeneration technique in 1915 *(1)* (**Fig. 31.8**). Denis Browne then modified the Russell method and extrapolated the "principle of buried urethral epithelium strip" for hypospadias patients. Tuner Warwick further refined this procedure many years later as a "scrotal inlay technique." In Hamilton Russell's 1915 seminal description of urethroplasty, he detailed his surgical technique and experience with urethral excision and primary anastomosis. At that time, Hamilton stated "excision of [urethral] stricture has never been generally practiced and is attempted only in a small number of cases …[because urethroplasty]… is difficult and uncertain in its results." Watson and Cunningham reviewed their experience in 1908 with EPA, noting short term success in only 5 of 13 patients. Despite the efforts of a small number of surgeons, the role of EPA remained poorly defined as late as the early 1970s, when perineal and scrotal flap procedures were popular and DVIU was just being introduced.

Shortly thereafter, a number of reports demonstrated excellent and durable results with EPA, so that by the mid 1980s, EPA was a well-established

as a superb method of reconstructing short bulbar strictures. By 1926, H. H. Young reported his experience with urethral reconstruction using the principle of urethral mucous membrane regeneration, and buried strip of intact epithelium. G Marion summarized in 1942, his 25-yr experience with anastomotic urethroplasty for defects up to 4 cm. This technique often resulted in ventral chordee that did not resolve spontaneously. Urethroplasty surgeries with tubular autologous grafts, utilizing saphenous vein, appendix, peritoneum or ureter have also been reported over time. Not surprisingly, they failed uniformly.

Bengt Johanson, a Swedish surgeon, further adapted the staged Denis Browne technique from hypospadias back to urethral strictures (*see* Fig. 18.7 in Chapter 18 by Coburn in this volume). First reported in 1953, the first stage of the procedure entailed the strictured urethra being opened ventrally and left open as a buried skin strip for roughly 6 mo *(6)*. Because hair will continue to grow on the scrotum lining the new deep urethra, epilation needs to proceed months before the second stage. In the second stage, the urethra is not tubularized because there remains only a buried skin strip, on top of which is sutured penile of scrotal skin.

In Johanson's seminal paper, he also noted that excessive proximal and distal urethral mobilization and primary anastomosis for long urethral stenoses resulted in severe ventral penile curvature. After Johanson's staged urethroplasty, the next great advances in urethral reconstruction came in with the patch grafting techniques of Devine. For the next two decades, patch grafting was the most commonly used method for reconstruction. Subsequently, the popularity of perineal and scrotal flaps flourished. Later followed penile skin flaps for single stage urethral reconstruction, as initially described by such urologic surgeons as Orandi (a longitudinal and ventral flap in 1968). After further advances by Quartey (a transverse flap and Turner-Warwick, McAninch popularized the circular subcoronal fasciocutaneous flap in 1993. Onlay flap urethroplasty thus replaced grafts as the reconstruction method of choice for another decade or so, until the report by El-Kasaby of successful buccal mucosa patch graft urethroplasty in 1993.

The pendulum has shifted again to grafting, when possible, as the method of choice. For the future, tissue engineering and regenerative medicine will lead the way for urethral reconstructive surgery.

Appendix

Preferred Instruments of EL Keys (circa 1905)

Conical steel sounds, Nos. 15 to 33, preferably double taper from 24 up
Several whalebone filiform guides
Conical woven french bougies, sizes 5 to 18
Set of bulbous or blunt sounds, or a Urethrometer
Instillation syringe and Aspirator
Conical woven olivary catheters, small and large
One silver catheter, No 6, tunneled
Steel sounds
Otis or Maisonneuve urethrotome
Soft rubber catheter and a female catheter
Blunt pointed straight bistoury
Heavy soft –rubber perineal tube
Bottle of 10% nitrate of silver solution.
Clover's crutch.

(From: Keyes EL, (1905) The Surgical Diseases of the Genitor-urinary Organs, New York and London, D Appleton and Co, pgs. 226–227.)

References

1. Murphy LJT (1972) The urethra, in The history of urology. Springfield IL, Charles C Thomas, pp 453–482.
2. Bell C (1816) A system of operative surgery founded on the basis of anatomy (vol 2). Hartford, CT, George Goodwin and Sons
3. Amussat JZ (1840) Amussat's Lectures on Retention of Urine Caused by Strictures of the Urethra and on Diseases of the Prostate. Translated by James P Jervery edited by A Petit, Philadelphia, Haswell, Barrington and Haswell.
4. Ducamp T (1827) A treatise on retention of urine caused by strictures in the urethra. Translated by William M Herbert, New York, NY, Samueal Wood and Sons
5. Schultheiss D, Truss MC, Jonas U (1999) History of direct vision internal urethrotomy (Erratum in: Urology 53:456). Urology 52:729–734
6. Johanson B (1953) Reconstruction of the male urethra in strictures. Application of the buried intact epithelium tube. Acta Chir Scand 176 (suppl):1

Index

A

Abdominal sepsis, in RUF, 252
Abdomino-perineal approach
  for bladder neck injury and rectal injury, 192
  for RUF, 264
  for urethral identification, 198
Abdomino-perineal resection and pelvic
        radiotherapy, prostatoperineal urinary
        fistula after, 265
Abscess, periurethral, 58–59, 78
ACA. *See* Acrodermatitis chronica atrophicans
Acellular tissue matrices, as biomaterial for engineering
        of urethral tissues, 339–340
Acrodermatitis chronica atrophicans, 22
Acute urinary extravasation, in anterior anastomotic
        urethroplasty, 219
Adductor brevis, 179
Adductor longus
  course of, 264
  fascia of, 177
  freed of, 263
  medial fascia of, 179
Adductor magnus, 177
Adjunctive flaps, for tissue transfer in plastic surgery,
        51–52
Advancement flaps sliding, for tissue transfer in plastic
        surgery, 48–49
Aged
  prone to recurrence of urethral strictures in, 73
  urethroplasty tolerance in elderly, 324
Allium bulbar urethral stent(s)
  clinical experience with, 93
  insertion technique of, 92–93
  for recurrent urethral stricture, 91
  stent characteristics, 91–92
Alopecia areata, with LS, 21
American Urological Association symptom score,
        282, 324
  obstructive voiding complaints on, 306
American Urological Association symptom severity
        index, 315, 317, 319

and peak urinary flow rate, 318
Amplatz dilators, 280
Anal sphincter
  function of, 254
  and rectum, anatomy of, 254–255
Anastomotic urethroplasty, 328–329
  advantage of, 116
  anterior, complications in
    acute urinary extravasation, 219
    chordee, 220
    erectile dysfunction, 220
    postvoid dribbling, 219–220
    recurrence, 220–221
    UTI, 221
  for bulbar urethral stricture, 154
  complications after, 330 (*see also*
        Anastomotic urethroplasty; anterior,
        complications in)
  for management of urethral strictures, 55
  vascular principles of, 16
Anastomotic urethroplasty, augmented, 142
  bulbar urethral stricture disease by, management
        of, 144
    graft location for, 144–145
    preoperative evaluation for, 145–146
  postoperative complications of, 150
    donor-site complications in, 150
    sexual function in, 150
    stricture recurrence in, 150
  rational for uses of, 142–144
  results of, 150
  stricture factors important in procedure selection
        of, 144
  surgical technique for, 146
    graft obtaining in, 148
    graft placement in, 148–149
    postsurgical follow-up in, 149–150
    urethral exposure in, 146–147
Anemia, 44
  pernicious, vitiligo associated with, 99
Anesthesia, for urethral strictures, 70

Antegrade cystoscopy, 333
Antibiotics, for urethral strictures, 70
Apoptosis, 21
Arterial plexuses of penile skin, cross-sectional
    view of, 12
Artificial urinary sphincter (AUS)
    placement of, 235
    for urinary incontinence, 234
AUA-SSI. *See* American Urological Association
    Symptom Severity Index
Auricular skin, posterior, for substitution
    urethroplasty, 137
Autoimmunity, and genetic susceptibility for etiology
    of LS, 21
Autologous fascia, alternative source for, 308
Axial flaps
    example of, 156
    extragenital, for local genital skin
        substitution, 171
    subdivisions of, 47

B

Back pain, severe lower, in positioning-related
    complications, 223
Bacteremia, 33
Balanitis xerotica obliterans, 20
    with characteristic patchy white plaques, 99
    glanular urethral stricture disease caused
        by, 98
    management of, 100
    related strictures of fossa navicularis, 272
    strictures caused by obliterative effects of, 207
Balloon dilation, 65
Barotrauma, 247
Bartholin glands, 2
"Bear claw" retractor, 265
Benique sound, in Europe, 194
Biliary cirrhosis, vitiligo associated with, 99
Bladder
    filling, Hypaque enema for, 262
    poor function, supravesical urinary diversion
        for, 252
Bladder flap, 308–309
Bladder mucosal graft, in reoperative hypospadias
    surgery, 290
Bladder neck
    beaked, 191
    closure, transvaginal, 311–312
    cystoscopy for location of fistula in, 252
    incision, principles of, 232
    injury
        adominoperineal approach for, 192
        urinary incontinence in patients with, 223
    RT effects on, 243

strictures, consequence of prostatic carcinoma
    treatment, 189
    voiding cystourethrography for continence
        evaluation, 122
Bladder neck contracture
    after RT, development of, 243
    after TURP, occurrence of, 230
    cystoscopic appearance of, 233
    enterocystoplasty for, 246
    for patients with failed dilation, electrosurgical
        incision of, 233
    recurrent, TUIBN with resectoscope for, 237
    treatment of, 232
Bladder neck-rectal fistula, after salvage radical
    prostatectomy, 256
Bladder neck stenosis, after TURP, endourethral
    brachytherapy in patients with, 77
Bladder tube, post-RRP stricture reconstruction by, 235
Bladder tumor, cystoscopy for discover of, 67
Bladder urothelium, visual appearance of, 254
Blandy flap, for perineal urethrostomy, 13
Blandy two-stage urethroplasty, with posteriorly based
    scrotal inlay flap, 204
Bleeding diathesis, suspicion of, 64, 78
BMG. *See* Buccal mucosal grafts
BMU. *See* Buccal mucosal urethroplasty
BNC. *See* Bladder neck contracture
Borrelia burgdorferi, ACA associated with, 22
Botulinum toxin, for prevention of urethral strictures
    recurrence, 77
"Bougie a ventre," 349
Bougienage, and endoscopy for clarification of
    stricture, 166
Bougies a boule, 307, 328
Brachytherapy
    and EBRT, RUF caused by, 252
    I^{125}, for prostate cancer, 247
    for prevention of recurrence of urethral strictures, 77
    prostate
        achievement of, 242
        prostatic and membranous urethral strictures after, 245
    urethral stricture after, rate of, 244
Brodney clamp, 324
BT. *See* Brachytherapy
Buccal grafts. *See also* Buccal mucosal grafts
    completed, to prostatic fistula, 260
    and gracilis muscle, dorsal placement of, 174–175
    to prostatic fistula, parachuting in, 265
    for urethral trauma, placement of, 203
    urinary fistula by, closure of, 264
    ventral skin island flap and, obliterated urethral
        reconstruction with, 170
Buccal graft urethroplasty, 172
    flaps in, use of, 164

Buccal mucosa, 330
    patch onlay, for stricture and prostatic fistula,
        placement of, 185
    as sources of tissue for reconstruction, 109
Buccal mucosal graft onlay, with gracilis support,
    technique of, 173
Buccal mucosal grafts, 273. *See also* Buccal grafts
    advantages of, 101
    bilateral
        for panurethral strictures, 165
        for surgical reconstruction of panurethral
            strictures, 166
    for bulbar urethral stricture repair, 131, 154
    from cheeks, retrieval of, 174
    on corpora cavernosa, application of, 121
    for distal portion of bulbar stricture, 181
    dorsal, for urethral plate salvage, 273
    for male urethral reconstruction, 310
    for pendulous reconstruction, 273
    for penile and bulbar urethral strictures, 120
        surgical techniques for, 121
    vs. penile skin graft, discussion for, 130–131
    for prostatic fistula, 183
    in reoperative hypospadias surgery, 290–291
    for urethral stricture, 184, 214
Buccal mucosal urethroplasty
    and complications in
        erectile dysfunction, 216
        fistula, 214–215
        oral complications, 217
        postvoid dribbling, 216
        recurrence, 215–216
        urethral sacculation, 216–217
        urine leak, 214
        UTI, 216
Buccal urethral grafts, for fossa navicularis and meatal
        reconstruction, 101–102. *See also* Buccal grafts;
        Buccal mucosal grafts
Bulbar strictures
    Memokath 044 for, 90
    short, anastomotic urethroplasty for, 142
Bulbar urethra
    for BMG urethroplasty, preparation of, 122–124
    within bulbospongiosus muscle, exposure and
        mobilization of, 193
    natural curve of, straightening of, 328
    opening of, 125
    in reconstruction of failed urethroplasty, 273–274
    traumatic strictures of, 108
Bulbar urethral stents, allium, in treatment of recurrent
        urethral stricture, 91–93
Bulbar urethral strictures
    BMG onlay urethroplasty for, 131
    by BMG, surgical techniques for, 121

disease, by augmented anastomotic urethroplasty,
        management of, 144–145
    perineal artery fasciocutaneous flap for, 180
Bulbar urethroplasty, fistula formation in complication
        of, 214
Bulbomembranous disruption, 37
Bulbospongiosus muscle
    bulbar urethra within, exposure and mobilization of,
        193
    urethra at distal margin of, approach of, 111
Buried strip regeneration technique, 353
Burrow's triangles, and island advancement skin flap, 49
Bursitis, trochanteric, in positioning-related
        complications, 223
BXO. *See* Balanitis xerotica obliterans

C
Cancer(s)
    abdominoperineal resection of rectum for, 182
    complex urinary fistulas in patients with, 266
    prostate
        radiation beams for treatment of, 242
        surgery for, 229
    urethral, 59, 309
Candida, 122
Candywrap effect, 91
Capener's gouge, 195
Carcinoma. *See also* Cancer(s)
    prostatic, 189
    urethral, suspicion of, 64, 78
Cardiovascular disease (CVD), in radiation
        complications, 242
Catheterization
    after endoscopic incision, duration of, 79
    as risk factor for recurrence of urethral strictures, 75
    self
        for BNC, 246
        CISC for prevention of urethral strictures
            recurrence, 76
        for long-term stricture management, 271
        and urethrotomy, 241, 245
    for urethral strictures, 70–71
    urethral strictures caused by, 99
Charriere urethrotome, 352
Childhood perineal trauma, causing idiopathic
        stricture, 59
Children
    after laser DVIU, urethralgia and urethral
        diverticulum in, 71
    pubectomy for rerouting of urethra in, 199
Chordee
    in anterior anastomotic urethroplasty, 220
    correction of, 291
    iatrogenic, correction of, 329

Chordee (*continued*)
  penile, 282
  persistent, as reoperative hypospadiac complication, 286–287
  as specific urethral stent complication, 279
Cigarette smoking, effect on fistula repair, 254
Circumcision
  LS management by, 25
  meatal stenosis, as long-term complication of, 99
CISC. *See* Clean intermittent self-catheterization
Civiale urethrotome, 352
Clean intermittent self-catheterization, 76
Clutton's sound, in UK, 194
Cobb's collar, 108
Coccygectomy, for fistula exposure, 265
Collagen matrix, rehydration of, 341
Collins' knife, bladder neck incision by, initiation of, 233
Colo-anal pull through
  for management of nonradiated fistulas, 252
  Turnbull-Cutait, for RUF, 264
Color Doppler ultrasound
  for evaluation of stricture length and diameter, 68
  for fibrosis assessment, 55
  for spongiofibrosis assessment, 56
Colostomy, for fecal diversion, 254
Compartmental syndrome, lower extremity, in positioning-related complications, 223
Computed tomography
  angiography, for pudendal artery occlusion, 204
  of pelvis, 262
    for diagnosis of fistula, 253
  urethrography, voiding, of male urethra, 39
  for visualization of target organ, 242
Contrast radiography, for urethral obstruction, 191
Core-through urethrotomy, 72
Coronary artery, drugeluting stents to prevent restenosis in, 94
Corpora cavernosa, injection of fibrin glue over albuginea of, 128
Corpus spongiosum
  blood supply of, 14
    arterial, 14–17
    venous, 17–18
Cowper's ducts, 270
Cowper's glands
  bulbar urethral stricture with filling of, 35
  ducts of, 6
  with urethral stricture disease, opacification of, 32
  urethral stricture with filling of, 34
Crohn's disease
  RUF caused by, 252
  trans-sphincteric RUF of, 253
Crura, in exposure of inferior pubic symphysis, 197

Cryotherapy
  complex fistulas due to, 252
  for prostate cancer, prostato-rectal fistula after, 253
CT. *See* Computed tomography
CTU. *See* Core-through urethrotomy
Cystitis
  post-procedure, incidence of, 71
  radiation, component of, 245
Cystogram
  combined, and urethrogram for stricture length, 191
  for demonstratoin of vesico-rectal fistula, 253
  and flowrate study for stricture postoperative follow-up, 197
  micturating, for urethral obstruction, 190
Cystography, contrast, for absence of extravasation, 236
Cystoprostatectomy, salvage, for BNC, 246
Cystoscope, pediatric
  for degree of spongiofibrosis, 100
  for vision of urethral stricture, 67
Cystoscopy
  antegrade, 333
  for diagnosis of strictures, 243
  flexible, 326
    for bladder neck obstruction, 191
    for recurrent stricture, 270
  intraoperative, 326
    for detection of eggshell calculi, 274
  for investigation of stones or bladder tumor, 67
  for location of fistula in bladder neck, 252
  for patients with iatrogenic stricture post-TURP or RRP, 231
  radiation urethral strictures on, 241
  in urethral stricture treatment, 319
Cystostomies, suprapubic, management of, 203
Cystourethrogram, voiding. *See* Voiding cystourethrogram
Cystourethrography (CUG), voiding. *See* Voiding cystourethrography

D
Dartos pedicle flaps, 288
Dartos pedicle interposition, 286
Debakey forceps, 333
Denonvier's fascia, 255
Dermal grafts, 46–47
Diabetes mellitus
  failed urethroplasty due to, 270
  insulin-dependent, vitiligo associated with, 99
  LS association with, 21
  poor wound healing in, 154
  in radiation complications, 242
Dilation
  clinic, for prevention of recurrence of urethral strictures, 76–77

complication of urethral strictures in, 71
first stricture recurrence after, risk of, 73
for management of stricture, 86
or DVIU for urethral strictures, indications for, 77–78
for recurrent stricture, 270
stricture-free rate after, 73, 75
stricture length and stricture recurrence after, association between, 74
for treatment of recurrent strictures, 218
urethral, for fossa navicularis and meatal reconstruction, 100
for urethral strictures, 64–66
for vesicourethral anastomotic strictures after RRP, 232
Dilators, of Oberlander and Kollmann, 350
Direct vision internal urethrotomy, 76, 352–353
  cold-knife, for vesicourethral anastomotic stricture, 234
  complication of urethral strictures in, 71–72
  endoscopic treatment of recurrent stricture by, 222
  fibrosis after, MMC for prevention of, 77
  and filiform dilation in men with urethral strictures, comparison of, 65
  for fossa navicularis and meatal reconstruction, 100
  or dilation for urethral strictures, indications for, 77–78
  predictor of outcome of, 74
  single, for ring recurrence strictures, 216
  success rate of, 72
  for treatment of recurrent strictures, 218, 220
  for urethral strictures, 60, 66–68
Distal urethral stricture, 290
  and repair, 310
DM. See Diabetes mellitus
Doppler, hand-held, for gracilis vessels, 262
Drugeluting stents, for prevention of restenosis in coronary artery, 93
Ducamp's dilating bougies, 349
Ducamp's porte impreinte, 351
DVIU. See Direct vision internal urethrotomy
Dysesthesia, 129
Dysuria, prevention of, 277

E
Ecchymosis, occurrence of, 167
ED. See Erectile dysfunction
Eggshell calculi, by cystoscopy, removal of, 275
Ejaculatory dysfunction, in fasciocutaneous urethroplasty complications, 218
Electrocautery, 286
  use of, 271
  bipolar, 327
    use of, 159
    Pesky bleeding control by, 331

monopolar
  initiation of bladder neck incision by, 233
  in surgical mangement of stricture, use of, 232
  for omental hemostasis, 301
Electrocautery fulguration, use of, 205
Embolization
  for complex urinary fistulas, 266–268
  for urethral-internal pudendal artery fistula, 71
Endoscopic deployment device, of allium bulbar urethral stent, 92
Endoscopic laser urethrotomy, 353
Endoscopic litholapaxy, for stent encrustation, 89
Endoscopic urethroplasty, for urethral strictures, 70
Endoscopy
  and bougienage for clarification of stricture, 166
  Nitze endoscope, 351
  for visual assess of urethral mucosa and associated scarring, 324
Endourethral prosthesis
  for radiation induced urethral strictures, 241
  for urethral stricture, 85–86
Endourethroplasty, after CTU in patients with strictures, 70
EPA. See Excision and primary anastomosis
Epididymitis, 59
  post-procedure, incidence of, 71
  UTI with, occurrence of, 270
Epitheliazation, 277
Erectile dysfunction
  in anterior anastomotic urethroplasty, 220
  as BMU complication, 216
  as DVIU complication, 71
  as fasciocutaneous urethroplasty complication, 219
  as posterior urethroplasty complication, 222–223
  urethral obstruction in patients with, 191
Estrogen deficiency, 304
Excision and primary anastomosis, 353
  for bulbar stricture reconstruction, 274
  for urethral strictures, clinical outcomes of, 114–116
  urethroplasty, for radiation induced urethral strictures, 241
Excision vs. augmentation, of stricture, discussion for, 133
Extracellular matrix (ECM), 338
Eyelid reconstruction, PAG for, 139

F
Fascial pedicle, completed flap mobilization with preservation of, 103
Fasciocutaneous flap
  and buccal grafting for urethral trauma, placement of, 203
  circular penile, for stricture reconstruction, 273
  posterior thigh, 175
  for urethral trauma, placement of, 203
  versatile, example of, 51

Fasciocutaneous island flap, of penile skin for midbulbar
   urethral stricture, 248
Fasciocutaneous onlay flaps, circular
   mobilization of, 168
   for panurethral strictures reconstruction, 166–168
Fasciocutaneous urethroplasty
   complications, 217
      ejaculatory dysfunction in, 218
      erectile dysfunction/diminished penile sensation
         in, 219
      penile skin necrosis in, 219
      postvoid dribbling in, 218
      rate of, 215
      recurrent stricture in, 217–218
      urethral diverticulum in, 218
      urethrocutaneous fistula in, 219
      urinary extravasation in, 219
Fasciocutaneous ventral penile transverse island flap,
      for fossa navicularis and meatal reconstruction,
      102–104
Fecal and urinary diversion
   anal sphincter and rectum for, anatomy of, 254–255
   indications for, 254
   in rectourinary fistulas, 254–255
   York Mason technique for, 256
Fecal diversion, trans-abdominal approach for, 264
Fecal incontinence, prevention of, 257
Fecaluria, in RUF, 252
Female urethral reconstruction, 303
   bladder neck, transvaginal closure of, 311–312
   outcomes of, 311
   preoperative evaluation, 305–306
   technical principles of, 311
   urethra
      anatomy of, 303
      function of, 304
   urethral injury, pathology of, 304–305
   urethral injury, treatment for, and incontinence
      urethral loss, surgery for, 306–309
      urethral stricture reconstruction, 309–311
Fibrin glue
   dorsal onlay BMG urethroplasty by, 127–128
   in graft revascularization, role of, 132
Fibrosis
   after DVIU, MMC for prevention of, 77
   due to chronic effects of radiation, 242
   site of, 194
   urethroscopy and ultrasonography for assessment
      of, 55
Fibrous ring strictures, etiology of, 132
Filiform dilation
   and DVIU in men with urethral strictures, comparison
      of, 65
   for immature anastomotic stricture, 78

Fistula(s)
   in BMU complications, 214–215
   complex rectourinary and vesicoperineal, 251–252
   complex urinary, 266
      embolization costs and outcomes of, 268
      embolization technique for, 266–268
   etiology of, 252
   large and complex, 258
      gracilis muscle flap for, 260–264
      transabdominal approaches of, 264
      trans-perineal approaches of, 258–260
   prostatic radiation, exposure of, 178
   radiation prostatocutaneous, retrograde urethrogram
      in patient with, 177
   rectourinary, 252
      diagnosis of, 252–254
      preoperative assessment and decision-making for, 254
      signs and symptoms of, 252
      specific reconstruction methods for, 255–257
      urinary and fecal diversion in, 254–255
   rectovesical and urinary-perineal, 265–266
   urethral strictures associated with, 58
   urethrocutaneous, in fasciocutaneous urethroplasty
      complications, 219
Flap(s). See also specific flaps
   in buccal graft urethroplasty, 164
   combined with graft, for panurethral strictures
      reconstruction, 168–169
   dorsal vs. ventral vs. lateral pedicle, for urethral
      reconstruction, 157
   fasciocutaneous, development of, 44
   genital skin, for LSA, 26
   vs. grafts, in penile urethroplasty, discussion for, 131
   harvest, in technique for urethral reconstruction,
      158–161
   longitudinal vs. transverse, for urethral reconstruction,
      156–157
   penile skin, for urethral reconstruction, 153–154
   proximal vs. distal penile skin, for urethral
      reconstruction, 157
   reconstruction, in management options of tissue
      transfer techniques, 47–48
   urethral closure with ventral onlay island skin, for
      urethral reconstruction, 161–162
   for urethral reconstruction, types of, 155–156
   ventral onlay vs. tube flap vs. combined tissue
      transfer, for urethral reconstruction, 158
Flap techniques
   adjunctive, for tissue transfer in plastic surgery, 51–52
   free, for tissue transfer in plastic surgery, 51
   pedicled muscle, for tissue transfer in plastic surgery,
      50–51
   rotation/transposition, for tissue transfer in plastic
      surgery, 49–50

sliding advancement, for tissue transfer in plastic
        surgery, 48–49
    for tissue transfer in plastic surgery, 48
    tubed, for tissue transfer in plastic surgery, 50
Flap tubularization, alternative to, 273
Flap urethroplasty, for fossa navicularis and meatal
        reconstruction, 102–104
Foley catheter, 127
    for BNC, 246
    for distal urethral stricture, 310
    16-French silicone, 334
    insertion of, 123
    in retrograde urethrography, uses of, 100
    for site of obliteration of urethra, 193
Foreskin, as tissue source for reconstruction, 109
Fossa navicularis
    BXO-related strictures of, 272
    in patients with LS, reconstruction of, 25
    related urethral strictures, 208, 272
    strictures, discreet, penile skin flap for, 272
Fossa navicularis and meatal reconstruction
    complications of, 104
    etiologic factors of, 98
        iatrogenic, 99
        inflammatory, 98
    management consideration of, 100
    minimally invasive techniques for, 100
        DVIU in, 100
        meatotomy in, 101
        urethral dilation in, 100
    patient evaluation of, 99–100
    reconstructive techniques for, 101
        flap urethroplasty in, 102–104
        graft urethroplasty in, 101–102
Fournier's gangrene, 59
Fracture, pelvic. See Pelvic fracture
Free flaps, for tissue transfer in plastic
        surgery, 51
Free skin graft
    for anterior urethral reconstruction, 120
    and rectus flap, post-RRP stricture reconstruction
        by, 236

G
Gallaudet's fascia, 192
Gastroepiploic artery, 298
    middle omental artery from, 300
    omental mobilization based on, 299
Gastrostomy tube, 302
Genital reconstruction
    flaps for
        extragenital axial flaps for skin substitution, 171
        in genital skin and urethra, 14
        peninsular skin flaps, 156

        skin flaps, for LSA, 26
        tubed flaps and muscle flaps, 50
    gracilis muscle for, 172
Genital skin
    female, 1–3
    flaps, for LSA, 26
    male, 3–5
    substitution, extragenital axial flaps for, 171
    and urethra, for implications of urethral
        reconstruction, vascular anatomy of, 9
Genital tissues, adjacent/extra-, in reoperative
        hypospadias surgery, 288–290
Glansplasty, 286, 290
Glanular reconstruction, fasciocutaneous ventral penile
        transverse island flap for, 103–104
Glanular torsion, as complication in fossa navicularis
        and meatal reconstruction, 104
Glanular urethral strictures, characterization of, 99
Glanuloplasty, glans-cap, for glans reconstruction, 102
Glaucoma, bulbar urethral stricture in man with, 247
Gluteal muscles, course of, 186
Gluteus maximus
    elevation of inferior half of, 185
    inferior, for impaired wound healing, 182
    muscle flap
        anatomy and clinical applications, 183
        for bulbomembranous urethral reconstruction,
            182–183
    repair of perineal-urethral strictures (and fistulas),
        techniques of, 183–186
Gonococcal inflammation, acute, of paraurethral glands
        of Littre, 57
Gonococcal urethritis, posterior urethral strictures
        caused by, 221
Gonorrhea, 348
    anterior urethral strictures due to, 108
Gorget, and needle to facilitate suture placement, 196
Gout, prostatic urethral stricture in man with, 247
Gracilis fascia, 179
Gracilis (muscle) flap
    anatomy and retrieval for urethral stricture disease, 172
        buccal graft and gracilis muscle, dorsal placement
            of, 174–175
        buccal mucosal graft onlay with gracilis support,
            technique of, 173
        short gracilis flap, 173–174
        skin and gracilis flap reconstruction, prefabricated
            combined, 175–176
    anatomy of, 260–261
    buttressed with, for prostate-rectal fistulas, 255
    for fistula repair, 258
    for genital reconstruction, 50
    interposition, buttressed with, for management of
        nonradiated fistulas, 252

Gracilis (muscle) flap (*continued*)
　　for large and complex fistulas, 260–264
　　surgical dissection of, 262–264
　　vascular anatomy of, 261
Gracilis myofasciocutaneous flap
　　for urethral stricture disease, 176–178
　　　operative technique for transfer of, 178–180
Graft reconstruction
　　in management options of tissue transfer techniques,
　　　45–47
　　of tubular structure, 47
Graft(s)
　　bilateral buccal mucosal, for panurethral strictures
　　　reconstruction, 166
　　characteristics of, 137
　　flap combined with, for panurethral strictures
　　　reconstruction, 168–169
　　vs. flaps, in penile urethroplasty, discussion
　　　for, 131
　　location, for management of bulbar urethral stricture
　　　disease, 144–145
　　loss, in BMU complications, 217
　　placement, in surgical technique, 148–149
　　for urethral reconstruction, use of, 142
Graft urethroplasty, 310–311
　　dorsal onlay, development and evolution of, 120
　　for fossa navicularis and meatal reconstruction,
　　　101–102
　　ventral vs dorsal bulbar onlay, discussion
　　　for, 131–133
Groin reconstruction, gracilis muscle for, 172
G tube. *See* Gastrostomy tube
Guillemin's technique. *See* Direct vision internal
　　urethrotomy
GYN malignancy, 309

H
Halofuginone, for prevention of recurrence of urethral
　　strictures, 77
HBO. *See* Hyperbaric oxygen
Head and neck reconstruction, 178
Hematoma
　　formation of, 45
　　pelvic, MRI for location of, 39
Hematuria, 304
　　penis in patient with, images of, 39
Herpes virus, 122
Heyman dilators, 280
Hockey stick extension, of circular penile skin flap, 157
Hockey stick-shaped flap, illustration of, 167
Holmium (HO) laser, 280–281
Hormone ablation therapy, for man with
　　hypertension, 247
Human leukocyte antigen (HLA), LS with, 21
Hypaque enema, for bladder filling, 262

Hyperbaric oxygen
　　therapy
　　　for ischemia, 246
　　　for urethral stricture, 247
Hyperplasia
　　prostatic, bladder neck strictures due to treatment
　　　of, 189
　　as specific urethral stent complication, 279
Hypertension
　　failed urethroplasty due to, 270
　　hormone ablation therapy for man with, 247
　　prostatic urethral stricture in man with, 247
　　in radiation complications, 242
Hyperthyroidism, vitiligo associated with, 99
Hyponatremia, risk of, 67, 72
Hypospadias
　　failed, multistage urethroplasty for patient with, 120
　　patients with
　　　collagen-based acellular matrix for reconstruction, 342
　　　reconstructive problems for, 338
　　surgery
　　　childhood, 120
　　　failed, panurethral strictures due to, 169
　　urethroplasty with skin graft to pendulous urethra in, 208
Hypothyroidism, vitiligo associated with, 99

I
Iatrogenic chordee, correction of, 329
Iatrogenic etiologic factors, of fossa navicularis and
　　meatal reconstruction, 99
Iatrogenic injuries
　　anterior urethral strictures due to, 108
　　posterior urethral strictures caused by, 221
Iatrogenic posterior urethral strictures, algorithm for
　　clinical evaluation of, 232
Ichthyosis, vulvar and oral, 20
IDDM. *See* Insulin-dependent diabetes mellitus
Ileal-vesicostomy, for management of obliterative
　　stricture, 248
Ileostomy, temporary loop, for fecal diversion, 254
Imaging. *See also* Computed tomography; Magnetic
　　resonance imaging
　　for preoperative assessment in urethroplasty surgery,
　　　324–325
Impotency, in patients with bilateral pudendal complex
　　injury, 16
Incision(s)
　　cold knife, 232
　　　with DVIU for iatrogenic bulbar strictures, 76
　　　for iatrogenic posterior urethral strictures, 233
　　electrosurgical, of BNC for patients with failed
　　　dilation, 233
　　endoscopic
　　　catheterization after, duration of, 79
　　　for mature anastomotic stricture, 78

paracoccyxygeal, for prostatic fistula exposure, 265

risk factors for recurrence of urethral strictures, 75

Incontinence, in posterior urethroplasty complications, 223

Infection, perioperative, risk factor for recurrence of urethral strictures, 75

Inflammatory bowel disease, with urethrocutaneous fistulas, gracilis myofasciocutaneous flap for, 176

Ingual mucosa and posterior auricular skin grafts, 138–139

Injury(ies)

to female urethra due to pelvic fracture, 305

posterior urethral distraction

indication of staged procedure for, 203–204

staged procedure for, technical approaches to, 204–205

urethral, incidence of, 190

Instrumentation, urethral

iatrogenic stricture caused by, 58

ischemic urethral strictures from, locations of, 59

panurethral strictures due to, 169

urethral stricture due to, 99

Insulin-dependent diabetes mellitus, vitiligo associated with, 99

Internal urethrotomy

otis, for dilation of urethral strictures, 66

stricture-free rate after, 73, 75

International prostate symptom score, 317

Intestinal submucosa (IS), 70

Intraoperative cystoscopy, 274, 326. *See also* Cystoscopy

Intrastent bulbar stricture, through urolume, 282

IS. *See* Intestinal submucosa

Island skin flaps

advancement, Burrow's triangles and, 49

genital skin, for anterior urethral reconstruction, 14

for reconstruction of radiated stricture, 246

for urethral reconstruction, 156

urethral closure with ventral onlay, 161–162

IU. *See* Internal urethrotomy

K

Kartenblattförmige sklerodermie, 20

Koebner phenomenon, in LS etiology, 20

Kraske laterosacral approaches, for repair of RUF, 255

L

Lamina propria, 3–4

of penile urethra, 7

Laser

ablation, for urethral stricture, 230

CTU, for obliterative posttraumatic urethral strictures, 69

DVIU, urethralgia and urethral diverticulum in children after, 71

fulguration, use of, 205

IU, for patients with untreated strictures, 69

Nd:YAG laser, 292

urethrotomy

for patients with posterior urethral strictures, 233

for urethral strictures, 68–69

Leukoplakia, 24, 98

erythroplasia of, 24, 98

Lichen planus, 24

Lichen sclerosus, 19, 272

clinical presentation in, 23–24

etiology of, 20

genetic susceptibility and autoimmunity for, 21

infections for, 22

Koebner phenomenon for, 20

oxidative stress for, 21–22

extensive perimeatal, in fossa navicularis stricture, 272

histology of, 22–23

historical aspects of, 20

management of, 24–25

medical, 25

surgical, 25–26

multistage urethroplasty for patient with, 120

and SCC, 22

Lichen sclerosus *et* atrophicus

classification scheme for, 56

genital skin flaps for, 26

panurethral strictures induced by, 169–170

penile skin in patients with, uses of, 154

phimosis due to, 58

related urethral strictures, 208

strictures caused by obliterative effects of, 207

Lingual (mucosal) grafts, 137, 273

technique for, 138–139

for urethroplasty, 273

Lip mucosa, 331

Litholapaxy, endoscopic, for stent encrustation, 89

Lithotomy position

exaggerated, 110

social, for access of perineum, 192

with table fixed Bookwalter retractor, patient in, 146

Littre's glands

acute gonococcal inflammation of paraurethral glands of, 57

filling of glands of, urethra stricture with, 34

musculus compressor nuda and filling of glands of, 36

in penile urethra, 6–7

with urethral stricture disease, opacification of glands of, 32

Littritis, 58

secondary, 169

Lonestar retractor system, 332

self-retaining, 271

LS. *See* Lichen sclerosus

LSA. *See* Lichen sclerosus *et* atrophicus
Lupus erythematous, LS association with, 21

M
Magnetic resonance angiography, for pudendal artery
      occlusion, 204
Magnetic resonance imaging
   for diagnosis of stricture, 245
   for evaluation of spongiofibrosis, 29
   of male urethra, 37–39
   for urethral obstruction, 191
Maisonneuve urethrotome, 352
Male sling surgery, for urinary incontinence, 234
Malignancy, urethral, ruling out, 271
Malnutrition, failed urethroplasty due to, 270
Martius flap, 306
   fat pad flap, 307–308
   labial fat pad flap, over bladder neck closure, 312
McAninch flaps
   onlay anastomosis of, 162
   for panurethral strictures, 165
   rotation of, 162
   technique of harvest of, 160–161
McCarthy panendoscope, 353
Meatal atrophy, due to vitiligo, 99
Meatal dilation, repeated, for management of LS, 25
Meatal retraction, manual, fossa navicularis stricture
      diagnosed by, 100
Meatal stenosis
   in complication of circumcision, 99
   development of, 24
   due to paraurethral stricture, 169
   meatotomy for, 129
   recurrent urethral, occurrence of, 272
   resultant, LS in man with, 23
   urethral, 286
Meatal strictures, 54
   due to vitiligo, 99
   pathognomonic of, 100
Meatotomy
   for fossa navicularis and meatal reconstruction, 101
   for management of LS, 25
   for meatal stenosis, 129
   for treatment of distal strictures, 309
Meatus
   in patients with LS, reconstruction of, 25
   related urethral strictures, 208
   strictures of, etiology of
   urethral, in reconstruction of failed urethroplasty, 272
Meatus reconstruction, 98
   complications of, 104
   etiologic factors of, 98
      iatrogenic, 99
      inflammatory, 98

management consideration of, 100
minimally invasive techniques for, 100
   direct visual internal urethrotomy in, 100
   meatotomy in, 101
   urethral dilation in, 100
patient evaluation of, 99–100
reconstructive techniques for
   flap urethroplasty in, 102–104
   graft urethroplasty in, 101–102
Meissner's corpuscles, 2
Melanocytes, absence of, 23
Memokath 028, for prostatic obstructions, 90
Memokath urethral stent
   for treatment of post prostate surgery, 90
   for treatment of recurrent urethral stricture
      disease, 89
Memotherm, 87
Mercier urethrotome, 352
Meshed graft urethroplasty, 206
Microvascular free flaps, 48
Micturition, 304
Mitomycin-C (MMC), for prevention of recurrence of
      urethral strictures, 77
Morphea, pathogenesis of *B. burgdorferi* role in, 22
Mosquito clamps, for suture orientation, 334
MRA. *See* Magnetic resonance angiography
MRI. *See* Magnetic resonance imaging
Mucosal grafts, for context of urethral reconstruction, 46
Muscle flaps, for genital reconstruction, 50
Musculocutaneous flap, for urethral strictures in patients
      with prior procto-colectomy, 186
Musculus compressor nuda
   and Littre glands, 32
   filling of, normal appearance of, 36
Myofibroblasts
   action of, 46
   proliferation of, 244

N
Nasal reconstruction, skin grafts for, 44
Nd:YAG laser, 292
Neourethra
   formation of, 210
   tubularization of, 209
   tubularized pedicle skin flaps for creation of, 207
Neourethral prolapse, in complication of fossa
      navicularis and meatal reconstruction, 104
Neo-urethras, immunocytochemical analyses of, 342
Nephrostogram, antegrade, for lumen occlusion, 266
Nephrostomy
   drainage
      for management of refractory urinary
         incontinence, 266
      for patients with complex urinary fistulas, 266

tube
    after ureter embolization, placement of, 267
    bilateral percutaneous, for urine divertion, 266
Neurogenic dysfunction, ED caused by, 222
Nitze endoscope, 351
North American Multicenter Urolume Trial (NAUT), 278
Nutritional deficiency, 44

O

Obstetrical trauma, of urethra, 305
Omental mobilization, into colic gutter, 301
Omental vascularity, variations in, 299
Omentum
    anatomy of, 299–300
    surgical mobilization of, 300–302
    use in urethral reconstruction, 297
Onlay flaps, 50
    for midbulbar urethral stricture, 248
    for reconstruction of radiated stricture, 246
    urethroplasty, for radiation induced urethral
        strictures, 241
Onlay graft urethroplasty
    dorsal, development and evolution of, 120
    ventral *vs.* dorsal bulbar, discussion for, 131–133
Onlay urethroplasty, dorsal, development and evolution
        of, 120
Open urethroplasty
    for treatment of urethral stricture disease, 269
    vaginal flap urethroplasty, 307
    vaginal wall urethroplasty, 307–308
Orandi flaps
    cartoon of rotation and onlay anastomosis of, 160
    for panurethral strictures, 165
    technique of harvest of, 159
Osteomyelitis, skeletal muscles in, role of, 172
Otis IU, for dilation of urethral strictures, 66
Oxidative stress, for etiology of LS, 21–22

P

PAG. *See* Posterior auricular grafts
Pain. *See also* Back pain
    chronic, and/or chordee, as specific urethral stent
        complication, 279
    penile, 282
Panurethral strictures, 165–166
    evaluation of, 166
    patient positioning for, 166
    surgical reconstruction of, 166
        with areas of complete lumen obliteration in, 170
        bilateral buccal mucosal grafts for, 166
        circular fasciocutaneous onlay flaps, "Q flap" for,
            166–168
        flap combined with graft for, 168–169
        LSA-induced panurethral stricture in, 169–170

proximal buccal graft and distal staged
    urethroplasty for, 169
Parachute-style anastomosis, 199
Paracoccyxygeal incision, for prostatic fistula
    exposure, 265
Paraplegic patient, with bulb stricture, dorsal placement
    of BMG and gracilis muscle for, 174
Parasthesia
    in BMU complications, 217
    lower extremities, in positioning-related
        complications, 224
Paraurethral glands, 58
Patch-graft urethroplasty, for fossa navicularis
    strictures, 101
Pedicled muscle flaps, for tissue transfer in plastic
    surgery, 50–51
Pelvic arteriography, for pudendal artery occlusion, 204
Pelvic fracture
    associated with vascular injuries, 15
    DVIU for urethral strictures after, 78
    incidence of, 190
    injury to female urethra due to, 305
    patient with urethral disruption injury, MRI
        for, 29
    posterior urethral defect after, combined cystogram/
        retrograde urethrogram for, 275
    posterior urethral disruption in patients with, 221
    posterior urethral strictures caused by, 189
Pelvic hematoma, MRI for location of, 39
Pelvic radiation
    penile dry gangrene and urinary retention after, 243
    prostatoperineal urinary fistula after, 265
    radiation-induced urethral stricture in, management
        of, 245–247
    urethral stricture in, 241
        evaluation of, 245
        grading of radiation morbidity of, 242
        histology of, 244–245
        illustrative cases for, 247–249
        incidence, risk factors, and presentation of,
            242–243
        radiobiology of, 241–242
Pelvic sepsis, in RUF, 252
Pelvic trauma
    panurethral strictures due to, 169
    pericatheter RUG in patient with, 37
    posterior urethral injuries due to, 274
Pelvis
    CT of, 262
    for diagnosis of fistula, CT of, 253
Pendulous urethra, in reconstruction of failed
    urethroplasty, 272–273
Penile anatomy, for implication of urethral
    reconstruction, 9–10

Penile cancer/carcinoma, association between LS and, 20, 22

Penile cordee or deformity, in BMU complications, 217

Penile defect, thigh and lower abdominal skin for, 50

Penile dry gangrene, and urinary retention after pelvic RT, 243

Penile flaps
  use of, 131
  for bulbar reconstruction, 274
  fasciocutaneous flap, 273

Penile hemorrhage, post-procedure, 71

Penile LSA, 100

Penile MRI, normal, 40

Penile sensation, diminished, in fasciocutaneous urethroplasty complications, 219

Penile shaft skin, for recurrent penile urethral strictures, 269

Penile shortening
  in anterior anastomotic urethroplasty complication, 219
  complaints of, 274

Penile skin
  arterial blood supply of, 10–12
  blood supply and lymphatics of, 5
  distal, for urethral reconstruction, 157
  for midbulbar urethral stricture, fasciocutaneous island flap of, 248
  as sources of tissue for reconstruction, 109
  venous drainage of, 13

Penile skin flaps, for urethral reconstruction, 47–48, 153–154, 330, 353
  desirable flap characteristics of, 154–155
  for discreet fossa navicularis strictures, 272
  editorial comment on, 163
  fascial and vascular anatomy of penis for, 155
  longitudinal ventral, with lateral pedicle, harvest of, 159
  patient selection for, 154
  repairs, 272
  results of, 163
    complications in, 163
    success rates in, 163
  technique for, 158
    flap harvest in, 158–161
    patient positioning in, 158
    preoperative preparation in, 158
    urethral closure, 161–163
  transverse circular, with primarily dorsal pedicle, harvest of, 160–161
  types of, 155–156
    dorsal vs. ventral vs. lateral pedicle in, 157
    longitudinal vs transverse in, 156–157
    proximal vs. distal penile skin in, 157
    ventral onlay vs. tube flap vs. combined tissue transfer in, 158
  for urethral reconstruction, 47–48, 153–154

Penile skin island flap, ventral, for obliterative strictures, 158

Penile skin necrosis
  in BMU complications, 217
  in fasciocutaneous urethroplasty complications, 219
  in surgical technique complications, 163

Penile skin vs. buccal mucosal graft, discussion for, 130–131

Penile torsion
  in complication of fossa navicularis and meatal reconstruction, 104
  prevention of, 167

Penile transverse island flap, fasciocutaneous ventral, for fossa navicularis and meatal reconstruction, 102–104

Penile urethra
  anatomy of epithelium and glands of, 7
  strictures of, 108

Penile urethral strictures
  by BMG, surgical techniques for, 121
  recurrent, penile shaft skin for, 269
  UroCoil for, 90

Penile urethroplasty, graft vs. flap in, discussion for, 131

Penis
  arterial supply and venous drainage of, 156
  cross section and distal portion of, 4
  fascial and vascular anatomy of, 155
  medial retraction of left crus of, 198
  in patient with hematuria, images of, 39
  revascularization of, 17
  venous drainage of, 18

Perineal approach
  anterior, for RUF repair, 259–260
  and exposure of prostaterectal fistula, 260
  for repair of RUF, 255

Perineal artery fasciocutaneous flap. See Singapore flap

Perineal flaps, placement of, 203

Perineal prostatectomy, transection of central tendon with, 259

Perineal reconstruction, gracilis flaps for, 172

Perineal tourniquet, 352

Perineal trauma
  childhood, idiopathic stricture caused by, 59
  external, anterior urethral strictures due to, 56

Perineal-urethral strictures/fistulas, gluteal maximus repair of, 183–186

Perineal urethrostomy
  with inverted "U" flap, after Blandy, 207
  for pendulous urethral stricture, 205

Perineal urinary fistulas, salvage prostatectomy for, 258

Perineal vein, course of, 13

Perineo-abdominal approach, for pediatric posterior urethroplasty, 275

Perineum
  closure of, 182
  section of central tendon of, 125
  social lithotomy position for access of, 192
  watering pot, 202
Peripheral vascular disease
  poor wound healing caused by, 154
  prostatic urethral stricture in man with, 247
Periurethral abscess, 59
  urethral strictures associated with, 58
Periurethral fibrosis, 36
Periurethral scarring, in risk factors for recurrence
    of urethral strictures, 74
Permanent stents. See also Wallstent
Pernicious anemia, vitiligo associated with, 99
Peroneal nerve neuropraxia, as positioning-related
    complication, 223
Pesky bleeding, 331
Petrequin urethrotome, 352
Peyronie's disease surgery, 10
Pfannenstiel incision, 308–309
PGA. See Polyglycolic acid
PHB. See Polyhydroxybutyric acid
Phimosis, due to LSA, 58
PLA. See Polylactic acid
Plastic surgery
  assessment of tissue transfer techniques in, 44
  flap techniques for tissue transfer in, 48
    adjunctive, 51–52
    free, 51
    pedicled muscle, 50–51
    rotation/transposition, 49–50
    sliding advancement, 48–49
    tubed, 50
  management options of tissue transfer techniques
      in, 44
    flap reconstruction in, 47–48
    graft reconstruction in, 45–47
    primary repair in, 45
    secondary intention in, 44–45
  for urologist, tissue transfer techniques
      in, 43–44
PLGA. See Polylactic-co-glycolic acid
Pneumaturia, in RUF, 252
Polyglactin sutures, 195
Polyglycolic acid, as biomaterial for engineering of
    urethral tissues, 339–340
Polyhydroxybutyric acid, use in urethral
    reconstruction, 340
Polylactic acid
  as biomaterial for engineering of urethral tissues,
      339–340
  PLA stent, in patients after prior failed
      urethrotomy, 94

Polylactic-co-glycolic acid, as biomaterial for
    engineering of urethral tissues, 339–340
"Porte impreinte," 348
  Ducamp's, 351
Positioning, patient
  for panurethral strictures, 166
  posterior urethroplasty, positioning-related
      complications in, 223–224
  technique for urethral reconstruction, 158
Posterior auricular grafts, 139
Posterior transsphincteric approaches. See York-Mason
    approaches
Posterior urethroplasty, 328–329
  positioning-related complications in, 223–224
Postprostatectomy strictures
  editorial comment on, 236–238
  endourological surgical management of, 232
    after RRP, 233–234
    after TURP, 232–233
  epidemiology of, 229–230
  evaluation and preoperative management
      of, 230–231
  management of strictures in, 231–232
  mechanisms and risk factors of, 230
  open surgical management of, 234
    after RRP, 235–236
    after TRUP, 234–235
Postvoid dribbling
  in anterior anastomotic urethroplasty, 219–220
  in BMU complications, 216
  in fasciocutaneous urethroplasty complications, 218
  as specific urethral stent complication, 279
Priapism, high flow, in complication of DVIU, 71
Proctectomy, for management of nonradiated
    fistulas, 252
Procto-colectomy, prior, urethral strictures in patients
    with, musculocutaneous flap for, 186
Proctoscopy, for identification of fistula, 252
Prostate brachytherapy (BT), prostatic and membranous
    urethral strictures after, 248
Prostate cancer
  high-dose BT for, 244
  prostato-rectal fistula after cryotherapy for, 253
  radiation beams for treatmento of, 242
  radiotherapy for, radiation induced urethral stricture
      after, 248
  surgery for, 229
  urethral strictures after management of, 236–237
Prostatectomy
  perineal, transection of central tendon with, 259
  radical
    BNC after, 230
    DVIU for anastomotic stricture after, 68
  salvage

Prostatectomy (*continued*)
  with anastomotic urethrovesical urethroplasty
    for radiation induced urethral strictures, 241
    for prostato-rectal fistulas, 258
  salvage radical, bladder neck-rectal fistula after, 256
  stricture reconstruction after, exposure of bladder
    neck region for, 234
Prostatectomy anastomotic stenoses, post, 91–92
Prostate gland
  MRI for location of, 39
  RUG imaging of, 32
Prostate liquefaction, 245
Prostaterectal fistulas
  perineal approach and exposure of, 260
  transanal rectal advancement flap for, 255
Prostate surgery, post, Urocoil and Memokath stent for
    treatment of, 90
Prostatic carcinoma, bladder neck strictures due to
    treatment of, 189
Prostatic fistula
  BMG for, 183
  buccal graft to
    completed, 260
    parachuting in, 265
  buccal mucosa patch onlay for, placement of, 185
Prostatic hyperplasia (PH), benign, TURP for, 229
Prostatic radiation fistula, exposure of, 178
Prostatic urethra
  due to treatment of prostatic carcinoma, strictures of, 189
  obliteration of, 203
Prostatitis
  chronic, 59
  signs or symptoms of, 54
  tuberculous, urethral strictures associated with, 58
  UTI with, occurrence of, 270
Prostatocutaneous (urethral) fistulas
  occurence of, 182
  radiation, retrograde urethrogram in patient with, 177
Prostato-membranous stricture, Singapore flap for, 180
Prostatoperineal urinary fistula, after abdomino-perineal
    resection and pelvic radiotherapy, 265
Prostato-rectal fistulas
  after cryotherapy for prostate cancer, 253
  salvage prostatectomy for, 258
Prosthetic graft sepsis, skeletal muscles in, role of, 172
Psoriasis, LS association with, 21
Pubectomy
  abdominoperineal approach for, 200
  inferior, for safe bulboprostatic anastomosis, 144
  and transabdominal urethroplasty, 301
  wedge, for rerouting of urethra, 198
Pubic symphysis
  inferior, crura to expose, separation of, 197
  wedge resection of inferior part of, 198

Pubovaginal sling, for associated stress incontinence, 308
Pudendal artery
  pelvic arteriography for occlusion of, 204
  superficial external
    blood supply of, 11
    relative areas of arborization of, 10
Pudendal artery fistula, urethral-internal, in
    complication of DVIU, 71
Pudendal vein, internal, 13
Pulmonary embolism, in positioning-related
    complications, 223

Q
Q-flap
  for panurethral strictures reconstruction, 166–168
  penile skin, for panurethral strictures, 165
  for strictures reconstruction, 169
Queyrat, erythroplasia of, 22, 24, 98

R
Radiation, complex fistulas due to, 252
Radiation morbidity, of urethral stricture and
    urethroplasty, grading of, 242
Radiation therapy
  adjunctive, prostatocutaneous urethral fistulas and
    strictures associated with, 182
  fistulas due to, 251
  pelvic, penile dry gangrene and urinary retention
    after, 243
  poor wound healing caused by, 154
Radical retropubic prostatectomies
  bladder neck strictures after, 230
  BNC after, 232
  endourological surgical management after, 233–234
  open surgical management after, 235–236
  post, combined RUG and VCUG of stricture of, 231
  vesicourethral anastomotic strictures after, dilation
    for, 232
Radiotherapy
  pelvic, prostatoperineal urinary fistula after, 265
  for prostate cancer, radiation induced urethral
    stricture after, 248
Recalcitrant stricture, rapid dilation method for opening
    of, 350
Rectal-colon pathology, proctoscopy for, 252
Rectal injuries
  adominoperineal approach for, 192
  RUF due to, 252
Rectal pain, in RUF, 252
Rectourethral fistula, 252
  approaches for repair of, 255
  complex vesicoperineal and, 252
  diagnosis of, 252–254
  due to Crohn's disease and tuberculosis, 252

preoperative assessment and decision-making for, 254
specific reconstruction methods for, 255–257
urinary and fecal diversion in, 254–255
Rectovesical fistulas, urinary-perineal and, 265–266
Rectum
and anal sphincter for fistula repair, anatomy of,
254–255
cancer, abdominoperineal resection of, 182
Rectus abdominus muscle, for genital reconstruction, 51
Rectus flap, and free graft, post-RRP stricture
reconstruction by, 236
Recurrent epididymitis, as symptom of urethral
stricture, 54
Recurrent prostatitis, as symptom of urethral stricture, 54
Recurrent stenosis, 281
Recurrent stress incontinence, 304
Recurrent stricture
in fasciocutaneous urethroplasty complications,
217–218
as specific urethral stent complication, 278–279
Reoperative hypospadias surgery, 285
complex reoperative hypospadias techniques
adjacent genital tissues, 288
bladder mucosal graft, 290
buccal mucosal graft, 290–291
extragenital tissues, 288–290
squamous epithelium, 290
urethral plate retubularization, 287–288
postpubertal and adult complications, 291
urethral hair, 292–294
surgical complications
chordee, persistent, 286–287
urethral diverticulum, 286
urethrocutaneous fistula, 286
treatment algorithm for, 292
Resectoscope loop, 280
Retrograde urethrography
use of, 351
for diagnosis
of fistula, 253
of stricture, 245
use of Foley catheter in, 100
of male urethra, 31
pericatheter, in patient with pelvic trauma, 37
retrograde urethrogram, use of, 270
and VCUG
for posterior urethral stricture, 231
for urethral stricture, 33
Rhabdomyolysis, in positioning-related complications, 223
Rheumatic polymyalgia, LS association with, 21
Rhomboid flap, 50
Ricord coarctotome, 352
Rotation/transposition flaps, for tissue transfer in plastic
surgery, 49–50

RRPs. See Radical retropubic prostatectomies
RT. See Radiation therapy; Radiation therapy
RUF. See Rectourethral fistula
RUG. See Retrograde urethrography

S
Sachse urethrotomy, 67
Sacrectomy, for fistula exposure, 266
Saphenous vein, 13
Sartorius, 177
SC. See Self-catheterization
Scar formation, MMC for prevention of, 77
Scarring, periurethral, in risk factors for recurrence
of urethral strictures, 74
SCC. See Squamous cell carcinoma
Schreiter urethroplasty, with tubularization of matured
grafted skin, 207
Sciatic nerve, location of, 184
Scleroderma, 99
Scrotal edema, 72
Scrotal flaps, placement of, 203
Scrotal inlay flap, posteriorly based, Blandy two-stage
urethroplasty with, 204
Scrotal inlay technique, 353
Turner-Warwick two-stage, procedure of, 206
Scrotal skin, arterial blood supply of, 12–13
Scrotal skin flap, near recurrent stricture, sacculation
of, 273
Scrotum
blood supply and lymphatics of, 5
venous drainage of, 13
Self-catheterization
for BNC, 246
CISC, for prevention of urethral strictures
recurrence, 76
for long-term stricture management, 271
and urethrotomy
for bulbar urethral stricture, 245
for radiation induced urethral strictures, 241
Semitendinosis, 177, 179
Seroma, formation of, 45
Sexual function
in complications of augmented anastomotic
urethroplasty, 150
in urethral surgery, impact of, 115
Silicone catheters
after DVIU, uses of, 70
uses of, 75
Singapore flap
for bulbar urethral stricture, 180
flap design, and technique of elevation for onlay
patch urethroplasty, 180–182
Single-stage reconstruction, for complex anterior
urethral strictures, 154

Skene's glands, 2–3
"Ski" needle, 333
Skin flaps. *See also* Skin island flaps
    classification of, 48
    genital, for LSA, 26
    island advancement, 49
        Burrow's triangles and, 49
    penile, for single stage urethral reconstruction, 353
    peninsular, for genital reconstruction, 156
    reconstruction, combined with gracilis flap
        reconstruction, prefabricated, 175–176
    repairs, penile, 272
    tubularized pedicle, for creation of neourethra, 207
Skin grafts
    for fossa navicularis and meatal reconstruction, 101
    free, for anterior urethral reconstruction, 120
    for nasal reconstruction, 44
    subdivisions of, 46
Skin graft urethroplasty, muscle assisted
        full-thickness, 172
Skin island flaps, 330
    and dorsal buccal graft, obliterated urethral
        reconstruction with, 170
Skin, layers of, 46
Small intestinal submucosa (SIS), as onlay patch graft
        for urethroplasty, 340
Smith's Compressor. *See* Perineal tourniquet
Sonography, for evaluation of strictures length, 109
Sonourethrography
    for degree of spongiofibrosis, 100
    for determination of stricture length, 245
    limitations of, 100
    of male urethra, 34–37
    for stricture characteristics, 122
    for true bulbar urethral stricture length, 29
Sphincter, poor function, supravesical urinary diversion
        for, 252
Sphincter strictures, treated by urethral dilation, 189
Spinal cord injuries (SCI), failed urethroplasty
        due to, 270
Spongiofibrosis, 324
    color Doppler for assessment of, 56
    degrees of, 54
    minimal, epithelial scar with, 55
    periurethral inflammation in patients with, 37
    sonourethrography for degree of, 100
    ultrasound and MRI for evaluation of, 29
Spongiosum, 274, 281, 324
SP tube, for management of obliterative stricture, 248
Squamous cell carcinoma
    BXO and, relationship between, 98
    LS and, 22
    urethral stricture due to, 42
    with vulvar lichen sclerosus, incidence of, 20

Staged urethroplasty, proximal buccal graft and, for
        panurethral strictures, 169
Stem cell injury, due to chronic effects of radiation, 242
Stenosis. *See* Recurrent stenosis; *specific stenosis*
    of membranous urethra, 35
Stenotic scar, development of, 86
Stensen's duct damage, in BMU complications, 217
Stent encrustation
    prevention of, 277
    as specific urethral stent complication, 279
Stent migration, prevention of, 92
Stents
    allium bulbar urethral
        clinical experience with, 93
        insertion technique of, 92–93
        in treatment of recurrent urethral stricture, 91–93
    bioabsorbable, for urethral stricture, 94
    biodegradable urethral, 94
    limitations of, permanent and temporary, 91
    in treatment of recurrent urethral stricture, 86–87
        permanent stents, 87–89
        temporary stents, 89–91
    urethral
        biodegradable, 94
        complications and methods for explantation
            (*see* Urethral stents)
Steroids, for prevention of recurrence of urethral
        strictures, 77
Stone(s)
    cystoscopy for diagnosis of, 67
    formation
        hair in urethra leads to, 154
        nidus/wick for, 279
        prevention of, 277
        risk of, 203
Stress incontinence
    associated, pubovaginal sling for, 308
    recurrent, 304
Stricture chair, 351
Stricture(s)
    augmentation *vs.* excision of, discussion for, 133
    casts of, 348
    diagnosis, objective criteria for, 316
    disease (*see also* Urethral stricture disease)
        and substitution urethroplasty, 329–332
    of fossa navicularis and meatus, etiology of, 98
    recurrence, 351
        in complications of augmented anastomotic
            urethroplasty, 150
        rapid, 350
    recurrence of, risk factor for
        length of, 74
        number of, 75
        site of, 74

Stricturotome, 352
Stricturotomy, ventral longitudinal, 103
Substitution urethroplasty
 complications after, 330
 and "stricture disease," 329–332
Surgery
 male sling, for urinary incontinence, 234
 post prostate, Urocoil and Memokath stent for
  treatment of, 90
 for prostate cancer, 229
 and surgical reconstruction
  of distal urethral stenoses, 208
  for glanular urethral strictures, 100
  for panurethral strictures, 166–170
 and techniques
  for BMG urethroplasty, 122
  for repair of penile or bulbar urethral strictures by
   BMG, 121
 urological reconstructive, buccal mucosa for, 119–120
Surgical anastomosis, and excision for treatment of
 anterior urethral strictures, 107
Surgical dissection, of gracilis muscle flap, 262–264
Surgical management
 endourological
  after RRP, 233–234
  after TURP, 232–233
 open
  after RRP, 235–236
  after TRUP, 234–235
Surgical trauma, prostatocutaneous urethral fistulas
 occur from, 182
Syme's operation, 351

T
Techniques, for fossa navicularis and meatal
 reconstruction, 101
Tensor fascia lata, as alternative source of autologous
 fascia, 308
Thigh flap, anterolateral, use of, 51
TIP. See Tubularized incised plate
Tissue engineering of urethra, 337
 with acellular matrices, 340–343
 biomaterials for, 338
  acellular tissue matrices, 339–340
  selection, 339
  synthetic polymers, 340
  tissue–regeneration strategies, 340
 with cell-seeded matrices, 343
 use of cells for, 338
Tissue expansion, in utility and range of flap, 51
 drawbacks of, 52
Tissue–regeneration strategies, 340
Tissue transfer techniques
 flap, in plastic surgery for urologist, 48

 adjunctive, 51–52
 free, 51
 pedicled muscle, 50–51
 rotation/transposition, 49–50
 sliding advancement, 48–49
 tubed, 50
 in plastic surgery for urologist, 43
  assessment of, 44
  management options of, 44–48
 urethral closure in combined, for urethral
  reconstruction, 162–163
 for urethral trauma, 203
Tobacco abuse, failed urethroplasty due to, 270
Transabdominal approach
 of large and complex fistulas, 264
 for repair of RUF, 255
Transanal approach
 for management of nonradiated fistulas, 251–252
 for repair of RUF, 255
Transanal rectal advancement flap, for prostate-rectal
 fistulas, 255
Transperineal approach
 complications of, 260
 of large and complex fistulas, 258–260
 for prostate-rectal fistulas, 255
Trans-sphincteric anterior approach, for fistulas,
 258–259
Transurethral incision of bladder neck, with
 resectoscope for recurrent BNC, 237
Transurethral resection, 278–279
 of fibrous callus for prevention of recurrence of
  urethral strictures, 75–76
 of scar tissue after DVIU, complication of urethral
  strictures in, 72
Transurethral resection of prostate
 bladder neck stenosis after, endourethral
  brachytherapy in patients with, 77
 BNC after, occurrence of, 230
 BNC with prior, development of, 243
 for BPH, 229
 endourological surgical management after, 232–233
 open surgical management after, 234–235
 otis IU for prevention of urethral stricture after, 66
Trauma
 acute urethral, staged urethroplasty for, 202–203
 anterior urethral strictures due to, 108
 pelvic
  panurethral strictures due to, 169
  posterior urethral injuries due to, 274
 perineal, anterior urethral strictures due to, 56
 posterior urethral, MRI for, 37
 surgical, prostatocutaneous urethral fistulas occur
  from, 182
 trans-sphincteric anterior approach for fistulas of, 258

Trauma (*continued*)
  urethral
    staged urethroplasty for management of, 201
    strictures caused by, 33
Tubed flaps, for tissue transfer in plastic surgery, 50
Tuberculosis
  RUF due to, 252
  of urethra, 58
Tubularization, of matured grafted skin, Schreiter urethroplasty with, 207
Tubularized incised plate, hypospadias repair, 287–288
Tubularized urethral repair, 343
TUIBN. *See* Transurethral incision of bladder neck
Tumescence, 332
Tumor, of bladder, cystoscopy for investigation of, 67
Tunica vaginalis flaps, 273, 292
TUR. *See* Transurethral resection
Turnball-Cutait colo-anal pull through, for RUF, 264
Turner-Warwick flap, technique of harvest of, 160–161
Turner-Warwick two-stage scrotal inlay, procedure of, 206
TURP. *See* Transurethral resection of prostate

U
UG. *See* Urethrogram: Urethrography
Ultrasound
  for assessing fibrosis, 55
  color Doppler, to evaluate length and diameter of stricture, 68
  for evaluation of spongiofibrosis, 29
Ureteric embolization
  for managing complex urinary tract fistula, 268
  for refractory urethro-rectal fistula and urinary incontinence, 267
Urethra
  abdomino-perineal approach for identification of, 198
  anatomy, 303
    and selection of surgical technique for BMG urethroplasty, significance of, 120–121
  anterior
    obliteration of, 207–208
    vascular insufficiency of, 203–204
  bulbar
    in reconstruction of failed urethroplasty, 273–274
    urolume stents in, 88
  at distal margin of bulbospongiosum muscle, approach of, 111
  endoscopic view of, 343
  female, 3
  flexible cystoscopy for obstruction of, 191
  Foley catheter for site of obliteration of, 193
  function of, 304
  genital skin and anatomy of, 1
  and genital skin, for implications of urethral reconstruction, vascular anatomy of, 9

  HBO for angiogenesis of, 246
  male, 5–7
    anatomy of, 5
    conventional urethrography of, 30
    DVIU for strictures of, 72
    imaging of, 29–30
    MRI of, 37–39
    RUG of, 31
    sonourethrography of, 34–37
    stricture characteristics and extent of, 33–34
    subdivision of, 189
    VCUG of, 31–33
    voiding CT urethrography of, 39
  membranous
    CTU for occlusion of, 69
    stenosis of, 35
  mobilization of, 192
  pendulous
    normal distention of, 38
    in reconstruction of failed urethroplasty, 272–273
  posterior, in reconstruction of failed urethroplasty, 274–275
  prostatic, obliteration of, 203
  reconstructed, within intercrural plane, 197
  RT effects on, 243
  switchblade transection of, 190
  tissue engineering of (*see* Tissue engineering of urethra)
  tuberculosis of, 58
  wedge pubectomy for rerouting of, 198
Urethra injury, pathology
  iatrogenic, 304–305
  trauma, 305
Urethral arteries, in bulbar and pendulous urethra, distribution of location of, 15
Urethral biopsy, for malignancy investigations, 42
  in refractory stricture cases, 270
Urethral calibration, and bouginage, 318
Urethral cancers, 59, 309
Urethral carcinoma, suspicion of, 64, 78
Urethral defect, thigh and lower abdominal skin for, 50
Urethral dilatation, 91, 232, 348
  for stent obstruction, 89
Urethral dilation, 348–350
  for anterior urethral stricture disease, 190
  for fossa navicularis and meatal reconstruction, 100
  for management of urethral strictures, 246
  for patients with urethral strictures, 60
  for recurrent urethral stricture, 247
  sphincter strictures treated by, 189
Urethral disruption, post-traumatic, patient with, 41
Urethral distraction injury
  complications after posterior urethroplasty for, 221
  impairment of male sexual function after, 222

posterior
  catheter-realignment techniques for, 203
  indication of staged procedure for, 203–204
  technical approaches to staged procedure for,
    204–205
Urethral diverticulum, 59
  in children after laser DVIU, 71
  in fasciocutaneous urethroplasty complications, 218
  post hypospadias surgery, 287
  as reoperative hypospadiac complication, 286
Urethral erosion, symptoms of, 304
Urethral exposure
  in surgical technique, 146–147
  using ventral subcoronal incision, 102
Urethralgia, in children after laser DVIU, 71
Urethral hair, 292–294
Urethral injury(ies). See also Urethral distraction injury
  common causes of, 304
  incidence of, 190
  pelvic fracture-related, posterior urethral strictures
    caused by, 189
  posterior, due to pelvic trauma, 274
  RUF due to, 252
  stress urinary incontinence in, 223
  traumatic posterior, MRI for patients with, 39
Urethral instrumentation, urethral stricture due to, 99
Urethral ischemic necrosis, 15
Urethral length, single stage anastomotic urethroplasty
    for deficiencies of, 203
Urethral loss, surgery for
  bladder flap, 308–309
  open urethroplasty
    vaginal flap urethroplasty, 307
    vaginal wall urethroplasty, 307–308
  pubovaginal sling for associated stress incontinence, 308
  urethral sling injury, 306–307
Urethral meatal stenosis, 286
Urethral meatus
  anterior, creation of, 208
  in reconstruction of failed urethroplasty, 272
  stenosis of, 72
Urethral mucosa, regeneration of, 120
Urethral obliteration
  catheter after CTU for, use of, 70
  complication rates of CTU for, 72
  CTU for, 73
  prostatic, 56
Urethral obstruction, retrograde urethrogram and
    micturating cystogram for, 190
Urethral occlusion, intrastent, temporary stent for, 89
Urethral plate
  dorsal buccal mucosa graft salvage of, 273
  mucosal, 123
  in patients with strictures, replacement of, 131

urethrography for evaluation of, 122
Urethral plate retubularization, as reoperative
    hypospadias technique, 287–288
Urethral reconstruction, 171. See also Tissue
    engineering of urethra
  anterior
    free skin graft for, 120
    genital skin island flaps for, 14
  collagen based inert matrix for, 342
  female (see Female urethral reconstruction)
  genital flap selection for implication of, 14
  gluteus maximus muscle flap
    anatomy and clinical applications, 183
    for bulbomembranous urethral reconstruction,
      182–183
    gluteal maximus repair of a perineal-urethral
      strictures (and fistulas), techniques of, 183–186
  gracilis flap, 172
    buccal graft and gracilis muscle, dorsal placement
      of, 174–175
    buccal mucosal graft onlay with gracilis support,
      technique of, 173
    gracilis myofasciocutaneous flap, 176–180
    short gracilis flap, 173–174
    skin and gracilis flap reconstruction, prefabricated
      combined, 175–176
  grafts for, use of, 142
  Johanson's original staged, 209
  lingual mucosa and posterior auricular skin for, 137
  male, buccal mucosa grafts for, 310
  for management of LS, 25
  mucosal grafts for context of, 46
  muscle assisted full-thickness skin and buccal graft
    urethroplasty, 172
  use of omentum in (see Omentum)
  penile anatomy for implications of, 9–10
  penile skin arterial blood supply for implication of,
    10–12
  penile skin flaps for, 47–48 (see also Penile skin
    flaps, for urethral reconstruction)
    patient selection for, 154
  perineal artery fasciocutaneous flap (Singapore flap)
    flap design, and technique of elevation for onlay
      patch urethroplasty, 180–182
  scrotal skin blood supply for implication of, 12–13
  staged urethroplasty for, 202
  tissues used for, 338
  urethra and genital skin, vascular anatomy of, 9
  urethra for implications of, blood supply of, 14
    arterial, 14–17
    venous, 17–18
  venous drainage
    of penile skin, 13
    of scrotum, 13

Urethral repair, tubularized, 343
Urethral restenosis
    in complication of fossa navicularis and meatal
        reconstruction, 104
    occurrence of, 163
Urethral sacculation, in BMU complications,
    216–217
Urethral sling injury, 306–307
Urethral sphincters, external, function of, 254
Urethral stenosis
    distal, surgical reconstruction of, 208
    in patients with post-traumatic strictures, 88
Urethral stents
    biodegradable, 94
    complications and methods for explantation, 277
    complications, specific
        chronic pain and/or chordee, 279
        hyperplasia, 279
        postvoid dribbling, 279
        recurrent stricture, 278–279
        stent encrustation, 279
    for treatment of urethral strictures, 85
    urolume explantation
        endoscopic methods, 279–281
        open surgical methods, 281–283
Urethral stricture
    after management of prostate cancer, incidence of,
        236–237
    anesthesia for, 70
    anterior, 34, 36
        associated with LS, 24
        clinical outcomes of excision and primary
            anastomosis for, 114–115
        combined tissue transfer techniques for
            obliteration, 162
        editorial comment on, 116
        etiology of, 108
        patient selection for excision and primary
            anastomosis for, 108–109
        postoperative care for, 114
        preoperative evaluation of, 109
        stricture excision and primary anastomosis for,
            107–108
        surgical technique for, 109–114
    antibiotics for, 70
    bioabsorable stents for, 94
    BMG for, 184
    bulbar
        BMG onlay urethroplasty for, 131
        with filling of Cowper's glands, 35
    catheterization for, 70–71
    caused by trauma, 33
    classification system of, 348
    complication of, 71

CTU, 72
    dilation, 71
    DVIU, 71–72
    TUR of scar tissue after DVIU, 72
core-through urethrotomy for, 69
with Cowper's glands and glands of Littre, 34
dilation for, 64–66
due to SCC, voiding urethrogram of, 42
due to urethral instrumentation, 99
DVIU for, 66–68
editorial comment on, 78–80, 93–94
endoscopic urethroplasty for, 70
endourethral prostheses for, 85–86
iatrogenic posterior
    algorithm for clinical evaluation of, 232
    cause of, 229
indications for dilation or DVIU for, 77–78
laser urethrotomy for, 68–69
meatal, submeatal, fossa navicularis, LSA-related, 208
minimally invasive interventions for, 64
obliterative posttraumatic, laser CTU for, 69
pendulous
    and bulbar, RUG and VCUG for, 33
    perineal urethrostomy for, 205
posterior, 189–190
    assessment of, 190–191
    classification of, 231
    complications of, 197
posterior urethroplasty
    postoperative follow-up, 196–197
    preparation of patient for, 191–192
    principles of, 192
    procedure of, 192–196
recurrence, prevention of, 75
    botulinum toxin for, 77
    brachytherapy for, 77
    CISC for, 76
    clinic dilation for, 76–77
    halofuginone for, 77
    hydraulic self-dilation for, 76
    mitomycin-C for, 77
    steroids for, 77
    TUR of fibrous callus for, 75–76
recurrence, risk factors for, 73
    age of patient in, 73
    caliber or diameter of stricture in, 74
    complications during procedure in, 75
    duration of catheterization in, 75
    etiology in, 73
    instrument used, number, and location
        of incisions in, 75
    length of follow-up in, 75
    length of stricture in, 74
    number of strictures in, 75

perioperative infection in, 75
periurethral scarring in, 74
previous stricture treatment in, 74
repeated treatment in, 75
site of stricture in, 74
symptoms at presentation in, 73
type of catheter used in, 75
recurrence, stents in treatment of, 86–87
allium bulbar urethral, 91–93
limitations of previous generations of permanent
and temporary, 91
permanent, 87–89
temporary, 89–91
recurrent epididymitis/prostatitis, as symptom of, 54
results of, 72–73
short, anastomotic urethroplasty for, 219
true bulbar, sonourethrography for, 29
urethroplasty for, 214
urethrotomy for, 64, 66
and wound healing, 86
Urethral stricture and management, history of
caustics and cauterization, 350
stricture diagnosis, 351
stricture etiology, 347–348
treatment methods, 348
alternative methods for, 351–352
urethral dilation, 348–350
urethroplasty, 353–354
urethrotomes, contemporary, 353
urethrotomy
external, 350–351
internal, 352–353
Urethral stricture and urethroplasty, in pelvic irradiated
patient, 241
evaluation of, 245
grading of radiation morbidity of, 242
histology of, 244–245
illustrative cases for, 247–249
incidence, risk factors, and presentation of, 242–243
radiation-induced, management of, 245–247
radiobiology of, 241–242
Urethral stricture disease
anterior
indication of staged procedure for, 205–208
technical approaches to staged procedure for, 208–210
bulbar
augmented anastomotic repair for, 143
by augmented anastomotic urethroplasty,
management of, 144–145
primary anastomotic repair for, 142
complex, staged urethroplasty for management of, 201
consequences of untreated strictures in, 59–60
Cowper's glands with, opacification of, 32
economic impact of, 60–61

epidemiology of, 53–54
demographics, 53
incidence, 54
signs and symptoms of urethral stricture, 54
glands of Littre with, opacification of, 32
glanular, due to BXO, 98
gracilis flap for, 172
buccal graft and gracilis muscle, dorsal placement
of, 174–175
buccal mucosal graft onlay with gracilis support,
technique of, 173
short gracilis flap, 173–174
skin and gracilis flap reconstruction, prefabricated
combined, 175–176
histology of, 54–55
open urethroplasty for treatment of, 269
pathology of, 54–55
pre-and post-operative imaging of, 30
stricture characteristics and etiology of, 56
etiology, 56–58
stricture etiology by location of stricture in, 58–59
stricture classification of, 55–56
Urethral stricture reconstruction, female
distal urethral stricture, 309–310
mid-urethral strictures
endoscopic repair, 310
graft urethroplasty, 310–311
Urethral stricture surgery
staged urethroplasty for, 202–203
subsequent, predictors of, 237
Urethral stricture treatment, follow-up strategies after
follow-up frequency, 319
invasive evaluations
cystoscopy, 319
urethral calibration and bouginage, 318
urethrography, 319
noninvasive evaluations
AUA symptom score and urinary flow
rate, 318
patient-reported symptoms, 317–318
urinary flow rate, 316–317
Urethral substitution, fasciocutaneous ventral penile
transverse island flap for, 103
Urethral surgery, sexual function in, impact of, 115
Urethral trauma
acute, staged urethroplasty for, 202–203
posterior, MRI for, 37
staged urethroplasty for management of, 201
Urethritis
anterior urethral strictures due to, 108
gonococcal, 57
prevention of, 277
Urethrocele, in fasciocutaneous urethroplasty
complication, formation of, 218

Urethrocutaneous fistulas
    in complication of surgical technique, 163
    in fasciocutaneous urethroplasty, 219
    inflammatory bowel disease with, gracilis
        myofasciocutaneous flap for, 176
    as reoperative hypospadiac complication, 286
Urethrogram
    combined, and cystogram for stricture length, 191
    and flowrate study for stricture postoperative
        follow-up, 197
    for long bulbar urethral stricture with affected
        urethra, 145
    with patent bulbar urethra after augmented
        anastomotic urethroplasty, 149
    postoperative, reveal fistula closure, 179
    retrograde, 88 (see also Retrograde urethrography)
        for determination of recurrent stricture, 270
        in patient with radiation prostatocutaneous
            fistula, 177
        for surgical anastomotic repair, 109
        for urethral obstruction, 190
    voiding, of bulbar urethral stricture due to SCC, 42
Urethrography
    conventional, of male urethra, 30
    for evaluation of urethral plate, 122
    retrograde (see Retrograde urethrography)
    voiding CT, of male urethra, 39
Urethroplasty, 353–354
    anastomotic (see Anastomotic urethroplasty)
        augmented (see Anastomotic urethroplasty,
            augmented)
    endoscopic, for urethral strictures, 70
    fossa navicularis and meatal reconstruction
        flap for, 102–104
        graft for, 101–102
    for management of LS, 26
    mid-bulbar anastomotic, 113
    open surgical, for recurrent urethral stricture, 85
    patient posterior urethral strictures for, preparation of,
        191–192
    for patients with urethral strictures, 60
    in pelvic radiation
        evaluation of urethral stricture and, 245
        grading of radiation morbidity of urethral stricture
            and, 242
        histology of urethral stricture and, 244–245
        illustrative cases for urethral stricture and, 247–249
        incidence, risk factors, and presentation of urethral
            stricture and, 242–243
        radiation-induced urethral stricture and,
            management of, 245–247
        radiobiology of urethral stricture and, 241–242
        urethral stricture and, 241
    for pendulous strictures, 58

    perineal anastomotic, for urethral strictures, CTU
        with, 69
    perineal or transpubic, for posterior strictures, 78
    for posterior urethral strictures, 191
        principles of, 192
        procedure of, 192–196
    for recurrent urethral stricture, 86
    Schreiter-type, 210
    single stage anastomotic, for urethral length
        deficiencies, 203
    staged, 201–202
        for anterior urethral stricture disease, 205–210
        history and rationale of, 202–203
        for posterior urethral distraction injuries, 203–205
    staged, skin grafting in, use of, 165
    substitution, lingual mucosa and posterior auricular
        skin for, 137
Urethroplasty, buccal mucosal graft, 119–120
    discussion for, 129
        excision of stricture vs. augmentation of stricture
            in, 133
        flap vs. graft in penile urethroplasty, 131
        penile skin vs. buccal mucosal graft, 130–131
        ventral vs. dorsal bulbar onlay graft urethroplasty,
            131–133
    dorsal onlay graft, development and evolution of, 120
    postoperative care and complications of, 128–129
    preoperative evaluation of, 121–122
    surgical techniques for, 122
        dorsal onlay buccal mucosal graft urethroplasty
            using fibrin glue in, 127–128
        penile one-stage dorsal inlay buccal mucosa graft
            urethroplasty in, 122
        preparation of bulbar urethra in, 122–124
        ventral onlay buccal mucosal graft urethroplasty in,
            124–127
    urethral anatomy and selection of surgical technique
        for, significance of, 120–121
Urethroplasty, complications, 214
    anterior anastomotic, 219
        acute urinary extravasation in, 219
        chordee in, 220
        erectile dysfunction in, 220
        postvoid dribbling in, 219–220
        recurrence in, 220–221
        UTI in, 221
    buccal mucosal, 214
        erectile dysfunction in, 216
        fistula in, 214–215
        oral complications in, 217
        other uncommon complications in, 217
        postvoid dribbling in, 216
        recurrence in, 215–216
        urethral sacculation in, 216–217

urine leak in, 214
UTI in, 216
fasciocutaneous, 217
ejaculatory dysfunction in, 218
erectile dysfunction/diminished penile sensation in, 219
penile skin necrosis in, 219
postvoid dribbling in, 218
recurrent stricture in, 217–218
urethral diverticulum in, 218
urethrocutaneous fistula in, 219
urinary extravasation in, 219
posterior, 221
erectile dysfunction in, 222–223
failure of repair in, 221–222
incontinence in, 223
positioning-related complications in, 223–224
Urethroplasty, failed, reconstruction of, 269
bulbar urethra in, 273–274
causes of, 270
evaluation of, 270–271
pendulous urethra in, 272–273
posterior urethra in, 274–275
preparation and general considerations of, 271–272
urethral meatus in, 272
Urethroplasty surgery, technical considerations and decision making in, 323
anterior urethroplasty, general concepts, 326–328
positioning
patient, 325
scrub tech, 325
preoperative assessment
imaging, 324–325
stricture vs. stricture disease, 324
timing of surgery, 325
specific methods
anastomotic urethroplasty, 328–329
posterior urethroplasty, 328–329
substitution urethroplasty and "stricture disease," 329–332
Urethro-rectal fistula, refractory, ureteral embolization for, 267
Urethrorrhagia, due to nocturnal erections, 129
Urethroscopy
for stricture characteristics, 122
for underlying fibrosis, 55
to visualize distal side of stricture, 109
Urethrostomy
perineal
Blandy flap for, 13
for pendulous urethral stricture, 205

Urethrotome(s)
contemporary, 353
of Oberlander, 350
pediatric, for urethrotomy, 78
Urethrotomy
bulbar, for bulbar urethral stricture, 160
core-through, for urethral strictures, 69
dorsal, repair of dorsal wall injuries by, 176
external, 350–351
first stricture recurrence after, risk of, 73
internal, 352–353
laser, for urethral strictures, 68–69
for management of stricture, 86
maximal bulbar urethral stricture length managed by, 79
and other minimally invasive interventions for urethral strictures, 64
for patients with urethral strictures, 60
pediatric urethrotome for, 78
for stent obstruction, 89
stricture length and stricture recurrence after, association between, 74
sutured full-thickness BMG into, 174
for urethral strictures, 66
ventral, for exposure of urethral stricture, 180
Urinary and fecal diversion
anal sphincter and rectum for, anatomy of, 254–255
indications for, 254
in RUF, 254–255
Urinary diversion surgery
suprapubic, for bulbar urethral stricture, 245
supravesical
for BNC, 246
for mangement of prostatic urethral strictures, 248
for poor bladder and sphincter function, 252
for radiation induced urethral strictures, 241
Urinary extravasation, acute, in fasciocutaneous urethroplasty complications, 219
Urinary fistulas
buccal graft closure of, 264
complex, 266
embolization costs and outcomes of, 268
embolization technique for, 266–268
Urinary incontinence
AUS for, 234
cause of, 232
refractory, embolization for management of, 266
salvage prostatectomy for, 258
ureteral embolization for, 267
Urinary-perineal fistulas, rectovesical and, 265–266
Urinary retention, and penile dry gangrene after pelvic RT, 243
Urinary sepsis, postoperative, 110

Urinary stream, in complication of fossa navicularis
    and meatal reconstruction, splaying of, 104
Urinary toxicity scale, modified RTOG, 242
Urinary tract fistula, ureteric embolization for
    management of, 268
Urinary tract infection
    in anterior anastomotic urethroplasty, 221
    rates of, 59
Urinary tract symptoms (UTS), lower, surgery
    for, 229
Urine
    divertion, bilateral percutaneous nephrostomy tube
        for, 266
    extravasation of, 44
    leak, in BMU complications, 214
UroCoil system
    clinical results of, 90–91
    for penile urethral strictures, 90
    stents
        for treatment of post prostate surgery, 90
        for treatment of recurrent urethral stricture
            disease, 89
Uroflowmetry, 317
Urography, retrograde, of allium bulbar urethral
    stent, 93
Urological reconstructive surgery, buccal mucosa
    for, 119–120
Urologist
    assessment of tissue transfer techniques in plastic
        surgery for, 44
    flap techniques of tissue transfer in plastic surgery
        for, 48
        adjunctive, 51–52
        free, 51
        pedicled muscle, 50–51
        rotation/transposition, 49–50
        sliding advancement, 48–49
        tubed, 50
    management options of tissue transfer techniques
        in plastic surgery for, 44
        flap reconstruction in, 47–48
        graft reconstruction in, 45–47
        primary repair in, 45
        secondary intention in, 44–45
    tissue transfer techniques in plastic surgery
        for, 43–44
UroLume complications, open surgical management
    of, 93
UroLume endourethral prosthesis, 277
Urolume explantation
    endoscopic methods, 279–281
    open surgical methods, 281–283
Urolumes, failed/sequential, graft and flap urethral
    reconstruction for, 283

UroLume stent, 277
    failures, 278
    overlapping, retrograde urography of, 279
    for recurrent urethral stricture, 247
    removal, 280–281
UroLume Wallstent, clinical outcome of, 87–89
Uropathy, obstructive, risk of, 203
Urosepsis, 216
UTI. See Urinary tract infection

V
Vaginal flap urethroplasty, 307–308
Vaginal wall urethroplasty, 307–308
Van Buren, in United States, 194
Varicellavirus, 122
Vascular insufficiency, of anterior urethra, 203–204
Vascularized flap urethroplasty, 289
Vascular stents, 87
Vastus medialis, 177
    medial fascia of, 179
VCUG. See Voiding cystourethrography
Venous thrombosis, deep, in positioning-related
    complications, 223
Verumontanum, 6
Vesicoperineal fistulas, complex rectourinary and, 252
Vesico-rectal fistula, cystogram for demonstratoin
    of, 253
Vesicourethral anastomotic strictures
    after RRP
        dilation for, 232
        men with, 235
Vesicovaginal fistula, radiation, perineal artery
    fasciocutaneous flap for, 180
Vicryl sutures, 342
Vitiligo
    disorders associated with, 99
    with LS, 21
    meatal stricture due to, 99
Voiding cystourethrogram
    for fossa navicularis and meatus, 100
    imaging modality for fossa navicularis and
        meatus, 100
    for proximal urethra and bladder neck strictures, 109
    revealing distal urethral stricture, 306
Voiding cystourethrography, 231, 305
    for diagnosis of fistula, 253
    for evaluating continence of bladder neck, 122
    of male urethra, 31–33
    and RUG
        for posterior urethral stricture, 231
        for urethral stricture, 33
Voiding urethrogram, of bulbar urethral stricture
    due to SCC, 42
Vulva, topography and squamous epithelium of, 2

W
Waldeyer's fascia, 255
Wallstent, for vascular disease, 87
Weissflecken dermatose, 20
Wound healing, 297
  extragenital flap for, 172
  impaired, inferior gluteus maximus
    for, 182

poor, caused by peripheral vascular disease
    and diabetes, 154
urethral stricture and, 86

Y
York-Mason approaches
  for management of nonradiated fistulas, 251–252
  for repair of RUF, 255–257

Printed in the United States of America